Handbook of Palliative Care

Yvonne Carter has been very much in our minds throughout the preparation of the third edition of the *Handbook of Palliative Care*. Sadly, she was not part of the team on this occasion. After many years living with cancer, she died in 2009 but her voice has been heard loudly by us, giving encouragement and direction throughout the process. We dedicate this edition to her.

Handbook of Palliative Care

EDITED BY

Christina Faull BMedSci, MBBS, MD, FRCP, PGCert Med Ed, Dip Clin Hypnosis
University Hospitals of Leicester and LOROS, The Leicestershire and Rutland Hospice, Leicester, UK

Sharon de Caestecker RN, BN, MA
LOROS, The Leicestershire and Rutland Hospice, Leicester, UK

Alex Nicholson MBBS, FRCP
South Tees Hospitals NHS Foundation Trust, Middlesbrough, UK

Fraser Black MD, CCFP, FCFP
International Network for Cancer Treatment and Research (Belgium/Canada); Victoria Hospice and InspireHealth, Victoria, Canada

3rd edition

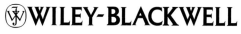

WILEY-BLACKWELL

A John Wiley & Sons, Ltd., Publication

For general information on our other products and services or for technical support, please contact our Customer Care Department within the United States at (800) 762-2974, outside the United States at (317) 572-3993 or fax (317) 572-4002.

Wiley also publishes its books in a variety of electronic formats. Some content that appears in print may not be available in electronic formats. For more information about Wiley products, visit our web site at www.wiley.com.

Library of Congress Cataloging-in-Publication Data:

Handbook of palliative care / edited by Christina Faull . . . [et al.]. – 3rd ed.
       p. ; cm.
    Includes bibliographical references and index.
    ISBN 978-1-118-06559-4 (pbk. : alk. paper)
    I. Faull, Christina.
    [DNLM: 1. Palliative Care–Handbooks. WB 39]
    616′.029–dc23

                                                            2012014815

Printed in Singapore

Cover Image: © The Map Foundation
Cover Design: Michael Rutkowski

10 9 8 7 6 5 4 3 2 1

Contents

List of Contributors

Debbie Allanson, RGN, HND
Lymphoedema Clinical Nurse Specialist
The Queen's Centre for Oncology and Haematology
Hull, UK

Megory Anderson, MA
Director
Sacred Dying Foundation
San Francisco, USA

Rachael Barton, MA MSc DM MRCP FRCR
Consultant Clinical Oncologist and Honorary Senior
Lecturer
The Queen's Centre for Oncology and Haematology
Hull, UK

Fraser Black, MD, CCFP, FCFP
Medical Director and Palliative Care Physician, Victoria
Hospice, Canada InspireHealth, Integrative Cancer
Center, Victoria, Canada
Clinical Professor, University of British Columbia,
Canada International Network for Cancer Treatment
and Research (Belgium/Canada)

Deb Braithwaite, MD, CCFP, FCFP
Community Lead and Palliative Care Physician Victoria
Hospice
Victoria, Canada

Camara van Breemen, MN, CHPCN(c)
Nurse Practitioner (F)
Canuck Place Children's
Hospice, Vancouver, Canada

Sharon de Caestecker RN, BN, MA
Director of Education and Training
LOROS, The Leicestershire and Rutland Hospice
Leicester, UK

Rodger Charlton, MD, FRCGP
Associate Clinical Professor, Division of Primary Care,
Nottingham Medical School
Honorary Professor
College of Medicine
Swansea University
Swansea, UK

Andrew Chilton, MBBS, FRCP
Consultant and Honorary Senior Lecturer
Gastroenterologist and Hepatologist
Kettering General Hospital Foundation Trust
Kettering, UK

Monica Compton, BS, AAS
Nutrition Team Dietitian and Lead Dietetic Prescribing
Advisor
Kettering General Hospital
NHS Foundation Trust
Kettering, UK

Rachael E. Dixon, MBBS, BSc, MRCP
Consultant in Palliative Medicine
Dove House Hospice
Hull, UK

Joanna Dunn, MBBS, MRCP, MA
Specialist Registrar in Palliative Medicine
UCLH,
Camden and Islington Palliative Care Team
London, UK

Jacqueline Edwards, RGN, RSCN, MSc, BSc (Hons)
Head Nurse, Children, Quality and Governance Heart of
England NHS Foundation Trust Bordesley Green East
Birmingham, UK

Christina Faull, BMedSci, MBBS, MD, FRCP, PGCert Med Ed, Dip Clin Hypnosis
Consultant in Palliative Medicine
University Hospitals of Leicester and LOROS
The Leicestershire and Rutland Hospice
Leicester, UK

Liz Grant, PhD
Deputy Director
Global Health Academy
University of Edinburgh
Edinburgh, UK

Jo Griffiths, MBChB, MRCPCH, Dip Pall Med (Paeds)
Consultant in Paediatric Palliative Medicine &
Community Child Health Abertawe Bro Morgannwg
Health Board, Swansea, Wales, UK

Christine Hirsch, BPharm, PhD
Lecturer in Clinical Pharmacy
Medical School
University of Birmingham, Birmingham, UK

Christine Jones, MD, CCFP, FCFP
Palliative Medicine Physician
Victoria Hospice Society
Vancouver Island Health Authority
Victoria, Canada

Daniel Kelly, PhD, MSc, BSc, RN, PGCE, FRSA
Royal College of Nursing Chair of Nursing Research
School of Nursing & Midwifery Studies
Cardiff University
Wales, UK

Victoria Lidstone, BM, FRCP
Consultant in Palliative Medicine & All Wales Clinical
Lead for transition in Palliative Care
Department of Paediatric Palliative Care
University Hospital of Wales
Cardiff, UK

Ryan Liebscher, MD, CCFP
Palliative Care Physician
Victoria Hospice
Victoria, Canada

Maria McKenna, MBBS, MRCP
Newcastle upon Tyne Hospitals NHS Foundation Trust,
UK

Daniel Munday, MBBS, FFARCSI, DRCOG, MRCGP, Dip Pall Med, PhD, FRCP
Associate Clinical Professor/Honorary Consultant in
Palliative Medicine
Division of Health Sciences, Warwick Medical School
Coventry, UK

Alex Nicholson, MBBS, FRCP
Consultant in Palliative Medicine, South Tees Hospitals
NHS Foundation Trust, Visiting Fellow, University of
Teesside School of Health and Social Care,
Middlesbrough, UK

David Oliver, BSc, FRCP, FRCGP
Consultant in Palliative Medicine
Wisdom Hospice
Rochester, UK
And
Honorary Reader
Centre for Professional Practice
University of Kent
Kent, UK

Wendy Prentice, MBBS, FRCP, MA
Consultant/Honorary Senior Lecturer in Palliative
Medicine
King's College Hospital NHS Foundation Trust
Cicely Saunders Institute
London, UK

Aziz Sheikh, BSc, MBBS, MSc, MD, DRCOG, DCH, FRCGP, FRCP
Professor of Primary Care Research & Development
Director of Research Centre for Population
Health Sciences
University of Edinburgh
Edinburgh, UK

Harold Siden, MD, MHSc, FRCPC
Medical Director
Canuck Place Children's Hospice
Clinical Associate Professor, Pediatrics
University of British Columbia
Vancouver, Canada

Surinder Singh, BM, MSc, FRCGP
Senior Clinical Lecturer in General Practice
Research Department of Primary Care & Population
Health
UCL Medical School
London, UK

Neil Small, BSc (Econ), MSW, Phd.
Professor of Health Research
School of Health Studies
University of Bradford
Bradford, UK

Sue Taplin, BA (Joint Hons), MA/PgDipSw, DSW
Education Facilitator, LOROS The Leicestershire and
Rutland Hospice
Leicester, UK

Nick Theobald, MA, MSc, MBBS
Clinical Lecturer and Associate Specialist
St Stephen's Centre
Chelsea and Westminster Hospital
London, UK

Elizabeth Thompson, DMOxon, MBBS, MRCP, FFHom
Lead Clinician/Consultant Homeopathic Physician and
Honorary Senior Lecturer in Palliative Medicine
University Hospitals Bristol NHS Foundation Trust
Bristol Homeopathic Hospital
Bristol, UK

Mary Walding, RGN, BSc (Hons), PGDip
Clinical Nurse Specialist Palliative Care
Katharine House Hospice
Banbury, UK

Richard K.M. Wong, MA, MD, FRCP
Consultant Geriatrician
University Hospital of Leicester NHS Trust
Leicester, UK

Catherine Zollman, BA(Oxon), MBBS, MRCP, MRCGP
GP
Bristol and Lead Doctor
Penny Brohn Cancer Care
Bristol, UK

Foreword

Every minute over 100 people die in the world but far too many people still do not get the palliative and end-of-life care they need or want. Even patients in countries with well-developed health-care systems such as Europe, Australasia, and North America, who could benefit from the full range of palliative care support and services, never have that opportunity. The consequence is that many die with the distress of uncontrolled symptoms and with relatives and carers who are unsupportive. A difficult time may be made worse because no one has established the wishes of the patient, and they die in a place they would not have chosen and are perhaps subject to inappropriate and futile interventions, such as resuscitation, that they would have declined. Furthermore, it is still unfortunately true that access to palliative care services varies according to age, diagnosis, gender, and geography, and the basic levels of palliative care that are available are of inconsistent quality. The time has come to change this and to change it for good.

My vision is for a "good death" to be the norm. We only get one chance to get it right for people living in the late stages of incurable illness and those who are dying. I believe the *Handbook of Palliative Care* will undoubtedly contribute to achieving this vision by providing evidence-based knowledge for doctors and nurses, and for other members of the multiprofessional team. This new edition is highly impressive and should be required reading for all those involved in delivering palliative care at any level wherever they work in the world. As a practicing general practitioner, I know on a daily basis how a clinician can be faced with complex clinical and ethical dilemmas in patient management. I would find a resource like this book very reassuring, providing as it does a wide range of trusted knowledge, experience, and expertise.

An ageing population with complex health and social care needs requires a new caring approach and a new deal for the dying. All health-care systems need to effect a change in clinical practice to recognise the dying patient earlier and improve access for these patients to the palliative care and hospice approach—for example, through use of supportive and palliative care registers—particularly for patients with conditions other than cancer. The development of better generalists is a must, as is implementing comprehensive evidence-based guidelines for palliative care. Key to grasping this opportunity is development of the workforce.

And we need to achieve fundamental changes in public and professional attitudes. A society that is more comfortable with talking about death, dying, and bereavement is much needed. I am therefore delighted that the handbook includes a chapter on communication skills. I also welcome the new chapter on spirituality in this edition. Spirituality is often the missing piece in palliative care plans, even though meeting the individual spiritual needs of a patient is an important part of that person's journey at the end of life.

In 2008, readers of the British Medical Journal voted "palliative care beyond cancer" as the area of health care in which doctors could make the most improvement. This is an outstanding book that is to be thoroughly commended for its broad range of clinical issues and particularly for its focus on noncancer palliative care. All clinicians will recognise that the noncancer patient presents challenges when we are trying to determine the starting point for the last few months of life, but this is critical if we are to identify those patients who need palliative attention and for whom we should be starting advance care planning discussions. I am glad to see practical guidance on this area of practice.

We know that there is still considerable room for improvement in palliative care. Although maybe 70% of people would prefer to die at home, more than half currently die in hospital in the United Kingdom. This is replicated in many countries in the developed world. The realities of living and dying well are at the heart of palliative care, an important clinical area that deserves to be more widely understood.

I restate my ambition to reduce the fear of dying and make a "good death" the norm. The authors of this book share their expertise, experience, and wisdom in guiding us towards these goals. I am confident that good progress will be made and I invite readers of *The Handbook of Palliative Care* to join me in making good end-of-life care not only a priority but also a reality.

Prof. Mayur Lakhani, CBE, FRCGP, FRCP (Edin), FRCP

Practicing GP and Chairman of the
National Council for Palliative Care and the
Dying Matters Coalition (www.ncpc.org.uk and
www.dyingmatters.org)

Past Chairman, Royal College of General Practitioners
National Council for Palliative Care
London, UK

Preface to the Third Edition

In preparing the third edition of the *Handbook of Palliative Care*, we are encouraged and grateful that the previous editions have been so well received. However, both the specialty of palliative care and the place it occupies in modern health and increasingly social care continues to evolve. The third edition seeks not only to retain the strengths of the previous editions but also to prove responsive to feedback and to have been adapted with additional content and chapters reflecting relevant developments in palliative care practice and scope.

Our main aim has been to provide a handbook that is informative and practical, thereby supporting the care professional delivering palliative care in any setting and enhancing the quality of both everyday and unusual clinical practice. Thus, the content on assessment and symptom management, communication skills, and ethics remains key and emphasises the essential nature of a holistic, patient-centred approach to care. We have also included sections that allow more expansion into some philosophical and historical background in order to provide breadth and balance in a handbook about a type of care that is wide-ranging and deeply rooted. For example, the chapters *User Voices, Palliative Primary Care*, and *Spirituality in Palliative Care* support this ambition. These dual approaches are intended to improve the understanding of what really "makes palliative care work" as well as increasing the confidence and skills of those working to support patients and their families. As in previous editions, emphasis is placed throughout on the importance of teamwork and highlighting the multidisciplinary nature of palliative care. Never forgetting that "the team" must include the patient and those who are important to them.

Taking a global perspective, the need for palliative care remains great. Estimates suggest that more than 100 million people worldwide would benefit from palliative care provision every year, yet only a small fraction of those individuals in need actually receive the necessary support. Worldwide we know that close to three-quarters of people diagnosed with cancer and other life-limiting illnesses present late with incurable disease and that this is accompanied by a burden of significant symptoms and suffering that is both physical and nonphysical.

There continues to be an expanding knowledge and recognition of how palliative care can benefit not only patients with cancer but also those with noncancer illnesses, and the updated chapters include significant new content in the areas of heart failure, renal failure, advanced respiratory diseases, and HIV and AIDS. We have also added a new chapter *Palliative Care for People with Advanced Dementia,* arguably the biggest issue on the horizon. The chapter *Palliative Care for Adolescents and Young Adults* now includes the important issue of transition from children's to adult palliative care for the growing number of young people with life-limiting diseases surviving to their early adult years.

Advance care planning is another area that is recognised increasingly to be fundamental to sound holistic patient-centred palliative care provision, and a new chapter gives the reader a sure grounding in key considerations.

In this third edition, a decision was made to expand the remit of the text beyond the perspectives of the United Kingdom, and the result has been a book that has been authored and edited by a team drawn from the United Kingdom and North America. Contributing to this edition are new authors from two longstanding hospice palliative care programmes in Canada. Victoria Hospice was among the early hospice palliative care programmes established in Canada, and Canuck Place Children's Hospice in Vancouver was the first free-standing children's hospice in North America.

There is so much to learn from one another in making progress to address the need for increased access to palliative care worldwide, and we hope that this collaboration has added a richness and variety to the handbook's content that will appeal to all readers. Naturally, there are some differences in terminology and language and we have tried to accommodate these as far as possible while leaving the content intelligible to all. We recognise that

Table P.1 Drug names used in Handbook of Palliative Care.

Recommended International Non-proprietary Name (rINN) (European market)	British Approved Name (now replaced by rINN)	United States Adopted Name (used in USA in preference to rINN)
Aspirin		Often known as aspirin but also **Acetyl salicylic acid**
	No UK equivalent	**Benzonatate**
Calcitonin	Salcatonin	**Calcitonin**
Chlorphenamine	**Chlorpheniramine**	**Chlorpheniramine**
Colestyramine	Cholestyramine	
	Not marketed in UK	**Desipramine**
Furosemide	Frusemide	**Furosemide**
Glitazones		**Thiozolidinediones**
Guaiphenesin		**Guaifenesin**
	Not marketed in UK	**Hydrocodone**
Hyoscine		Scopolamine
	No UK equivalent	**Levodropropizine**
Levomepromazine	**Methotrimeprazine**	
Levothyroxine	**Thyroxine**	
	No UK equivalent	**Miltefosine** (hexadecylphosphocholine)
Paracetamol		**Acetaminophen**
Pethidine		**Meperidine**
Phenobarbital	Phenobarbitone	
Rifampicin		Rifampin
Riluzole		
Risperidone		
S		
Senna		
Sertraline		
Silver sulphadiazine		
Sodium citrate		
Sodium cromoglicate	**Sodium cromoglycate**	Cromolyn sodium and Sodium cromoglycate

This table lists drugs which may be known by different names in Europe and North America. Names shown in **bold** appear in the text.

drug names vary in different countries—sometimes subtly, sometimes significantly—and have included a list of drugs used in the handbook to aid the reader to align their European and North American names (see Table P.1). For important drugs that are mentioned often in the text, both names are used. Spellings have followed the British tradition. Where terminology varies, we have tried to explain this within the text of the relevant chapter. An interpretation of abbreviations also appears in the front of the book (page xvi).

It is our hope that this third edition will succeed in its aims of keeping prominent those parts of hospice and palliative care that we know make a difference to patients and families while also incorporating new knowledge and approaches that will help improve the provision of palliative care to patients and families worldwide. Thank you for your efforts in this regard by using this handbook and by providing the care that you do to patients, families, and communities around the world.

Acknowledgements

This book has only been made possible by the hard work of many contributing colleagues and we hope that this edition does justice to the efforts of all the individuals who have given so much of their time over and above their normal duties and responsibilities. We are aware of how much personal complexity some of the writing team have been dealing with and we should like to pay tribute not only to their determination in fulfilling their commitment to this book but also to their efforts in trying to ensure that high-quality palliative care is available to those who need it. We would particularly like to acknowledge Richard Woof who contributed so much to the first edition and whose legacy lasts in this third edition.

Acknowledgement: Cover illustration

A water-colour titled *Between Night and Day* (1995) reproduced with kind permission of the artist Michele Angelo Petrone who sadly died in 2007. It is reproduced with kind permission of the MAP Foundation, an arts in health organization founded by Mr. Petrone to promote expression, communication, and understanding for people affected by life-threatening illness. Michele painted and wrote of his experience during treatment for Hodgkin's disease:

'As time goes by, night follows day and day follows night- a natural cycle without beginning, without end and without gaps. Life's cycle continues without interruption, or at least it should do. Suddenly illness arrives, uninvited, unexplained. I found myself caught between life and death, light and dark, banished to an unknown place- between night and day. The illness forced itself into my life where there was no place for it. The arrival of the illness stole a place and time that should have been destined for better things.'

List of Abbreviations

AIDS	acquired immune deficiency syndrome		MSCC	malignant spinal cord compression
ADL	Activities of Daily Living		MLD	manual lymphatic drainage
ACP	advance care planning		MCA	Mental Capacity Act
ADRT	advance decision to refuse treatment		MR	modified release
AD	advance directive		MND	motor neuron disease
ADA	After Death Analysis		MNDA	Motor Neurone Disease Association
AND	allow natural death		MDT	multidisciplinary team
ALS	amyotrophic lateral sclerosis		MS	multiple sclerosis
BPI	Brief Pain Inventory		MSA	multiple system atrophy
CPR	cardiopulmonary resuscitation		MD	muscular dystrophies
CVD	cardiovascular disease		NG	nasogastric
CP	care professional		NHS	National Health Service
CKD	chronic kidney disease		NICE	National Institute for Health and
COPD	chronic obstructive pulmonary disease			Clinical Excellence
CNSs	clinical nurse specialists		NPSA	National Patient Safety Agency
CHF	congestive heart failure		NMDA	N-methyl-D-aspartate
CDs	controlled drugs		NIPPV	noninvasive positive pressure ventilation
DNACPR	do not attempt cardiopulmonary resuscitation		NIV	noninvasive ventilation
			NSAID	nonsteroidal antiinflammatory drug
DNAR/PND	do not attempt resuscitation/permit natural death		NR	normal release
			OT	occupational therapy
EoLCS	end-of-life care strategy		PO	oral
ESRD	end-stage renal disease		PD	Parkinson's disease
EAPC	European association for palliative care		PCT	primary care trust
GI	gastrointestinal		PEG	percutaneous endoscopic gastrostomy
GMC	General Medical Council		PPI	proton pump inhibitor
GP	general practitioner		RFA	radiofrequency ablation
GFR	glomerular filtration rate		SSRI	selective serotonin reuptake inhibitor
GSF	Gold Standards Framework		SNRI	serotonin noradrenaline reuptake inhibitors
HF	heart failure			
HIV	human immunodeficiency virus		SLD	simple lymphatic drainage
HD	Huntington's disease		SC	subcutaneous
IV	intravenous		SVC	superior vena cava
LPA	lasting power of attorney		TENS	transcutaneous electrical nerve stimulation
LANSS	Leeds assessment of neuropathic symptoms and signs		TCA	tricyclic antidepressant
LLCs	life-limiting conditions		WHO	World Health Organization
LCP	Liverpool Care Pathway			

1 The Context and Principles of Palliative Care

Christina Faull

University Hospitals of Leicester and LOROS, The Leicestershire and Rutland Hospice, Leicester, UK

Introduction

Palliative care touches almost every health and social care professional. Irrespective of their particular specialty, most professionals will encounter people with advanced illness, and the care of people in the last months and weeks of life is an important part of their work [1]. This can be an extremely rewarding area of practice, and professional satisfaction is enhanced by confidence in core skills and knowledge of basic physical and nonphysical symptom management [2,3].

Palliative care should not be seen as an alternative to other care. It is a complementary and vital part of total patient management that should be integrated, in people with advanced illness, alongside appropriate care to reverse illness or prolong life. The challenges of the parallel approaches of trying to improve physical well-being and prolong life while also addressing the realistic probability of deterioration and death are significant, especially in those illnesses characterised by episodes of acute deterioration. Perhaps one of the biggest challenges we face in medicine and indeed in society is balancing the clinical and ethical "pros and cons" (weighing the burdens, benefits, and risks) of investigation and intervention in those with advanced illness and in the frail elderly. In the United Kingdom, the General Medical Council (GMC) has recommended that death should be an explicit discussion point when patients are likely to die within 12 months [4,5]. Box 1.1 identifies the mandated expectations in this guidance [5].

The majority of care received by patients during the last year of life is delivered by general practitioners (GPs) and

> **Box 1.1 Mandated expectations of the GMC guidance—Treatment and care toward the end of life: good practice in decision making [4,5]**
>
> - Identification of patients approaching the end of life.
> - Provision of information on this matter.
> - Determination of preferences regarding life-sustaining treatment including cardiopulmonary resuscitation (CPR).
> - Documentation of the above in an unambiguous and accessible format.
> - Communication of decisions within relevant health-care teams.

community teams. A systematic review of GP involvement in this care reported the following [3]:

- GPs value this work and it is appreciated by patients.
- Palliative care is sometimes delivered less well in the community than in other settings.
- Some GPs are unhappy with their competence in this field.
- With specialist support, GPs demonstrably provide effective care.
- The confidence of GPs and the understanding of the potential of team members increase through working with specialist teams.

Of course, many patients spend significant time in hospitals during their last year of life, and it has been estimated that 20% of hospital beds are occupied by patients near the end of life who often do not need, or want, to be there [6]. Despite the majority wishing to die at home, almost 60%

of patients still die in a hospital in the United Kingdom [7]. The lack of recognition of the fact that patients are nearing the ends of their lives and open discussion of this with the patients and their families is the major barrier in achieving better outcomes including enabling people to die where they would most want to [6,8,9].

Palliative care is more than just end-of-life care. Some of the newest challenges are in providing effective support for those living with cancer, or other advanced illness, for long periods of time who are suffering from a complex mix of effects of the cancer or human immunodeficiency virus (HIV) or other condition. There is considerable unmet need in supporting people with the effects of the treatments for the disease and the psychosocial and psychospiritual impacts of facing not only the fear of recurrence and death but also the ongoing symptoms such as fatigue, disability, and change of role and social and family dynamics [10,11].

There is a broad range of challenges in delivering high-quality palliative, end-of-life, and terminal care including professional competence and confidence, teamwork and organisational factors, and access to resources. Patients with advanced disease can present some of the most challenging ethical, physical, psychological, and social issues, and it is vital to have a grasp of the communication skills required to explore these issues effectively. It is also important to be able to identify when referrals to specialists and other services are needed.

This chapter outlines the development of palliative care, defines the principles that underpin effective care, and presents an overview of the attainment and assessment of quality in palliative care.

What are hospice, palliative care, and end-of-life care?

Much of our understanding and knowledge of the philosophy, science, and art of palliative care has developed and grown through the work of the hospice movement. Dame Cicely Saunders worked with patients suffering from advanced cancer and undertook systematic narrative research to understand what patients were experiencing and needed. The bedrock of the hospice philosophy, in Western society at least, is that of patient-centred holistic care focusing on quality of life and extending support to significant family and carers:

> What links the many professionals and volunteers who work in hospice or palliative care is an awareness of the many needs of a person and his/her family and carers as they grapple with

---

> **Box 1.2 Etymology**
>
> The word "hospice" originates from the Latin *hospes* meaning host; *hospitalis*, a further derivative, means friendly, a welcome to the stranger. The word *hospitium* perhaps begins to convey the vital philosophy of the hospice movement: it means the warm feeling between host and guest. Hence, a hospice denotes a place where this feeling is experienced, a place of welcome and care for those in need.
>
> The word "palliative" derives from the Latin *pallium*, a cloak. Palliation means cloaking over, not addressing the underlying cause but ameliorating the effects.

all the demands and challenges introduced by the inexorable progress of a disease that has outstripped the possibilities of cure [12].

Hospice has perhaps become thought of as solely a place of care. It is, however, much more than this and in essence is synonymous with palliative care. Both have a philosophy of care not dependent on a place or a building but on attitude, expertise, and understanding. The term "palliative care" was coined by Canadian urological cancer surgeon, Balfour Mount, as a term to apply hospice principles more broadly including within the hospital setting. More recently, the term *specialist palliative care* has been used to represent those professionals and services that concentrate on this area of health care as their main role and expertise, recognising that almost all health-care professionals provide elements of palliative care for patients as part of their practice (see Box 1.2).

Palliative care has been defined as:

> an approach that improves the quality of life of patients and their families facing the problems associated with life-threatening illness, through the prevention and relief of suffering by means of early identification and impeccable assessment and treatment of pain and other problems, physical, psychosocial and spiritual [13].

Palliative care [13]:
- provides relief from pain and other distressing symptoms;
- affirms life and regards dying as a normal process;
- intends neither to hasten nor postpone death;
- integrates the psychological and spiritual aspects of patient care;
- offers a support system to help patients live as actively as possible until death;
- offers a support system to help the family cope during the patient's illness and in their own bereavement;

• uses a team approach to address the needs of patients and their families, including bereavement counselling, if indicated;
• will enhance quality of life and may also positively influence the course of illness; and
• is applicable early in the course of illness, in conjunction with other therapies that are intended to prolong life, such as chemotherapy or radiation therapy, and includes those investigations needed to better understand and manage distressing clinical complications.

To this end palliative care is a partnership between the patient, carers, and a wide range of professionals. It integrates the psychological, physical, social, cultural, and spiritual aspects of a patient's care, acknowledging and respecting the uniqueness of each individual:

> You matter because you are you, and you matter until the last moment of your life. We will do all that we can to help you not only to die peacefully, but to live until you die [14].

End-of-life care

End-of-life care is the care needed by everyone as they approach the end of their lives. It is usually regarded as a focus on the last 6–12 months of life. It is of course difficult to define the last 12 months of life prospectively and much thought has been given to how indicators may help identify people. Figure 1.1 shows an example of how such indicators can be incorporated in to guidance to help identify appropriate people, which has been developed in Scotland.

The End-of-Life Care strategy (EoLCS) in England and Wales defined a pathway to optimise the quality of care in the last months of life (Figure 1.2) [7]. Many other countries have had similar initiatives.

All patients in the last months, weeks, and days of life need support from primary care. Many, because they are ill, will have contact with secondary care specialists including elderly care services and many of the more elderly patients (85 years+) (who, by 2030, will be 44% of the people that die every year in the United Kingdom) will live in care homes. Only a minority of those that die every year will need direct contact with specialist palliative care services.

The Gold Standards Framework (GSF) [15] provides a quality framework for end-of-life care in primary care and is explored in Chapter 2, *Palliative care in the community*.

Specialist palliative care

Specialist palliative care came into focus with the founding of St Christopher's hospice in London in 1967 by Dame Cicely Saunders. It was here that an approach that formed the basis for the role of specialist services was developed:
• High-quality care for patients and their relatives, especially those with complex needs.
• A range of services to help provide optimum care: whether the patient was at home, in hospital, or required specialist in-patient care.
• Education, advice, and support to other professionals.
• Evidence-based practice.
• Research and evaluation.

The subsequent, mostly unplanned, growth of specialist palliative care services has led to a wide variety of models of service provision, distribution and funding, with some areas, and therefore patients, being better served than others.

Issues in palliative care worldwide

Fifty-six million people die across the world each year, 80% of deaths occurring in developing countries. The world population is estimated to increase by 50% in the next 50 years and almost all of this increase in population will be in the developing world. In addition, there will be a huge shift in age of the population with a two- to threefold increase in population aged over 60 years in both the developed and the developing world. In the United Kingdom, it is estimated that by 2030 the percentage of deaths over 85 years of age will increase by almost a third to 44% of all deaths, around 255,000 people [16].

The Barcelona declaration on palliative care in 1996 [17], like the World Health Organization (WHO) in 1990 [18], called for palliative care to be included as part of every governmental health policy. Recent studies suggest that palliative care is integrated with wider service provision in only 15% of countries [19]. Although not enshrined in the Human Rights Act, most would agree that every individual has the right to pain relief. Inexpensive, effective methods exist to relieve pain and other symptoms. The *Life Before Death* campaign together with the International Association for the Study of Pain shows, in documentary films, the shocking and profound issues about pain management for people throughout the world, especially in the developing world [20]. Analgesics are inexpensive, and cost need not be an impediment to pain control. It is estimated that globally a hundred million people would currently benefit from the availability of palliative care. We are a long, long way from achieving this. Tens of millions of people die each year in unrelieved suffering [21].

Identifying patients with advanced illness

NHS
Lothian

Supportive & Palliative Care Indicators Tool (SPICT)

1. Look for two or more general clinical indicators

Two or more unplanned hospital admissions in the past 6 months.

Performance status deteriorating
(needs help with personal care, in bed or chair for 50% or more of the day).

Unplanned weight loss (5–10%) over the past 3–6 months and/or body mass index < 20.

A new event or diagnosis that is likely to reduce life expectancy to less than a year.

Persistent symptoms despite optimal treatment of advanced illness.

Lives in a nursing care home or NHS continuing care unit; or needs a care package at home.

2. Now look for two or more clinical indicators of advanced, progressive illness

Advanced heart/ vascular disease

NYHA Class III/IV heart failure, or extensive coronary artery disease:
- Breathless or chest pain at rest or on minimal exertion.

Severe, inoperable peripheral vascular disease.

Advanced respiratory disease

Severe chronic obstructive pulmonary disease (FEV1<30%) or severe pulmonary fibrosis
- Breathless at rest or on minimal exertion between exacerbations.

Meets criteria for long-term oxygen therapy (PaO$_2$ < 7.3 kPa).

Has needed ventilation for respiratory failure.

Advanced kidney disease

Stage 4 or 5 chronic kidney disease (eGFR < 30 ml/min).

Kidney failure as a recent complication of another condition or treatment.

Stopping dialysis.

Advanced liver disease

Advanced cirrhosis with one or more complications in past year:
- Diuretic resistant ascites
- Hepatic encephalopathy
- Hepatorenal syndrome
- Bacterial peritonitis
- Recurrent variceal bleeds

Serum albumin < 25 g/l, INR prolonged (INR > 2).

Liver transplant is contraindicated.

Advanced cancer

Performance status deteriorating due to metastatic cancer and/ or co-morbidities.

Persistent symptoms despite optimal palliative oncology treatment or too frail for oncology treatment.

Advanced neurological disease

Progressive deterioration in physical and/or cognitive function despite optimal therapy.

Speech problems with increasing difficulty communicating and/or progressive dysphagia.

Recurrent aspiration pneumonia; breathless or respiratory failure.

Advanced dementia/ frailty

Unable to dress, walk or eat without help; unable to communicate meaningfully.

Needing assistance with feeding/ maintaining nutrition.

Recurrent febrile episodes or infections; aspiration pneumonia.

Urinary and faecal incontinence.

Fractured neck of femur.

3. Ask

Would it be a surprise if this patient died in the next 6–12 months?   **No**

4. Assess and plan

Assess patient and family for unmet needs.

Review treatment/care plan; and medication.

Discuss and agree care goals with patient and family.

Consider using GP register to coordinate care in the community.

Handover: care plan, agreed levels of intervention, CPR status.

SPICT Version 21, October 2011

Figure 1.1 The supportive and palliative care indicators guidance used in Lothian National Health Service (NHS), Scotland. (Reproduced with permission from NHS, available at www.palliativecareguidelines.scot.nhs.uk)

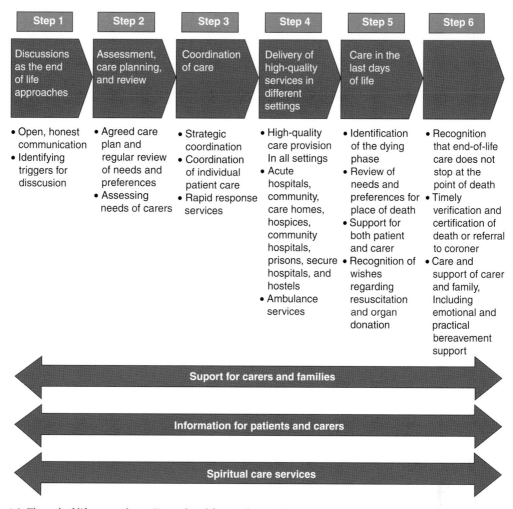

Figure 1.2 The end-of-life care pathway. (Reproduced from Reference 7)

The challenges for palliative care in developing countries

A multiplicity of challenges faces the development of palliative care globally, but the issues are more pronounced in the developing world for several reasons—principally, poverty, the ageing population, the high prevalence of smoking, and the increase in cancer and acquired immune deficiency syndrome (AIDS)-related deaths. It is estimated that in the Western world, deaths from cancer will increase by approximately 25% by 2020, but in China cancer deaths will increase by 145%, in India by 158%, in the Middle East by 181%, and in Africa by 149% [22]. The developing world has only 5% of the world's total resources for cancer control, although it must cope with almost two-thirds of the world's new cancer patients [23].

Globally the annual number of tobacco-related deaths is expected to rise from three million to ten million by the year 2025 [24]. Much more than half of this increase will occur in the developing world, three million in China alone. The developing world is currently suffering from an epidemic of lung cancer, making this cancer the most common worldwide. By 2015 approximately one million deaths in China will be from lung cancer.

Since the second edition of this book, the experience of HIV infection and AIDS has been transformed for those who can access antiviral medications. In 2009 some 33 million people were living with HIV/AIDS, of whom half are women, but during that year 1.8 million people died. It is estimated that deaths might rise to 6.5 million by 2030. Of those living with HIV/AIDS, 98% are in the developing world. The sociological effect of AIDS deaths in the developing world is catastrophic, especially in sub-Saharan Africa where the adult prevalence rate may be as high as 35% (although decreasing in some countries). AIDS affects those most likely to be breadwinners for the extended three-generation family and leaves many children orphaned. In 2009 there were estimated to be 16.6 million children orphaned through AIDS.

Availability of opioids

Under the international treaty, *Single Convention on Narcotic Drugs* [25], governments are responsible for ensuring that opioids are available for pain management. The 2010 report from the International Narcotics Control Board showed that opioids are still not widely available for medical needs [26]. More than 90% of the global morphine is used in ten industrialised countries. Over 80% of the world population will have insufficient analgesia, or no analgesia at all if they suffer from pain, including 5.5 million people with terminal cancer.

The main impediments to opioid availability, even in Europe, are government concern about addiction; insufficient training of health-care professionals; and restrictive laws over the manufacture, distribution, prescription, and dispensing of opioids [27]. There is also considerable prescribing reluctance on the part of the health-care profession, due in part to concerns about legal sanctions. This is made worse by the burden of regulatory requirements, the often insufficient import or manufacture of opioids, and the fear of the potential for diversion of opioids for nonlegitimate use. Most recently the Global Access to Pain Relief Initiative, a multiagency collaboration, is tackling the lack of access for the majority of people in need [28].

International observatory on end-of-life care

This is an invaluable resource for anyone wishing to learn more about global issues in palliative care. The website http://www.lancs.ac.uk/shm/research/ioelc provides research-based information about hospice and palliative care provision internationally, presenting public health and policy data, as well as cultural, historical, and ethnographic perspectives.

Unmet need and continued suffering in the developed world

The hospice movement and palliative care have come a long way in the past 45 years. There is a considerable body of knowledge and expertise, and services have grown enormously in number and character. There is, however, still a major unmet need. The majority of people are not living and dying with the comfort and the dignity that it is possible to achieve for most patients. Identified areas for improvement include:

- explicit recognition of patients in the last months, weeks, and days of life [4,8,9];
- management of pain in advanced cancer [27,29–33];
- management of other symptoms [29,33,34];
- information and support for patients and carers [35];
- attention to comfort and basic care for those dying in hospitals [9,36];
- the needs of patients dying from nonmalignant illness [37–43]; and
- the needs of patients who call for help out of "normal" working hours [44–47].

The major challenge for those who seek to improve the care for patients with advanced disease is to ensure that all health-care professionals consider palliative care an important part of their role and have adequate skills, knowledge, and specialist support to undertake it effectively. This is of crucial importance in the 70% of the week that occurs "out-of-hours" when patients are especially vulnerable to the deficits in health-care systems.

There are defined groups of patients who have poor outcomes, who underutilise specialist palliative care services, who have insufficient access to services and for whom service models need to develop to meet their needs in an appropriate way. Patients with illnesses other than cancer are considerably disadvantaged compared to those with cancer, and chapters later in this book discuss these issues in some depth and provide information on how to tackle them.

Health professionals in the world over recognise the fundamental human right to die with dignity. However, the notion of what constitutes a "good death" may vary considerably between and within cultures. While it has been shown that there are often greater similarities than differences between cultures when living and dealing with cancer [48], we know that it is more difficult for people from ethnically diverse communities to access or obtain information, support, and services that will meet their needs. Issues of communication, cultural diversity, appropriateness of information, organisational and staff attitudes, and discrimination are contributing factors across the spectrum of health and illness contexts, and having cancer is no exception to this experience [49–54]. For example, services such as counselling and psychological interventions in appropriate languages may not be available [48]. There may be difficulties in accessing self-help and support groups, Asian or African Caribbean wig types or prostheses and holistic pain control [54]. Greater understanding of cultural and individual variations in concepts of disclosure, patient autonomy, and patient-centeredness is needed. The extent to which these concepts may be ethnocentric and lack universality deserves wider consideration [49].

Compounding this disadvantage and poor quality of life is that people from diverse ethnic communities are more likely to be poor and have financial and housing difficulties. In addition, evidence, although limited by inadequacy of ethnicity monitoring, suggests that people with cancer from diverse ethnic communities have poorer survival than others [55]. In these conditions, it is not surprising that people from ethnically diverse communities with cancer consistently wish for [56]:

- more information about cancer, cancer treatments, and cancer care services;
- improved open communication and awareness about their condition;
- reduced feelings of stigma, isolation, and fear;
- greater control and choice in their care; and
- more effective care.

Migrant communities often have proportionately higher death rates from diseases not related to cancer, compounding their disadvantage in accessing palliative care. Gatrad and colleagues [57] suggest that realising high-quality palliative care for all will need fundamental changes on at least three fronts:

1. Tackling institutional discrimination in the provision of palliative care.

2. Progress in incorporating transcultural medicine into medical and nursing curriculums.

3. A greater willingness on the part of health-care providers to embrace complexity.

In doing these we shall develop a richer appreciation of the challenges facing people from minority communities in achieving a good end to their lives. These themes are explored further in Chapter 4, *Palliative care: choice, equality, and diversity.*

Enabling people to be at home

The EoLCS for England and Wales [7] has identified the key things that need to be in place to achieve the best possible care for people in the last months of life. These include:

- identifying people approaching the end of life;
- care planning;
- coordination of care;

- rapid access to care; and
- delivery of high-quality care by trained and competent practitioners in all service sectors.

These facets of care are discussed in depth in other chapters of this book, and Chapter 21, *Terminal care and dying*, focuses specifically on enabling people to die in the place of their choice.

Thomas [58,59] has developed seven standards (Box 1.3) to help primary care providers and teams improve their delivery of palliative care. Benefits have been demonstrated that include better communication and co-working and increased staff morale; however, the impact on patient outcomes especially achieving death in place of choice is less clear [60]. This is explored further in Chapter 2, *Palliative care in the community*. Communication with, and the quality of, out-of-hours primary care services is of critical importance in achieving the goals of care [44–47]. In more closed health systems such as the hospice programme in the United States, achievement of care and death at home is almost a prerequisite criterion of entry to the programme and therefore self-fulfilling; however, 80% of deaths in America are in hospital and only 7% die at home under hospice care.

Box 1.3 The seven "C's": gold standards for palliative care in primary care

Communication: Practice register; regular team meetings for information sharing, planning and reflection/audit; patient information; patient-held records.

Coordination: Nominated coordinator maintains register, organises meetings, audit, education symptom sheets, and other resources.

Control of symptoms: Holistic, patient centred assessment and management.

Continuity out-of-hours: Effective transfer of information to and from out-of-hours services. Access to drugs and equipment.

Continued learning: Audit/reflection/critical incident analysis. Use of continuing professional development time.

Carer support: Practical, financial, emotional, and bereavement support.

Care in the dying phase: Protocol-driven care addressing physical, emotional, and spiritual needs. Care needs around and after death acted upon.

The principles of palliative care

Knowing how to approach patients with advanced illness is the first step in achieving effective care. Six key principles underpin effective, holistic care:

1. Consider the patient and their family/carers as the unit of care while respecting patient autonomy and confidentiality and acknowledge and encourage their participation.
2. Perform a systematic assessment of physical, psychological, social, and spiritual needs.
3. Communicate findings to the patient, providing information and support at all stages.
4. Relieve the patient's symptoms promptly: "*There is only today.*"
5. Plan proactively and thoroughly for potential/ anticipated future problems.
6. Use a team approach listening to suggestions and views and involving resources for extra support at an early stage.

What do patients and their carers need?

The uniqueness of each individual's situation must be acknowledged and the manner of care adapted accordingly. The essence of what patients and their carers may need is outlined in Box 1.4.

It should be clear from this that communication skills (see Chapter 6) play a fundamental role in achieving good palliative care and quality of life for the patient:

> Almost invariably, the act of communication is an important part of the therapy; occasionally it is the only constituent. It usually requires greater thought and planning than a drug prescription, and unfortunately it is commonly administered in subtherapeutic doses [61].

Achieving good symptom management

Twycross, among others, has done much to ensure an evidence-based, scientific rigor in palliative care [62]. The management of any problem should be approached as follows:

- Anticipation
- Evaluation and assessment
- Explanation and information
- Individualised treatment
- Re-evaluation and supervision
- Attention to detail
- Continuity of care.

Anticipation

Many physical and nonphysical problems can often be anticipated and in some instances prevented. Failure to anticipate problems and to set up appropriate manage-

---

Box 1.4 The rights and needs of patients and their carers

Patients have a right to confidentiality, pain control, and other symptom management and, wherever possible, to choose the setting of death and the degree of carer involvement. They also have a right to deny the illness.

Information
The patient has a need for sensitive, clear explanations of:
- the diagnosis and its implications;
- the likely effects of treatments on activities of daily living and well-being;
- the type and extent of support that may be required and how it may be addressed; and
- expected symptoms and what may be done about them.

Quality of life
The patient has a need for life that is as normal, congenial, independent, and as dignified as possible.

An individual's quality of life will depend on minimising the gap between their expectations and aspirations and their actual experiences. This may be achieved by:
- respect, as a person as well as a patient, from properly trained staff who see themselves as partners in living,
- effective relief from pain and other distressing symptoms,
- an appropriate and satisfying diet;
- comfort and consolation, especially from those who share the patient's values and beliefs and/or belong to the same cultural community;
- companionship from family and friends and from members of the care team;
- continuity of care from both the primary care team and other services;
- consistent and effective response to changes in physical and psychosocial discomfort; and
- information about support and self-help and other groups and services.

Support for carers
The patient's family or other carers have a need for support at times of crises in the illness and in their bereavement. These needs include:
- practical support with financial, legal, housing, or welfare problems;
- information about the illness (with the patient's consent) and the available support;
- respite from the stress of caring;
- involvement of carers in the moment of death and in other aspects of care;
- bereavement support; and
- special support where the patient's death may directly affect young children or where the patient is a child or adolescent.

Box 1.5 Applying an understanding of the natural history of a disease and psychosocial awareness to care planning

A 45-year-old woman has recently been found to have spinal metastases from her breast cancer. Potential issues that could be anticipated are:

- Pain—due to the boney origin; this may need nonsteroidal anti-inflammatory drug (NSAID), opioids, and radiotherapy.
- Constipation—start laxatives when opioid is prescribed.
- Spinal cord compression—examine neurology if unsteady or complains of numbness.
- If she has young children—may need help, practically and in telling the children.
- Work—may she need financial and benefit advice?
- Hypercalcaemia—check blood if nauseated or confused.
- Psychospiritual—how is she coping with the impact?

ment strategies (e.g., who should they call?) is a common source of dissatisfaction for patients [63]. Understanding the natural history of the disease with specific reference to an individual patient, awareness of the patient's psychosocial circumstances and identification of risk factors allows planning of care by the team. For an example of applying this in practice, see Box 1.5.

Evaluation and assessment

An understanding of the pathophysiology and likely cause(s) of any particular problem is vital in selecting and directing appropriate investigations and treatment. Deciding what treatment to use is based on consideration of the evidence of the mechanism of the symptom and of the treatment's efficacy, safety, and appropriateness in the situation. This is illustrated by the following specific examples:

- Sedation for an agitated patient with urinary retention is not as helpful as catheterisation.
- Antiemetics for the nausea of hypercalcaemia are important but so too is lowering the serum calcium (if appropriate).
- A patient who is fearful of dying may be helped more by discussing and addressing specific fears rather than taking benzodiazepines.
- Pain in a vertebral metastasis may be helped by analgesics, radiotherapy, orthopaedic surgery, transcutaneous electrical nerve stimulation, and acupuncture. A decision as to which to prescribe is made only by careful assessment.

Comorbidity is common and should always be considered. For example, it is easy (and unfortunately common) to assume that the pain in a patient with cancer is caused by the cancer. In one series almost a quarter of pains in patients with cancer were unrelated to the cancer or the cancer treatment [64].

The multidimensional nature of symptoms, such as pain, means that the use of drugs may be only one part of treatment. A holistic assessment is vital in enabling the most effective management plan. This includes eliciting the patient's concerns and focusing on their feelings.

Explanation and information

Management of a problem should always begin with explanation of the findings and diagnostic conclusions. This usually reduces the patient's anxieties, even if it confirms their worst suspicions—a monster in the light is usually better faced than a monster unseen in the shadows. Further information may be useful to some patients. A clear explanation of the suggested treatments and follow-up plan is important for the patient to gain a sense of control and security. Allow plenty of space for questions and check that what you meant to convey has been understood (see Chapter 6).

Some real examples:

Mr H, with advanced liver disease, was very anxious in the outpatient department. He told me he had developed a tender lump on his chest. On examination this turned out to be gynaecomastia, most probably, I thought, due to the spironolactone. With this explanation, and the relief of his anxiety, he chose to continue the drug rather than have recurrence of his ascites.

Mrs S looked worried and was angry. We discussed the scan results she had had 6 months earlier, before her chemotherapy and surgery. "So what does that mean?" she asked. "I'm afraid that means the cancer cannot be cured," I said. She dissolved in tears and said "Thank you doctor. I have been thinking this but no one would tell me."

Individualised treatment

The individual physical, social, and psychological circumstances of the patient and their views and wishes should be considered in planning care. For example, lymphoedema compression bandages may be unused unless there is someone available to help the patient to fit them daily.

Treatment options need to be shared with the patient and their perspective on choices be explored. For example, Mr K developed arterial occlusion in his leg. Because of his other symptoms, he was thought to have recurrent bladder cancer, but this was not confirmed by scans. He needed to consider whether to have an amputation. It appeared most likely that he would die from his disease within the next weeks to months. He decided that he would only have the amputation if he had 6 months or more to live and declined the operation.

Re-evaluation and supervision: be proactive

The symptoms of frail patients with advanced disease can change frequently. New problems can occur and established ones worsen. Interventions may be complex (many patients take more than 20 pills a day), and close supervision is vital to ensure optimum efficacy and tailoring to the patient.

Attention to detail

The quality of palliative care is in the detail of care. For example, it is vital to ensure that the patient not only has a prescription for the correct drug but also can obtain it from the pharmacy, have adequate supplies to cover a weekend, and understand how to adjust it if the problem worsens.

Continuity of care

No professional can be available for 24 h and 7 days a week, but patients may need support at all hours of the day. Transfer of information within teams and to those that may be called upon to provide care (e.g., out-of-hours services) is one way of ensuring continuity of care. Patient-held records, clear plans in nursing care records at the patient's house, team handover/message books, and formalised information for out-of-hours services [65] are all ways to achieve this.

Limits of symptom control

There is always something more that can be done to help a patient, but it is not always possible to completely relieve symptoms. Specialist advice should usually have been sought for help in the management of intractable symptoms. This extra support is in itself an important way of helping the patient.

In such situations an acceptable solution must be found to provide adequate relief of distress for the patient. For the management of a physical symptom and sometimes of psychological distress, this may be a compromise between the presence of the symptom and sedation from medications. It is hard for a team to accept suboptimal relief of symptoms, and discussions with the patient and the family may be very difficult. It is important for the team

to remember the great value of their continuing involvement to the patients and their carers, to acknowledge how difficult the situation is, and not to abandon the patient because it is painful and distressing for the professionals:

> Slowly, I learn about the importance of powerlessness.
> I experience it in my own life and I live with it in my work.
> The secret is not to be afraid of it—not to run away.
> The dying know we are not God.
> All they ask is that we do not desert them [66].

Attaining quality in palliative care

The quality of palliative and end-of-life care is an area of increasing focus. A key challenge is the integration of palliative care alongside treatments of curative intent and in the care of many more patients [67]. Discussion of treatment benefits and burdens and of end-of-life choices is an important feature of quality in advanced disease. Guidance from the National Institute for Health and Clinical Excellence (NICE) in the United Kingdom interprets the evidence base for achieving high-quality palliative and supportive cancer care [68] (see the key recommendations for primary care in Box 1.6) and has recently developed a Quality Standard for end-of-life care for adults [69]. The EoLCS in England and Wales has defined an array of quality outcomes markers [70]. Similar initiatives are in place in many countries across the world [71–74].

Box 1.6 Recommendations of the NICE guidance for Supportive and Palliative Care 2004, which are key for primary care

12: Mechanisms need to be implemented within each locality to ensure that medical and nursing services are available for patients with advanced cancer on a 24 h, 7 days a week basis and that equipment can be provided without delay. Those providing generalist medical and nursing services should have access to specialist advice at all times.

13: Primary care teams should institute mechanisms to ensure that the needs of patients with advanced cancer are assessed and that the information is communicated within the team and with other professionals as appropriate. The *GSF* provides one mechanism for achieving this.

14: In all locations, the particular needs of patients who are dying from cancer should be identified and addressed. The *Liverpool Care Pathway for the Dying Patient* provides one mechanism for achieving this.

Source: Reproduced from Reference 68.

Quality assurance

The GSF for palliative care described above [15,58,59] is one possible method for assuring high-quality palliative care and is partially embedded in the quality and outcomes framework for primary care in England and Wales. The practical use of frameworks such as the GSF is discussed further in Chapter 2, *Palliative care in the community*. The use of a care pathway is another method of quality assurance, and two such pathways have been developed for care in the last days of life [75,76]. Standards for palliative care have also been developed for community hospitals and nursing homes.

Clinical governance systems are a key component of quality assurance, and examples relating to palliative care within this framework are shown in Box 1.7. In the future, commissioners may develop novel enhanced level services in palliative care, driving up the quality in areas of poor performance.

Audit of quality

In some countries, measurement and benchmarking of outcomes of specialist care is quite advanced [77], but none as yet measure quality or outcome in whole health systems.

Quality assurance frameworks such as the GSF and Dying Care Pathway are relatively easily audited with respect to goals of care. For example, a standard could be set by a commissioner or service or practice that the place of choice for death should be known for at least 80% of patients and a death at home should be achieved for at least 80% of those desiring this. Various measures of outcomes in palliative care has been developed, with a breadth of validation work [78,79]. Only two, however, have validation in primary care: the Palliative Care Outcome Scale [80] and the Cambridge Palliative Audit Schedule: CAMPAS-R [81]. Chapter 2, *Palliative care in the community*, explores the use of the After Death Analysis tool of the GSF.

References

1. Gott M, Seymour J, Ingleton C, et al. That's part of everybody's job: the perspectives of health care staff in England and New Zealand on the meaning and remit of palliative care. *Palliat Med* 2011; doi: 10.1177/0269216311408993.
2. Redinbaugh EM, Sullivan AM, Block SD, et al. Doctors' emotional reactions to recent death of a patient: cross sectional study of hospital doctors. *BMJ* 2003; 327: 185.

3. Mitchell GK. How well do general practitioners deliver palliative care? A systematic review. *Palliat Med* 2002; 16: 457–464.

4. General Medical Council. *Treatment and Care Towards the End of Life: Good Practice in Decision Making.* London: GMC, 2010

5. Bell D. GMC guidelines on end of life care. *BMJ* 2010; 340: c3231.

6. Lakhani M. Let's talk about dying. *BMJ* 2011; 342: d3018.

7. Department of Health. *End of Life Care Strategy.* London: DH, 2008

8. Boyd K and Murray SA. Recognizing and managing key transitions in end of life care. *BMJ* 2010; 341: c4863.

9. National Audit Office. *End of Life Care.* London: Stationary office, 2008.

10. Department of Health. *National Cancer Survivorship Initiative.* London: Vision, DH, 2010

11. Armes PJ, Richardson A, Crowe M, et al. Patients' supportive care needs beyond the end of treatment: a prospective and longitudinal survey. *J Clini Oncol* 2009; 27: 6172–6179.

12. Saunders C. Foreword. In: Doyle D, Hanks GWC and Macdonald N (eds), *Oxford Textbook of Palliative Medicine.* Oxford: Oxford University Press, 1993, pp. v–viii.

13. *National Cancer Control Programmes: Policies and Managerial Guidelines,* 2nd edition. Geneva: World Health Organization, 2002.

14. Saunders C. Care of the dying—the problem of euthanasia. *Nursing Times* 1976; 72: 1049–1052.

15. Shaw KL, Clifford C, Thomas K, et al. Review: improving end-of-life care: a critical review of the gold standards framework in primary care. *Palliat Med* 2010; 24(3): 317–329.

16. Gomes S, Higginson I, Gomes B, et al. Where people die (1974–2030): past trends, future projections and implications for care. *Palliat Med* 2008; 22: 33–41.

17. The Barcelona Declaration on Palliative Care. *Eur J Pall Care* 1995; 3: 15.

18. Cancer pain relief and palliative care. Technical report series: 804. Geneva: World Health organization, 1990.

19. Wright M, Wood J, Lynch T, et al. *Mapping Levels of Palliative Care Development: A Global View.* Lancaster: International Observatory for end of life care, 2008.

20. *The Lien Foundation: Conspiracy of Silence: Life before Death Moonshine Movies.* 2011. Available at: http://www.youtube.com/watch?v=01ˈISKV2eF0; www.lifebeforedeath.com (accessed on May 17, 2012).

21. Sternswärd J and Clark D. Palliative medicine—a global perspective. In: Doyle D, Hanks G, Cherny N and Calman K (eds), *Oxford Textbook of Palliative Medicine,* 3rd edition. Oxford: Oxford University Press, 2003.

22. Kanavos P. The rising burden of cancer in the developing world. *Ann Oncol* 2006; 17(Suppl 8): viii15–viii23.

23. Bulato RA and Stephens PW. Estimates and projections of mortality by cause: a global overview 1970–2015. In: Jamison DT and Mosley HW (eds), *The World Bank Health Sector Priorities Review.* Washington, DC: World Bank, 1991.

24. World Health Organization. Tobacco-attributable mortality: global estimates and projections. In: *Tobacco Alert.* Geneva: World Health Organisation, 1991.

25. United Nations. *Single Convention on Narcotic Drugs, 1961.* United Nations sales No. E62.XI.1. New York, NY: United Nations, 1962.

26. International Narcotics Control Board. *Availability of Internationally Controlled Drugs: Ensuring Adequate Access for Medical and Scientific Purposes.* New York, NY: United Nations, 2011.

27. Cherny NI, Baselga J, de Conno F, et al. Formulary availability and regulatory barriers to accessibility of opioids for cancer pain in Europe: a report from the ESMO/EAPC Opioids Policy Initiative. *Ann Oncol* 2010; 21: 615–626

28. Anderson T. Cancer doctors pledge to widen access to pain relief in developing countries. *BMJ* 2010; 341: c4645.

29. Kutner JS, Kassner CT and Nowels DE. Symptom burden at the end of life: hospice providers' perceptions. *J Pain Symptom Manage* 2001; 21: 473–480.

30. Rogers MS and Todd CJ. The "right kind" of pain: talking about symptoms in outpatient oncology consultations. *Palliat Med* 2000; 14: 299–307.

31. European Pain in Cancer (EPIC) survey. 2007. Available at www.epicsurvey.com (accessed on May 17, 2012).

32. Valeberg BT, Rustoen T, Bjordal K, et al. Self-reported prevalence, etiology, and characteristics of pain in oncology outpatients. *European Journal of Pain* 2008; 12(5): 582–590.

33. Addington-Hall J and McCarthy M. Dying from cancer: results of a national population-based investigation. *Palliat Med* 1995; 9: 295–305.

34. Valdimarsdottir U, Helgason AR, Furst CJ, et al. The unrecognised cost of cancer patients' unrelieved symptoms: a nationwide follow-up of their surviving partners. *Br J Cancer* 2002; 86: 1540–1545.

35. Livingston G, et al. Making decisions for people with dementia who lack capacity: qualitative study of family carers in UK. *BMJ* 2010; 341: c4184.

36. Mills M, Davies HTO and Macrae WA. Care of dying patients in hospital. *BMJ* 1994; 309: 583–586.

37. Jones RVH. *A Parkinson's Disease Study in Devon and Cornwall.* London: Parkinson's Disease Society, 1993.

38. Addington-Hall JM, Lay M, Altmann D, et al. Symptom control, communication with health professionals and hospital care of stroke patients in the last year of life, as reported by surviving family, friends and carers. *Stroke* 1995; 26: 2242–2248.

39. Department of Health. *National Service Framework for Coronary Heart Disease.* London: Department of Health, 2000.

40. Department of Health. *National Service Framework for Older People.* London: Department of Health, 2001. www.doh.gov.uk/nsf/olderpeople/pdfs/nsfolderpeople.pdf.

41. Tebbit P. *Palliative Care for Adults with Non-malignant Diseases: Developing a National Policy*. London: National Council for Hospices and Specialist Palliative Care Services, 2003.

42. Thorns A and Cawley D. Palliative care in chronic obstructive pulmonary disease. *BMJ* 2011; 342: d106.

43. Pinnock H, Kendall M, Murray SA, et al. Living and dying with severe chronic obstructive pulmonary disease: multi-perspective longitudinal qualitative study. *BMJ* 2011; 342: d142.

44. Fergus CJY, Chinn DJ and Murray SA. Assessing and improving out-of-hours palliative care in a deprived community: a rapid appraisal study. *Palliat Med* 2010; 24: 493–500.

45. Munday D, Dale J and Barnett M. Out-of-hours palliative care in the UK: perspectives from general practice and specialist services. *J R Soc Med* 2002; 95: 28–30.

46. Shipman C, Addington-Hall J, Barclay S, et al. Providing palliative care in primary care: how satisfied are GPs and district nurses with current out-of-hours arrangements? *Br J Gen Pract* 2000; 50: 477–478.

47. Thomas K. *Out of Hours Palliative Care in the Community*. London: Macmillan Cancer Relief, 2001.

48. Chattoo S, Ahmad W, Haworth M, et al. *South Asian and White Patients with Advanced Cancer: Patients' and Families' Experiences of the Illness and Perceived Needs for Care. Final Report to Cancer Research UK*. Centre for Research in Primary Care, University of Leeds, January 2002.

49. Kai J, Beavan J and Faull C. Challenges of mediated communication, disclosure and patient autonomy in cross-cultural cancer care. *Br J Cancer* 2011; 1–7. doi: 10.1038/bjc.2011.318.

50. Hill D and Penso D. *Opening Doors: Improving Access to Hospice and Specialist Palliative Care Services by Members of Black and Ethnic Minority Communities*. London: National Council for Hospices and Specialist Palliative Care Services, 1995.

51. Karim K, Bailey M and Tunna KH. Non-white ethnicity and the provision of specialist palliative care services: factors affecting doctors' referral patterns. *Palliat Med* 2000; 14: 471–478.

52. Firth S. *Wider Horizons: Care of the Dying in a Multicultural Society*. London: The National Council for Hospice and Specialist Palliative Care Services, 2001.

53. Gunarantum Y. Ethnicity and palliative care. In: Culley L and Dyson S (eds), *Ethnicity and Nursing Practice*. Basingstoke: Palgrave, 2001.

54. Faull C. Cancer and palliative care. In: Kai J (ed.), *Ethnicity, Health and Primary Care*. Oxford: Oxford University Press, 2003.

55. Selby P. Cancer clinical outcomes for minority ethnic groups. *Br J Cancer* 1996; 74: S54–S60.

56. Johnson MRD, Bains J, Chauan J, et al. *Improving Palliative Care for Minority Ethnic Communities in Birmingham*. A report for the Birmingham Specialist and Community NHS Trust and Macmillan Trust, 2001.

57. Gatrad AR, Brown E, Notta H, et al. Palliative care needs of minorities. *BMJ* 2003; 327: 176–177.

58. Thomas K. *Caring for the Dying at Home: Companions on a Journey*. Oxford: Radcliffe Medical Press, 2003.

59. Thomas, K. The gold standards framework in community palliative care. *Eur J Palliat Care* 2003; 10(3): 113–115.

60. Munday D, Mahmood K, Agarwal S, et al. Evaluation of the Macmillan gold standards framework for palliative care (GSF)—Phases 3–6 (2003–2005). *Palliat Med* 2006; 20(2): 134

61. Buckman R. Communication in palliative care: a practical guide. In: Doyle D, Hanks GWC and Macdonald N (eds), *Oxford Textbook of Palliative Medicine*. Oxford: Oxford University Press, 1993, pp. 47–61.

62. Twycross R, Wilcock A and Toller S. *Symptom Management in Advanced Cancer*, 4th edition. Oxford: Radcliffe Medical Press, 2009.

63. Blyth A. An audit of terminal care in general practice. *BMJ* 1987; 294: 871–874.

64. Twycross RG and Fairfield S. Pain in far advanced cancer. *Pain* 1982; 14: 303–310.

65. King N, Thomas K and Bell D. An out-of-hours protocol for community palliative care: practitioners' perspectives. *Int J Palliat Nurs* 2003; 9: 277–282.

66. Cassidy S. *Sharing the Darkness; the Spirituality of Caring*. London: Darton, Longman and Todd, 1988.

67. Spotlight: palliative care beyond cancer. *BMJ* 2010; 341: 644–662.

68. National Institute for Clinical Excellence. *Guidance on Cancer Services: Improving Supportive and Palliative Care for Adults with Cancer*. London: National Institute for Clinical Excellence, 2004.

69. National Institute for Health and Clinical Excellence. Quality standard for end of life care for adults, 2011

70. Department of Health. *End of Life Care Strategy: Quality Markers and Measures for End of Life Care*. London: DH, 2009.

71. National Consensus Project for Quality Palliative Care. 2009. *Clinical Practice Guidelines for Quality Palliative Care*, 2nd edition. Available at: http://www.nationalconsensusproject.org.

72. African Palliative Care Association Standards for Providing Quality Palliative Care Across Africa. APCA, 2010

73. *Standards for Providing Palliative Care for all Australians*, 4th edition. Palliative Care Australia, 2005

74. Canadian Hospice Palliative Care Association (CHCPA). A Model Guide to Hospice Palliative Care: Based on National Principles and Norms of Practice, 2002.

75. Ellershaw J and Ward C. Care of the dying patients; the last hours or days of life. *BMJ* 2003; 326: 30–34.

76. Fowell A, Finlay I, Johnstone R, et al. An integrated care pathway for the last two days of life: Wales-wide benchmarking in palliative care. *Palliat Nurs* 2002; 8: 566–573.

77. Eagar K, Watters P, Currow DC, et al. The Australian palliative care outcomes collaboration (PCOC)—measuring the quality and outcomes of palliative care on a routine basis. *Aust Health Review* 2010; 34: 186–192.

78. Hearn J and Higginson IJ. Outcome measures in palliative care for advanced cancer patients. *J Pub Health Med* 1997; 19:193–199.

79. Clinical Effectiveness Working Group. *The Which Tool Guide?* Southampton: Association for Palliative Medicine, 2002.

80. Hearn J and Higginson IJ. Development and validation of a core outcome measure for palliative care: the palliative care outcome scale. Palliative Care Core Audit Project Advisory Group. *Qual Health Care* 1999; 8: 219–227.

81. Ewing G, Todd C, Rogers M, et al. Validation of a symptom measure suitable for use among palliative care patients in the community: CAMPAS-R. *J Pain Symptom Manage* 2004; 27: 287–299.

2 Palliative Care in the Community

Daniel Munday[1], Rodger Charlton[2]

[1] Division of Health Sciences, Warwick Medical School, Coventry, UK
[2] Swansea University, Swansea, UK

Introduction

Patients who require palliative care as part of their illness management, whether they suffer from cancer or other long-term conditions, need to receive it where they live. In the community setting as elsewhere, for care to be effective, it is widely accepted that it should be delivered by a multidisciplinary team (MDT). In the United Kingdom and many other affluent countries, palliative care in the community is principally provided by the patient's general practitioner (GP) and district nurses, who in this context are the central members of the primary care team. The configuration of primary care services does vary from country to country, and it is impossible to give a detailed account of generic community palliative care that will apply to all settings, although many of the principles involved are transferable between countries with different health-care systems. This chapter is written from the perspective of the United Kingdom, as this is where both authors practice.

Currently, there is much debate about the small proportion of people who die at home compared to those dying in hospital, and it is easy to forget that dying at home, apart from in the past 50 years, used to be the norm. In fact, the debate in the early 1960s was around the lack of availability of hospital beds for dying patients, particularly the old [1,2]. At that time it was recognised that death could not always be effectively managed at home, and admission for symptom control and nursing care was sometimes necessary.

Although admissions to hospital have increased in frequency in recent decades, even now patients in their last year of life spend the majority of their time at home. Admissions to hospital accelerates toward the end of life (Figure 2.1) and more than 50% of deaths occur in hospital. However, currently more than a third of patients die in community settings under the clinical management of the GP and primary care team, either at home (20%) or in care homes (16%) [3].

On average a GP with a list size of 2,000 will have around 20 patient deaths in a year. Only about two of these will be sudden as a result of acute disease with no previous chronic condition or as a result of an accident, the vast majority dying from chronic illness of some form:

- Five deaths will be from cancer.
- Six from organ failure including heart failure, chronic obstructive pulmonary disease, and renal failure.
- Seven will be from diseases of old age, frailty, and dementia [5].

These illness types have been defined according to the typical trajectories that they follow (see Figure 2.2). Cancer patients frequently decline in a more predictable manner with a clear terminal phase, while death in the other two trajectories can be much more difficult to predict. This can lead to difficulty for the GP and primary care team knowing when to take a palliative and supportive care approach—leading to "prognostic paralysis," a term that has been used to describe why noncancer patients mostly fail to receive palliative and supportive care [6].

This chapter explores palliative care in the community and new developments that aim to improve its quality and extend its provision to all patients, irrespective of diagnosis. It examines the role of the GP and district nurse, community specialist teams, and the relatively new role in the United Kingdom of the community matron. It explores specialist services that have been developed to support community palliative care for patients with cancer and other conditions. Since patients may require health-care services 24 h a day and 7 days a week, out-of-hours care is

Handbook of Palliative Care, Third Edition. Edited by Christina Faull, Sharon de Caestecker, Alex Nicholson and Fraser Black.
© 2012 by John Wiley and Sons, Inc. Published 2012 by John Wiley & Sons, Inc.

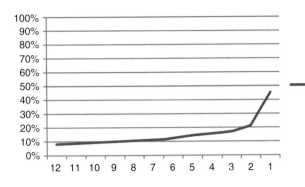

Figure 2.1 Hospital admissions at end of life [4].

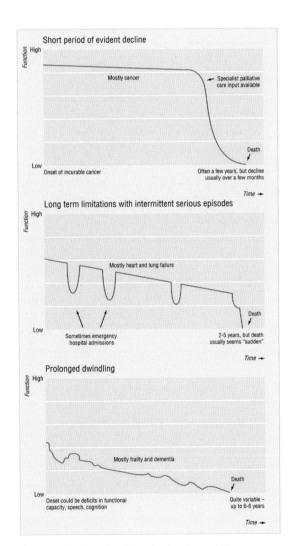

Figure 2.2 Trajectories of function in advanced illnesses. (Reproduced from Reference 7.)

an important aspect of community provision and can be particularly challenging. Therefore, the chapter explores important issues relevant in providing effective out-of-hours care and some of the recent developments that are designed to enhance its effectiveness.

Over recent years, several initiatives have been developed and implemented to support and improve community palliative care. We take a critical look at one, the Gold Standards Framework (GSF) that is now used by more than 60% of practices in the United Kingdom [8]. We explore some of the tools available to evaluate the effectiveness of community palliative care and discuss the aims of the End of Life Care Strategy (EOLCS) [9] as the main policy driver for palliative care in England.

Palliative care and the general practitioner

Care of the dying has always been central to the role of the GP, although few studies systematically explored this before the inception of hospice care 45 years ago [10].

Several of the original pioneers of hospice and palliative care were GPs [11], and the association between general practice and palliative care has continued since that time. Eric Wilkes, who established St Luke's Hospice in Sheffield (the first hospice to have a day unit) and became Professor of General Practice at the University of Sheffield in 1971, published a review of care of the dying in the community in 1967 [2]. Another early pioneer, Dewi-Rees, a GP in mid-Wales and later Medical Director at St Mary's Hospice, Birmingham, published a review of his practice in caring for the dying in the *BMJ* in 1972, which demonstrated the importance of community hospitals in care of the dying [12]. Several publications followed through the 1970s and 1980s, illustrating the growing focus on care of the dying among GPs [13–16].

"Terminal Care" was explicitly identified as a core service in the 2004 GP contract, although previously it had been clearly considered by many GPs as being such [17–19]. While, historically, specialist palliative care services have particularly focused on cancer patients, GPs will be involved in the care of all their patients at the end of life irrespective of diagnosis [20]. Commentators have argued that this indicates the importance of considering the GP and primary care team as the central providers of palliative care in the community. Many GPs will see palliative care as being a special part of general practice and an important aspect of its distinctive character, although a minority have indicated that they see it as being more appropriately delivered by specialist teams [21,22]. Recently the Royal College of General Practitioners (RCGP) has developed its own strategy for "End of Life Care" and has re-emphasised care of the dying as being a central aspect of general practice [23].

GPs have the special role of providing continuity of care to their patients over long periods of time, frequently many years. The distinctive doctor–patient relationship that develops over this time is central to high-quality general practice, and indeed palliative care patients particularly value this relationship [24]. Accessibility and attention to detail are consistently reported as the most important attributes of the "good" GP in international studies of palliative care [25,26].

Many studies of satisfaction with GP services have surveyed patients' carers some time after the death of the patient; these have reported high levels of satisfaction, with between two-thirds and three-quarters of bereaved carers reporting good or excellent care from their GP [27–29]. Frequent visiting of terminally ill patients has been particularly associated with high levels of satisfaction by bereaved carers [30] and willingness to make home visits, time taken to listen and discuss issues of importance to the patient and their carers, and making an effort to control symptoms are highly valued [28]. Grande and colleagues in a large qualitative study with bereaved carers highlighted that they were particularly satisfied with GPs who went "beyond their remit to make themselves available" [24, p. 775], such as giving their personal number, visiting when not on duty and attending without being summoned. In addition, they highlight the importance carers attach to GPs offering support for themselves, including information about the patient's illness and approaches to symptom control.

While overall satisfaction seems to be high, symptom control provided by GPs may not be always as effective as hoped [27,29,31], despite GPs being familiar with the modern approaches to pain management [31]. The adequacy of symptom control will depend on symptoms being appropriately identified, and this seems to be an area where there are some problems. In a sample of 150 GPs in Cambridgeshire, whose reporting of symptoms for patients was compared to patients' own reports, GPs were found to under-report all symptoms apart from loss of appetite, which they over-reported in comparison with patients. Under-reporting was greater for symptoms that GPs reported as more difficult to control, suggesting that GPs may be less likely to ask patients about symptoms for which they have no ready solution [32]. In addition, since patients may be less likely to consult about symptoms that they see as inevitable and untreatable [33], these issues combined may lead to a lack of effective symptom control in patients being cared for principally by their GP.

Studies of GPs' knowledge in palliative care have suggested that they might not possess all the knowledge or skills necessary for effective symptom control. While the majority of GPs demonstrate a good grasp of the basics of palliative pain control, fewer demonstrate this in more complex areas [31]. In addition a substantial number of GPs do express a lack of confidence in areas of symptom control [32] and wish for more education in palliative care particularly in symptom control for noncancer patients [34].

Training in palliative care for GPs

Palliative care teaching in medical school is frequently given relatively little time and prominence in the curriculum, and many newly qualified doctors feel unprepared to care for dying patients [35]. Lack of training for GPs has also been reported. Two surveys conducted by Barclay et al., one in East Anglia and the other in Wales [36,37], reported similar results. GPs had received very little training in palliative care in medical school or as junior hospital doctors, but had received more in the specific training time in practice as a GP registrar (GPR) and as GP principals. The majority of GPR training schemes do offer some training in palliative care, although the amount of time dedicated to it is often relatively short, and lack of resources has sometimes meant difficulty in finding experienced clinicians to teach or adequate hospice placements for trainees to gain experience [38]. Evidence from the West Midlands suggests palliative care training can be effective with GPR confidence increasing during the practice attachment year [39].

District nurses

As with GPs, district nurses have always been involved in caring for dying patients at home. Similarly there is little written about the role of the district nurse until the early 1990s. In the early days of the National Health Service (NHS), district nurses worked under the instructions of GPs although there was little understanding of teamworking as such, and it was quite common for GPs and district nurses never to meet apart from if they happened to visit the same patient at the same time [40]. District nurses were employed by local authorities and were not attached to particular practices.

The late 1960s and 1970s saw a marked change in the ways community nursing was provided, so that by 1977 84% of general practices had attached nurses [41]. Two large national studies of care of patients in the last year of life, one in 1967 and one in 1987, highlight some important changes in the way district nurses worked over this time. In 1967 district nurses were more likely to only be involved late in the patient's illness, providing frequent visits when the patient was dying, while in 1987 patients tended to be referred earlier, but were visited less frequently. As there was little research into district nursing at this time [42], it is not totally clear what brought about this change, although it is likely to be related to the increased awareness of palliative care and also the adoption into practice of continuous subcutaneous infusion devices (syringe drivers), which perhaps led to the need for less frequent visiting [43]. Now, the central role of district nurses in palliative care has been officially recognised and formalised in national strategy [44,45].

More studies into the role of the district nurse in palliative care have been undertaken since 1990, although this is still a relatively poorly researched area [46]. It has been estimated that around 40% of a district nurses' work is devoted to caring for patients with palliative care needs [47], and district nurses themselves describe palliative and terminal care as being a central part of their work [48–51], considering their principal role to be that of coordinator of care [50,52–54]. Patients and carers have identified that district nurses are the professionals who have the greatest regular contact with palliative care patients in the community [55]. District nurses have reported their work as being emotionally stressful, time consuming, and unpredictable. Although district nurses see their role in community palliative care as vital, they fear that this is not well recognised by their managers [56].

District nurses' role is highly practical and varied; wound dressing including pressure sores and complex fungating wounds in cancer patients, monitoring a patient's general condition, symptom control, bowel care, managing syringe drivers, organising packages of care for patients as they become increasingly frail and need regular nursing care at home, and providing emotional support for patients and families.

Grande et al. identified that the clinical skills of district nurses are complementary to that of GPs with district nurses demonstrating more confidence and skill in dealing with practical issues such as incontinence and pressure sores [32]. Many studies have highlighted district nurses' preference for early referral [49,51,57,58], even from the point of cancer diagnosis [48]. This is particularly important to enable close and supportive relationships not only to develop with patients and carers [52,57] but also to ensure that the patient is receiving a multidisciplinary approach to their care.

In postbereavement studies, levels of carer satisfaction with district nurses work has been high and consistently higher than for GP with dissatisfaction being related to the district nurse being rushed, the service being poorly coordinated or to a feeling that the district nurse was not knowledgeable [27,28,59].

District nurse self-expressed learning needs have been varied and include symptom control, bereavement care, training in breaking bad news, dealing with difficult situations, noncancer symptom control and nonpharmacological pain control [48,54,58,60].

Training of district nurses in palliative care was a key policy of the NHS Cancer Plan in which £6 million was invested in a training programme delivered by the 34 English cancer networks. This was the largest and most focused programme of its kind in palliative care and the evaluation reported that following training, the confidence of district nurses increased, particularly for those with little previous training in palliative care or no formal district nurse qualification. However, there was no change in either carer satisfaction or GP assessment of district nurse knowledge or skills [61].

Patients with end-stage cardiopulmonary disease have been reported as being less likely to receive input from a district nurse [56,62,63]. Goodman et al. proposed that the special role district nurses identified for themselves in caring for terminally ill cancer patients possibly has the detrimental effect of lessening the importance they place on nursing those with chronic nonmalignant illnesses [49]. In addition, patients with nonmalignant disease are less likely to receive care from specialist nurses, making the district nurse role all the more vital [20,53].

Community matrons and case mangers

Care of patients with chronic illness has changed in many areas since the introduction of "NHS case managers" or "community matrons" whose role is to coordinate care for patients with long-term conditions, particularly the ones at increased risk of emergency admission to hospital [64]. The community matron role was based on successful models developed in chronic disease management principally from the United States [65], and initially, it was projected that community matrons could reduce hospital admissions by 10–20% [64]. However, while studies have shown that patients are highly satisfied with the care they receive from community matrons, results from a pilot study showed that community matrons did not have an impact on admission rates [66,67].

The place of community matron in palliative care has not been well-defined. This reflects lack of clarity in their role in general, compounded by a lack of consistency in the way these posts have been established in different localities. King et al. exploring the contribution of community matrons to palliative care discovered a range of views among both matrons themselves and their district nursing colleagues. Some saw the community matron role as being valuable and providing an important addition to community palliative care provision; others believed they had no place in palliative care, with district nurses able to provide any care that might fall to community matrons [68]. Personal experience of one of us, working with a number of community matrons, is that their case management role with patients with advanced long-term conditions is evolving and their skills have become very valuable in delivering palliative care, particularly to patients with noncancer diagnoses approaching the end of life. Experience is likely to vary depending on the local conditions, other resources available, and how services co-evolve. As the role becomes increasingly established, further evaluations of their effectiveness in delivering palliative care will be required.

Specialist palliative care services in the community

Soon after St Christopher's hospice was established in London in 1967, Saunders and colleagues became increas-ingly aware of the need to provide hospice care within the patient's home. The first patients admitted to St Christopher's normally remained in the hospice and died there. It soon became clear that many patients following a period of admission when they received specific symptom-control measures wanted to return home. The St Christopher's home care service was established in 1969, two years after the inpatient unit was opened, with patients receiving the type and quality of care at home that they had received in the hospice. Teams of nurses supported by the hospice medical staff provided care. Baines recognised that the work undertaken in later years by community specialist palliative care clinical nurse specialists (CNSs) was being provided in nascent form by these teams [69].

In 1975 the National Society for Cancer Relief (now Macmillan Cancer Support) established their first community palliative care nursing services. "Macmillan nurses" have become synonymous with palliative care nursing since that time [70]. Palliative care CNSs provide direct patient care often managing complex symptom issues; support and advise district nursing colleagues and GPs; and provide emotional support and palliative care education to generalist colleagues [71,72].

Currently most areas within the United Kingdom have a palliative care CNS service, many, but not all of which have support from a consultant or other doctor in specialist palliative medicine [73]. Specialist palliative care services have often developed in rather an ad hoc manner often first established as a result of a local initiative and fund raising [74]. There is also no one model of community palliative care provision; hence, it is difficult to generalise on the type of services that are offered.

Palliative care and the primary care team

Teamwork is at the heart of delivering effective holistic palliative care in any setting. The aim of palliative care is to enable patients to live as well as possible until they die. That necessitates a holistic approach to provide psychosocial and spiritual care as well as symptom control and physical care. The wider palliative care team will therefore involve rehabilitation specialists (occupational therapy [OT] and physiotherapists), social workers and chaplains as well as nurses and doctors. The core team caring for patients in the community however is the GP and community nurse in the primary care team.

The primary care team started to emerge following the introduction of the GP Charter in 1966 that enabled GPs to employ nurses directly. Team working and a holistic approach to general practice was promoted by Balint, a Hungarian psychotherapist who published his observations of general practice in a book "The doctor, his patient and the illness" in 1957 [75], which became the seminal text for a generation of GP trainees [76]. Within 10 years of the GP charter, 84% of general practices worked within primary care teams that included practice nurses and district nurses [41]. Thus, primary care and palliative care as disciplines providing holistic care based on team working, developed simultaneously through the 1970s and 1980s.

In community palliative care, GPs and district nurses have been seen as having complementary roles, both of which are necessary to provide good quality care. Early on the primary care team had been recognised not just as a place to encourage good clinical care and a vital element for enabling a home death [77] but also as a forum to develop guidelines and protocols with a sense of shared ownership [78] and as an opportunity for education [79]. By the late 1990s many primary care teams had developed sophisticated systems for identifying terminally ill patients on registers (practice registers had become extensively used with the advent of GP clinical IT systems), using faxes to share information with out-of-hours services [80] and auditing palliative care practice [78]. From these early developments emerged the GSF for palliative care [81], designed and promoted in 2000 by Dr Keri Thomas, then a Macmillan GP advisor. GSF has become the most notable development in community palliative care in the past 10 years.

Gold standards framework for palliative care

History of gold standards framework

The development of GSF is quite remarkable in terms of its impact on community palliative care both in the United Kingdom and more latterly internationally [82]. It underwent rapid uptake in the United Kingdom, from small beginnings with a handful of practices in one area to a position where within 6 years more than half of practices randomly surveyed in England and Northern Ireland were involved with GSF [8].

GSF started initially as a pilot project with 12 practices in West Yorkshire, developed and facilitated by Keri Thomas, working with an advisory group of GPs and district nurses. The framework was based on best practice that had emerged and had been defined over previous years by a number of GPs and others working in palliative care [81]. The overall aims of GSF were and remain:

- to identify palliative care patients within the practice;
- to assess their needs; and
- to plan their ongoing care in a proactive way.

Practices agreed to focus improving care and processes in six domains (Table 2.1). The seventh domain, "care of the dying," was not one of the initial domains and was added later.

In each of the practices a coordinator and lead GP were appointed who worked with the area project facilitator to implement the framework within the practice. Central to the GSF then as now was a register of patients with palliative care needs developed by each practice, regular primary care team meetings to discuss patients, and a range of resources to assist in delivering effective care.

The evaluation of the initial pilot phase was by means of a longitudinal comparative study involving serial audit questionnaires completed by the 12 practices undertaking the GSF and by 12 matched practices that did not take part. Focus groups were also held with staff from participating practices to explore the benefits and drawbacks of taking part. Results showed that in comparison with the nonparticipating matched practices, the GSF practices improved processes in all six domains. In the focus groups, there was general agreement that care had improved since the introduction of the framework [83].

Following the success of the first phase, an extended pilot was established with 76 practices in 18 areas in England, Scotland, and Northern Ireland funded jointly by Macmillan Cancer Support and the NHS Modernisation Agency. In each area, there was a facilitator, frequently one of the established Macmillan GP facilitators.

Table 2.1 The seven domains of the GSF.

Communication (C1)
Palliative care register, primary care team meetings, patient-held record
Coordination (C2)
Nominated link person, ACP
Control of symptoms (C3)
Assessment of physical symptoms, psycho-social needs
Continuity of care (C4)
Handover forms, support services
Continuing education (C5)
Review audit meetings, significant event analysis
Carer support (C6)
Practical and emotional support, protocol for the bereaved
Care of the dying (C7)
Care of the dying pathway, anticipatory medication

The programme was evaluated qualitatively with a sample of participants from GSF practices and participants from matched practices being interviewed. It was reported that in practices implementing the framework, care had become more consistent with less chance that patients would be missed or fail to receive the care they required [84].

In 2003 GSF began to be rolled out to practices throughout the United Kingdom. Between 2003 and 2005 more than 1,300 practices enrolled for the GSF in England and Northern Ireland. Scotland ran a separate programme. Uptake of the framework was patchy, with some areas achieving uptake by all local practices and other areas with very few, or even no practices participating [85].

In 2004 GSF became one of four national tools adopted by the NHS End-of-Life Care Programme that had been established by the Department of Health to improve the care patients received, promote choice, and enable more people to die in their preferred place. Through the program, uptake of GSF continued to increase rapidly, so that by 2007 in a large random survey of general practices in the United Kingdom, 61% of respondents indicated that they had involvement in GSF [8].

GSF was approved by the RCGP in 2005 [86] and was promoted in the End of Life Care Strategy (EoLCS) [9] as a framework for achieving widespread improvement in end-of-life care in the community.

In 2004 following the successful implementation of GSF in primary care (GSFPC), a partner programme, GSF in care homes (GSFCH) was established, which sought to transfer the principles of identification, assessment, and care planning into the care home environment [87].

Effectiveness of gold standards framework

Evaluations of GSFPC (between 2000 and 2007) used serial questionnaires that had been developed from the original instrument used in phase 1. Results indicated that within a year of enrolling in the GSF programme, over 90% of participating practices were operating palliative and supportive care registers, had a GSF coordinator within the practice, and had regular team meetings in which patients on the register were discussed [85]. The majority of practices sent handover forms to out-of-hours providers for their palliative care patients, had a system for leaving anticipatory medication in the patient's home, used a systematic approach to assessing patients' physical symptoms, and routinely engaged in advance care planning (ACP) with patients including recording preferred place of death. Fewer practices followed a protocol for

dying patients, such as the Liverpool care pathway (LCP), or offered spiritual care for their patients.

While several studies have looked at the effectiveness of GSF on improving practice processes, few have explored outcomes for patients [82]. While it would have been desirable to explore whether patients had been more likely to die in their place of choice following implementation of GSF, it was clear from the questionnaire data that practices did not routinely record this before starting GSF, and therefore, it was impossible to judge whether this aspect had improved as a result of the framework. In response to this, researchers at the University of Birmingham, along with the GSF central team, have devised an online audit tool "After death analysis (ADA)" [88].

After death analysis tool

The GSF evaluation questionnaires sought to understand the extent to which practices had changed their policies and procedures in palliative care and the impact this had had on patient care. There were two problems associated with this approach: first, the questionnaires were self-completed by the practices, relying on the recall and objectivity of the respondents with the inherent bias that could affect the results. Second, it was likely that to some extent responders would report what they aspired to, rather than what they actually invariably did.

ADA sought to improve recall and focus on patient outcome by looking at five actual deaths that had recently occurred and reporting on those. ADA focuses on important clinical processes and outcomes for individual patients covering the key topic areas as highlighted in Table 2.2.

Specific questions for each patient are posed, for example:

- Were they on the palliative care register?
- Were they offered ACP discussions?
- Did they have an ACP?
- Where was their preferred place of care?
- Did they die in their preferred place?

ADA also enables the respondent to indicate why the patient did not achieve various aspects of care—for example, they were not on the register because it was not an expected death, they did not die at home (their preferred place) because they deteriorated rapidly in hospital where they had been admitted for treatment.

ADA that was based on the original GSF questionnaire was developed at the University of Birmingham and tested in one area in the West Midlands as part of a GSF project [89]. Following this initial phase, the tool was modified and an online version was developed and used in a national

Table 2.2 Key topic areas of the ADA.

Patient choice
  Numbers having ACP discussions
  Numbers dying where they chose or their usual place
    of care
  Reasons they might die elsewhere
Hospitalisation
  Hospital bed days and crisis admissions
Preplanning of care
  Anticipatory prescribing
  Out-of-hours forms sent
Local services
  Use of gaps in service provision
  Bereavement care offered
Systematic
  Benefits advice offered

Source: Reproduced from Reference 88.

audit of palliative care in the community. All the practices in 15 primary care trusts (PCTs) were invited to take part and 502 (57%) did so. The audit ran for 2 months in 2009 and practices were asked to record all deaths in this period. Altogether data on 4,487 deaths were collected.

As practices used the tool to input data, they were immediately able to see a comparison between their own practice and national averages. This was reported as being the most valuable aspect of the exercise. 80% found the tool easy to use and 66% were interested in using the tool on a yearly basis to audit their practice. Many practices agreed that the tool had helped them to reflect on how they delivered care at the end of life, and for 39%, this had resulted in changes being made.

The main challenge in using ADA reported was the time taken per patient, although the average time for completion was around 15 min. In addition, for patients who had died in hospital, all necessary data were not always available [90].

Following the national audit, the online version of the ADA is available for use by individual practices, services, or organisations through the GSF Central Team [88].

Gold standards framework and the multidisciplinary team

Team working is at the root of effective palliative care within the community setting. This has been confirmed and extended through the GSF programme as teams have become focused on delivering integrated care encouraged by the structured approach of the GSF. For many practices team working was already firmly established, together with other central aspects of primary palliative care (e.g., having a register of patients and sending summary faxes to out-of-hours providers). These practices saw the GSF as formalising the processes that they had already been utilising [84,91]. The *success* of the framework also depends on successful teamwork. In one study, those practices in which effective team work was in evidence seemed likely to implement the framework more effectively than in practices where this was not a feature [91].

While multidisciplinary meetings are a central feature of good palliative care in the primary care setting, they can take various forms. They can involve just the district nurse and GP, whereas others will involve a wider group of professionals, most commonly the community palliative care CNS [91]. Also the type of meeting may vary. In one study, district nurses were more likely to prefer structured, formal meetings, while GPs favoured informal "ad hoc" ones. The most successful teams were the ones where both formal meetings and informal communication were utilised. Working in such a flexible way may be a sign of more equality within the GP/district nurse relationship, although Mahmood-Yousuf et al. comment that even in the best-performing teams the hierarchical nature of the relationship remained [92].

Nurses in the primary care team have also used GSF as a way of engaging with GPs more in the effective delivery of community palliative care [93]. District nurses may sometimes struggle to establish effective multidisciplinary working with GPs, frequently because of the competing pressures of general practice [94]. This is also arguably because of the relative lack of power that nurses possess in comparison with their medical colleagues, encouraged by the hierarchical nature of the relationship of between the two disciplines [95]. In this context, GSF can provide the authority that a nurse might lack, to improve the communication between doctor and nurse through the establishment of "GSF" meetings within the practice [93].

Sustaining GSF involvement can also be problematic. King found that a key role maintaining GSF activity was vested in the coordinator. If the coordinator left, then the implementation of the project in a particular practice could be put at risk [84].

Many studies that have reported on the effectiveness of GSF were undertaken before the advent of the Quality and Outcomes Framework (QOF) points for palliative care. Through the QOF process, practices are rewarded for following predefined evidence-based processes that promote good care and beneficial outcomes for patients with chronic long-term conditions. Initially when introduced in 2004 the QOF programme did not include points for palliative care activity, these were added in 2007. Currently practices are rewarded three points for having a palliative care register and 3 for having team meetings at least once every three months, out of a total of 1,024 possible points. Currently 90% of practices achieve their QOF points for palliative care [96]. Whether QOF points lead to enhanced sustainability of GSF is unknown and needs further exploration.

Palliative and end-of-life care in care homes or residential facilities

Death in care homes is becoming increasingly common, a feature of an ageing population; the majority of deaths occurring in nursing home facilities in the over 85 year olds, with an average length of stay less than 1 year. Around 70% of care home residents have dementia [97].

In the past 10 years, much work has been done in exploring the end-of-life issues faced by residents of nursing homes and a number of initiatives to improve care have been devised; the most prominent of these has been the GSFCH. Many care homes may combine GSFCH with the LCP, and this seems to be particularly effective [98].

Since GSFCH was first introduced in 2004 over 1,500 care homes have enrolled in the programme. GSFCH highlights the same seven domains for development, but modified for the care home setting. Staff receive training in these areas in a series of workshops. There is a particular focus on:

• improving processes used within the home—to make ACP the norm with each patient, developing systems for working more effectively with GPs and for providing care in the last days of life (e.g., LCP).

• improving communication—awareness of how to discuss end-of-life care issues with residents and better communication with families and between staff;

• improved team working both within the home and with wider health and social care practitioners;

• decreasing hospitalisation: in using good processes to avoid hospital admission and receiving patients from hospital more rapidly; and

• providing high-quality care with a particular focus on patients with dementia [99].

Homes undertaking the training programme are able to gain a quality standard mark "Going for Gold" delivered by the GSF central team, which is supported by Age UK and endorsed by major care home providers nationally [99].

While robust evidence in primary care for GSF improving patient outcomes directly is lacking [82], GSFCH has been demonstrated to improve outcomes for patients, particularly in terms of reducing crisis admissions and increasing the proportion of residents who die in the care home, rather than being admitted to hospital and dying there [87,98].

Out-of-hours palliative care in the community in the United Kingdom

One feature of the illnesses from which people nearing the end-of-life suffer is that they are unstable. It is not uncommon that symptoms suddenly occur anew or worsen out of hours, and patients need to have access to high-quality care at these times.

Traditionally care was delivered by general practices to their own patients either as a single practice or on a rota with other local practices. Some practices particularly in city areas had for many years used deputising services where they paid commercial companies who employed GPs to provide out-of-hours care for their patients. As the demand for out-of-hours care increased there were increasing calls for GPs to be allowed to set up cooperatives to provide out-of-hours care, with large groups of practices working together (e.g., Birmingham was covered by a single cooperative). These cooperatives operated under different structures, but effectively, were companies own by the GP members [100].

There was great interest in palliative care in cooperatives, much of it generated by Macmillan GP facilitators, who were concerned that the care provided by such organisations might be of a lesser quality than that provided by the patient's own GP practice. Some of the concern centered around the lack of information to which cooperative GPs were likely to have access [101,102].

Many cooperatives developed systems for communicating information about individual patients to out-of-hours GPs, principally by using forms that could be faxed by the patient's own practice. A number of such forms were developed for patients who were receiving palliative care, who were in fact much more likely than other patients to need the services of the cooperative [80]. While this good practice was often aspired to by cooperative GPs, there was evidence that communication was often poor [103] and information can rapidly become out of date.

In 2004 a new GP contract was established that freed GPs from their previous 24-h responsibility for patient care. Out-of-hours care became the responsibility of

PCTs who might provide care by developing their own service, employing the cooperative to carry on delivering care (with many cooperatives becoming "for profit" companies) or by purchasing the services of deputising agencies.

There was much disquiet about what effect this might have on palliative care out of hours and that more patients might be admitted. It seems that there has been no firm evidence published to suggest that this has been the case, although one study found that response times for a GP to attend a patient had increased [104]. However, because of a lack of appropriate quality indicators for out-of-hours palliative care, it is difficult to judge whether quality of care has suffered.

GPs working out of hours still report that their ability to provide the best care for patients is hampered by lack of information, lack of time to address their problems, and poor access to medications and equipment [105,106] and that this increases the likelihood of them having to admit patients who otherwise might have been able to remain at home [106]. The national primary care audit (2009) confirmed that only 27% of patients who died were on the practice palliative care register and less than half of these had information sent by the practice to the GP out-of-hours provider [90].

Many patients at home at the end of life also require district nursing visits during out-of-hours periods and the provision of such a service 24 h a day has been recognised as essential for providing effective domiciliary palliative care [44]. Many areas, however, do not have such a service [47,107]. The EoLCS also recommends the provision of 24-h access to specialist advice for patients in any setting, although whether this is feasible given the lack of consistent provision of specialist services remains to be seen, and whether it is sufficient for this to be telephone advice for primary care professionals or direct face to face services also remains unclear [108].

Out-of-hours services in primary care may be improved by establishing protocols for good practice, including provision of information about patients that is accessible to health-care professionals, the use of anticipatory prescribing and provision of medication that may be needed out of hours [109]. Fergus et al. highlight the development of electronic summary records that can be updated directly from GP systems as a positive development to enable up to date information about patients at the end of life to be made widely available to out-of-hours providers [110]. Such a system is being rolled out through the whole of Scotland [111], and various similar systems have recently been piloted in England [112].

The future: planning and commissioning future palliative care

Focusing on delivering patient choice has been a hallmark of palliative care since the establishment of St Christopher's Hospice. Soon after the hospice was opened, they realised that many patients preferred to die at home, and hence, they established their home care service. Many surveys have indicated that given the choice, most people would prefer to die at home [113] but only around 20% do so in the United Kingdom at present (or 36% if a care home is accepted as the patients "home"). There is evidence that as death approaches many patients do change their minds and prefer an institutional death even where they are receiving high-quality hospice at home services [114]. While practitioners are encouraged to record a patient's "preferred place of death," this for many patients is not possible as preference for place of death may not be absolute, but rather leaning toward one place rather than another [115].

What is also unclear is how *important* achieving home death is to dying patients. Little research has explored this, although one study from the United States found that compared to other factors such as freedom from pain, being mentally aware and have control over treatment decisions, dying at home was relatively unimportant to terminally ill patients [116]. Whether this finding is generalisable or applicable in the British or other contexts is unclear, and further research is needed into this.

While hospital admission does increase rapidly toward death, recent audits have suggested that between 30% and 40% of patients could have been cared for in places other than hospital [117,118], and while it is likely that some of these hospital deaths would have been avoidable, interpreting data following a patient's death is problematic. Many patients who die in hospital have had several admissions before the final one from which they have benefitted and from which they have been discharged. Hospital might be a place of safety for patients and an appropriate place to die, particularly when a patient receiving treatment deteriorates rapidly, the relatives are unable to cope with caring (even when they are given community support) or where the patient lives alone [119].

Focusing on a preference for home death has been a particular feature of health strategy, however, another factor has been the acknowledgement of the need to contain the costs of health care and the need to find more cost effective ways of delivering end-of-life care. Projections have been made that more investment in home care services could substantially decrease hospital deaths to enable cost savings as well as allowing people the opportunity to die at home [118,120]. Whether this is feasible or how savings on hospital budgets would be transferred into community care is unclear [121].

Planners and commissioners of the future will need to recognise the complexity of providing high-quality palliative care in the community and the need to plan and commission care at all levels: primary, acute sector, and specialist palliative care. Outcome measures for effective palliative care have always been challenging to develop and use in practice, because there are no clear and robust quantitative markers available. Considerable work is ongoing in this area, and tools for measuring effectiveness of end-of-life care services are being developed. A new End-of-Life Quality Assessment Tool (ELCQuA) has recently been made available [122] and an End-of-Life Care Quality Standard was published in late 2011 by the NICE [123].

Conclusion

High-quality palliative care delivered in the community is essential. Care provision is traditionally the responsibility of primary care professionals, supported where necessary by multidisciplinary specialist palliative care services. Care for patients at the end of life has traditionally been the role of the GP and district nurse, and while surveys of patients have shown high levels of satisfaction, there is evidence that care can be suboptimal particularly out of hours. Aspects of care such as regular GP visiting and close therapeutic relationships with district nurses, which are highly valued by patients, seem to be increasingly under threat through pressures to increase efficiency and lack of time to commit to palliative care.

Patients' needs are also becoming more complex as new treatments for cancer become available and they survive for longer but with a high disease burden and a poor level of health. The health-care teams that care for them need to be more knowledgeable and skilled in symptom control and recognising and managing palliative care emergencies.

Palliative care needs to be delivered along with disease modifying treatment, particularly in patients with end-stage respiratory and heart disease. Lack of effective methods of making accurate prognostic predictions in these patients leads to difficulty in deciding when a palliative care approach should begin. However, studies have shown that these patients do have high levels of need for palliative care.

New tools, frameworks, and programmes are available to aid practitioners in delivering high-quality care and have demonstrated some success, but they have yet to make a major impact on the patient's experience of end-of-life care. Whether these initiatives will be able to produce the "step change" in the quality of end-of-life care delivered in the community remains to be seen. Commissioners will need to ensure that multidisciplinary, integrated care, delivered by a range of health-care providers with appropriate skills, is allowed to flourish if end-of-life care is going to be of high quality in the future. Simple solutions to the complex challenge of delivering effective community palliative care are unlikely to succeed.

References

1. Glyn Hughes H. *Peace at Last.* London: Calouste Gulbenkian Foundation, 1960.
2. Wilkes E. Terminal cancer at home. *Lancet* 1965; i: 799–801.
3. EoLCIN. 2011. *End of Life Care Intelligence Network. National End of Life Care Programme.* Available at: http://www.endoflifecare-intelligence.org.uk/home.aspx (accessed on May 21, 2012).
4. Bardsley M, Georghiou T and Dixon J. *Social Care and Hospital Use at the End of Life.* London: Nuffield Trust, 2010.
5. Murray SA and Sheikh A. Palliative care beyond cancer: care for all at the end of life. *BMJ* 2008; 336: 958–959.
6. Murray S, Boyd K and Sheikh A. Palliative care in chronic illness. *BMJ* 2005; 330: 611–612.
7. Murray S, Kendall M, Boyd K, et al. Illness trajectories and palliative care. *BMJ* 2005; 330: 1007–1011.
8. Hughes PM, Bath PA, Ahmed N, et al. What progress has been made towards implementing national guidance on end of life care? A national survey of UK general practices. *Palliat Med* 2010; 24: 68–78.
9. Department of Health. *End of Life Care Strategy.* London: DH, 2008
10. Loudon I, Horder J and Webster C. *General Practice under the National Health Service 1948–1997.* London: Clarendon Press, 1998.
11. Clark D, Small N, Wright M, et al. *A Bit of Heaven for the Few: An Oral History of the Modern Hospice Movement in the United Kingdom.* Lancaster: Observatory Publications, 2005.
12. Dewi Rees W. The distress of dying. *BMJ* 1972; iii: 105–107.
13. Reilly P and Patten M. Terminal care in the home. *J R Coll Gen Pract* 1981; 31: 531–537.
14. Woodbine G. The care of patients dying from cancer. *J R Coll Gen Pract* 1982; 32: 685–689.
15. Barritt P. Care of the dying in one practice. *J R Coll Gen Pract* 1984; 34: 446–448.

16. Wilkes E. Dying now. *Lancet* 1984; i: 950–952.

17. Charlton R. Palliative care is integral to practice. *BMJ* 1995; 311: 1503.

18. Fordham S, Dowrick C and May C. Palliative medicine: is it really specialist territory. *J R Coll Gen Pract* 1998; 91: 568–572.

19. Field D. Special not different: general practitioners accounts of their care of dying people. *Soc Sci Med* 1998; 46: 1111–1120.

20. Barclay S. Palliative care for non cancer patients: a UK perspective from primary care. In: Addington-Hall J, Higginson I (eds), *Palliative Care for Non Cancer Patients*. Oxford: Oxford University Press, 2001.

21. Burt J, Shipman C, White P, et al. Roles, service knowledge and priorities in the provision of palliative care: a postal survey of London GPs. *Palliat Med* 2006; 20: 487–492.

22. Shipman C, Addington-Hall J, Barclay S, et al. Educational opportunities in palliative care: what do general practitioners want? *Palliat Med* 2001; 15: 191–196.

23. Thomas K. *End of Life Care Strategy*. London: Royal College of General Practitioners, 2009.

24. Grande G, Farquhar M, Barclay S, et al. Valued aspects of primary palliative care: content analysis of bereaved carers' descriptions. *Br J Gen Pract* 2004; 54: 772–778.

25. Mitchell G. How well do general practitioners deliver palliative care? A systematic review. *Palliat Med* 2002; 16: 457–464.

26. Borgsteede S, Graafland-Riedstra C, Deliens L, et al. Good end-of-life care according to patients and their GPs. *Br J Gen Pract* 2006; 56: 20–26.

27. Addington-Hall J and McCarthy M. Dying from cancer: results of a national population-based investigation. *Palliat Med* 1995; 9: 295–305.

28. Lecouturier J, Jacoby A, Bradshaw C, et al. Lay carers' satisfaction with community palliative care: results of a postal survey. *Palliat Med* 1999; 13: 275–283.

29. Hanratty B. Palliative care provided by GPs: the carer's viewpoint. *Br J Gen Pract* 2000; 50: 653–654.

30. Fakhoury W, McCarthy M and Addington-Hall JM. Determinants of informal caregivers' satisfaction with services for dying cancer patients. *Soc Sci Med* 1996; 42: 721–731.

31. Barclay S, Todd C, Grande G, et al. Controlling cancer pain in primary care: the prescribing habits and knowledge base of general practitioners. *J Pain Symptom Manage* 2002; 23: 383–392.

32. Grande G, Barclay S and CJ T. Difficulty of symptom control and general practitioners' knowledge of patients' symptoms. *Palliat Med* 1997; 11: 399–406.

33. Cartwright A, Hockey L and Anderson JL. *Life Before Death*. London and Boston: Routledge and Kegan Paul, 1973.

34. Shipman C, Addington-Hall J, Thompson M, et al. Building bridges in palliative care: evaluating a GP facilitator programme. *Palliat Med* 2003; 17: 621–627.

35. Charlton R and Smith G. Perceived skills in palliative medicine of newly qualified doctors in the U.K. *J Palliat Care* 2000; 16: 27–32.

36. Barclay S, CJ T, Grande G, et al. How common is medical training in palliative care? A postal survey of general practitioners. *Br J Gen Pract* 1997; 47: 800–805.

37. Barclay S, Wyatt P, Shore S, et al. Caring for the dying: how well prepared are general practitioners? A questionnaire study in Wales. *Palliat Med* 2003; 17: 27–39.

38. Lloyd-Williams M and Carter Y. General practice vocational training in the UK: what teaching is given in palliative care. *Palliat Med* 2003; 17: 616–620.

39. Charlton R, Field S, Faull C, et al. The effect of the general practice registrar year on perceived skills in palliative care in the West Midlands. *Med Educ* 2000; 34: 928–935.

40. Hockey L. *Feeling the Pulse*. London: Queen's Institute for District Nursing, 1966.

41. Cartwright A and Anderson R. *General Practice Revisited*. London: Tavistock Publications, 1981.

42. Bergen A. Nurses caring for the terminally ill in the community: a review of the literature. *Int J Nurs Stud* 1991; 28(1): 89–101.

43. Doyle D. *Domiciliary Terminal Care: Handbook for Doctors and Nurses*. London: Churchill Livingston, 1987.

44. NICE. *Guidance on Cancer Services: Improving Supportive and Palliative Care for Adults*. London: National Institute for Clinical Excellence, 2004.

45. DH. *The NHS Cancer Plan: A Plan for Investment, A Plan for Reform*. London: Department of Health, 2000.

46. Walshe C and Luker KA. District nurses' role in palliative care provision: a realist review. *Int J Nurs Stud* 2010; 47: 1167–1183.

47. *First Assessment: A Review of District Nursing Services in England and Wales*. London: The Audit Commission, 1999.

48. Hatcliffe S, Smith P and Daw R. District nurses' perception of palliative care at home. *Nurs Times* 1996; 92: 36–37.

49. Goodman C, Knight D, Machen I, et al. Emphasizing terminal care as district nurse work: a helpful strategy in a purchasing environment. *J Adv Nurs* 1998; 28: 491–498.

50. Mcilfactrick C and Curran C. The perceived role of the DN in palliative care. *J Comm Nurs* 2001; 15: 46.

51. McHugh G, Pateman B and Luker K. District nurses experiences and perceptions of cancer patient referrals. *Br J Comm Nurs* 2003; 8: 72–79.

52. Dunne K, Sullivan K and Kernohan G. Palliative care for patients with cancer: district nurses' experiences. *J Adv Nurs* 2005; 50: 372–380.

53. Bliss J. Palliative care in the community: the challenge for district nurses. *Br J Comm Nurs*. 2000; 5: 390–395.

54. Mcilfactrick S and Curran C. District nurses perception of palliative care services: part 2. *Int J Palliat Nurs* 2000; 32–38.

55. Beaver K, Luker K and Woods S. Primary care services received during terminal illness. *Int J Palliat Nurs* 2000; 6: 220–227.

56. Burt J, Shipman C, Addington-Hall J, et al. *Palliative Care: Perspectives on Caring for Dying People in London.* London: Kings Fund, 2005.

57. Luker K, Austin L, Caress A, et al. The importance of "knowing the patient": community nurses constructions of quality in providing palliative care. *J Adv Nurs* 2000; 31: 775–782.

58. Seale C. Community nurses and the care of the dying. *Soc Sci Med* 1992; 34: 375–382.

59. Addington-Hall J, MacDonald L, Anderson H, et al. Dying from cancer: the views of bereaved family and friends about the experiences of terminally ill patients. *Palliat Med* 1991; 5: 207–214.

60. Addington-Hall J, Shipman C, Burt J, et al. *Evaluation of the Education and Support Programme for District and Community Nurses in the Principles and Practice of Palliative Care.* London: Department of Health, 2006.

61. Shipman C, Burt J, Ream E, et al. Improving district nurses' confidence and knowledge in the principles and practice of palliative care. *J Adv Nurs* 2008; 63: 494–505.

62. Exley C, Field D, Jones L, et al. Palliative care in the community for cancer and end-stage cardiorespiratory disease: the views of patients, lay-carers and health care professionals. *Palliat Med* 2005; 19: 76–83.

63. Edmond P, Karlsen S, Khan S, et al. A comparison of the palliative care needs of patients dying from chronic respiratory diseases and lung cancer. *Palliat Med* 2001; 15: 287–295.

64. Murphy E. Case management and community matrons for long term conditions. *BMJ* 2004; 329: 1251–1252.

65. Wagner E. The role of patient care teams in chronic disease management. *BMJ* 2000; 320(7234): 569–572.

66. Williams V, Smith A, Chapman L, et al. Community matrons – an exploratory study of patients' views and experiences. *J Adv Nurs* 2011; 67: 86–93.

67. Gravelle H, Dusheiko M, Sheaff R, et al. Impact of case management (Evercare) on frail elderly patients: controlled before and after analysis of quantitative outcome data. *BMJ* 2007; 334: 31.

68. King N, Melvin J, Ashby J, et al. Community palliative care: role perception. *Br J Comm Nurs* 2010; 15: 91–98.

69. Baines M. The origins and development of palliative care at home. *Prog Palliat Care* 2010; 18: 4–8.

70. Webber J. A model response. *Nurs Times* 1994; 90: 66–68.

71. Skilbeck J, Corner J, Bath P, et al. Clinical nurse specialists in palliative care. Part 1. A description of the Macmillan nurse caseload. *Palliat Med* 2002; 16: 285–296.

72. Seymour J, Clark D, Hughes P, et al. Clinical nurse specialists in palliative care. Part 3. Issues for the Macmillan nurse role. *Palliat Med* 2002; 16: 386–394.

73. NCPC. National Survey of Patient Activity Data for Specialist Palliative Care Services: MDS Full Report for the year 2009–2010.

74. Ahmed N, Bestall J, Ahmedzai S, et al. Systematic review of the problems and issues of accessing specialist palliative care by patients, carers and health and social care professionals. *Palliat Med* 2004; 18: 525–542.

75. Balint M. *The Doctor, His Patient and the Illness.* London: Churchill Livingston, 1957.

76. Hart J. The 60s: 50 years of the National Health Service. *Br J Gen Pract* 1998; 48: 1284–1285.

77. Thorpe G. Enabling more dying people to remain at home. *BMJ* 1993; 307: 915–918.

78. Robinson L and Stacy R. Palliative care in the community: setting practice guidelines for primary care teams. *Br J Gen Pract* 1994; 44: 461–464.

79. Jones R. Improving terminal care at home: can district nurses act as catalysts. *Eur J Cancer Care* 1995; 4: 80–85.

80. Thomas K. *Out of Hours Palliative Care in the Community.* London: Macmillan Cancer Relief, 2001.

81. Thomas K. *Caring for the Dying at Home: Companions on the Journey.* Oxford: Radcliffe Medical, 2003.

82. Shaw KL, Clifford C, Thomas K, et al. Review: improving end-of-life care: a critical review of the gold standards framework in primary care. *Palliat Med* 2010; 24: 317–329.

83. Thomas K and Noble B. Improving the delivery of palliative care in general practice: an evaluation of the first phase of the gold standards framework. *Palliat Med* 2007; 21: 49–53.

84. King N, Thomas K, Martin N, et al. "Now nobody falls through the net": practitioners' perspectives on the gold standards framework for community palliative care. *Palliat Med* 2005; 19: 619–627.

85. Dale J, Petrova M, Munday D, et al. A national facilitation project to improve primary palliative care: impact of the gold standards framework on process and self-ratings of quality. *Qual Saf Health Care* 2009; 18: 174–180.

86. Munday D and Dale J. Palliative care in the community. *BMJ* 2007; 334: 809–810.

87. Badger F, Clifford C, Hewison A, et al. An evaluation of the implementation of a programme to improve end-of-life care in nursing homes. *Palliat Med* 2009; 23: 502–511.

88. After Death Analysis Tool. 2011. *Gold Standards Framework.* Available at: http://www.goldstandardsframework .org.uk/GSFAuditTool (accessed on May 21, 2012).

89. Badger F, Shaw K, Clifford C, et al. Evaluation of a framework for end of life care in primary care: a report for the public health department, Walsall Primary Care Trust. Birmingham: School of Health Sciences, University of Birmingham, 2008.

90. OMEGA. *End of Life Care in Primary Care: National Snapshot Audit 2009.* Walsall: Omega: National Association for End of Life Care, 2009.

91. Munday D, Mahmood K, Dale J, et al. Facilitating good process in primary palliative care: does the gold standards framework enable quality performance? *Family Practice* 2007; 24: 486–494.

92. Mahmood-Yousuf K, Munday D, Dale J, et al. Interprofessional relationships and communication in primary palliative care: impact of the gold standards framework. *Br J Gen Pract* 2008; 58: 256–263.

93. Walshe C, Caress A, Chew-Graham C, et al. Implementation and impact of the gold standards framework in community palliative care: a qualitative study of three primary care trusts. *Palliat Med* 2008; 22: 736–743.

94. Walshe C, Todd C, Caress A-L, et al. Judgements about fellow professionals and the management of patients receiving palliative care in primary care: a qualitative study. *Br J Gen Pract* 2008; 58: 264–272.

95. Speed S and Luker K. Getting a visit: how district nurses and general practitioners "organise" each other in primary care. *Sociol Health Illn* 2006; 28: 883–902.

96. The NHS Information Centre, Prescribing and Primary Care Services. Quality and Outcomes Framework Achievement Data 2009/10: NHS Information Centre, 2010.

97. Seymour JE, Kumar A and Froggatt K. Do nursing homes for older people have the support they need to provide end-of-life care? A mixed methods enquiry in England. *Palliat Med* 2011; 25: 125–138.

98. Hockley J, Watson J, Oxenham D, et al. The integrated implementation of two end-of-life care tools in nursing care homes in the UK: an in-depth evaluation. *Palliat Med* 2010; 24: 828–838.

99. *The Gold Standards Framework*. Available at www.goldstandardsframework.nhs.uk (accessed on July 24, 2011).

100. Jessopp L, Beck I, Hollins L, et al. Changing the pattern out of hours: a survey of general practice cooperatives. *BMJ* 1997; 314: 199.

101. Munday D, Carroll D and Douglas A. GP out of hours cooperatives and the delivery of palliative care. *Br J Gen Pract* 1999; 49: 489.

102. Barclay S, Rogers M and Todd C. Communication between GPs and cooperatives is poor for terminally ill patients. *BMJ* 1997; 315: 1235–1236.

103. Burt J, Barclay S, Marshall N, et al. Continuity within primary care: an audit of general practice out of hours cooperatives. *J Pub Health* 2004; 26: 275–276.

104. Richards SH, Winder R, Seamark D, et al. Accessing out-of-hours care following implementation of the GMS contract: an observational study. *Br J Gen Pract* 2008; 58: 331–338.

105. Taubert M and Nelson A. "Oh God, not a palliative": out-of-hours general practitioners within the domain of palliative care. *Palliat Med* 2010; 24: 501–509.

106. Worth A, Boyd K, Kendall M, et al. Out-of-hours palliative care: a qualitative study of cancer patients, carers and professionals. *Br J Gen Pract* 2006; 56: 6–13.

107. Munday D, Dale J and Barnett M. Out of hours palliative care in the UK: perspectives from general practice and specialist services. *J R Coll Gen Pract* 2002; 95: 28–30.

108. Sheils R, Ankrett H, Edwards A, et al. Out-of-hours need for specialist palliative care face-to-face assessments. *Palliat Med* 2009; 23: 276–277.

109. King N, Thomas K and Bell D. An out of hours protocol for community palliative care: practitioners perspectives. *Int J Palliat Nurs* 2003; 9: 277–282.

110. Fergus CJ, Chinn DJ and Murray SA. Assessing and improving out-of-hours palliative care in a deprived community: a rapid appraisal study. *Palliat Med* 2010; 24: 493–500.

111. Electronic Palliative Care Summary (ePCS). 2011. *The Scottish Government*, Available at: http://www.scotland.gov.uk/Topics/Health/NHS-Scotland/LivingandDyingWell/ePCS) (accessed on August 8, 2011).

112. Ipsos MORI Social Research Institute. *End of Life Locality Registers Evaluation.* London: Ipsos MORI, 2011.

113. Higginson I and Sen-Gupta GJA. Place of care in advanced cancer: a qualitative systematic literature review of patient preferences. *J Palliat Med* 2000; 3: 287–300.

114. Hinton J. Can home care maintain an acceptable quality of life for patients with terminal cancer and their relatives? *Palliat Med* 1994; 8: 183–196.

115. Thomas C, Morris S and Clark D. Place of death: preferences among cancer patients and their carers. *Soc Sci Med* 2004; 58: 2431–2444.

116. Steinhauser KE, Christakis NA, Clipp EC, et al. Factors considered important at the end of life by patients, family, physicians, and other care providers. *JAMA* 2000; 284: 2476–2482.

117. Abel J, Rich A, Griffin T, et al. End-of-life care in hospital: a descriptive study of all inpatient deaths in 1 year. *Palliat Med* 2009; 23: 616–622.

118. Jackson K., McBride T., Ahmad S., et al. *End of Life Care.* London: National Audit Office, 2008.

119. Barclay S and Arthur A. Place of death: how much does it matter? The priority is to improve end-of-life care in all settings. *Br J Gen Pract* 2008; 58: 229–231.

120. Leadbeater C and Gadber J. *Dying for Change.* London: Demos, 2010.

121. Ellershaw J, Dewar S and Murphy D. Achieving a good death for all. *BMJ* 2010; 341: c4861.

122. End of Life Care Quality \ (ELCQuA). 2011. Available at: http://www.elcqua.nhs.uk/faq.php (accessed on August 8, 2011).

123. National Institue for Health and Clincial Excellence. *Quality Standard on End of Life Care*, 2011.

3 Public and Patient Involvement in Palliative Care

Neil Small

University of Bradford, Bradford, UK

Introduction

Public and patient involvement in health and social care has been promoted by governments and enshrined in legal systems in many countries. It has also been incorporated into professional protocols in the form of requirements to consult "lay" views, or in guidance that such consultation is integral to best practice. But a concern to promote public and patient involvement predates its recent induction into political orthodoxies. Across wide areas of health and social care, members of the public and patients have organised to identify shortcomings in care and to present alternatives. They have created new services, modified existing ones, transformed the way the public think about health concerns, and changed the way people with particular conditions are seen by others. Furthermore, the solidarities created through joint action have changed the self-perception of people living with a range of different health needs.

Examples of areas where public and patient involvement has challenged pre-existing orthodoxies about what can and should be provided, generated new services and have changed peoples' views include learning (intellectual) disabilities [1]; physical disabilities [2]; human immunodeficiency virus (HIV) and acquired immunodeficiency syndrome (AIDS) [3–5]; cancer [6]; mental health; women's health including childbirth [7]; the health of minorities; health in rural communities; and the health experiences of deprived city populations [8]. As this list illustrates, sometimes the focus is on specific conditions, sometimes it is on areas of experience that characteristically bring people into contact with health services, childbirth is one such area, and sometimes the focus is more about being in a category that seems to carry with it a generic health disadvantage, living in an economically deprived area, for example.

The modern hospice movement and palliative care deserve a central place in any history of public and patient involvement. Hospices offer examples of the development of new services and new ways of thinking about end-of-life care that emerged from vanguard professionals who acknowledged that patients' wishes should shape the services provided [9]. The remit identified by hospice pioneers included providing a setting that would meet the needs of the individual patient, developing a service to act as an exemplar for the sorts of care that could be achieved and, in so doing, seeking to influence the care of the dying in whatever setting they were to be found [10] and creating a change in social perceptions about the dying process in such a way that the dying would not be shunned [11,12]. Furthermore, hospices typically identified the patients' family as a legitimate subject for concern and, in so doing, became a key setting for the development of bereavement services. The broader community was also engaged through fund raising and in providing volunteers. Service developments that have closely adhered to the voices of patients and their families have made a huge contribution to improvements in end-of life care. Beyond the provision of services, there has also been strong, consistent, and long-lasting expressions of public preferences in terms of the services that are seen as desirable for end-of-life care. These preferences have been shaped by the sorts of care that are made possible by advances in hospice and palliative care.

This chapter takes two complementary approaches to examine public and patient involvement. In the first part, two specific areas are considered. The aspirations and experiences of the early modern hospice movement, exemplified by St Christopher's Hospice in the United

Handbook of Palliative Care, Third Edition. Edited by Christina Faull, Sharon de Caestecker, Alex Nicholson and Fraser Black.
© 2012 by John Wiley and Sons, Inc. Published 2012 by John Wiley & Sons, Inc.

Kingdom, are contrasted with a recent UK report, *Dying for Change* [13]. A second specific area concentrates on the impact legislation has had in the United States. A US Department of Health and Human Services report from 2008, *Advance Directives and Advanced Care Planning* [14], is considered, as are initiatives in La Crosse, Wisconsin. La Crosse provides an example of both public involvement and of a way to give voice to patient preferences through advance directives (ADs).

The second part of the chapter focuses more generally on the context in which a concern with public and patient involvement has arisen. Arguments as to why public and patient involvement is considered desirable will be presented as will an outline of the forms involvement has characteristically taken.

Exemplars of good practice in terms of listening to patients' voices in hospice and seeking, recording, and utilising patients preferences for treatment through ADs have had limited impact. Public and patient input can change the legal framework in which end-of-life care operates and can change individual practice; but to embed a different approach to end-of-life care requires a change in cultural responses to dying, death, and bereavement. For this, practice and legislative change are necessary but not sufficient. Initiatives discussed in this chapter from Australia that consider how palliative care can engage with health promotion and public health provide an example of one route for pursuing cultural change.

Part 1: Examples from end-of-life care

Listening to the patient

Developing services

Public and patient involvement can develop through "top-down" initiatives prompted by prevailing political agendas, by a "bottom-up" manifestation of unmet, or inadequately met, need generating protest and calls for action, or it can also be manifest in a more developmental interaction between patient experience, professional response, and incremental service development. An example of this latter sort of public and patient involvement is provided by the modern hospice movement. This has drawn on the experiences of the involved and the committed to initiate, shape, and develop services. The involved have included health and social care professionals (CPs), academics, and the clergy. Their work has been undertaken alongside the contribution of volunteers and with support, for example, by providing finance, from the public. But crucial to the nature of hospice care has been a

decision to listen to the voice of the committed, the patient and their family.

As with many examples of public and patient involvement, the motivation for seeking a change in end-of-life care was a recognition of shortcomings in services. This was combined with a vision of what alternatives might be possible. Dame Cicely Saunders, writing 34 years ago, argued that:

> [p]atients are not easily given appropriate care in a busy general ward. Often it is not the right place for them nor do their needs arouse the interest of many of the doctors who look after them [15: p. 158].

The response to these shortcomings was the development of a new sort of hospice with a clear agenda to develop care by building on the experiences of the patient, and to:

> [g]ive such people all the care that will help them to die easily and at peace, to spread knowledge . . . of its potential in special units or hospices, in general hospitals, and in the patients own home [15: p. 159].

Hospice care has looked to the best science while not forgetting the importance of listening to the subjective voice of those intimately involved. Evidence as to what was possible in end-of-life care has been combined with the testimony as to what was desirable. Two examples from the early years of St Christopher's illustrate this. Parkes was producing rigorous and innovative work, drawing on his clinical practice, in relation to family reactions to bereavement [16]. This was a work that helped set the agenda for bereavement research for many years [17]. At the same time he was involved in a patient group that met weekly and discussed life and death in the hospice, including the impact of loss and grief. But the patient group had a wider role:

> On other days they concentrate on learning from or instructing those who visit them. It is a coveted honour for staff or visitors to be invited to join in one of the meetings, and although small in number, this group has an impact on the life of the Hospice as well as on that of its members [15: p. 168].

Twycross [18] was researching the control of chronic pain and pioneering approaches to using diamorphine in advanced malignant disease. At the same time a conceptualisation of the multifaceted nature of pain was emerging from close attention to what patients were saying. This was most vividly captured by Cicely Saunders remembering the patient who, when asked, "what was the matter?" replied "all of me is wrong" [19]. It is a conceptualisation exemplified by the talismanic hospice mantra that emerged in response to such patient insights, "constant pain needs constant control" [20] and that total pain needs total care.

This approach combined the scientific and the subjective in a way that changed a prevailing relationship between medical staff and patients. That change was manifest in both the practical details of everyday interactions and the underlying assumptions about the nature of that relationship:

> Everybody on the ward round was given a chair, and talking to the patient didn't start until everybody was sitting down at eye-level with the patient (Dr Tim Lovel) [21: p. 22].
>
> You can't be with dying people and remain strict within boundaries, because there aren't any boundaries when you are dying (Dame Cicely Saunders) [21: p. 19].

By the 1990s, palliative care was developing beyond its hospice origins; it was being offered earlier in the disease trajectory, was seeking a role across different illnesses, and was grappling with the challenges of being assimilated into evidence-based medicine [22]. There was a widely recognised tension between hospice as a social movement, focused on both the improvement of the care of individual dying people, and seeking to shift social attitudes to dying, and palliative medicine, recognised as a specialty in 1987, which was seeking to be integrated into "mainstream health services" [21: p. 3]. These developments and tensions impacted on public and patient involvement in end-of-life care. While there has been a continuing engagement in hospices with listening to the patient what was now added was the need to engage with the structures and processes of public and patient involvement that were developing generically in health care.

Shortcomings in end-of-life care

More than 40 years after the birth of the modern hospice movement at St Christopher's in London (1967), and nearly 25 years after palliative medicine's recognition as a specialty in the United Kingdom (1987), we can see both advances in the quality of end-of-life care and continuing formidable challenges. Two recent reports, one from the United Kingdom and one from the United States, underline how difficult it is to either change the care of the individual, outside the centres of excellence that hospices constituted, or achieve a shift in the overall pattern of end-of life care. These reports illustrate that despite many examples of what constitutes best practice in end-of-life care, and despite legislative and legal changes, patient and family wishes, and public preferences, are far from being realised.

In the United Kingdom, Leadbeater and Garber [13], while acknowledging improvements in the way we die and accepting that the United Kingdom may be better placed than many countries, summarise the present position thus:

> the institutionalised ways we cope with dying are out of kilter with how most people aspire to live at the end-of-life. Most people want to die with family and friends nearby, cared for, free from pain, with medical support available when it is needed. Instead, most people will die in hospitals and care homes, often feeling cut off from friends and family, dependent on systems and procedures that feel impersonal, over which they have little control and which offer them scant sense of dignity. As things stand, many of us will die unnecessarily distressing deaths [13: pp. 13–14].

This summary is supported by both statistics and individual testimony. Together they remind us that the individual death is an irredeemable experience. We might improve what is the norm and achieve improvements in the actuarial probability of having a good death, but for the person who is dying and for their family you have to get it right *this* time.

Leadbeater tells us, movingly, of his father Bill's death in a hospital in the north of England in 2010:

> The drab room in which he died provided a measure of privacy but little else . . . . The room was a workplace for nurses and doctors rather than somewhere someone would choose to reflect on their life and be close to his family in his final days. Bill's wife Olive would struggle past chairs, push away stands and tubes, and stretch across the metal guards surrounding his bed to kiss him. The room was designed for medical procedures not for kissing. . . . When Bill's family met the consultant for the first time it was after his death and she revealed that she talked to patients' families only when they pestered her. . . . Establishing a relationship with (the nurses) was impossible: with every shift came a different nurse. . . . Often it seemed as if no one knew what was wrong with Bill. But that might be because no one was comfortable talking about the fact he was dying. . . . [None of Bill's family] were well prepared for a direct discussion with Bill about the fact he seemed to be dying. Everyone had an interest in skirting around the subject.

He concludes:

> Too often hospitals neglect the social, psychological and spiritual aspects of dying, which are vital to dying a good death. That social shortfall is why hospitals are rarely the best places in which to die [13: pp. 9–10].

Figures that help contextualise both his testimony and analysis are presented in the report; 66% of people in a recent UK poll said that they would prefer to die at home and 1% said that they would prefer to die in a care home. 58% of deaths currently occur in hospital. Given increases in longevity, and in the number of older people in the population, projections for the year 2030 are that 10% of people will die at home, 20% will die in a care home, and 65% will die in hospital [13: p. 13].

Leadbeater and Garber's report (2010) captures how the end-of-life care people receive differs from the preferences of families and from the views the public express. A US Department of Health and Human Services Report [14] identifies a similar situation:

> There is substantial evidence that the treatment people would choose at the end-of-life commonly is different from the treatment they receive. Too often individuals receive more aggressive care than they desire. However, some individuals, particularly those with disabilities, find that the health care system and sometimes their families undervalue their quality of life, and as a result, withhold life-prolonging treatments that these patients want [14: p. viii].

This report highlights two possible scenarios that set different agendas for palliative care and pose different challenges for those who seek to promote ADs. First, there is a need to counter neglect of the dying and ensure key services are in place and used. Second, there is a need to counter the possibility that there will be too much intervention, attempts to prolong life in ways that reflect the medically possible rather than the subjectively desirable. The US Department of Health and Human Services Report [14], and more recent controversies in the United Kingdom about patterns of care at the end of life, highlights that while for some people too much intervention is their primary concern, for others it is the danger of having their needs dismissed.

Consider these two examples. First, a study from New York published in 2004 reported that 51% of patients with advanced dementia received a new feeding tube during a terminal hospitalisation compared with 11% of patients with metastatic cancer and that both empirical data and expert opinion was clear that this intervention, "has no demonstrable health benefits in this population and may be associated with undesirable outcomes" [23: p. 325, 24: pp. 53–4]. Second, UK organisations representing the views of older people, such as Age UK, or of people with disabilities, for example, SCOPE who work with and for people with Cerebral Palsy, have highlighted a concern that there is too great a willingness to impose "do not resuscitate" (DNR) instructions on hospital staff when the patient is someone who is seen (by them) as having some impaired quality of life because of pre-existing conditions or old age [25,26].

The position in the United Kingdom is clear. Doctors cannot be required to give treatment against their clinical judgement, and patients can legally refuse medical treatment even if that leads to their death. In the narrow example of resuscitation, the clinical judgement of the doctor is final, although health authority guidance does recommend that patients be "sensitively informed" that resuscitation will not be attempted. The Director of Professional Activities at the British Medical Association (a doctor's organisation) summarised the position: families of mentally competent adult patients had "no right to anything in law but in practice we always try to talk to the family" [27]. A draft East of England Strategic Health Authority document captures the situation with regard to patients, "Opportunities to sensitively inform patients … (about a decision not to resuscitate) should be sought unless it is judged that the burden of such a discussion would outweigh the possible benefit for the patient" [28]. While it is unlikely that anyone will disagree that futile treatments should never be countenanced and that a final decision about what constitutes futility in any specific case has to be made by the responsible person who would have to administer treatment, there remain unresolved questions. If people with certain types of diagnosis receive considerable numbers of interventions and, conversely, if DNR orders occur disproportionately with people with disabilities, or with the very elderly, it would appear that judgements are being made that reflect beliefs about capacity and about worth that are not just case based but that reflect cultural constructs. Even if one wishes to retain clinical independence, there is a role for public and patient involvement in scrutinising, and calling to account, the collective result of these "individual" decisions. Furthermore, in a prevailing context that supports seeking public and patient views is it anomalous, in relation to DNR orders, that the British Medical Associations commitment is only to "try" to talk to the family and that Health Authorities say patients "should" be informed.

The cultural basis of decision making and structural differences in end-of-life care experience are also evident when we move from considering public and patient involvement in the context of interactions with health professionals and look at attempts to change practice through legislation.

Legislative initiatives to change end-of-life care

In the United States, the enactment of legislation and the interventions of the courts in end-of-life care have been evident since the mid-1970s. For example, the *Californian Natural Death Act* of 1976 sought to refocus end-of-life care by utilising living wills. There were also specific court cases relating to withdrawing life-sustaining treatments from individuals who were deemed to have lost decision-making capacity. In 1991, the US Congress enacted the *Patient Self-Determination Act* to encourage "competent adults to complete ADs." ADs are legal tools to state treatment preferences and name a proxy decision-maker in case of a loss of personal capacity to make health-care choices. In 1993, the *Uniform Health Care Decisions Act* promoted a national model where a link was made between reimbursement systems, Medicaid and Medicare, and the incorporation of ADs into medical records. Also in the 1990s, State legislation focused on ensuring ADs and DNR instructions were transferred between treatment settings as the patients circumstances changed.

But changing the law and establishing new legal precedents did not, in themselves, create a widespread change in practice. Seventeen years after the initial Act, it was clear that, "this Act did not reduce unwanted aggressive treatment" [14: p. viii]. Furthermore:

- "Only" 18–36% of the adult population had completed an AD.
- Rates of completion of an AD for those with serious medical conditions were only slightly higher.
- Physicians were often unaware that their patient had completed an AD.
- Most end-of-life decision making was made through ad hoc interactions between patients, family members, and doctors.
- Much of the care in intensive care units (where many of the challenges underpinning the legislation like DNR instructions are most likely to be manifest) did not conform to patients ADs.
- Residents of nursing homes were most likely to have ADs but a process of transfer from an established nursing home placement to another treatment setting, a characteristic of many peoples' end-of-life care experience, was accompanied by a possibility that the new setting did not know about, or act upon, the AD that was in place.

Legislative and legal changes also did not impact on equity issues. Those social characteristics that are generally predictive of poor health-care outcomes including nonwhite race and low socioeconomic status are also evident in the lower proportion of people in these groups with ADs [14: pp. x–xi].

Increasing the use of advance decisions

There have been a number of initiatives to increase the numbers of people who make ADs and to increase the chance that they are implemented. In the United States, two initiatives are considered to have been successful. One, the Physician Order for Life-Sustaining Treatment (POLST), began in Oregon and offers "a mechanism to elicit patients' care preferences, translate them into a set of medical orders addressing several high probability interventions relevant to the patients' current condition, document them on a highly visible form, and ensure their portability across care settings" [29].

The second successful intervention is a communitybased approach, *Respecting Choices*, based in La Crosse, Wisconsin. This sustained intervention, began in 1993 in a county of 110,000 people, has demonstrated nearly a sixfold increase in the proportion of the population reported to have some sort of written AD. In 1991, like reports from other parts of the country, the rate was about 15% [30: p. 383]. By 2010, Hammes and colleagues reported prevalence of ADs in the medical record at the time of death of 99.4%. Furthermore, the clarity and specificity of ADs compared with a previous review in 1998 had been enhanced, and there was evidence from examining medical treatment and place of death to indicate that end-of-life care was consistent with the patients AD [31].

Respecting Choices is a collaborative effort involving health-care providers in La Crosse. It is championed by an advance care planning (ACP) "microsystem," a group who work together to "elicit, understand, document and honour a patients preferences about future medical care" (31: p. 1250). Six specific goals are now part of routine care: (1) adult patients are invited to understand, to reflect on, and to discuss plans for future health care; (2) they are given assistance in planning what they want; (3) written plans are developed, using accessible terminology; (4) these plans are stored and retrieved whenever and wherever the patient is cared for; (5) plans are updated and become more specific as illnesses progress; and (6) plans are honoured at the appropriate time [31: pp. 1249–1250]:

> Ultimately, what needs to be created is a healthcare culture in which knowing and honouring a patient's preferences is given a priority similar to knowing and documenting: a patient's allergies to medications, what medicines a patient is taking, and what medical problems a patient has. These are challenging but not impossible improvements to make. If a high value is truly put on knowing and honouring a patient's preferences, an effective ACP system can be realized [31: p. 1254].

Hammes and colleagues have demonstrated that it is possible to develop a widely used ACP system. This combines public and patient preferences in that it collects preferences before illness and allows these to be modified if the person so wishes. The La Crosse project identifies the need to create a change in health-care culture such that patients' preferences are prioritised and concludes that such a change will follow a shift in individuals' values. But the La Crosse initiative to change end-of-life care is notable because it is unique. More than 35 years of state and national legislation in the United States have neither created a system-wide shift in practice nor modified inequalities in whose voice is sought and whose requests are honoured.

As with initiatives to change end-of-life care that focus on listening to the voice of patients, the overall picture of seeking to change practice through legislative initiative shows only limited areas of success and highlights system-wide stasis. It is possible to set up a new approach to care. An alliance between professionals and patients can create a culture shift that will mean the experience of large numbers of individuals cared for in such settings is more likely to closely reflect their wishes. But what the Leadbeater and Garber study shows is that, even after more than 40 years of providing examples, the value shift and the diffusion of this culture into broader health-care provision that is needed has not occurred to any great extent. By themselves, examples of good practice have not created a paradigm shift. Likewise sustained efforts in particular locations, using teams of workers with clear aims, can change the extent to which people identify their preferences for end-of-life care and have those preferences honoured. But, as the *Advance Directives and Advance Care Planning* [14] report demonstrates, making laws and even seeking to bolster them through financial encouragements does not lead to systemic change. It is a conceit of representative democratic systems that making laws changes lives. Our examples here illustrate that there are many mediating steps between the intention and the implementation, between what the philosopher Habermas calls the system world and the life-world [24: pp. 10–12,32].

In the next section, the underlying changes that underpin a rise of interest in public and patient involvement are examined as are details of how public and patient involvement has been implemented. This consideration of both context and practicalities helps illuminate the paradox of why there is apparent enthusiasm but only localised, rather than system wide, change in end-of-life care.

Part 2: Why public and patient involvement?

Both the growth of palliative care and a concern with how to seek out and respond to public and patient views have occurred in the context of significant shifts in general social attitudes in the West. Consider what public and patient involvement is seeking to replace. If services are guided by patient views, then a precondition is a shift in personal value systems away from deference to "experts." If health services are to reflect public views, a pre-existing political and social culture that has been characterised by delegation of powers has to change.

Preconditions for public and patient involvement

Changing attitudes to experts

The US Department of Health and Human Services report discussed earlier [14] identified a change, beginning in the 1970s, in what had been a traditional assumption that physicians acted in the best interests of the patient and were the appropriate persons to make decisions about end-of-life care. This change not only questioned a previous long-standing deference to the profession of medicine but assumed that a personal involvement in the subject under discussion constituted a qualification to contribute to decisions about what services were provided. This change in the position of medicine was both prompted by and evidenced in a number of influential critiques of the shortcomings of professional knowledge in health [33,34]. These critiques achieved more prominence because they were presented in the context of a changing intellectual landscape that was engaging in a sustained examination of the assumptions underpinning science, including medicine. This new landscape drew on structuralism and its criticisms of linear cause and effect explanations and postmodernism with its incredulity toward over-arching explanatory systems [35].

Changing attitudes to the state and society

The promotion of public and patient involvement has also occurred in the context of two other significant changes in social attitudes. One is the growth of the idea of governmentality. This is the move from seeing governing as something that goes on among a few people in centralised institutions to a way of thinking that sees it in, "a myriad of practices that proliferate throughout society" [36]. This different way of thinking about the relationship between the individual, civic society, and the state was first linked, in the United Kingdom, to the "New Labour" politics of Prime Minister Tony Blair's administrations [37] but is now also evident in the "Big Society" ideas of the contemporary Conservative government [38]. The second change in social attitudes is evident in the idea of consumerism and of the market as a legitimate, or even a pre-eminent, mechanism to determine resource allocation in society. In the market, the empowered consumer is the archetypal actor, and in governmentality it is the active citizen.

These changes in social attitudes elevate the truth claims of personal experience alongside the scientific views of experts and seek to encourage individual agency, either as a person taking responsibility or as a person making choices. Their impact helps frame a more detailed examination of public and patient involvement.

Voice and choice

There are two main arguments about the merits of public and patient involvement in health care, an intrinsic and an instrumental argument. The intrinsic argument is that if a person is likely to be effected by something they have a right to be involved in decisions about it. Involvement is not inherently linked to any idea that it will produce "better" health care. The instrumental argument is that one should promote involvement because it brings benefits, either immediately or eventually, in terms of better health care.

The intrinsic and instrumental arguments have been linked to democracy and consumerism. It is argued that public and patient involvement enhances the democratic nature of the way health care is planned, delivered, and evaluated. If it does this, then we can either consider that this is a good thing in itself or say that an enhanced democracy is likely to improve health care because it will increase the possibility that it better reflects public and patient needs. In consequence the democracy argument can be linked to both intrinsic and instrumental positions. Consumerism is more likely to be linked with an instrumental argument. It is epitomised by the idea of being able to develop and act on preferences, by having a choice. Consumerism therefore requires reliable information and realistic alternatives to be available. It then assumes that more desirable options flourish, because they are preferentially chosen.

There have always been links to ideas about democracy and consumerism in health care. In state-run systems like the United Kingdom's National Health Services (NHS), the idea of representative democracy has been the prevailing one. People present themselves for election with manifestos of their intentions once in office, including their intentions in relation to health policy. Voters select them and hold them to account for their actions at the next election. Between elections the citizen has the right of redress under the law and has the right to organise to lobby for changes in the law, or for changes in what services are provided. In privately funded or insurance-based systems, there is an assumption that the citizen makes provision for their own health care through balancing their resources, anticipated needs, and available options. But while representative democracy and choice of provider are manifestations of voice and choice, neither readily enables you to achieve changes in the sorts of services you get, subsequent to shifts in your individual circumstances.

For voice and choice to be effective, there would need to be changes in the sort of democracy we practise and changes in the capacity of the market to respond to rapid change in individuals, circumstances. Representative democracy is too passive. An alternative is a "deliberative approach to democracy [which] aims to develop citizens capacity to engage in critical reflection" [39]. Applied to health services this would see managers and clinicians held to account as they delivered services by the enhanced critical acumen of citizens/patients. When applied to the market, a more dynamic expression of voice and choice would need consumers to have timely information that allows them to identify their preferences. They then need to be able to seek out providers who will meet these preferences from a range of available and affordable options [40].

Given that we have seen, above, that it is difficult to change the generality of health provision and that shifting our stance toward political engagement or changing the responsiveness of markets might be a reasonable aspiration but not a goal likely to be quickly achieved, ways of enhancing voice and choice in the shorter or medium term are needed, or ways of thinking about public and patient involvement other than as voice or choice.

Limitations in thinking of public and patient involvement as voice or choice

In this section the focus on ideas of responsive markets and of active citizenry, which are depictions of an ideal state, is left behind to concentrate on the complexities of seeking public and patient involvement in the current health-care environment.

We can see involvement as a continuum rather than an all-or-nothing process. There might be different degrees of involvement, from consultation to user-initiated and user-led projects [41]. Sometimes initiatives stay at one level of involvement, and sometimes they develop from a low-intensity involvement into a more wide-ranging contribution. As well as its being a continuum the process of developing public and patient involvement is rarely smooth. Characteristically, there are likely to be changing needs and preferences in the individual involved, dynamic interactions within patient groups and changes in their relationship with professionals, bureaucrats, and politicians [42]. As well as the complexities of what we can see as involvement, voice and choice can be complementary approaches. Some aspects of public and patient involvement may be better furthered by voice, strategic decisions on resource allocation perhaps. Other aspects favour a focus on choice, types of care setting, for example.

Operationally, involvement is a nuanced term, and its pursuit can involve varied agendas. It also has to grapple with some more general conceptual challenges.

Differences between the public and the patients

While public and patients are not exclusive categories, all patients are members of the public and all members of the public are possible patients, there may be differences in priorities between those who are contemplating the best configuration of end-of-life care as members of the public and those who are making immediate demands on services as patients. Furthermore, palliative care accepts as part of its domain a concern with the patients' family, and they may prioritise different things. There is then a need to address how one balances the views of these three different constituencies.

One might take an ethical position that closeness to a situation is a justification for one's views being prioritised. That is, having your central interests engaged gives you priority over others whose considerations are focused on the needs of others or on hypothetical futures. Such a position would see the patients' wishes followed, not the families if they differed. For example, the patient may be more concerned to maintain a level of awareness, so that they can continue to engage with the world around them, and the family member may be distressed by what they see as excessive pain and prefer greater sedation. While following the patients' wishes may seem uncontroversial in theory, we have seen that it is often not evident in practice. From post Second World War England when Cicely Saunders was encouraged to study medicine by a mentor, Dr Barrett, because "It's the doctors who desert the dying" [43: p. 63], to 2010 England where no one knew what was wrong with Bill Leadbeater because they were not "comfortable about talking about the fact he was dying" [7: pp. 9–10], to a contemporary United States where physicians were unaware of patients' wishes and ad hoc interactions with patients, family members, and doctors made decisions [14], there are examples of the patients wishes neither being sought or acted upon. Furthermore, when seeking patients' wishes becomes more difficult, perhaps they are mentally incapacitated or not fully conscious, we can see many examples of their wishes being subsumed by a prevailing ethos of care, high levels of intervention in people with dementia [23], and decisions not to resuscitate in people with pre-existing disabilities for example [26].

But if we prioritise patients' views, how do we change the overall pattern of palliative care? The public, when they are involved, might want to pursue greater equity. For example, they may want greater geographic spread of specialist facilities, or they may want to shift care to conditions other than cancer [44]. But seeking greater equity might necessitate some loss of quality in those services that are currently in place. If this is done, then there may not be the services, or the quality of service, the member of the public, now reconfigured as the patient, would wish to have as he or she approaches their own end of life.

The challenge then is to recognise what sorts of decisions can be left to the public, the involved, and how you stop the choices they make restricting the patient, the committed, from getting what they need. Conversely, how can prioritising the committed be achieved without stopping change in the overall pattern of care provision?

Social divisions and involvement

Some people will be better able to become involved and to express their voice or choice. For example, there are barriers experienced by older people. Abbott and colleagues reported a reduction in civic participation as people get older due to increased dependency, the construction of older people as passive by others and by themselves and by a preference of the older people interviewed in their study to focus on everyday decision making [45]. Some barriers to older people's participation are practical ones; economic disadvantage, transport, and accessibility of buildings and meeting rooms. Lack of Internet access and IT skills also increases the social exclusion of the older population [46]. Some barriers link to health problems more prevalent in older people; greater morbidity, reduced mobility, and a combination of hearing, visual, or cognitive impairments [47]. Reduced levels of stamina and tiredness can also affect involvement [48,49].

More generally, US research reported above, shows that those factors that are generally predictive of one's health status, ethnicity, and socioeconomic class shape the likelihood that one will exercise one's voice and made clear one's choice through an AD [14: pp. x–xi].

Involvement and a history of activism

Equating public and patient involvement with consumerism, or with the active citizen imagined in governmentality, does not capture that narrative in public and patient involvement that sees it as a bottom-up push for change, as a manifestation of dissatisfaction—an oppositional movement. As introduced earlier, public and patient involvement has been demanded and has been taken, as well as being encouraged or given. This is not the incorporation of the citizen into the expanded civic sphere of governmentality, nor is it captured in the idea of an empowered consumer in the health market place. This is a noisier history made by "troublesome" people working together often to seek to redefine a particular social problematic, the nature of mental illness, or the difference between disability and handicap [2] for example, or to say, "we will provide what we need ourselves" [50]. Its driving force comes from a wish to improve the experiences of repressed or neglected groups and its central explanatory construct lies in an analysis of differentials in power in society.

Discussion

Public and patient involvement in health care is one manifestation of an overall societal change in which the status of the professions and the authority of a particular sort of scientific knowledge has been challenged. It is a social change that has also made possible the emergence of governmentality and of market approaches to the provision of health care. Both of these have been encouraged by governments. Markets, for example, are perceived to have the potential to stimulate change in patterns and quality of health care. They are approaches whose success is predicated on the presence of active citizens and empowered consumers, although these active citizens and empowered consumers are envisaged as contributing to established structures rather than confronting or replacing them. Top-down public and patient involvement, while not necessarily tokenism, is instrumental in serving established systems.

But public and patient involvement is neither new nor is it only something given at the behest of government. Active citizens are not a government invention. Involvement has been something that has been demanded by dissatisfied patients, their families, friends, and sometimes sympathetic health professionals. Critiques of existing attitudes and practice have engendered solidarity among people with the same sorts of needs, led to new mobilisations including the development of new sorts of services, and generated a critique of prevailing social attitudes. Bottom-up public and patient involvement has the potential to both change services and change minds and cultures.

We have discussed two examples of public and patient involvement. The first, St Christopher's Hospice provides a bottom-up example of building on an alliance between professionals and patients to address shortcomings in existing services and implement new approaches to meeting patient need. Talking about the inspiration for opening St Christopher's, Dame Cicely Saunders was clear that it was:

> the impact of listening to individual patients which was my own initial impetus and certainly was so for many of the other hospice pioneers [51: pp. 1363–1364].

Furthermore, it was widely seen at the time that it was important that the modern hospice movement developed outside the NHS. Taylor has argued that this facilitated their development of different models of care, and Saunders was clear that St Christopher's moved out of the NHS:

> [s]o that attitudes and knowledge could move back in [52: p. 4].

The example of St Christopher's and the other pioneer modern hospices has been influential in stimulating the further growth of hospices, in influencing more mainstream services, and in engaging with cultural attitudes about pain, dying, death, and bereavement.

The second example, from the United States, concentrates on top-down initiatives to ensure the patient voice was heard in end-of-life care. The interventions of the legislature and the courts led to a requirement that patients' views about present care and about hypothetical scenarios for their future be sought, recorded, and acted upon. But to move beyond a policy and legal intention to deliver the sorts of engagement of all involved in end-of-life care that was envisaged in various AD policies required a major and sustained engagement over many years in Oregon and in La Crosse. In the latter, it was the existence of "microsystems" championing the patients' voice that allowed the system change necessary to embed AD as the normal practice in this community. Hammes and colleagues identify the need to create a health-care culture in which patients' preferences are sought and acted on. The work they report from La Crosse has taken many years and involved a broad range of people; some committed to the project of championing the patient voice through ACP, and many others involved in making ACP the standard practice in their institutions [31]. It has taken this sort of sustained implementation to embed a legislative requirement as the default position in this community. In so doing, it has changed the culture of practice in end-of-life care into one that better reflects patients' views. It seems reasonable to assume that in so doing it has also changed attitudes to dying and death in this Mid-West community. At the very least, patients, families, and health-care professionals are talking more explicitly about future care needs and about dying.

The sustained intervention in La Crosse has led to the effective implementation of legal requirements. It impacts on practice and is embedded in a wider cultural project. It illustrates what ought to be axiomatic, that sending an instruction, or even passing a law, does not change practice in a complex system like that of health care. There are mediating stages that require further mobilisations if cultures of practice are to be changed [53]. There are also established cultural practices and belief systems on the part of the public, patients, and their families that have to be recognised and engaged if change in any area is to be achieved and especially in an area of such emotional and cultural resonance as end-of-life care.

The examples from the United Kingdom and United States are both of long-standing and much praised projects. Two reports, one from a UK "think-tank" [13] and one from the Federal Government in the United States [14], have illustrated how having examples of good practice from hospice and palliative care services, or having clear requirements in the legislative, legal, and reimbursement system, have not changed the prevailing experience of end-of-life care in key areas in each country, although they have changed individuals experience. Despite the hospice example of being conscious of the need to properly engage with the patient; sitting at eye-level, talking about all aspects of any pain, being flexible about which member of the team does what, as "there aren't any boundaries when you are dying"; despite the dissemination of these practices in publications, and through training, we see, more than 40 years later, that Cicely Saunders arguments that hospitals are not the right place to die and that the needs of the dying do not "arouse the interest of many of the doctors who look after them" still captures the end-of-life experience of many. Bill's death in 2010 saw the paraphernalia of technological care being a barrier to the personal, "The room was designed for medical procedures not for kissing," there was no continuity of care and "no-one knew Bill" [13: pp. 9–10]. The consultant in charge of Bill actively avoided talking to his family.

If "bottom-up" learning from the patient has not changed the end-of-life care experience for most, neither has "top-down" law making. Living wills, patient self-determination, and ADs have been promoted in the United States but even when they were requirements, did not change most peoples' experience.

Furthermore, changes in attitudes toward professions and government encouragement for new sorts of rela-

tionships between citizen and state, or citizen and health service provider, do not eradicate social divisions. These changes might diffuse or obscure differentials in social power but do not remove them. We have seen, for example, how involvement is harder for older people because of structural, attitudinal, and practical barriers and how sustained attempts in the United States to encourage the use of ADs results in a pattern of take-up that replicates existing social divisions.

It might be that the sustained examples of listening to the patient and the long-running attempts to change practice through legislation have not made the widespread changes they sought because the sorts of public and patient involvement they have fostered have been ill-chosen. It might be that there are other agendas that have competed with public and patient involvement and have defeated or diverted it. Or it might be that the scale of the task has been underestimated.

In the United Kingdom much of the activity in the area of public and patient involvement has focused on routes by which patients can make their views heard in health-care provision through the creation of administrative structures that require and support this [54] or through support for the expression of the subjective views of "Expert Patients" in planning and evaluating care [55]. But experience so far shows how resistant structures, and the people within them, are.

There are however approaches to patient and public involvement that start from the opposite end of this continuum of change. These approaches seek to engage with community understandings of end-of-life care.

Community development and cultural change

In recent years, work by Kellehear and colleagues has argued for an expansion of what is perceived as the domain of the social within palliative care. Kellehear [56] has developed the World Health Organisation (WHO) *Healthy Cities* framework [57] to highlight the potential of linking palliative care with other public and private services and with communities themselves. This is an approach that builds on health promotion ideas [58] through emphasis on:

- creating supportive environments;
- strengthening community action;
- developing personal skills; and
- reorienting health services toward partnership with communities.

The case is being made here for an approach to palliative care that is both remedial, responding to the impact of loss in individuals, and formative in developing social competencies [59]. Kellehear offers a new way of thinking about public involvement in palliative care. He is suggesting that we can enhance end-of-life care experience through making discussion of dying and death more commonplace. This will facilitate better social support and increase the chances of the dying person receiving the sorts of care they wish to have.

An example from Australia saw members of the hospital palliative care team initiating "cafe conversations" with members of their community. As the name suggested these were held in a local cafe and saw small groups of people discussing questions set by the team including: "Imagine you had twelve months to live. What does this mean for you and for your community?" and, "Is it OK to die?" Participants reported an increase in comfort and confidence in talking about death, and Kellehear and O'Conner conclude that this can enhance the possibility of "meaningful social support for the person with a life-threatening illness and enhance the quality of all our lives" [60].

Kellehear and O'Connor are suggesting then that it is not just the dying person who benefits from this change to a more open discussion of death. Communities' own ideas about support develop, and this fosters its own resilience, a characteristic that is transferrable to other challenges it faces [60: p. 112]. The proposed direction of change for palliative care then is summarised thus:

> The current interpretation of hospice and palliative care as clinical care at the end-of-life, although appropriate and worthy in its own terms, is not community care. Palliative care must develop a public health approach to end-of-life care if it is to embrace health promotion activities that draw it towards community partnerships beyond volunteer programs and towards broader collaborations . . . [61: p. 321].

A changing palliative care

The involvement agenda has impacted on clinical specialties less prepared that palliative care to have to examine how to reconcile expert knowledge, evidence-based medicine, and lay views. The history of hospice, palliative care, and palliative medicine leaves its practitioners, who have experience of engaging with the scientific and the subjective, in a position to help lead the discussions across medicine as to what public and patient involvement can contribute. But, as noted above, by the 1990s, palliative care was grappling with the challenges of being assimilated into evidence-based medicine [22]. Tension between seeing changing end-of-life care as a social movement and alternatively as something to be integrated into "mainstream health services" [21: p. 3] creates a scenario

in which different agendas are competing. Edward Said describes change as "contrapuntal," different things happen at the same time, it is never simple and one cannot be sure which will become the dominant [62]. Perhaps the challenge of public and patient involvement is not in harmony with other, agendas in palliative care. These other agendas might include a wish to ally palliative care more closely with a medical model and seek, as a priority, alliances with doctors rather than with patients. This would see as resurgence of the scientific rather than the subjective, of the system world not the life world:

Commonplace and unique death

> So many people now die who never died before (Viennese saying; quoted in Feifel) [63: p. viii].

What Feifel calls "a sardonic Viennese saying" reminds us that death is both commonplace and unique. It is a social and an individual event, discussed both through considerations of "group norms and actuarial statistics" and a subjectivity that allows each of us "to grasp the concept of a future—and [our] inevitable death" [63: p. xiv]. Surely the potency of the subjective encounter with death helps explain why, in that UK hospital in 2010, no one was comfortable about talking to Bill about dying; why his doctor, his nurse, his family, and even Bill himself avoided the subject, right up to the end. Until we can change this it does not matter how many examples there are, how many laws are passed and committees are set up. The unique experience of each persons' death, and of each professional's engagement with it, will risk-generating fear that will drown out the benefits of accumulated experience about how things can be done better.

Conclusions

The experience of St Christopher's and the developments in La Crosse present us with examples of culture change. Both show how such change can be achieved and the gains that can be realised. Both also show that such change takes time and coordinated effort. Culture change can also be pursued by emphasising the social dimension of palliative care through a community and health promotion approach. No one would suggest that having "cafe-conversations," or linking those concerned with end-of-life care and those involved in receiving or providing other sorts of social support, will transform things. It is argued only that it is likely to foster solidarities, to develop individuals' sensitivities and skills, and perhaps most importantly, to link dying and death into the life of communities.

Bringing death and dying into the everyday can contribute to the development of communities, and of the individuals that make them up, so that they are more resilient. Then they can overcome the inertia created by the fear of the dying and draw on the creativity that has been generated through public and patient involvement as it has shaped a new kind of end of life care.

References

1. Goodley D. *Self-advocacy in the Lives of People with Learning Difficulties.* Buckingham: Open University Press, 2000.

2. Oliver M. *The Politics of Disablement.* London: Macmillan. See also, Campbell J and Oliver M. *Disability Politics: Understanding Our Past, Changing Our Future.* London: Routledge, 1996.

3. Kayal PM. *Bearing Witness. Gay Men's Health Crisis and the Politics of AIDS.* Boulder, Colorado: Westview Press, 1993.

4. King E. *Safety in Numbers.* London: Cassell, 1993.

5. Watney S. *Practices of Freedom. Selected Writing on HIV/AIDS.* London: Rivers Oram Press, 1994.

6. Fallowfield L and Clark A. *Breast Cancer.* London: Routledge, 1991.

7. Graham H and Oakley A. Competing ideologies of reproduction: medical and maternal perspectives on pregnancy. In: Currer C, Stacey M (eds), *Concepts of Health, Illness and Disease.* Leamington: Spa, Berg, 1986.

8. Small N. User voices in palliative care. In: Faull C, Carter Y, Daniels L (eds), *Handbook of Palliative Care*, 2nd edition. Oxford: Blackwell Publishing Ltd, 2005, pp. 61–74.

9. Small N. The modern hospice movement. In: Bornat J, Perks R, Thompson P, Walmsley J (eds), *Oral History, Health and Welfare.* London: Routledge, 2000, pp. 288–308.

10. Mount B. The Royal Victoria hospital palliative care service : a Canadian experience. In: Saunders C, Kastenbaum R (eds), *Hospice Care on the International Scene.* New York: Springer, 1997, pp. 73–85.

11. Sudnow D. *Passing On: The Social Organisation of Dying.* Englewood Cliffs, NJ: Prentice-Hall, 1967.

12. Prior L. *The Social Organisation of Death.* Basingstoke: Macmillan, 1989.

13. Leadbeater C and Garber J. *Dying for Change.* London: Demos, 2010. Available at www.demos.co.uk (accessed on September 1, 2011).

14. US Department of Health and Human Services. 2008. *Advanced Directives and Advanced Care Planning: Report to Congress.* Available at: http://aspe.hhs.gov/daltcp/reports/2008/ADCongRpt.htm (accessed on March 18, 2011).

15. Saunders C. Dying they live: St. Christopher's hospice. In: Feifel H (ed), *New Meanings of Death.* New York: McGraw-Hill, 1977, pp. 153–179.

16. Parkes CM. Evaluation of a bereavement service. In: DeVries A, Carmi A (eds), *The Dying Human.* Ramat Gan, Israel: Turtledove, 1979, pp. 389–402.

17. Small N. Theories of grief: a critical review. In: Hockey J, Katz J, Small N (eds), *Grief, Mourning and Death Ritual.* Buckingham: Open University Press, 2001, pp. 19–48.

18. Twycross RG. Clinical experience with diamorphine in advanced malignant disease. *Int J Clin Pharmacol Ther Toxicol* 1974; 9: 184–198.

19. Saunders C. The symptomatic treatment of incurable malignant disease. *Prescribers J* 1964; 4(4): 68–73.

20. Saunders C. Drug treatment of patients in the terminal stages of cancer. *Curr Med Drugs* 1960; 1(1): 16–28.

21. Clark D, Small N, Wright M, et al. *A Bit of Heaven for the Few.* Lancaster: Observatory Publications, 2005.

22. Clark D and Seymour J. *Reflections on Palliative Care.* Buckingham: Open University Press, 1999.

23. Mitchell SL, Kiely DK and Hamel, MD. Dying with advanced dementia in the nursing home. *Arch Intern Med* 2004; 164(3): 321–326.

24. Small N, Froggatt K and Downs M. *Living and Dying with Dementia.* Oxford: Oxford University Press, 2007.

25. Owen T. (ed.) Dying in older age: reflections and experiences from an older persons' perspective. Available at: http://www.ageuk.org.uk/professional-resources-home/policy/health-and-wellbeing/ (accessed on August 30, 2011).

26. ComRes, Scope Assisted Suicide Survey. Available at: http://www.scope.org.uk/news/poll-on-assisted-suicide/ (accessed on August 30, 2011).

27. Dr Vivienne Nathanson. *The Guardian*, August 27, 2011, p. 20.

28. East of England Health Authority. *The Guardian*, August 27, 2011, p. 20.

29. Cantor MD. Improving advance care planning: lessons from POLST. Physician orders for life-sustaining treatment. *J Am Geriatr Soc* 2000; 48(10): 1343–1344.

30. Hammes BJ and Rooney BL. Death and end-of-life planning in one midwestern community. *Arch Intern Med* 1998; 158: Feb 23, 383–390.

31. Hammes BJ, Rooney BL and Gundrum JD. A comparative, retrospective, observational study of the prevalence, availability, and specificity of advanced care plans in a county that implemented an advance care planning microsystem. *JAGS* 2010; 58(7): 1249–1255.

32. Habermas J. *Legitimation Crisis.* Boston, MA: Beacon Press, 1975.

33. Illich I. *Medical Nemesis: The Expropriation of Health.* London: Marion Boyars, 1975.

34. Kennedy I. *The Unmasking of Medicine.* London: George Allen and Unwin, 1981.

35. Best S and Kellner D. *Postmodern Theory.* London: Macmillan, 1991.

36. Marinetto M. Who wants to be an active citizen? *Sociology* 2003; 37(1): 103–120.

37. Seldon A. *The Blair Effect.* London: Little Brown and Co., 2001.

38. Norman J. *The Big Society: The Anatomy of the New Politics.* Buckingham: University of Buckingham Press, 2010.

39. Barnes M. The same old rocess? Older people, participation and deliberation. *Ageing Soc* 2005; 25: 245–259.

40. Small N. The changing National Health Service, user involvement and palliative care. In: Monroe B, Oliviere D (eds), *Patient Participation in Palliative Care.* Oxford: Oxford University Press, 2003, pp. 9–22.

41. Arnstein S. A ladder of citizen participation. *J Am Inst Plann* 1969; 35: 216–224.

42. Tritter JQ and Mccallum A. The snakes and ladders of user involvement: moving beyond Arnstein. *Health Policy* 2006; 76: 156–168.

43. du Boulay S. *Cicely Saunders.* London: Hodder and Stoughton, 1984.

44. Gunaratnam Y. *Widening Access to Hospice Care.* London: Help the Hospices, 2006.

45. Abbot S, Fisk M and Forward L. Social and democratic participation in residential settings for older people: realities and aspirations. *Ageing Soc* 2000; 20: 327–340.

46. Help the Aged. *Learning for Living: Helping to Prevent Social Exclusion among Older People.* London: Help the Aged, 2008.

47. Clare L and Cox S. Improving service approaches and outcomes for people with complex needs through consultation and involvement. *Disabil Soc* 2003; 18(7): 935–953.

48. Comes M, Peardon J, Manthorpe J *et al.* Wise owls and professors: the role of older researchers in the review of the National Service Framework for Older People. *Health Expect* 2008; 11(4): 409–417.

49. Postel K, Wright P and Beresford P. Older people's participation in political activity—making their voices heard: a potential support role for welfare professionals in countering ageism and social exclusion. *Practice* 2005; 17(3): 173–189.

50. Sutherland AT. *Disabled We Stand.* London: Condor Books, 1981.

51. James N and Field D. The routinization of hospice: charisma and bureaucratization. *Soc Sci Med* 1992; 34: 12: 1363–1375.

52. Taylor H. *The Hospice Movement in Britain: Its Role and Its Functions.* London: Centre for Policy on Ageing, 1983.

53. Small N. *Politics and Planning in the National Health Service.* Buckingham: Open University Press, 1999.

54. Department of Health. *Health and Social Care Act.* London: Department of Health, 2001.

55. Department of Health. *The Expert Patient.* London: Department of Health, 2001.

56. Kellehear A. *Compassionate Cities.* London: Routledge, 2005.

57. World Health Organisation. 1997. *Twenty steps for developing a Healthy Cities project.* WHO Regional Office for Europe. EUR/ICP/HSC 644(2).

58. Kellehear A. *Health Promoting Palliative care.* Melbourne: Oxford University Press, 1999.

59. Small N and Sargeant A. User and community participation at the end-of-life. In: Gott M, Ingleton C (eds), *Living with Ageing and Dying.* Oxford: Oxford University Press, 2011, pp. 90–101.

60. Kellehear A and O'Connor D. Health-promoting palliative care: a practical example. *Crit Public Health* 2008; 15(1): 111–115.

61. Kellehear A. Third-wave public health? Compassion, community and end-of-life care. *Int J Appl Psychoanal Stud* 2004; 1(4): 313–323.

62. Said E. *Orientalism.* New York: Vintage Books, 1979.

63. Feifel H. *The Meaning of Death.* New York: McGraw-Hill, 1959.

4 Palliative Care: Choice, Equality, and Diversity

Liz Grant[1], Joanna Dunn[2], Aziz Sheikh[1]

[1] University of Edinburgh, Edinburgh, UK
[2] Camden and Islington Palliative Care Team, London, UK

Introduction

The word palliative comes from the Latin, *palliare*, meaning "to cloak" (*pallium*) or "to conceal." The quintessential role of palliative care is thus the ability not only "to cover" physical pain with appropriate and effective pain relief but also to care for the person as a whole and relieve the many additional dimensions of distress that may be experienced during the process of dying. But is there a danger that there is a very different form of "cloaking" going on at present?—a cloaking of the huge local and global disparities in the access to and quality of palliative care determined by, for example, age, disease type, ethnicity, religion, social class, and geography. While this is of major impact to people globally, this chapter focuses primarily on reviewing the evidence for disadvantage, exclusion, and poor access to palliative care and explores some of the reasons that lie behind these inequalities in the developed world, largely the United Kingdom.

Supportive and palliative care is both multidimensional and complex. It is an approach to care, a care delivery service, and a system of care for those living with, and dying from, life-limiting illness. Holistic palliative care is responsive to the different stages of illness as experienced by patients; the differing needs associated with various illnesses; patients' and their families' and carers' cultural, social, spiritual beliefs about illness and death, but which also remains cognisant of the range of health and social services that are available in any place or time [1–3]. The spectrum of palliative care, from supportive and generalist palliative care, rehabilitative palliative care to specialist palliative care, should create a continuum, though this continuum is much less linear and more circuitous than is often assumed [4]. Therefore, it is not surprising that within this complex and comprehensive care domain there are often inequalities in the identification of the need for palliative care, in palliative care provision, including its availability, accessibility, appropriateness, and the extent to which it embraces the different facets of need, be they physical, psychological, social, or spiritual [5]. That inequalities exist is not surprising; this recognition should not, however, be interpreted as meaning that they are acceptable.

There is increasing evidence from a large number of research studies and from commissioned reports of significant inequalities across a number of palliative care domains. Examples include [6–9]:

• discrimination on the basis of race, age, social status;
• culturally, traditionally, and religiously inappropriate care;
• lack of understanding of services; and
• lack of, or reduced opportunities to access, enter, or negotiate services.

In a systematic review of the effects of age on the referral to and use of specialist palliative care services in adult cancer patients, Burt and Raine highlighted growing inequalities related to age, with the elderly 18–63% less likely to use specialist palliative care than those who were younger [10]. Importantly, while recognising that unequal use of health care between different populations is not necessarily inequitable (if, e.g., it reflects an unequal need for such care), Burt and Raine have raised the issue that the lack of a common understanding of how needs are defined and of how responses to these needs are operationalised lies at the heart of the problem of inequalities. As Raine commented in a later interview:

Handbook of Palliative Care, Third Edition. Edited by Christina Faull, Sharon de Caestecker, Alex Nicholson and Fraser Black.
© 2012 by John Wiley and Sons, Inc. Published 2012 by John Wiley & Sons, Inc.

Specialist palliative care is a very slippery service as it is more difficult to determine who needs what and when. GPs need explicit understanding as to who will benefit, yet nobody knows where the inequities lie. The system needs repackaging [11].

Inequalities in both access to and in delivery of appropriate palliative care are not inevitable nor do they just randomly happen. Inequalities can affect not only the patient and their family network but also other informal carers and service providers, creating pockets of burdens of care. Understanding the processes that lead to these inequalities and tracing back their origins can provide insights into where there are opportunities to change systems to reduce these inequalities. Such process mapping can also help to identify those areas that may be out with the realm of policy makers, palliative care practitioners, and primary care providers to change—areas where wider societal change is a prerequisite to improving health outcomes for all sections of society.

The environment that breeds inequalities

There are multiple ways of looking at how national health and social care systems are established, sustained, and managed. One way is to understand how interrelated and frequently interlocked structures create and sustain the units of care that are delivered, and in consequence, create the environment where inequalities in palliative care or WHO provision can emerge. Marmot's influential report on the social determinants of health, *Closing the gap in a generation: health equity through action on the social determinants of health* [12], put into the public, and the public health domain, what Tudor Hart and countless other protagonists of "community care" had been saying for years, namely, that well-being owes far less to medicine and to health services than to the systems and structures in which these health services function [13,14]. Understanding how the societal determinants of health and the determinants of the health system sit together provides a new matrix in considering inequalities. Box 4.1 shows the different structures that together determine how palliative care is delivered and received.

The current context of care: the model in the United Kingdom

Palliative care has been divided into two areas: generalist palliative care seen as the care provided by, among oth-

Box 4.1 Structures shaping care

Institutional structures: The way that care systems are built and maintained. This includes both the physical space and place of care, and also the delivery processes and the packages of care managed by institutions. Once in place, packages of care, like buildings, are often difficult to deconstruct and reshape.

Educational structures: The way that skills are taught and transferred, the premises on which health-care teaching is delivered, and the foundational knowledge base that determines the type of care that is presented as the standard "normative" care within communities and national systems.

Economic structures: The way in which care is costed, and the drivers to greater cost efficiency and productivity. Alongside the very direct care costings, economic structures determine the benefit systems and drive decision making for carers and for relatives. Once a night-time carer's allowance has been put in place, or a benefit granted, few feel able to make changes.

Societal structures: The ways in which society establishes its norms and values. There is an overriding emphasis on unity within our health systems, with established patterns and processes and systems of health care that veer away from complexity and multidimensional "untidy" diverse approaches to care and encourage an endless move toward uniformity.

Identity structures: Potentially the most fluid of all of the structures, they can also be the most set in stone. Identity structures refer to the way that each of us experience and interpret the world around us, influenced by religious, social, emotional beliefs and traditions, family and cultural normative behaviours and expectations.

ers, a patient's general practitioner (GP), linked nursing services, and health-care teams in the hospital setting; and specialist palliative care delivered by palliative care teams in hospital wards or community settings, and by hospices. Generalist palliative care should be provided by everyone who is caring for patients with life-limiting illnesses. Generalist palliative care should encompass basic pain and symptom management, social, psychological, and spiritual support for those patients with life-limiting illnesses, often alongside other treatment. For example, it would be expected that a nonspecialist in palliative care would be able to initiate a patient who is suffering from severe pain on morphine or other strong opioid analgesia. However, the specialist should be available to support the delivery of palliative care, through training, and by providing clinical care for those patients with complex symptoms unable to be managed by nonspecialists. This should operate in a similar way to many other aspects of health-care provision, whereby GPs are able to manage core aspects of conditions such as hypertension and heart disease, but refer patients to secondary or tertiary care when the conditions are require particular technical expertise or services. Guidelines have been produced for the expected competencies of specialist and nonspecialists in palliative care, and training of health-care professionals should be undertaken to ensure these competencies are achieved [15,16]. In recent years, training in palliative care has been included in many undergraduate and postgraduate curricula, but the knowledge and skills may take some time to be fully disseminated to make a difference to patient care. While the majority of palliative care in the United Kingdom is delivered by generalists, the majority of designated funding and tools to support palliative care delivery are still confined to specialist services.

Understanding inequalities

Perhaps the best way of understanding and tackling inequalities is to, first of all, focus on a set of suggested principles that encapsulate the best in palliative care (both generalist and specialist) and to explore situations in everyday service where these principles have been compromised.

Principle 1: The most equitable palliative care resonates with different communities' meta-narratives (the issues, preferences, choices, and experiences) of death and dying

The narratives, related to advanced, progressive illnesses, that define and shape the cultures of different people groups within our increasingly multicultural societies are harder to hear. They are pushed to the side by a death-defying, death-ignoring meta-narrative of successfulness and life-sustaining medicine. All the grand religious meta-narratives recognised the inspiration of the sacred beyond the grave, the possibilities of passing places between this world and the "next," and acknowledged that the essence of life was that it was physically finite, yet spiritually eternal. Aging and death were understood and accepted within the religious and social frameworks that constituted a community's culture and traditions. As new secular paradigms have emerged that provide alternative premises to explain and indeed manage life's beginnings

and endings, one of the major consequences is an uncertainty of talking about death and dying, coupled with a belief that success lies in cure and fending off death rather than in ensuring a good death. Who suffers the most in such situations? Is it the patient receiving aggressive treatments when treatments are futile? Or the family hanging onto hope that death is still somewhere in the future and thus failing to say goodbye properly? Or the clinician who feels that they have failed when nature has taken its course?

Principle 2: The most equitable palliative care is responsive and adaptive to a person's beliefs, tradition, language, culture, and way of life

Closely connected to the dissolution of the grand narratives that provided the opportunities to talk about death and dying is the disappearance of the expertise, and the comfortableness, to respond actively to religious and cultural community needs concerning dying and the confidence to speak about spiritual issues, especially among health professionals. Respect for the religious and spiritual beliefs of others is an essential competency for GPs but for many patients this respect has not actually resulted in recognition of their particular spiritual issues and needs, nor has it been translated into active engagement with them to meet these particular and often highly sensitive needs [17]. Studies conducted in Edinburgh uncovered considerable anxieties about discussing spirituality and supporting the spiritual needs of patients. For example, when asked about the palliative care needs of a patient who was a Muslim, one health professional commented:

> Social [needs] I obviously enter into. Spiritual things I don't because I am an atheist myself and I don't enter into any of this nonsense whatsoever. People go and see their priests or preachers or whatever . . . I don't discuss that at all [18].

Members of minority ethnic communities have found themselves struggling to access care and to find support that respects and honours their particular traditions and views, and this has had significant negative consequences for those nearing death and for their families. Equitable palliative care must ensure that all patients and their families are able to carry out the traditions and rituals important to them, in a space and place where they feel comfortable and respected (Box 4.2).

Inequalities in care can arise that are specifically associated with migration. Patients newer to the health system frequently lack awareness of what services are available and lack an understanding of the cost of services. An early study by Hill et al. in 1995 [19] concluded that "some black

Box 4.2 Case study—Dealing appropriately with cross-cultural issues

Daniel was admitted with advanced carcinoma of the lung. He is 42 years old and of Nigerian origin but has lived away from Nigeria for many years. He was originally admitted for control of severe pain, but his condition has deteriorated and he is now bedbound. He has a large family and an argument has developed between the patient's family and a care assistant looking after him. The family brought in some food that they wished the patient to have and the care assistant has said they are unable to use facilities to heat the food due to health and safety regulations. The care assistant is very unhappy about too many relatives being around and upsetting other patients and their relatives in the neighbouring rooms by making noise, particularly praying very loudly.

The case is discussed at the multidisciplinary team (MDT), and one of the nurses caring for Daniel explains that his family members are scared about what is happening to him. They believe that if he has the right food to eat, he will become stronger and will be able to have more treatment to cure his cancer. She has spoken to Daniel separately who wants to go along with whatever his family members want, although he is aware that he is dying and wants to go back to Nigeria to die. The team agrees that the doctor, the nurse, and the social worker caring for Daniel will hold a family meeting.

The outcome of the meeting is that the ward agrees to let Daniel's family prepare his meals; they also look into the possibility of him flying to Nigeria, including access to palliative care services in the country.

and Asian patients and their carers are very disadvantaged, as they do not know what they are entitled to and hence what to ask for by way of benefits and services." Fifteen years later similar findings are still emerging. In a number of studies exploring issues of access to and experience of palliative care, members (across all minority communities and across generations of migrancy) have reported personal racial and religious discrimination from health staff, sometimes recognising that the discrimination was probably unintentional, at other times knowing that it was purposeful.

Thoughtful and sensitive communication with patients and relatives is an essential aspect of good palliative care provision. A common barrier to good care is that of language. Language difficulties with insufficient spoken English to communicate effectively, coupled with anxieties about the right to care (e.g., because of uncertainty about legal status), has resulted in cases where there is a lack of adequate interpretation services. This can result in barriers to provision of adequate care. Alongside those who struggle to communicate in English because it is a second or third language, many patients (even those who speak English as their mother tongue) feel they lack the "medical English speak" to communicate properly with doctors and nurses, or they may lack the "audacity" to challenge the professional narrative of palliative need that the health professional pronounces for them. Additionally, it is important to engage the services of an interpreter and include them as part of the interdisciplinary team where possible. Allowing family members to interpret can lead to nondisclosure of potentially important information because of family members not wanting to cause distress to patients or vice versa. There may also be a role for interpreters in promoting cultural understanding and insight for the CPs as well as providing language interpretation [20]. Chapter 6, *Communication skills in palliative care*, provides practical guidance on working with interpreters to facilitate good communication.

Principle 3: The most equitable palliative care is person rather than disease focused

Different diseases trigger different care responses, irrespective of patient need or likely prognosis. The diseases that stirred up great fear in the past have arguably become the "best" to die from. For example, those living with cancer in the United Kingdom and those living with human immunodeficiency virus (HIV) in urban areas of Africa have diseases that have been prioritised above almost every other disease by the health system. Cancer in the United Kingdom has a well-understood "public story" incorporated within its narrative. It is a death conversation, even if the threads of that conversation are about "fighting death," "not giving in," and "not losing the battle." Those with cancers in the United Kingdom are in addition relatively well served with services that meet their needs, living and dying on a relatively predictable course made explicit by significant research. About 90% of UK specialist palliative care is provided for those with cancer, although only 25% of people die from a neoplastic condition. It is hard to argue that this inequity is appropriate on grounds of either patient need or complexity.

Those living with advanced diseases or organ failure, or physical frailty, have far fewer services available, and what services are available are much less likely to deal with all dimensions of need. Murray and Sheikh have argued for the need to apply the lessons learned from cancer to the growing number of people dying from nonmalignant illnesses:

> People dying from cancer usually have needs lasting for weeks or months, whereas those dying from organ failure or old age often have unmet needs that extend over many months or years. It is little wonder, then, that people dying of the "wrong" condition and their carers, whether family, social, or professional, are increasingly frustrated by the major obstacles to accessing appropriate care [21,22].

Having the "wrong disease" can thus create great inequalities in care as it can reduce someone's chances of getting benefits appropriate to their condition. Having a disease that is not boxed into a set time, with a set expected journey, causes health service difficulties as palliative structures are set up to manage, and be managed within a time line. For example, in some health systems those not expected to die in 6 months may not be in a position to have their health-care costs covered for hospice care. The "wrong diseases" can in some cases be financially crippling, leading families into a spiral of poverty.

Box 4.3 Case study A—Holistic decision making

Tom, a 74-year-old man, with chronic obstructive pulmonary disease (COPD) has been increasingly breathless for the past 2 years and is now housebound. He lives with his wife Pauline who is 72 years old and is his main carer. Pauline is also unwell, suffering from diabetes and chronic leg ulcers. They are receiving some assistance from social services, who help with shopping and cleaning, but despite this are still struggling to manage. The district nurses visit regularly and suggest referring Tom to the local hospice for assistance with symptoms of breathlessness and pain. Tom and Pauline are reluctant for referral to the hospice, as they see the service as being only for patients with cancer who are dying. After some further discussion with the community respiratory nurse—who they know well—they agree to a joint visit from the palliative care community nurse together with the respiratory nurse.

After undertaking a holistic assessment of Tom and his wife's needs, the palliative care nurse refers Tom to the physiotherapist for advice on nonpharmacological management of his breathlessness. She also starts him on oral morphine to control his pain and breathlessness. She refers him to hospice day care that he will be able to attend once a week in order to give his wife some rest from caring for him. She also arranges for the occupational therapist to visit to assist with adaptations to their home to enable Tom and Pauline to care for themselves more easily. The palliative care nurse and respiratory nurse arrange to visit again in 2 weeks time to review the situation.

To challenge these inequalities, a number of tools such as the Gold Standards Framework (GSF) (discussed in Chapter 2, *Palliative care in the community*) [23] and the Supportive and Palliative Care Indicators Tool (SPICT) (shown as Figure 1.1 in Chapter 1, *The context and principles of palliative care*) [24] have been developed in the United Kingdom. Lying behind these tools is a recognition of the need to ensure that a palliative care approach as well as curative care is in practitioners' minds as they make care decisions with patients. One useful question that practitioners should consider asking is if they would be surprised if their patient died within the next year. If the answer is "no," consideration should be given to placing such patients, irrespective of diagnosis, onto a palliative/supportive care register. Box 4.3 provides a small case study of good practice in decision making. Rather than providing a definitive prognostication index, this approach enables the practitioner to adjust the focus of care from curative/life prolonging to supportive/palliative care to ensure that they consider the likely needs and choices of the patients and consequent provision of care, ensuring that patients are able to achieve excellence in end-of-life care, including discussions around advance care planning (ACP), do not resuscitate (DNR) decisions, and prevention of unnecessary hospital admissions.

Principle 4: The most equitable palliative care is initiated at the most appropriate time for the patient

In aiming to address "total pain" and suffering across all dimensions, palliative care seeks to affirm life and equip patients with the tools not just to die well but to live as well as possible well until death. Therefore, palliative care should start not at the end point of this journey, just before death, but at the stage when the patient, their carers, and clinicians recognise and accept that the patient is living with an illness that is life limiting. But knowing how and what and when to provide such care remains difficult for many practitioners. Too early and angst may be exacerbated especially in a culture that is socially death denying; too late and blame is apportioned for delays in starting to administer palliative care. In a cure-focused environment, where hope is pinned to retaining life and getting better, there is often a huge reluctance among practitioners to raise discussions about death and dying.

As noted earlier, much palliative care, as currently constructed, is disease focused rather than person focused, and certain diseases trigger the idea of palliative care for professionals, and indeed patients, more readily than others. While the cancer journey facilitates a conversation about palliation, other diseases such as COPD provide no such ready trigger. Looking at the question from the other side gives some clues. Studies from Edinburgh's Primary Palliative Care Research Group, longitudinal qualitative study of people with end-stage COPD identified the way in which COPD was a "disease with no beginning," "a middle that is a way of life," and "an unpredictable and unanticipated end." Pinnock et al. provide a telling description of the difference in approach to patients with COPD that have a fundamental influence on equity. In contrast to consultations with people with cancer where it seems to come up more naturally to talk about death, a familiar and comfortable pattern of consulting prevented initiating an unlooked for discussion about the future:

> Interviewer: I was going to ask you whether you have talked to him at all about what might happen in the future and how things might progress?
>
> GP: No, not really. He usually has got his own [agenda in the consultation]. It's more reassurance about how he is and chatting generally and he just likes a bit of social discourse I think [25].

Principle 5: The most equitable palliative care is fluid and adapts to suit the changing physical needs of patients and their carers

Palliative care needs to recognise both the linear journey element of living toward death (i.e., the inevitability of death) and the potential circular nature of this journey (the uncertainty of timing of death, the ups and downs of the disease journey, and the remissions and relapses). The majority of health services are constructed along linear models, and once patients are on the treadmill of a linear approach to care, it is extremely difficult to move off it.

Inequalities result when the care that is being given is not the care that is needed. There are various reasons why both professionals and patients struggle to make the care changes that would better serve the needs of patients. Patients can lack the right information about the nature of the care they can expect to receive, especially patients not familiar with the health system, or they may lack the confidence to challenge the nurse or the doctor when prescriptions are repeated, or advice given that was suitable a year ago, but has been overtaken by events. Patients may fear that describing an improvement may result in care being withdrawn, or a change in the routine of care. Box 4.2 captures best practice in dealing with a pertinent cultural and social issue.

Those least likely to challenge the routine are those most at risk of receiving a form of care that does not actually meet their current needs. Alongside the multiple patient-

initiated reasons for continuing with the status quo, there are an equally large number of reasons that are linked to professional reluctance or indecision around change. Nurses feel inhibited to speak out in support of change especially if senior doctors have made decisions. Services, once started that cannot easily be stopped, include social care benefits, meals provided for people at home, or intensive home care.

Principle 6: The most equitable palliative care is accessible and responsive to those whose lifestyle choices or lifestyle circumstances have placed them in vulnerable positions on the edges of communities

There are multiple reasons why people are, or feel they are, on the margins of society or feel that communities have pushed them to their edges. Among many, these include those with significant psychiatric illnesses; those with pronounced learning disabilities; those with disabilities such as blindness or deafness, or those who suffer from aphasia disorders; those whose lifestyle choices place them on the outside of settled community structures such as the travelling communities; those who are homeless; and those whose behaviours and needs are viewed as socially unacceptable, such as substance users.

Providing palliative care to those on the outside or the margins of "society" is challenging, not least because palliative care, as a service, is dependent on the concept of continuity of health care. Current palliative care referral structures have been so designed as to require practitioners to establish beginnings, to identify changes that transition a person from one form of supportive and palliative care to another form of specialist palliative care, and much palliative (and indeed health) care assumes a stable address, the availability of the patient to attend appointments, and to be in the "right place" at the "right time" for the service to function.

Barriers to accessing health care and palliative care in particular for the homeless include:
- anticipating that this group may be antisocial, violent, or have addiction problems;
- difficulties with access due to inconvenient appointments and opening times; and
- financial disincentives for practitioners [26].

Initiatives have been undertaken to improve access to palliative care for patients in such situations. One example of an effective intervention was a project undertaken in Ottawa in Canada where a 15-bed shelter-based hospice was set up. Input was given from specialist nursing staff, care workers, general medical input from physicians, as well as specialist palliative care physician support. The evaluators of the programme estimated that 68% of patients given care through the project would not have accessed palliative care and would have died homeless, without pain or symptom management [27].

Palliative care provision for prisoners is also an area that needs to be improved. Several studies have identified issues that make such provision challenging, in particular access to pain relieving medications due to a fear of diversion of controlled substances within the prison environment, and lack of facilities to adequately integrate and manage family support [28].

Principle 7: The most equitable palliative care has no age barriers

The majority of palliative care services have been established with a specific population in mind: an adult population, often between the ages of 40 and 70, the majority of whom have cancer. Children's palliative care has made huge advances in recent years leading to it being recognised as a speciality in its own right. But what about those in their teenage years, and those whose years are making them frail, with fragile memories? What sort of palliative care requirements do they have, and are their needs being equitably met?

Getting the place of care right for teenagers is difficult. Services have often assumed that their palliative care needs are those of adults, but their social and emotional care needs are those of children, and so teenagers can find themselves the oldest on wards where the seats are tiny, and cartoons run on television from morning to night, or the youngest on wards where others are much older.

The Teenage Cancer Trust, a charity specifically set up to provide support for young people, has identified three specific research challenges where more work needs to be done, and these research areas give us a window into some of the issues of appropriate choice that is needed, namely:

- Why are there delays in diagnosing teenagers and young adults with cancer?
- Can symptoms be managed by mobile phone as the most frequently used "meeting space" of youth?
- Why do organisers of cancer clinical trials frequently neglect teenagers and young adults from their trials?

A Macmillan survey (Box 4.4) reported by the Teenage Cancer Trust highlighted the issues for teenagers with cancer, especially the isolation felt by teenagers, whose peer group knew about cancer, but certainly did not want to talk about it.

Box 4.4 Macmillan teenage cancer survey

Four hundred 12–19-year-olds across the United Kingdom were asked about cancer, and the survey found that cancer is a big issue for teenagers:

- 70% know someone who has, or has had, cancer.
- 74% say they would not know what to say to a friend with cancer.
- 50% say they would avoid talking to them about it.
- 37% think that cancer could be caused by knocks and bumps.
- 12% think that cancer could be catching.

What are the issues raised by teenagers? Though overwhelmingly grateful for all the expert clinical care, many have talked about how difficult it is to be in a ward with no one else of their age and hence no one to talk to. Teenagers have noted how few resources there are that cater for the questions that teenagers have such as how can I change my appearance to look "normal again"?; how can I talk to my friends?; will I ever have a boyfriend or a girlfriend?; is sex possible?

Getting the place of care right for the frail elderly is equally challenging. Are nursing or care homes set up as palliative care providers? Staff in care homes may be less aware of the need for palliative care and the requirements to consider issues such as end-of-life care planning. Box 4.5 provides an illustration of a case managed well. However, frequently there may be little discussion with the patient and their relatives about what should happen if the patient's condition changes. Again in this group of patients, there is a disparity in the standard of palliative care between those with a diagnosis of cancer and those with other chronic, life-limiting conditions (LLCs) such as dementia. The long period of decline that the frail elderly experience often does not fit with a hospice care model. Until recently, palliative care has had relatively little dialogue with geriatricians, many of whom do provide good holistic care, although often with limited emphasis on planning for dying. Often end-of-life care for the frail elderly is triggered by crises admissions followed by weekend and night-time referrals to community crises care teams to provide a care cover until "something can be done, somewhere can be found" for the patient. Innovative work carried out in nursing homes in Midlothian, Scotland, by Jo Hockley has laid an excellent blueprint of new ways of embedding a palliative care approach within nursing home [29]. This work has led to new training initiatives for care home staff being organised, the use of

---

Box 4.5 Case study—Best practice in care of those who are elderly

Nora is a resident in a care home. She is 88 years old with advanced cancer of the breast and has been bedbound for the last 2 weeks. She has severe pain in her back and a decreased appetite. She has a very supportive family, although they live some distance from the nursing home so visit infrequently. Nora is referred by her GP to the palliative care team who see here together with her daughter to assess her pain and other symptoms. Nora wishes to remain in the residential home as she has lived there for 10 years and knows the carers well, her daughter is in agreement with this, and the advice of the palliative care team supports this.

However, the manager in charge wants to admit Nora to the local hospice for terminal care, as the care home staff are unhappy to give the patient morphine and are very reluctant for her to die in the home. They say they are not set up for caring for patients who are dying.

A meeting is arranged with the patient's GP who provides medical support to the home, the patient's daughter, the palliative care nurse, and the manager in charge of the home. After some discussion about how best to manage Nora's situation, it is agreed that the palliative care nurse will arrange a training sessions for the care assistants about palliative care. The GP arranges for the district nurses to visit Nora alternate days to support the care staff in the home, and the palliative care nurse agrees to visit weekly, with support out of hours provided by the on-call service at the local hospice and the GP out-of-hours service.

Nora remains in the home with her pain well controlled until her death 3 weeks later. The palliative care nurse returns to the home afterward to provide support to the care staff who have cared for Nora.

---

the Liverpool Care Pathway (LCP) in nursing homes, and a new investment in research into the palliative care needs of patients with diseases such as dementia.

International dimensions and global disparities

The need for palliative care in all countries, and especially in low-income countries, has never been greater. Increasing numbers of people are living with life-shortening chronic diseases in low- and middle-income countries. Despite living in the twenty-first century where technology has practically connected every geographical region in the world, regardless of its rurality through mobile phones, many still die in the most excruciating pain simply because they cannot access cheap and effective pain relief. The need has never been more of a social justice issue given the availability in the world today of vast numbers of treatments that can enable a person to live and die with dignity and comfort.

The Quality of Death Report [30] argues for the importance of palliative care in creating an environment where not only quality of life counts but also quality of death matters. They recognise that how a country cares for its dying defines the quality of its care system. A poor death is a failure of the whole system to accept its duty of care for all its citizens. Not living well with chronic illness and not dying well affects not only the patient but also those around them. Children carry the scars of their parents' poor dying experience, the impact of which are not as yet fully understood, but which are at least recognised by services that have over the last decade developed care structures such as memory books to help children remember and parents say goodbye. Families can bear huge financial cost, often for years afterward, of a poor and often lengthy dying experience, with patients requiring constant oversight, and being admitted for long futile treatments to hospitals far away from local homesteads. Financial costs, costs in time away from fields or work, costs in searching for anything that will reduce the severity of pain, and costs in endless travel to hospital and clinics and traditional healers seeking treatments before a delayed diagnosis is made that recognises that the illness has no cure.

There has been a shift in attitude at a global level toward palliative care, with the recognition that such care is not simply a small add-on specialist, or luxury optional service suitable for a small group of people suffering from particular illnesses, to a new awareness that palliative care is a human rights issue based in equity and justice. In 2006, a World Health Assembly resolution was passed that called for the provision of palliative care for all individuals in need to be treated as an urgent, humanitarian responsibility. Much has happened, but given the huge disparities there is still a long way to travel [31].

The Diana, Princess of Wales Memorial Fund, is one of the major investors in palliative care in Africa through its Palliative Care Initiative. This is an independent grant-giving charity established in September 1997 to continue the humanitarian work of the late Princess Diana in the United Kingdom and overseas. The Palliative Care Initiative has a vision to see a world where high quality of palliative care is accessible to all. It seeks to increase the availability of palliative care throughout Africa by building the capacity of palliative care programmes, by nurturing palliative care champions, and by fostering palliative care research that builds a strong evidence base. Key to this vision is to ensure that palliative care becomes fully integrated into national health policies and systems.

Conclusions: Building choice, equality, diversity, and responsiveness into comprehensive supportive and palliative care service

To improve choice and reduce inequalities both globally and locally, there needs to be a better understanding of, and recording of, vulnerability in all communities, and a heightened awareness of the silo nature of care systems that travel along individual disease continuums.

Awareness about the multiple inequalities that exist in palliative care is not enough. Systems need to be put in place that create pathways of action. One recommended course of action that has worked in various settings is active case management of the most vulnerable patients and carers. Social workers can be in excellent positions to identify those experiencing vulnerability and exclusion. Often this active case management can best be achieved through a coordinator, or through working alongside an advocate who understands the issues of vulnerability, the service issues and constraints and the social, religious, and cultural traditions that the patient and their carers live within. Examples of innovative interaction can be gleaned from other specialties and other contexts and situations such as the role of a community link worker providing the bridge between formal and informal services, between patient and professional.

Palliative care requires both a generalist service that should be integrated into all areas of health care and a specialist service available for situations where complexity of clinical needs require additional specific service and treatment interventions. One of the barriers that can prevent patients from accessing palliative care is the assumption that a palliative care service is only a very specialised service and patients should only be cared for by specialists, and only considered for palliative care when all else has failed. There is a need to consider which are the essential all encompassing components of palliative care--those that should be provided for all in need, and which aspects of care are technically challenging and therefore require some additional technical expertise.

Palliative care services have been traditionally provided mainly to those with cancer, those who are middle aged, and from particular cultural groups. These groups of patients are now thankfully able to access a high-quality

standard of palliative care encompassing all the add-ons of hospice care such as easy access to in-patient hospice care, 24-h care at home and access to complementary therapies (CTs). It will be possible for health services to provide this intensive level of palliative care to all those in need due to financial constraints within the health sector. There is nonetheless an overwhelming need to open up access to palliative care to everyone, and this may require learning from approaches adopted in Africa or Asia where communal care, and an understanding of the expert value of volunteers and health-care assistants is recognised.

The question that every health-care service needs to ask is this. Will a wider remit for palliative care across the ages, across illnesses and across socially constructed divides mean that the high-quality intensive and holistic care so much associated with traditional palliative care is no longer possible, or will it mean that this level of care becomes a common good, shared by all as a health-care right, and understood much more as a transition care, a facilitator to stabilise and normalise conditions so that care in the community can continue?

For most patients and carers the need for care is often in the here and now. Real-time support where professionals can obtain advice specific to the needs of the patient and the family can be immensely valuable. Lack of inclusion into services or failure to find the most appropriate service is often not through intention, but through lack of knowledge, a loss as to what to do next.

Getting end-of-life care "right" lies at the heart of what it means to be an equitable society. Prioritising this area needs no apologies.

References

1. Boyd KJ, Worth A, Kendall M, et al. Making sure services deliver for people with advanced heart failure: a longitudinal qualitative study of patients, family carers, and health professionals. *Palliat Med* 2009; 23: 767–776.
2. Grant L, Murray SA and Sheikh A. Spiritual dimensions of dying in pluralist societies. *BMJ* 2010; 341: 659–662.
3. Kendall M, Murray SA, Carduff E, et al. Use of multiperspective qualitative interviews to understand patients' and carers' beliefs, experiences, and needs. *BMJ* 2009; 339: b4122.
4. Boyd K, Mason B, Kendall M, et al. Advance care planning for cancer patients in primary care: a feasibility study. *Br J Gen Pract* 2010; 60: e449–e458.
5. Sheikh A. Ethnic minorities and their perceptions of the quality of primary care. *BMJ* 2009; 339: b3797.
6. Shipman C, Gysels M, White P, et al. Improving generalist end of life care: national consultation with practitioners,

commissioners, academics, and service user groups. *BMJ* 2008; 337: a1720.

7. Addington-Hall J and Altmann D. Which terminally ill cancer patients in the United Kingdom receive care from community specialist palliative care nurses? *J Adv Nurs* 2000; 32: 799–806.

8. Walshe C, Chew-Graham C, Todd C et al. What influences referrals within community palliative care services? A qualitative case study. *Soc Sci Med* 2008; 67: 137–146.

9. Callahan D and Topinkova E. Age, rationing and palliative care. In: Morrison RS and Meier DE (eds), *Geriatric Palliative Care*. New York: Oxford University Press, 2003.

10. Burt J and Raine R. The effect of age on referral to and use of specialist palliative care services in adult cancer patients: a systematic review. *Age Ageing* 2006; 35: 469–476.

11. Raine R. *Palliative Care Inequalities: Interview Pulse Magazine*, June 29, 2006

12. CSDH. Closing the gap in a generation: health equity through action on the social determinants of health. *Final Report of the Commission on the Social Determinants of Health*. Geneva: WHO, 2008. Available at: http://www.who.int/social_determinants/thecommission/finalreport/en/index.html (accessed on May 11, 2012).

13. Tudor Hart J. The inverse care law. *The Lancet* 1971; 297: 405–412.

14. Mclean G, Sutton M, and Guthrie B. Deprivation and quality of primary care services: evidence for persistence of the inverse care law from the UK quality and outcomes framework. *J Epidemiol Community Health* 2006; 60: 917–922.

15. National End of Life Care Programme. Core Competencies and Principles for health and social care workers working with adults at the end of life. Department of Health, 2009.

16. Association for Palliative medicine of Great Britain and Ireland. Palliative medicine Curriculum for specialists in other files and general practitioners. Association for Palliative Medicine, 2004.

17. Gatrad AR, Brown E, and Sheikh A (eds), *Palliative Care for South Asians: Muslims, Hindus and Sikhs*. London: Quay Books, 2006.

18. Worth A, Irshad T, Bhopal R, et al. Vulnerability and access to care for South Asian Sikh and Muslim patients with life limiting illness in Scotland: prospective longitudinal qualitative study. *BMJ* 2009; 338: b183.

19. Hill D and Penso D. Opening doors: improving access to hospice and specialist palliative care services by members of the black and ethnic minorities communities. Occasional paper 7, National Council for Hospice and Specialist Palliative Care Services, London, 1995.

20. Norris WM, Wenrich MD, Nielsen EL, et al. Communication about end-of-life care between language-discordant patients and clinicians: insights from medical interpreters. *J Palliat Med* 2005; 8: 1016–1024.

21. Murray SA and Sheikh A. Care for all at the end of life. *BMJ* 2008; 336: 958–959.

22. Murray S, Boyd K, and Sheikh A. Palliative care in chronic illnesses: we need to move from prognostic paralysis to active total care. *BMJ* 2005; 330: 611–612.

23. Gold Standards Framework. Available at: http://www.goldstandardsframework.org.uk/TheGSFToolkit/Identify (accessed on May 17, 2011).

24. Lothian NHS Supportive and Palliative Care Indicators Tool. Version 21, October 2011. Available at: www.palliativecareguidelines.org.uk (accessed on November 11, 2011).

25. Pinnock H, Kendall M, Murray SA, et al. Living and dying with severe chronic obstructive pulmonary disease: multiperspective longitudinal qualitative study. *BMJ* 2011; 342: d142.

26. Wright NMJ and Tomkins CNE. How can health care systems effectively deal with the major health care needs of homeless people? World Health Organisation Regional Office for Europe Health Evidence Network Report, 2005.

27. Podymow T, Turnbull J, and Coyle D. Shelter-based palliative care for the homeless terminally ill. *Palliat Med* 2006; 20: 81–86.

28. Lin JT and Mathew P. Cancer pain management in prisons: a survey of primary care practitioners and inmates. *J Pain Symptom Manage* 2005; 29: 466–473.

29. Hockley J, Watson J, and Dewar B. 2004. Developing quality end of life care in eight independent nursing homes through the implementation of an integrated care pathway for the last days of life. St. Columba's Hospice. Available at: http://www.stcolumbashospice.org.uk (accessed on May 11, 2012).

30. EIU. 2010. *The Quality of Death: Ranking End of Life Care Across the World*. London: Economist Intelligence Unit.

31. Grant L, Downing J, Namukwaya E, et al. Palliative care in Africa since 2005: good progress, but much further to go. *BMJ Support Palliat Care* 2011; 1: 118–122.

5 Ethical Issues in Palliative Care

Sharon de Caestecker

LOROS, The Leicestershire and Rutland Hospice, Leicester, UK

You won't find ethics in the rule books

David Seedhouse, 2007 [1]

Introduction

Why bother?

Why bother at all with ethics? It could be argued that ethics is just a series of circular arguments that are of little help to those involved in the real clinical care of patients. In the first part of the chapter, the argument is advanced that the discipline of ethical reflection has an everyday presence and has practical value in supporting decision making and best practice, combining both ethical reasoning and emotion. Second, the use of ethical principles in the context of palliative care, together with examples of common challenges, is presented with consideration given to the promotion of an ethically sound decision-making process. In summary, the following points are elaborated:

• Ethics is restricted neither to an expert body of knowledge nor to complex issues that arise infrequently. As social beings, ethics affects each and every one of us, regardless of our professional position, and therefore, we all have some experience of ethics.

• Patients need to be able to trust Care professionals (CPs) and ethics is concerned with defining moral practice as the basis of that trust.

• Practitioners should be aware of the need to respect a patient's autonomy, balancing this with other ethical principles.

We are all ethics practitioners

Ethics, simply defined, is the study of what we may classify as a good or a bad action and provides a framework for us to weigh that action. Ethics also concerns itself with what the character of a "moral person" should be. Hence, in the case of medical ethics, what would we class as a "good

action" for a CP and who would we class as a "good" health or social care practitioner?

Ethics is everywhere and concerns everybody [1]. As we stand waiting for a bus or queue in the supermarket, we are surrounded by moral issues: is it acceptable for somebody to jump the queue waiting for the bus? Should we be pleasant to everyone we meet as we make our way around the supermarket? We have a choice over how to respond in all such everyday matters. Our response to these issues may be values or principles based and may be taken in the moment; they do not generally arise through systematic ethical analysis. Our response may well be inconsistent or contradict a previously held position; in the world of everyday ethics, such variables are tolerable. However, in the world of health and social care, there is a need to overcome unpredictability and inconsistencies in favour of coherence, although this may be at the cost of flexibility and pragmatism [1].

Some might argue that ethics is irrelevant or of secondary concern to those involved in the real care of patients. Such a view may be held because ethics seems removed from everyday practice, its consideration appears elitist and requires specialised knowledge and wisdom to make sense of. If you feel that ethics belongs in the realm of the Ethics Committee and is not something that we as care providers should be concerned with, you may be surprised by Seedhouse's assertion that "*ethics is not an expert body of knowledge nor is it objective.*" Additionally, you may be relieved to hear that the ethics expert does not exist:

> Some people can think more efficiently than others, and some people have more experience than others, but no one has privileged access to the "right values" [1].

Instead, ethics is a thought process, involving reflection that combines both values and evidence and requires action; the choice of which action to commit to is the ultimate challenge for all of us. Above all, ethics is personal. Principles and theories have their place in helping us to

Handbook of Palliative Care, Third Edition. Edited by Christina Faull, Sharon de Caestecker, Alex Nicholson and Fraser Black.
© 2012 by John Wiley and Sons, Inc. Published 2012 by John Wiley & Sons, Inc.

think. However, without self-awareness and integration of our personal experiences, they are limited as they encourage us only to think using ideas that are not our own [1], devoid of life experience and the riches that it offers.

Whatever approach we adopt to confront ethical issues, be it one based on principles, rights, virtues, consequences, or duties, we do not get very far before we realise that full consideration of the issues requires us to go beyond merely one area. Other questions should also form part of the deliberation process: what will happen if I do this rather than that? Who will benefit? Who will suffer? Is my chosen action morally and legally justifiable? Could my action be applied to others? Do my actions stand up to public scrutiny, for example, would I be happy to have my story featured as a newspaper headline? Simply put, good ethics is thorough deliberation of the pros and cons of action [1].

Ethical deliberation in the context of care should also include consideration of the clinical, social, and philosophical basis of ethical dilemmas [1,2]. Standard approaches to ethics may not take account of emotion inherent in human thinking particularly when faced with emotive situations that resonate personally. Such situations lead to an instinctive response that may bear little relation to principles, codes, rules, and academic theory:

> Ultimately ethics is about making an emotional commitment to ways of living and acting—and to make this commitment we have to be open to our feelings and goals; to other people's feelings and goals; to the physical environment and to social contexts we inhabit; and we have to think carefully too. All these elements are necessary for anyone to become proficient at ethics. Reason and emotion are an essential part of ethical reflection [1].

The "commitment" we make will be different for each of us. As individuals each with our own landscape/experiences, we will hold different opinions and values to others, often a challenge in the context of multidisciplinary team (MDT) working. We may seem to possess some irreconcilable views, but this does not mean we have completely isolated outlooks. Rather than being a source of conflict, such differences should encourage us to explore each other's preferences, to visit each others' "landscapes" that enables an appreciation of the wider context.

Gestalt switch analogy offers a means of further explaining these challenges [1]. Take a look at Figure 5.1—what do you see? There are two possible ways of seeing the image (two faces in side silhouette or a vase), but it may

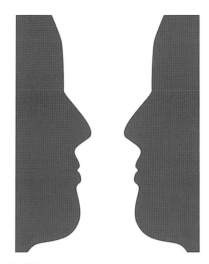

Figure 5.1 What do you see? Are you prepared to see more?

be that only one image stands out, and you are unable to see a second image. Similarly in ethical dilemmas we may only feel able to see one perspective while failing to appreciate others, but such challenges can be overcome; the way to do so is to show and explain both alternatives together. Instead of seeing just one thing—either a vase or two face profiles—you want to be able to say "I can see them both and I can therefore decide which I prefer." It is the same with ethical choices—we need to be open to seeing all the options in order to make a considered and therefore ethical decision [1].

Ethics in the context of palliative care

What about the case of palliative care? Surely no one could doubt that those involved in care of the dying are altruistic through and through and are good moral people? Whether we choose to admit it or not, our relationships with patients always have a power imbalance. Even more so for patients with palliative care needs who are particularly dependent on their doctors, nurses, and allied specialists. We provide advice, therapy, and often the very basics of care to people at a vulnerable time of their lives. Such dependence and vulnerability requires patients to place a great deal of trust in their care provider and should lead us to consider how we might best help patients and their families to navigate what feels like an ethical challenge or tension.

There may be an assumption that ethical challenges are less of an issue in the hospice setting when compared with the hospital or surgery setting because hospices restrict themselves purely to the provision of palliative care. Conversely, it could be argued that the holistic framework of palliative care can create additional challenges to those associated with just the medical aspects of end-of-life care [3]. Additionally, the hospice setting is regularly exposed to the intense feelings of patients and families as they face the end of life together with issues such as withdrawing life-sustaining treatments, artificial hydration, etc. all of which may give rise to "ethical tensions."

The fiduciary relationship

The term for such a professional relationship founded on trust is a *fiduciary relationship*. If the patient cannot guarantee to himself or herself the ethical nature of the care providers' practice, they will not trust them, and a fiduciary relationship therefore cannot exist. The very basis of care is therefore undermined.

The perceived morality of the care provider may therefore be called into question, which begs another question: what is meant by morality? Moral values can be viewed as a fundamental part of moral judgement. Studies suggest that there is wide variation in the perception of what might be classed as a moral value that could include respect for human dignity, empathy, respect for others, love, self-awareness, and an avoidance of attempts to religious or other conversions at the end of life. These values are commonly seen as absolute or eternal values, although the issue of moral relativism challenges such beliefs, evidenced through a perceived value shift in modern society with values varying at different times according to the situation [4].

This fiduciary relationship can also be looked at in another way. Palliative care involves a differing mindset to that of other areas of medicine. The focus of attention is not solely on the patient's cure and often involves withdrawing rather than just starting treatment. It can also involve using drugs where there may be a fine balance between beneficial and potentially harmful effects, such as the use of high-dose opioids without appropriate titration. A success in palliative care is not a patient "cured" but a patient who has had a "good" (comfortable and dignified) end to his or her life. This differing focus can make people feel uncomfortable and may be a particular struggle for those who do not work in the specialty full time. To work within an ethical framework in all areas of care including palliative care ensures that we act in the patient's, society's, and our profession's interest while maintaining transparency in our actions.

Ethics is at the heart of how care personnel treat their patients and stemming from this is the reason that a trusting relationship can exist between therapist and patient.

It is therefore at the heart of every clinical decision made and aspect of care delivered and is particularly relevant within the palliative care setting, which involves caring for very vulnerable people and providing symptom control rather than cure. If you still remain unconvinced, the reductivist argument might sway you—if you do not understand ethics, you may be more liable to get sued!

Principles of ethical decision making

A summary of some established ethical theories now follows, as a useful starting point from which to base an ethically sound decision-making process. In the Western world, autonomy might seem to take precedence with individual rights seen as having priority over all other considerations. However, autonomy is only one of the four "prima facie" principles (see Box 5.1): Prima facie means that the principle is binding unless it conflicts with another moral principle. It is important to weigh *each* principle in equal measure in an effort to reach a position where an appreciation of the implications of each principle has been met. It could be argued however that care workers can still be thoughtful and morally conscious and yet not have any knowledge of ethical theory; self-awareness, a readiness to respect the values and decisions of others, together with experiential learning may be more or at least equally important [1].

Autonomy—"deliberated self-rule" [5]

The patient's autonomy is not always viewed as an important factor in the clinical setting. A few decades ago, it could be argued, it was felt by the medical profession that responsibility for ethical decisions regarding health care rested solely with health-care professionals, who made their decision based on what they felt was appropriate for their profession to practise. This is part of what is termed *professional autonomy*, that is, a particular profession determines its role, policing, and disciplining its own members independently. However, present day society would recognise the individual patient as having a major part in deciding what is done to him/her, that is,

---

Box 5.1 The four prima facie principles of ethics:

1. Autonomy (personal, professional)
2. Beneficence
3. Nonmaleficence
4. Justice

individual autonomy—in other words *my* ability to make *my* own decisions for *my* life and *my* treatment, assisted, rather than instructed, by a professional. *No decision about me without me is a current mantra in the UK National health Service (NHS).*

Difficulties often arise where the autonomy of one of these groups is given prominence to the detriment of the other. Perhaps like many things in life, the "truth" is that the middle ground between these two often-polarised viewpoints is the most helpful. Doctors should have some freedom and right to decide how they practice, but patients should also have a say in what is done to them. Examples of issues relevant to autonomy are given in Box 5.2.

The eighteenth-century philosopher, Immanuel Kant argued that an individual's ability to self-determine and self-govern was the essence of personhood. He emphasised the importance of acting in terms of laws that were universally valid for all because they were based on reason and rationality. The fact that human beings possess a unique ability to act in a rationale manner warrants respect for all *persons in relation to their unique capacity to be self-governing.*

A common modern understanding of autonomy that sets out an expectation that respecting a person's dignity is merely doing what the patient wants is misplaced, incorrect, and an objectionable foundation for healthcare ethics. Individual choice is important but need not be unconditionally accepted in order to show respect for an individual's autonomy: what an individual may choose may not always be appropriate or realistic from a practitioner's or society's perspective [6].

Beneficence and nonmaleficence

The principles of beneficence (to do good) and nonmaleficence (to do no harm) should be considered together in recognition of the fact that the risk of harm is an integral part of attempts to help people or to do good. Examples are given in Box 5.3. This is the essence of moral engagement: the care worker needs to consider what he or she

aims to achieve and how he or she aims to achieve it. Ultimately, we should aim at producing net benefit over harm. To achieve this, we must also consider the principle of autonomy since each individual patient will have a different view of what constitutes harm—what is an acceptable risk to one may be unacceptable to another. It behoves the practitioner to be competent to provide any alleged benefits, including having received the necessary training to deliver this.

Evaluation of harm and benefits should include risk and probability. Here it is apparent that a low probability of harm is of less ethical significance in the context of nonmaleficence than a high probability, while a high probability of great benefit is of more ethical significance than is a low probability [5]. This is where the evidence base should inform practice by providing information about the probabilities of harms and benefits associated with intervention.

Justice

Often described in terms of fairness and equity, Gillon defines justice as "*the moral obligation to act on the basis of fair adjudication between competing claims*" and can be divided into three categories [5]:

1. *Distributive justice*: the fair distribution of scarce resources.
2. *Rights-based justice*: the respect for people's rights.
3. *Legal justice*: the respect for morally acceptable laws.

Integral to justice is equality yet people can still be treated unfairly even if they are treated equally; therefore, it becomes clear that there is more to justice than equality alone. In the context of health care, this is challenging as conflict arises between several competing moral concerns: to allow people choice in their care and place of care, to provide adequate care to meet the needs of all who require it, or at least to apportion resource according to need, to respect the autonomy of care providers *and* those in receipt of care. Examples are given in Box 5.4. All the above can be morally justified but cannot necessarily be met concurrently [5].

> **Box 5.4 Examples of issues with relevance to justice:**
>
> - Distribution of resources: "Postcode lottery."
> - Increased patient choice versus lack of money
> - Futility.

Additional perspectives

Deontology and consequentialism, the two major pillars of Western moral philosophy, are distinguished by their views of how the "right" (action) relates to the "good" (outcome).

Consequentialist theory

Consequentialism holds that decisions should be based on a calculation of likely future consequences with the aim of achieving the greater good—the greater good referring to the best possible outcome for the greater number of people. It may commonly be applied in the care setting in the form of a cost–benefit analysis. Focusing on consequences of decisions supports that a situation be considered in terms of how it will affect everyone that may be involved, that actions are deemed "right" that produce the greatest total amount of human well-being. To put another way, the ends (the outcome) justify the means (the action).

What are the limitations of consequentialist theory?
- Difficult to predict actual consequences of actions. There may be many possibilities.
- Can reduce ethics to economics, that is, is it "right" because it costs less in the long run?
- The argument that any action that leads to a "good" outcome is right, even if the intention of the practitioner was bad may at times seem difficult to justify.
- People have differing views of what makes them happy.
- Ends do not always (or ever?) justify the means if the means are morally objectionable.
- As with most classical ethics, there is no attention to life other than human.

Deontological theory

In contrast to consequentialism, deontology advocates that it is the fact that a person acted according to a perceived duty rather than the result of an action, regardless of the consequences, that is important. Some actions are inherently "wrong" and simply cannot be justified by predicted "good" consequences that will result from them. Deontology may also be referred to as duty ethics: some actions are right because there is a duty to follow them, for example, "I should always respect a patient's wish for confidentiality." While confidentiality is generally seen as

a good principle to uphold, one's duty always to maintain confidentiality may be called into question in the case of a patient with a communicable disease who asks for his or her disease to be kept secret; this situation has an obvious conflict with one's duty to protect the wider public.

Kant's Categorical Imperative defined morality as acting from rules that can be universalised to all people who are considered as valuable in themselves and worthy of moral respect. A simple summary would be:
- Do unto others, as you would have them do unto you.
- If you cannot desire that everyone follow the same rule, your rule is not a moral one.

What are the limitations of deontological theory?
- Difficult to form intentions into a rule and then test it for universality.
- Difficult fully to know intentions.
- Deontology fails to recognise that human feelings and emotions may have a role to play.
- Sometimes consequences do matter (and perhaps override our initial duties).
- As with most traditional ethics, there is no attention to life other than human.

In no sense is it suggested that the whole of ethical thought can be summarised in the short statements above although all offer a useful starting point for personal and team reflection.

Ethical issues in practice

Particular clinical situations will now be examined and discussed in respect of the roles of a fiduciary relationship and ethical principles of relevance to palliative care. Unless otherwise stated, the scenarios are fictitious. Where the example is a legal case, the case reference is provided. Please refer to the end of the chapter for an explanation of legal referencing, if required.

Truth or dare

Mrs. Taylor's daughter, who is also your patient, asks to see you before you visit her mother at home. She states that she knows her mother has breast cancer. However, she insists that you do not inform her mother of this diagnosis, as she knows that her mother will not cope with the information. You meet Mrs. Taylor later that day, who asks you what the tests showed when she was in hospital.

This is a fairly common scenario. It is tricky to deal with as one does not wish to alienate or disregard the relatives of the patient. Furthermore, part of the holistic mindset that palliative care encourages involves caring for the family as well as the patient. However, if one considers the fiduciary relationship of doctor and patient and the right of people to make autonomous decisions, it can change the emphasis of such ethical dilemmas. If telling a lie is well meaning, even if it is meant to protect a patient from information perceived to be harmful, there is the potential to harm the relationship with that patient for the future: if the patient learns he/she has been lied to, why should they trust the CP in the future? It may be that their loss of trust means that they can no longer form a therapeutic relationship with the CP.

Who does this information belong to in the first place? Obviously the answer is to the patient and therefore it is for them to decide who does and does not know their diagnosis and also how much of that diagnosis they wish to know about. The control of the information should rest with the patient. Therefore, if Mrs. Taylor asks what her diagnosis is, the CP is duty-bound to respect her question, despite what her daughter might say to the contrary.

There are two provisos to what may seem like a fairly strident position. We have to respect both a patient's right to know and right not to know. If patients do not wish to know their diagnosis but are given this information against their wishes, their autonomy has not been respected. The guidance as to how much and in what way their information is presented must come from patients themselves.

Such a position is easier if the patient is well known to the CP, who in these circumstances may have already gained insights into how the patient wants to have information given to them. Sometimes CPs meet a patient for the first time and have no idea of how this particular person may want their information given to them. A relative may be able to help guide this decision. This is not to say that the relative has a right of veto over what the patient is told but can act as an aid in doing this. The UK GMC guidelines [7] for example, are clear on this point. In their opinion, it is the patient who ultimately decides on treatment and on how much information is given, but that it is good practice to involve relatives in this process:

• The patient has the right to know the truth if they ask for it
• The best guide for how much information to give is the patient himself or herself
• The relatives can assist with this but do not have a right of veto.

The above situation does, and should, give rise to ethical consideration but to view it purely in this light misses another key issue: communication! While it is ethically objectionable to share information belonging to a patient with someone else without permission, we also have to remember that care of the relatives is an important part of our role. Acknowledging the difficulties for the relative and eliciting through sensitive and empathic communication any particular concerns they may have is an important role we have to play (see Chapter 6, *Communication skills in palliative care*, for further information).

The right to refuse

Ms B was a social worker who was tetraplegic and eventually required ventilation. The lady no longer wished to have the ventilator sustain her and requested that the ventilator be turned off. She had her case heard at the high court in order to decide that she was competent to make this decision. She was found to be competent and the ventilator was switched off. [*Ms B vs. An NHS Hospital Trust* (2002) All England Law Reports (All ER) 449]

Consent must first be obtained from a patient for any procedure to occur. To respect a patient's autonomy, sufficient information should be provided for the patient to be able to weigh the potential benefits and harms and make an informed decision. It is also necessary to ensure that the patient is not pressurised into making the decision that the CP feels is the correct one. It is important to note that under the English legal system CP are not duty bound to tell the patient absolutely everything—just the information that the patient needs in order to make the decision. This is what is meant in England by "informed consent." This still allows the patients to say that they do not want to know all the side effects or consequences but still be consenting. In this country the benchmark as to what is adequate information for consent is still the average practitioner "Bolam." This is in contrast to America where it is the average patient who is taken to be the guide in law. "Bolam" states that it is what the "reasonable medical practitioner" would have done in similar circumstances, which is taken as standard practice.

If a patient does not give consent for an intervention to happen, and a practitioner performs this despite the patient's wishes, then in law "battery" has occurred. Or, to put this in ethical terms, a patient's autonomy has not been respected. For example, if a person who is a Jehovah's Witness wishes not to have blood, then that decision must be respected. Therefore, before proceeding with interventions we are duty-bound to gain consent from the patient, having provided both the amount and detail of information requested by the patient. A patient does have the ethical and legal right to refuse treatment provided that they do not have reduced competence to do so.

The Mental Capacity Act (MCA) of 2005 [8] was implemented in England and Wales in 2007 and seeks to empower people to make their own decisions wherever possible and legally safeguard this right to do so. It provides a flexible framework based on the stipulation that individuals' best interests are integral to the decision-making process and thereby serves to protect people who lack capacity. The term "capacity" refers to:

> the ability to make a decision about a particular issue at the time the decision needs to be made or to give consent to a particular act [9].

In addition to capacity being assessed on a decision-specific basis, CP must also recognise that capacity may fluctuate over time in relation to those decisions.

Two key statutory principles of the MCA (2005) [8] are:

1. A person must be assumed to have capacity unless it is established that they lack capacity.
2. A person is not to be treated as unable to make a decision unless all practicable steps to help them to do so have been taken without success.

To be deemed competent to make the decision, the person must be able to:

• understand the information—The CP has a responsibility to make this information as clear and accessible as possible;
• retain the information—This need only be long enough to use and weigh up the information;
• use and weigh up the information relevant to this decision;
• communicate their decision in some way—The CP must try every method possible to enable this.

If the person is unable to do any one of the above, then they are deemed to lack capacity for that particular decision.

It is not enough to say that a patient suffers from a medical condition and therefore is incompetent to make a decision. Rather it must be proved that the medical condition inhibits the patient's ability to satisfy the four-pronged test described above. It is therefore conceivable that a patient may competently request for a treatment not to occur or to be withdrawn even if this treatment or procedure may result in their death. Put another way, a competent patient is allowed to make a decision that may be considered by the clinician as unwise. In the above case, Ms B was deemed to be competent to make an informed decision; therefore, her ventilation was discontinued.

This is all very well if patients are able to communicate their wishes to us, but very often patients may be deeply unconscious or confused, particularly in the last days of their life. How is it possible to know what to do in these circumstances? Advance care planning (ACP) that identifies individual preferences should they lack capacity to make decisions about their care in the future is a significant step

in addressing future challenges that may arise; dilemmas commonly associated with issues such as withdrawing or withholding treatment may well be avoided as a result of ACP. If ethically driven practice is concerned with promoting patient autonomy, then providing opportunity for patients to be involved in ACP, should they choose, would seem to be an obligation for CPs (see Chapter 8, *Advance Care Planning*, for further information).

If a competent patient refuses to continue with treatment, then there is a strong legal and ethical argument supporting the patient's stance. However, this does not mean that the CP is duty-bound to always provide the treatment that a patient requests. Patients cannot demand that a doctor or nurse does exactly as they wish them to do. This highlights one of the tensions that can often exist in care situations. Not only does the patient have autonomy that should be respected, but to some extent, the professional also has some amount of autonomy and duty to decide what is appropriate. Or to put this in a different way, a job that is termed professional does have some right to limit what the people involved in that job can do. The UK GMC recognises that life has a natural end. Their guidelines on good practice in end-of-life care state that:

> there is no absolute obligation to prolong life irrespective of the consequences for the patient, and irrespective of the patient's views, if they are known or can be found out [7].

It is recognised by the UK GMC that sometimes there may be conflict between the opinion of doctors (for whom the guidelines are expressly written) and that of patients. To use the terms that we have been using, sometimes the autonomy of the patient and the autonomy of the doctor may clash. It is recommended by the UK GMC that in such circumstances legal help should be sought.

It is difficult to give a definitive answer to all the eventualities that could occur in practice because there isn't one! Life, or even death, is never that simple. However, we have seen that some general guidelines are as follows:

• Competent patients have the right to refuse treatments.
• ACP has some ethical and legal standing.
• CPs also have some level of autonomy.

Live and let die

Diane Pretty was a lady who suffered from Motor Neurone Disease (MND). She was concerned that she had become so incapacitated that she was not [have been] able to take her own life. She went to the UK and then the European Courts to ensure that should her husband assist her in trying to take her own life that he would not be prosecuted. Her case and subsequent appeal were turned down, the court deciding that if this

were to happen, then a criminal act would have occurred*.
[*R. vs. Director of Public Prosecutions* (2002) 1 All ER 1].

The terminology associated with euthanasia and assisted suicide can be confusing; hence, let us begin by being clear about some of the definitions.

Assisted suicide

This is when the individual who wants to die requires assistance to kill themselves; the patient undertakes the action to kill themselves, a lethal dose of drugs, for example, aided by somebody else.

Involuntary euthanasia

This occurs when the individual who dies actually wants to live but is killed anyway and is usually classed as murder; someone commits an act, for example, giving a lethal injection.

Voluntary euthanasia

This is where euthanasia is carried out at the request of the person who dies. The act of killing is undertaken by another person.

In English law, a person assisting someone in an act of suicide may be prosecuted for murder. The UK DPP has produced guidance that provides further clarity.

Prosecution is more likely, for example, under the following conditions:
• The victim had not reached a voluntary, clear, settled, and informed decision to commit suicide.
• The victim had not clearly and unequivocally communicated his or her decision to commit suicide to the suspect.
• The suspect pressured the victim to commit suicide.
• The suspect did not take reasonable steps to ensure that any other person had not pressured the victim to commit suicide.
• The suspect had a history of violence or abuse against the victim.
• The victim was physically able to undertake the act that constituted the assistance himself or herself.
• The suspect was unknown to the victim.
• The suspect was paid by the victim or those close to the victim for his or her encouragement or assistance.
• The suspect was acting in his or her capacity as a medical doctor, nurse, other health-care professional, a professional carer (whether for payment or not), or as a person in authority, such as a prison officer, and the victim was in his or her care.

• The suspect was aware that the victim intended to commit suicide in a public place where it was reasonable to think that members of the public may be present.

Prosecution is less likely under the following circumstances:
• The suspect was wholly motivated by compassion.
• The victim had reached a voluntary, clear, settled, and informed decision to commit suicide.
• The actions of the suspect, although sufficient to come within the definition of the crime, were of only minor encouragement or assistance.
• The suspect had sought to dissuade the victim from taking the course of action that resulted in his or her suicide.
• The actions of the suspect may be characterised as reluctant encouragement or assistance in the face of a determined wish on the part of the victim to commit suicide.
• The suspect reported the victim's suicide to the police and fully assisted them in their enquiries into the circumstances of the suicide or the attempt and his or her part in providing encouragement or assistance.

The risk of prosecution stands even if the patient is competent and is expressing this wish as part of an autonomous decision. There is therefore a definite limit to how much a patient may dictate about their care. Space does not allow a full discussion of this area but includes the issues of fiduciary relationship, autonomy, beneficence, justice, and nonmaleficence. If a patient's relationship with his or her CP depends on a trusting relationship, will that trust be eroded if the patient is aware the professional can take a decision that could harm them? Specifically if doctors develop the power to prematurely end someone's life, will this reduce a patient's trust and faith in their doctor? Under existing UK law, a patient can guarantee that their doctor will never give them something intentionally that will kill them. This is a powerful guarantor of trust. There is debate about whether legalising assisted suicide or euthanasia would destroy that basis for trust.

We have seen how there is a balance of autonomy between patient and caregiver. The patient cannot demand everything they want of the carer, and the carer cannot expect the patient to do everything that they want either. There is a balance to be negotiated in the relationship. A profession can decide for itself what its absolute limits are. For a group of people dedicated to caring, it would seem sensible that this absolute would be not taking a life. It may therefore limit a caring profession's autonomy

---

*This has subsequently been clarified by the Director of Public Prosecution (DPP). See below for further information.

and trustworthiness if they were expected to perform actions that would harm their patient.

A further argument used is that if euthanasia becomes mainstream practice then an associated risk or harm is that it may become expected rather than chosen as an alternative to being a burden to the family, for example.

Summary of ethical stances in relation to assisted suicide and euthanasia

See Box 5.5.

Box 5.5 Ethical stances related to assisted suicide and euthanasia

Ethical principle	For	Against
Autonomy	Competent patients have the right to make their own decisions	• Autonomy does not include the right to engage others, for example, CPs • Honouring the sanctity of life takes precedence over the right of individuals to choose how and when they die
Justice	Cost reductions leading to increased opportunity and access to care services for others	There is a risk of vulnerable groups such as the elderly to feel obliged to opt for euthanasia to avoid being a burden to others
Beneficence	Enabling a patient to choose how and when to end their suffering is a compassionate act	To assist somebody to die is to desert them at a time of need
Nonmaleficence	Inability to relieve symptoms and other forms of suffering destroys trust between the patient and CP	Assisting somebody to die destroys trust and breaches the historical underpinnings of CPs

Current global position in relation to assisted suicide and euthanasia

Around the world, different countries, even different states within countries, have alternate views on assisted suicide (see Box 5.6).

Box 5.6 Global position on assisted suicide and euthanasia in 2011

Country	Assisted suicide	Euthanasia
United Kingdom	Illegal	Illegal
Canada	Illegal	Illegal
The Netherlands	Legal since 2001	Legal since 2001
Australia	Illegal	Illegal (legalised in the northern territory in 1995 and overturned in 1997)
Switzerland	Legal since 1942	Illegal
Belgium	Legal since 2002	Legal since 2002
Germany	Legal since 1751	Illegal
United States	Illegal across the United States with the exception of the states of Oregon, Montana, and Washington	Illegal

Ethical issues in hydration

Mr. Williams is a 74 year old patient in the advanced stages of dementia who is admitted to hospital because he has not been eating or drinking for a week. Clinical assessment finds him to be bedbound and incapable of any verbal communication but with no evidence of any complicating process such as an infection. The assessing clinician feels that Mr. Williams is in the terminal stages and is expected to die within the next few days. Mr. William's daughter expresses concern over her father's inability to drink and requests that he is provided with artificial hydration.

The debate around artificial hydration at the end of life is complex and includes clinical, emotional, and ethical issues. Food and drink is the essence of life, and its provision is viewed as compassionate care. Beyond this, there seems to be very little consensus. Indeed, there is not a universal clarity as to whether the administration of artificial fluids (and food) constitutes a medical intervention or an act of basic care [10] and is further complicated by the entrenched beliefs regarding food and drink held by families and care staff [11]. Some studies suggest a relationship between the nurse's attitude and the decision taken regarding how care is delivered, that is, the individual view of a nurse may be the reason why one particular decision is taken over another. Such an approach may lead to an ad hoc decision-making process that lacks structure, transparency, and methodology [11,12].

There is a lack of agreement (and indeed clear evidence) regarding the perceived benefits and burdens of artificial hydration meaning a lack of clarity with regard to both informed consent and best interests decision making. It seems that for every argument to support the use of artificial hydration, there is another to counter it. This topic is discussed in Chapter 21, *Terminal care and dying*. How then can CPs make a judgement call? In this grey sea of uncertainty what seems certain is the need for CPs to separate the facts (e.g., the law, clinical issues) from values and feelings.

The guidance issued by the UK GMC on end-of-life care summarises these current uncertainties [7]:

> Providing nutrition and hydration by tube or drip may provide symptom relief, or prolong or improve the quality of the patient's life; but they may also present problems. The current evidence about the benefits, burdens and risks of these techniques as patients approach the end of life is not clear-cut. This can lead to concerns that patients who are unconscious or semi-conscious may be experiencing distressing symptoms and complications, or otherwise be suffering either because their needs for nutrition or hydration are not being met or because attempts to meet their perceived needs for nutrition or hydration may be causing them avoidable suffering.

Let us now reflect on these issues using an ethical framework.

Autonomy and best interests

The law is clear in that patients with mental capacity are able to make their own decisions. However, in this particular case where Mr Williams clearly does not have mental capacity and in the absence of an advance decision or a legally appointed proxy decision-maker, CPs must act in the best interests of Mr Williams.

In the United Kingdom, the MCA [8] states that consideration of best interests requires us to take reasonable steps to ascertain:

- the person's past and present wishes and feelings (and, in particular, any relevant written statement made by him when he had capacity);
- the beliefs and values that would be likely to influence his decision if he had capacity; and
- the other factors that he would be likely to consider if he were able to do so.

The views of significant others should also be consulted where practicable and appropriate in helping the CP to identify the above steps and reach a decision on what constitutes best interests for this particular patient. The GMC [7] also provides useful guidance in this respect:

> Nutrition and hydration provided by tube or drip are regarded in law as medical treatment, and should be treated in the same way as other medical interventions. Nonetheless, some people see nutrition and hydration, whether taken orally or by tube or drip, as part of basic nurture for the patient that should almost always be provided. For this reason it is especially important that you listen to and consider the views of the patient and of those close to them (including their cultural and religious views) and explain the issues to be considered, including the benefits, burdens and risks of providing clinically assisted nutrition and hydration.

Mr William's daughter should therefore be asked her opinion of what she thinks her father would want. It should be made clear, gently and sensitively, during the conversation that the decision is not her responsibility (not least so that she will not feel the burden of what can seem like making a life or death decision about someone she loves): has he previously expressed an opinion about how he would like to be cared for in such circumstances? Ultimately is she able to help us to understand more about Mr William's past beliefs, values, and wishes and is she aware of any previously written statement by him? The duty of the CP to act in the best interests is clearly outlined and supported in law; if the decision of the clinical team is deemed to be in the best interests of the patient even if it goes against the wishes of the family, then that is the decision that stands.

Beneficence and nonmaleficence

A weighing up of the perceived harms and benefits to assess overall benefit should still be undertaken even in the absence of any conclusive evidence to support or negate the use of artificial hydration in terminal care. Harms should be considered in relation both to the patient and also his daughter. It is beyond the realms of this chapter to consider the numerous physiological-based arguments in relation to hydration and dehydration, and readers are directed to alternative sources of information (see also Chapter 21, *Terminal care and dying*). A wider appreciation of potential harms is however advocated including the concerns of the daughter. What are her particular concerns about withholding fluids? Does she have sufficient information? Is she struggling to accept the imminent death of her father? What is the significance of fluids to her? The provision of artificial fluids may provide reassurance to relatives that their loved one is not suffering from the effects of dehydration although it may also serve as a visual sign of hope, albeit unrealistic, that recovery is possible.

A key question to ask when faced with such decisions is "what are we trying to achieve?" In making a decision to withhold fluids, we may feel that our aim is to achieve a "good" death for Mr Williams. Conversely a decision to provide fluids may be with the intention of avoiding further conflict between his daughter and the care team. However difficult the decision not to start artificial fluids is, it is considered more challenging and of higher emotional impact to stop fluids once started, especially for the family [13].

Regardless of the overall decision made, the ongoing comfort of the patient and support of the family remains paramount; the UK GMC [7] clearly states doctors' responsibilities in this area:

> You should make sure that patients, those close to them and the healthcare team understand that, when clinically assisted nutrition or hydration would be of overall benefit, it will always be offered; and that if a decision is taken not to provide clinically assisted nutrition or hydration, the patient will continue to receive high-quality care, with any symptoms addressed.

Double effect

Are there actions that are always inherently wrong or is there ever a case for justifying a bad action for a good outcome?

> Dr Cox was a hospital physician responsible for the care of a lady who was suffering from rheumatoid arthritis. This lady was in intractable pain from her medical condition. Dr Cox

felt that he had tried everything to help this lady become pain free. He therefore decided that, in his opinion, the most compassionate thing to do was to give this lady a lethal dose of potassium chloride. He did this and the lady died. He was later taken to court and was tried for murder. He had his sentence reduced to manslaughter, and was sent to prison. [*R vs. Cox* (1992) Butterworth's Medico-Legal Reports (BMLR) 38]

The law, at least in the United Kingdom, has a fairly strong position concerning euthanasia and assisted suicide. Such a strong position can often make CPs quite circumspect about performing or prescribing certain therapeutic procedures. For example, in palliative care, morphine is commonly given for the treatment of pain. It could be that, in giving morphine in a sufficient dose to control very severe and complex pain, a person's life is prematurely shortened. In other words, in trying to make a good action occur, one may cause a bad action to happen. In these circumstances one would know that such consequences are possible. There is an ethical and legal phrase—"*the doctrine of double effect*"—that recognises that this dilemma exists. The doctrine can be broken down into the following elements:

- The original action intended is a good one in itself.
- The sole intention of the action is good.
- The good effect is not produced as a consequence of the bad effect.
- The required outcome is significant enough to permit the chance of the bad outcome occurring.

What does all that actually mean? Let us use the example of the patient who is in pain. The relief of pain, particularly in the terminal stages of life, is a good and necessary action that is also significant enough, it could be and indeed is argued, to justify the possibility of premature and unintentional shortening of life. However, what cannot be justified is intentionally causing someone's death as a method of pain control. The intention has to be, to fit with the doctrine, not to kill the patients but to make them pain free. The intention must not be to make them pain free by terminating their life. Dr Cox could not justify his actions using the doctrine of double effect, as he intended to end the patient's suffering by terminating life. In addition the only possible use of potassium chloride in the dose under the circumstances used was to end the patient's life as it has no analgesic effect.

This may seem just semantics, but the law and ethics recognise that *intention* is important. One large proviso—this doctrine does not excuse malpractice.

Guidelines and agreed standards of practice should be followed. Morphine and other drugs with significant adverse potential but established benefits must be used at the correct dose that should be titrated to the individual patient. A group of senior palliative care clinicians in the United Kingdom recently warned against the doctrine of double effect with opioids as "a perennial myth that has been used to defend unsafe prescribing" arguing that a lethal dose of opioid is never required to manage suffering, and therefore, the doctrine of double effect, as an argument to justify practice, need never be invoked [14].

The reason for the doctrine existing is to reassure CPs that if they treat their patients correctly and with good practice and appropriate intention, then they have no reason to fear prosecution. It would be unethical for a patient to be left in pain with a CP unable or unwilling to give them pain control. One of the largest factors that can return a patient's autonomy is giving them the necessary medication to allow them to be pain free:
- Patients have a basic human right to be pain free.
- Some medications may cause harmful effects.
- The doctrine of double effect can be used in these circumstances.
- This has four elements, all four of which must apply for the doctrine to be used.
- To intend to cause death is illegal in most countries.

Summary

This chapter began by emphasising how important ethics is in everyday practice. The crux of ethics in clinical practice is about preserving the relationship between clinician and patient. This relationship is vital not only for individual therapeutic relationships but also for the standing of CPs in the community. Some basic principles pertaining to ethical decision making have been described (autonomy of individuals and of professionals, beneficence/nonmaleficence, justice, consequentialism, and deontology) and some examples discussed to show how these principles need to be weighed with one another in reaching an ethical decision. The examples presented contain grey areas for which the ethical decision will be different for different patients, depending on their views, background, and exact circumstances. Readers should appreciate that emotion and life experience as well as principles will inform ethical decision making—and indeed should do so, since such decisions are not meant to be the province of the "expert." How-

ever, there are some situations in which support can be helpful—including patient advocates (where capacity is lacking), exploring views of family, enlisting views of colleagues and co-workers, and in the most difficult cases professional bodies, clinical ethics committees, or even specialist legal help.

This chapter cannot hope to act as either a philosophical or legal textbook and space does not allow for the details required to fully explore the issues involved. Further reading is suggested below. Indemnity organisations and/or professional bodies are helpful in clarifying specific legal situations.

Legal references and standard abbreviations

In this chapter citation has been made of several legal cases. Standard practice for a legal reference is that the title in italics refers to the actual case name while the title in bold refers to the year and name of legal report where the case can be found.

All ER—All England Law Reports

BMLR—Butterworth's Medico-Legal Reports

The number before the legal report title is the volume number and the number after the legal report is the page number.

References

1. Seedhouse D. *Ethics: The Heart of Health Care*, 3rd edition. Chichester: Wiley-Blackwell, 2009.
2. Sokol D, McFadzean WA, Dickson WA, et al. Ethical dilemmas in the acute setting: a framework for clinicians. *BMJ* 2011; 343: d5528.
3. McGrath P. Autonomy, discourse and power: a postmodern reflection on principlism and bioethics. *J Med Philos* 1998; 23: 516–532.
4. Salloch S and Breitsameter C. Morality and moral conflicts in hospice care: results of a qualitative interview study. *J Med Ethics* 2010; 36: 588–592.
5. Gillon R. Medical ethics: four principles plus attention to scope. *BMJ* 1994; 309: 184.
6. Randall F. *End of Life Choices: Consensus and Controversy.* Oxford: Oxford University Press, 2010.
7. General Medical Council. General Medical Council Treatment and care towards the end of life: good practice in decision making. July 2010.
8. *Mental Capacity Act.* Office of Public Sector Information, London. 2005. Available at: http://www.legislation

.gov.uk/ukpga/2005/9/contents (accessed on May 5, 2012).

9. *National End of Life Care Programme Capacity, care planning and advance care planning in life limiting illness: A Guide for Health and Social Care Staff 2011*. Available at: http://www.endoflifecareforadults.nhs.uk/publications/pubacpguide (accessed on May 11, 2012).

10. Casarett D, Kapo J and Caplan A. Appropriate use of artificial nutrition and hydration—fundamental principles and recommendations. *N Engl J Med* 2005; 353: 2607–2612.

11. Bryon E, Dierckx de Casterlé B and Gastmans C. Nurses' attitudes towards artificial food or fluid administration in patients with dementia and in terminally ill patients: a review of the literature. *J Med Ethics* 2008; 34: 431–436.

12. Clamp C. Learning through critical incidents. *Nurs Times* 1980; 2: 1755–1758.

13. Fox E. IV hydration in the terminally ill: ritual or therapy? *Br J Nurs* 1996; 5: 41–45.

14. Regnard C, George R, Grogan E, et al. So, farewell then, doctrine of double effect. *BMJ* 2001; 343.

Useful resources

http://www.lawtel.com. Lawtel gives details of all case and statutory law in this country and Europe (subscription required).

http://www.values-exchange.com. Seedhouse has developed an on line resource which offers the opportunity to debate social issues from a variety of perspectives.

Acknowledgement. I acknowledge the work of Derek Willis for the previous edition of this chapter.

6 Communication Skills in Palliative Care

Sharon de Caestecker

LOROS, The Leicestershire and Rutland Hospice, Leicester, UK

Introduction

Communication is an integral part of every day life; it is something that should come naturally to us. Why then is it that many of us find it so difficult to communicate with patients in the context of life-threatening illness? For many there may be a fear of getting it wrong, of causing further harm and distress to a patient and his family already burdened with suffering. The desire to "get it right" is endemic among the caring professions: consequently fear of making mistakes can engender uncertainty, anxiety, and paralysis [1].

Yet good communication is fundamental to all health and social care, particularly in the arena of palliative care. Effective, open, and honest communication improves both patient and carer experience and has been shown to have a positive impact on emotional health, symptom management, and a reduction in reported pain and drug use [2]. Good communication is the basis of high-quality end-of-life care: it facilitates patient choice and engagement thereby promoting patient-centred care. It also creates immense satisfaction and motivation for the professional.

Conversely, poor communication can have far-reaching negative consequences for patients, carers, and Care professional (CP). Poor communication is cited as the reason for over half of all end-of-life care–related complaints in the United Kingdom [3].

There is evidence that poor communication creates psychological distress and morbidity, results in poor treatment compliance [4], reduced quality of life and increased dissatisfaction with care [3].

Insufficient training in communication is a major factor contributing to stress, lack of job satisfaction, and emotional burnout in health-care professionals [5,6].

This chapter considers some of the issues that may undermine open communication in the context of end-of-life care. Behaviours that actively block open dialogue will be presented as a prompt to recognise such behaviours in ourselves and as a means to encourage a more positive and facilitative response. Communication skills that facilitate open and sensitive communication will be considered and finally some examples of situations commonly perceived to be challenging will be explored with some useful strategies offered for practice.

Barriers to effective communication

Example

Patient: I'm worried about having the chemotherapy—I have heard that some of the side-effects are dreadful.

CP: Everybody reacts differently, you may find that you the side effects aren't that bad. Besides, there are lots of things we can do to help with the side-effects.

In the above scenario, the patient alludes to some concern about undergoing chemotherapy treatment. The CP attempts to alleviate the concerns through reassurance; undoubtedly an attempt to make the patient feel better and worry less. However well intended, the CP's response serves to act as a block to further discussion and exploration of the patient's specific concerns and feelings. The reassurance offered in relation to the likelihood of side-effects in unfounded side-effects may well be the experience of this particular patient. In essence, the concerns of this patient, which are actually unknown to the CP, are minimised. Instead of the desired effect of reducing patient distress, the opposite may in fact be created, and the patient may be left unheard and frustrated:

> In fact, the specific concern of this patient was hair loss and the impact that may have on her children—will they be frightened? When and how should she explain this to her children? These are the real concerns and issues that lay behind her initial statement.

While palliative care offers many rewards, it also presents certain challenges. The impact on us as CPs can take its toll, and at times, we may find it difficult, preferring instead to find ways of avoiding or minimising the emotion involved. In communication, this avoidance manifests as blocking behaviours, which serve to inhibit patient disclosure of feelings or concerns [7].

There are many reasons why both patients and CPs may adopt blocking behaviours, either consciously or unconsciously, and it is interesting to reflect upon the similarities between CPs and patients. Table 6.1 shows some of these reasons.

There are a number of reasons why blocking behaviours may be adopted:
• As a result of a misplaced sense of care based on a concern that the patient may be "damaged" as a result of open and honest communication [8].
• The impact of the patient's emotional distress on the CP is such that they feel unable to tolerate is expression [9].

Having some awareness of our own responses to patients' experiences, particularly where emotions and distress are exhibited, can be useful. It is worth considering how such experiences impact on us, how they make us feel and how we might react. Table 6.2 outlines some blocking behaviours. Take a moment to consider them in relation to your own practice. Are there times when you may adopt these behaviours consciously or unconsciously? Are you able to identify what triggers such responses?

Table 6.1 Reasons why blocking behaviours may be adopted.

Patient	Care professional
Fear of upsetting the CP	Fear of upsetting the patient or causing further harm/distress
Feeling that CP doesn't have time	Takes too much time
Belief that it is not within the role of the CP to discuss emotional issues	Belief that "it's not my role"
Belief that their concerns are inevitable so why bother?	Belief that emotional concerns are inevitable when facing the end of life
Belief that nothing can be done about it	Futility: Belief that nothing can be done about emotional concerns
Belief that treatment may rely on being compliant, uncomplaining, and/or undemanding	Saying the wrong thing; risking a complaint
	Unleashing strong emotions such as distress, anger-opening up a "can of worms"
	Fear that patients will not handle the truth
	Fear of being asked difficult or unanswerable questions
	Fear of raising false expectations in relation to issues that "can't be resolved"
	Lack of follow-up support for patients and staff, for example, clinical supervision
	Lack of skills/confidence in dealing with certain communication situations such as breaking bad news, dealing with emotions, etc.

Table 6.2 Blocking behaviours.

Behaviour	Example
Overt blocking: complete change of topic	Pt: I've been worried about what the future might hold
	CP: I wanted to talk to you today about your pain
Distancing strategies: change of time frame, person, removal of emotion	Pt: I was anxious about being ill
	CP: And how does your wife feel? (change of person)
	Are you anxious now? (change of time frame)
	How long were you ill for? (removal of emotion)
Premature reassurance	Pt: I'm worried about having the treatment
	CP: You'll be fine . . .
Giving advice; attempting to problem solve. While offering some "solutions" to problems raised may be required at some stage during the consultation, it is important not to do this before all patient's concerns have been elicited and prioritised	Pt: I'm worried about what this pain might mean and feel anxious about the future
	CP: So I will prescribe some pain killers and I will ask the social worker to arrange some financial benefits advice . . .
Asking closed questions that generally lead to a yes or no–type answer meaning that patients are unable to elaborate	"Did you sleep well last night?" Instead of "How did you sleep last night?"
Asking leading questions suggesting a desired response within the question	"You don't have any pain do you?"
Giving information too early in the consultation too much or inappropriately reduces likelihood of further patient disclosure [10]	"Well I'm sorry to say the investigations have shown that you have cancer. This can be treated however using a variety of treatments including chemotherapy, radiotherapy and surgery"
While discussion of treatment may be appropriate, introducing this too early before the impact of a serious diagnosis has been allowed to sink in may inhibit the patient from bringing up concerns	
Minimising	"You say you're worried but I've seen many more patients cope even without the support your family give"
Normalising—this may serve to undermine the patient's situation/distress	"Many people in your situation feel anxious"
While it may be helpful for patients to know that what they are experiencing is quite normal that may reduce some anxieties, the key is to be able to explore what the situation means to this particular patient in front of you	The addition of "Tell me how it feels for you" would encourage further disclosure and generate greater insight of the patients perspective
Asking physical questions	Pt: I have a worrying pain . . .
While it is important to undertake a thorough physical assessment, it is also important to pick up on the cue offered by the patient—for example, what is it that is "worrying" about the pain?	CP: Can you describe the pain to me?
Asking multiple questions leading to confusion and uncertainty within the patient as to which question he should answer	"You say you haven't been sleeping well, how long has this been going on, do you take any medication to help you sleep, have you tried taking a warm drink before bed?"
"Passing the buck"	"It's not my role-You will have to ask the nurse/Dr/social worke r. . ."
Jollying along	"Come now, there's still lots to look forward to, you don't want to spend your time worrying when you could be enjoying this lovely weather . . ."
Defending	"We are all so busy, it's very difficult to get everything right all of the time . . ."

Facilitative skills

It may be suggested that communication skills are innate: some have this "gift" while others do not. However, there is compelling evidence that communication skills can be learnt; even the most experienced CPs can continue to develop communication skills and those that find it more of a challenge can definitely make improvements [11].

The list that follows highlights some key facilitative skills though is far from exhaustive. Indeed, 71 communication skills have been identified that are beyond the realms of this chapter to cover. However, the work of Silverman and colleagues is well worth exploring to gain more in-depth understanding of communication skills and the associated evidence base [11].

While highlighting key skills, it is also important to highlight that they need to be used with intent. Random interspersion of "skills" throughout the consultation will offer little benefit; rather, purposeful use of skills at appropriate times throughout the consultation will promote mutual understanding, satisfaction, and a patient-centred approach.

Listening: Active listening is listening in such a way that enables the patient's message to be heard and acknowledged. It is an active skill and one that requires great concentration. However, active listening is often compromised; time spent formulating the next question or response, distractions, either our own or external, and a belief that we need to say something are all ways in which listening is compromised, and as a result, the message that the patient is trying to express may be missed. Although active listening is an essential skill, alone it is not enough.

Summarising: Stopping at intervals throughout the consultation (and at the end) to summarise what has been said is a useful means of checking that you and the patient have an agreement and shared understanding. Summarising also demonstrates to the patient that you have been listening and they have been heard. If in doubt as to how to proceed, summarising gives you and the patient some additional time in which to think; summarising rather than asking another question or giving more information is likely to lead to further patient disclosure.

> ### Example
>
> CP: So what I've heard is that your chest pain wakes you at night between 4 and 6, you take the GTN but it doesn't work.
>
> Patient: Yes but it's also that it seems very different then and I'm quite frightened about it. . . .

Paraphrasing: Paraphrasing is saying back to the patient the gist of what they have said to you using your own words. By paraphrasing what the patient has said, you demonstrate active listening and also allow opportunity for the patient to correct any inaccuracies or misunderstandings. The patient is often encouraged to continue with further disclosure, removing the need for the professional to ask another question and promoting a patient-centred consultation.

> ### Example
>
> Patient: I've had trouble sleeping lately. My concentration at work is poor, I feel tired all of the time, I don't have the energy to meet up with my old friends and I find it difficult to talk to others about the way I am feeling.
>
> CP: You're not sleeping well and that's having a big impact on your life. . . .
>
> Patient: Yes. I feel completely overwhelmed and out of control.

Reflection: Like paraphrasing, reflection also demonstrates active listening and interest. As with a mirror, reflecting back an image, the professional simply repeats back exactly what the patient has said. This could be a phrase or one or two words used by the patient.

> ### Example
>
> Patient: I have had trouble sleeping lately. . . .
>
> CP: Trouble sleeping. . . .

Empathy: Empathy has often been described as the "experience of walking in another person's shoes." It is a way of attempting to recognise how another person may be feeling. Additionally, and perhaps even more importantly, it is about conveying to the other that we are trying to gain some appreciation of how it feels for them. It isn't a sense that we "understand" what another is feeling, perhaps because we have experienced something similar ourselves or we have cared for a patient in a similar situation; we cannot possibly understand how another is feeling. It is also important to recognise the difference between sympathy and empathy, and for this I will build on an analogy offered by Tschuden [12]:

Mr Sympathy is walking along the riverbank and notices that somebody is in difficulty in the river, at risk of drowning and in obvious distress (acknowledgement of situation). Recognising that he must act to help this person he jumps in alongside the drowning man (Sympathetic action) and they both sink to the bottom of the river.

Mr Empathy, on the other hand, is walking along the riverbank and notices that somebody is in difficulty in the river, at risk of drowning and in obvious distress (acknowledgement). Recognising that he must act to help this person he secures himself firmly on the riverbank, pulls out a rope, which he throws to the drowning man and pulls him to safety (empathic action).

This analogy can be transferred to the clinical context in how we convey our attempt to appreciate how the patient might be feeling. Here, the catch phrase of the Irish comedian Roy Walker "say what you see" may be helpful, for example, "I can see this must be difficult for you." This can also be taken a step further in that we can also "say what we feel," for example, "I imagine this must be very frightening for you." It may be that we wrongly label the emotion, perhaps suggest it might be very frightening when in fact what the patient is feeling is shock. The potential to get it wrong may inhibit an empathic response. However, what is important, and what is appreciated by patients, is that we care enough to attempt to understand. If we have got it wrong, the patient will correct us and thus deepen their disclosure, while appreciating our acknowledgment and efforts to try and understand.

Clarifying: The use of a clarifying question serves to ensure clarity about what has been said and that the meaning has been accurately understood by the professional. It also offers a useful opportunity for the patient to reflect on what they have said and to make sense of their situation.

Example

Patient: I've been feeling a little wobbly lately.

CP: What do you mean by wobbly?

Silence: Silence can be uncomfortable for many of us, and we may feel an urge to fill the silence when it arises in a consultation; often this is through giving more information to the patient or by asking another question. It is useful, however, to consider what may be going on for the patent in the silence. Given the difficulty of their situa-tion, the amount of information they are required to take on board, and the potential for high levels of uncertainty and anxiety, it is understandable that they may appreciate some time in which to take stock of the conversation and their situation. A silence within the consultation allows this opportunity for quiet reflection, to attempt to make some sense of what is happening to them and to form their next question or response.

Silence or minimal prompts, rather than further information or another question, are powerful tools, which commonly immediately precede disclosure [13].

Acknowledgement: Acknowledgement refers to those words, expressions, and intonations that demonstrate interest and understanding, for example, "mmm," "u-uh," "yes," or a nod of the head.

Encouragement: Phrases such as "Could you tell me more about that?" "Please go on," or "Help me to understand . . ." positively encourage the patient to continue, thus promoting the possibility of further disclosure and increasing the awareness and insight of the professional.

Open questions and, by contrast, closed questions: Open questions are those that encourage further disclosure from patients. For example, instead of asking "Are you sleeping well?" which may simply elicit a yes or no response, ask "How are you sleeping?" Closed questions of course do have a role to play, for instance, where a speedy factual response is required. It is therefore important to consider carefully which type of question best fits the situation and be aware when use of a closed question may actually block patient disclosure.

Picking up on cues: A cue is defined as "a verbal or nonverbal hint which suggests an underlying unpleasant emotion which needs clarifying by the professional" [14]. The "hint" can come in a number of forms:
- Reference to a psychological symptom such as "I worry."
- Description of physiological states that suggest an underlying issue such as sleep disturbance, loss of libido, etc.
- Words or phrases that suggest unclear or indeterminate emotions such as "It felt strange" or "I manage."
- Neutral reference to a significant or possibly stressful life event such as "My wife left me" or "I had surgery."

The use of facilitative questions linked to patient cues enhances the likelihood of further cues and are key to a patient-centred consultation [10].

While there may be concern that responding to cues may lengthen consultation times, the opposite has been demonstrated. 20% shorter consultation time was the experience of oncologists who responded to more than 90% of patient cues [4]. General practitioners (GPs) who responded to at least one emotional cue demonstrated consultation times shortened by 12.5%, while among surgeons consultations were shorter by 10.7% [15].

Educated guess: Sometimes, we have a sense of what the patient is telling us without them having specifically articulated it. An educated guess is when the professional can suggest what the patient may be saying or feeling.

Example

Patient: Since the treatment, I look nothing like I used to. I can't bear to look in the mirror anymore.

CP: Are you saying that you feel repulsed by what you see?

The concern here is that we may have guessed wrongly. Perhaps the patient isn't feeling repulsed at all and our suggestion may indicate that perhaps they should be. What generally happens is that the patient appreciates our attempts to understand their situation. If we have got it wrong, they will correct us. A simple apology followed by thanks for clarifying usually adds to the consultation rather than detracts.

Challenging: This allows for any discrepancies to be clarified thereby reducing the risk of misunderstanding. Verbal and nonverbal inconsistencies may be challenged.

Example

CP: You say you are fine but you look upset.

CP: You said earlier that you are not worried about starting the chemotherapy treatment and yet you have just told me that you are worried about possible side-effects.

Screening, Parking, and Prioritising: In our desire to respond to a patient's concerns and to improve the situation for them, there is a temptation to respond too quickly (see blocking behaviours above). The problem here is that if we were to pick up on and respond to the first concern raised by the patient, we forfeit the opportunity to discover what else is of concern. Often the greatest concern held by the patient is not necessarily the first concern they share. Equally, we may make assumptions that a particular concern holds the greatest impact for the patient. The use of

screening, that is, eliciting all the patient concerns, parking them to one side in order to continue eliciting concerns, and then encouraging the patient to prioritise concerns in order of greatest impact offers a valuable means by which we can identify a fuller picture and thereby promote a patient-centred approach. There could be a perception that parking of concerns that may be the cause of great distress to patients may seem insensitive, indicating failure to recognise their significance. The use of empathy, therefore, is of great importance in order to demonstrate an appreciation of the difficulties. Summarising (mentioned earlier) also demonstrates active listening, as well as the opportunity to check for accuracy.

Interestingly, differences have been demonstrated in outcomes through subtle choice of words. For example, the term "Is there something else?" rather than "Is there anything else?" more than doubles the likelihood of eliciting further concerns [16].

The example below demonstrates screening, parking, and prioritising. Note there is a range of facilitative skills used with purpose (empathy, paraphrasing, educated guesses, summarising) throughout the example in order to gain a full understanding of the patient's concerns.

Example of screening, parking, and prioritising

CP: How have things been for you since you started the chemotherapy?

Patient: I must admit I have been feeling very tired and I've not been able to keep up my evening class.

CP: That sounds tough—I remember you've told me how important your evening class is to you. Perhaps we can come back to think about your sleeping pattern a little later. Is there something else?

Patient: Yes, I've also had difficulty eating; I'm not enjoying my food because it just seems to taste differently.

CP: So not only are you not sleeping which has already got in the way of your evening class, you are also not enjoying food in the way you used to. Is there something else?

Patient: I worry about what my husband is thinking—he looks worried but he seems to find it difficult to talk about things.

CP: I sense that you would value being able to chat things through with your husband so this must feel quite isolating. . . .

Patient: Yes, I do feel alone at times.

CP: Yes I can hear that. Is there something else?

Patient: No, I think those are my biggest worries at the moment.

CP: Thank you for sharing that with me. Can I check that I have understood correctly? You say that you're not sleeping well and that is getting in the way of your usual interests, such as the night class. You are having trouble eating particularly because food seems to taste differently. You are worried about how your husband may be feeling and because he seems to find it difficult to share his thoughts, you feel alone at times. Would that be a fair summary of what we have discussed so far?

Patient: Yes that's exactly it.

CP: It all sounds very difficult for you at the moment. Which of those worries, would you say causes you the greatest concern?

Patient: I think the eating—I used to love my food but now it just seems to taste awful—it gets me down—my husband and I used to enjoy eating out together.

CP: Ok, well we have about 10 min today. Shall we spend that time discussing the problems you are having with eating? I also have a few questions I'd like to ask you as part of our assessment—would that be ok?

Patient: Yes that's fine.

The process of screening, parking, and prioritising enables the professional to get to the core of the patient's concerns in a timely and efficient manner, thereby promoting a patient-centred approach and making best use of time. It is worth remembering that the majority of patients prefer a patient-led or patient-centred approach while recognising that a significant minority prefer a "doctor"-led consultation [17].

Beginning the assessment by focusing on the patient's concerns (their agenda) generally means that you are more likely to achieve your own agenda that is negotiated as part of the consultation. Given that patients may well be sharing numerous concerns with you, it is a good practice to gain the patient's consent for you to take notes as you listen.

Structuring an assessment

One of the most commonly heard concerns about changing our style of communication to be patient-centred is that consultations will then take too long. Time is something that we do not have enough of, and suggesting anything that may create further time burdens is generally rejected. However, just as the use of effective communication skills can reduce the length of consultations, so too can the use of a structure. All too easily, consultations, particularly those that are emotionally charged, can appear to lack purpose and direction, leading the patient to feel dissatisfied and unsupported and the CP confused and uncertain how to move things forward. An overt structure to any consultation or meeting can provide order, yet flexibility, involves and encourages patient involvement, ensures an accurate understanding of the issues, and makes most efficient use of time [11].

The Calgary-Cambridge model [11] (see Figure 6.1) provides an organised approach to patient assessment, which incorporates structure, together with relationship building as a continuous thread throughout the consultation. Both are considered essential to the achievement of the following five sequential tasks:
- Initiating the session
- Gathering information
- Physical examination
- Explanation and planning
- Closing the summary.

Strategies for specific challenging scenarios

Breaking bad news

Before considering how to break bad news, it is important to define what is meant by the term. Often, bad news is the term reserved for imparting the presence of a life-limiting diagnosis. However such a view undermines the experience of many other losses associated with palliative care, such as loss of independence, no longer being able to share a bed with a long-term partner due to the need for a hospital bed being placed at home; bad news can relate to many events, and therefore, the term "significant news" may be more useful:

Bad news is "any news that adversely and seriously affects an individual's view of his or her future" [18].

Buckman [19] describes the impact of bad news as a "gap between the patient's expectations of the situation and the medical reality of it." Until we know the patient's perception of their situation, we cannot assume their reaction to significant news; "Ask, before you tell" is therefore a valuable starting point.

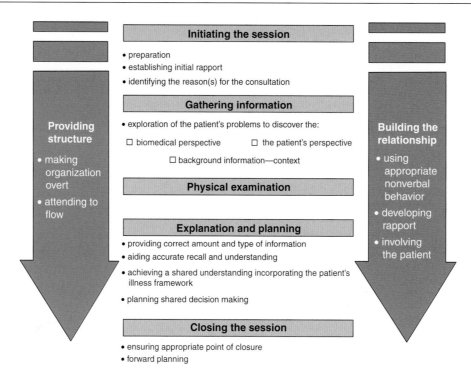

Figure 6.1 Calgary-Cambridge model [11]. Further information, particularly regarding application in practice can be found at www.gp-training.net/training/communication_skills/calgary/index.htm.

Imparting significant news is a challenge that can be stressful for the CP [20]. The distress of another can be difficult, sometimes bringing professionals in touch with their own mortality. A lack of subsequent support for the CP is not uncommon and may serve to increase reluctance to engage with the distress of the patient. Professionals may also experience a sense of helplessness, particularly if unable to offer active treatment options.

Despite the regularity with which some CPs have to convey significant news, many have not received training nor do they have a planned strategy for the way they do this [19]. However, evidence demonstrates the importance of a structured consultation in that [21]:

• Facts imparted at the start of a consultation are more likely to be remembered by patients than those given later.

• Patients are more likely to accurately remember something of importance to them, rather than an issue identified by the CP.

• Patients recall a smaller proportion of information if the CP imparts a large number of statements.

• Information that patients are able to recall tends to stick (and is less likely than other memories to be lost with time).

The SPIKES strategy for breaking bad news (Buckman)

Setting (S)

The environment where significant news is to be discussed is an important consideration; a private room, free of distractions, and where you are unlikely to be disturbed is advocated. Enlist the support of colleagues in "protecting" you from external distractions—hand over bleeps to others, switch off mobile phones, etc. Ask the patient whether he/she would like anybody else to be present—they may well appreciate the support of a family member or close friend.

Nonverbal body language can be powerful, and it is therefore important to use it with volition. Sitting down, preferably alongside the patient and not behind a desk or other physical obstacle, creates an impression of "partnership," is less intimidating for the patient, and also allows for good eye contact.

Although the CP may be feeling nervous, which may be demonstrated through behaviours such as fidgeting, it is important to display a sense of calm—the patient needs to see and hear that you are attentive to their needs and interested in their situation.

Perception (P)

Gaining insight into the patient's understanding of their situation is key to help you to gauge the gap between the patient's expectations and the reality of the situation. A question such as "Can you tell me what you have been told so far?" can be used.

Invitation (I)

The evidence shows that the majority of patients want full disclosure, but a small minority do not want to know. Giving information to those who would prefer not to know can cause serious psychological distress and therefore it is important to explore how much information this particular patient in front of you would want. A simple question such as "Are you the kind of person who prefers to know all the details about what is going on?" will be useful in indicating their preferences.

Knowledge (K)

A "warning shot" that "bad" news is to follow is valuable in allowing the patient to prepare for what is to follow. For example, "I'm afraid I have some bad news for you" or "I'm sorry to have to tell you...." The information to be shared should then be discussed in nontechnical terms, which avoids jargon. "Chunking" information into small sections allows for the checking of understanding and to modify the pace of information giving.

Example

CP: Treatment will start on Monday and will take 8 weeks, during which time you will need to attend the radiotherapy department twice a week. Does that make sense so far?

CP: I've given you a lot of information and I'd like to check that I have explained things clearly for you. It would help me if you could repeat back to me what we have said so far so I can check we are on the same page.

Empathy (E)

Empathy is an important and powerful aspect of how significant news is broken. Emotions should be acknowledged and addressed as they arise in the consultation with an empathic response—see earlier in this chapter. Validation of the emotions, for example, "I can see how you might feel that way" should then follow.

Strategy and summary (S)

A summary of the information should be given before the consultation ends. This enables understanding to be checked and also allows the patient to ask any questions or raise any concerns they may have. A clear plan should then be identified, which states the role of both practitioner and patient in taking it forward.

Dealing with strong emotion, for example, anger, distress

Often strong emotions such as anger and distress can have a significant impact on us as CPs. We can feel threatened by the presence of anger, feel the anger is directed at us personally and become defensive. The presence of distress, crying, and an outpouring of emotions can have an equally strong impact, perhaps by putting us in touch with our own distress at the situation or a similar one, we may have experienced in our personal lives. This can potentially lead to inappropriate and unhelpful reactions from the CP. A strategy for dealing with strong emotions can be of great benefit as it promotes an objective, patient-centred response:

- Recognise the presence of the emotion.
Example: I can see you're angry.
- Legitimise the emotion through permission.
Example: It's ok to feel this way—many people would feel angry in your situation.
- Gain the patient's perspective and gain as much information as possible.
Example: Can you tell me what has been happening?
- Focus on the patient's emotions and convey empathy.
Example: This all sounds very difficult for you. Can you bear to tell me how it leaves you feeling?
- Apologise if appropriate.
- Give reasons for the situation if appropriate though take care not to adopt blocking behaviours by becoming defensive or giving too much information.
- Negotiate a way forward together if appropriate.

Future care planning: initiating end-of-life care discussions (see also Chapter 8, Advance Care Planning)

Many practitioners find talking about end-of-life care challenging and may choose to avoid these discussions with patients. However, such discussions are important in promoting patient choice and ensuring individual wishes are known. Ensuring that patients, and their families, where appropriate, are central to the decision-making process is key to achieve care that is consistent with the patients' wishes.

While there may be a belief that some patients are unable or unwilling to talk about their own death, there is evidence that most patients look to their GP to initiate such discussions. Additionally patients would prefer to talk with a GP with whom they have an established trusting relationship rather than a stranger or nominated "advance care planning (ACP) professional" in the hospital setting [22,23].

Early discussions about end-of-life care are advocated before advanced illness makes discussion difficult [24]. Indecision, uncertainty, and conflict associated with end-of-life care can delay decisions and create additional suffering.

Before approaching an end-of-life care discussion, it is useful to have some understanding of the patient's cultural, familial, and religious beliefs as they will affect the family's readiness to talk about and engage in end-of-life care planning [25].

End-of-life care discussions should generally take place over a number of consultations and should not be an isolated conversation. In this way rapport and trust can be built and the patient, together with his/her family, has opportunity to reflect and make further contributions to the discussion and ask further questions. Don't worry if after offering an opportunity for the patient to discus the future, it becomes apparent that they would rather not. The fact that you have introduced the topic demonstrates that you are willing to discuss such sensitive issues. The patient is then aware that should they wish to discuss it at a future date, you will be supportive.

The acronym "PREPARED" [26] offers a useful structure to end-of-life care discussions:

Prepare for the discussion
> Ensure you have as much information as possible.
> Find a quiet room free of interruptions.
> Invite others to be present according to patient preference.

Relate to the person
Create rapport and show empathy, compassion and sensitivity.

Elicit patient and caregiver preferences
Establish the reason for the consultation and elicit the patient's (and the family's) expectations.
Clarify their understanding of the situation, and establish how much detail and what they want to know.
Consider cultural and contextual factors that may influence information preferences.

Provide information
Tailor information to the patient's and family understanding, preferences, and circumstances.

Check understanding and impact frequently.
Use clear, jargon-free language.
Be honest about the limitations of prognostic information and avoid being too exact with timeframes. Acknowledge the impact of such uncertainties on the patient and family.

Acknowledge emotions and concerns
Check understanding of what has been discussed and the emotional impact.
Respond empathically to distress.

(Foster) **R**ealistic hope
> Be honest without being blunt.
> Do not give more information than that required by the patient.
> Provide reassurance that ongoing support and symptom management will be offered.
> Identify what is important to the patient and what they would realistically hope to achieve in the time remaining.

Encourage questions
> Provide opportunity for any questions or clarification.
> Reassure patient that they are able to discuss things again in the future.

Document
Document a summary of the discussion and communicate the decisions to other members of the MDT as appropriate.

Collusion

The definition of collusion is *a secret or illegal cooperation or conspiracy in order to deceive others* [27]. In the context of palliative care, collusion often relates to a request from another, usually a family member, to withhold certain information from the patient. Such information commonly relates to discussing a diagnosis or informing the patient of prognosis or perhaps the transition from a curative to palliative phase of care.

In some instances, the withholding of information is culturally based, centred on the belief that the family hold primacy. Across Western systems of health and social care (for instance, those of the United States, United Kingdom, Canada, Australia, and Northern Europe), patient autonomy is widely acknowledged—the individual is the first consideration and patient ownership of information accepted. However, in many traditional cultures, such as in India and Japan, it is the well-being of the family, which takes priority. For example, there is an expectation that Korean or Japanese families be informed of the patient's situation and that it will be they who make treatment decisions for the patient with the family's best interests paramount. Often, the oldest male will make decisions for a family member or the husband will make decisions for the wife. One means of fulfilling obligations to patient, culture, and ethical standards is to ask the patient to whom information should be given and who should make decisions. In such situations family members should not translate [28].

In other situations the pretext of collusion is often to "protect" the patient *Please don't tell him he's dying—he would never cope,*" on the assumption (often erroneous) that the patient is in the dark about his/her illness, or out of concern for his/her physical or psychological well-being. There is a cost to collusion: lack of trust that is likely to strain relationships within the family, together with anger toward those suspected of colluding and suspicion the part of the patient if they feel information is being withheld [29].

Studies in Western cultures have shown that collusion can lead to regret about lack of openness among family members [30]. While falsely based optimism may initially appear helpful, once it becomes clear (as the illness progresses) that this optimism was illusory, the opposite is the case. Indeed as death approaches, it hinders preparations for what is inevitable, such as saying goodbye. Clearly collusion and the unrealistic expectations engendered prevent sensible, open discussion and decision making in the final phases of terminal illness.

Dealing with collusion

- Focus on relatives feelings with empathy.

    This must be very difficult for all of you—before we talk about your wife/father etc, can you tell me how all this makes you feel?

- Clarify the reasons for wishing to withhold information and identify any concerns.

    I understand that you are worried about me talking to.... About what is going on at the moment. We certainly wouldn't want to tell ... about the situation either if he/she doesn't want to know. What is it that you think will happen if we do have this conversation? [31]

- Do not challenge reasons but support them.

    I can appreciate why that might be a concern for you

- Identify any "costs" of withholding information such as a strain on the relationship between patient and family, inability to have open conversations, make future plans, etc.

What do you think might happen if we don't tell ... what is happening at the moment? [31] have you thought about how not telling ... may affect the relationship between the two of you?

- Explore if there is any evidence of the patient having raised the issue of the illness or asking questions.
- Propose that the patient may have some awareness— a "window on knowledge."

    Do you think ... knows that all is not right at the moment? What must that be like for ... to suspect but not know? [32]

- Ask for permission to assess the patient's current knowledge and desire for further information.
- Assure relative that unwanted information will not be given but further discussion will take place if the patient requests it.
- Negotiate a plan.

    We could talk to ... together and find out what he/she thinks is happening and what else he/she would like to know.

    I could talk to ... find out what he/she already knows and what else he/she would like to know. Perhaps we could then all talk together afterwards.

Dealing with denial or unrealistic expectations

Denial can be considered as "an unconscious mechanism aimed at negating a disease-orientated threat to the integrity of personhood and daily life." As CPs we may feel we have a responsibility to challenge such denial in an attempt to ensure that the patient is fully informed of their situation and therefore an integral part of the decision-making process. However denial is only problematic if it has a negative effect on the patient in terms of accessing appropriate care or guidance or quality of life. Indeed, denial has been shown to reduce psychological morbidity [33], acting as a coping mechanism and serving as a useful tool in enabling the patient to gradually acknowledge and work through their situation in their own time, rather than within the imposed timeframe of professionals. As such, denial is usually shortlived, but it is important that the CP explores the extent of the denial in order to determine if it is an absolute barrier or if there is evidence of inconsistencies. Forcing unwanted information could undermine the patient's coping mechanism and could cause severe psychological distress.

Of course, denial may not be the only cause of a patient's reluctance to talk, and it is valuable to explore if there are other reasons. For example, the patient may not be able to process information due to low intellect, sensory impairments, misconceptions, misunderstanding, incorrect or inadequate information, or temporary issues such as intermittent hypoxia or effects of fluctuating levels of medication. Depression, cognitive impairment, and disengagement may be other possible causes or else the patient may have already addressed their situation and feel that they now want to "move on."

Responding to denial and unrealistic expectation

• Check for evidence that the denial is not ABSOLUTE, which might provide a "window" in which to discuss the situation realistically.

Now: How do you feel things are at the moment?

Past: Have you ever thought that things might not go the way you are expecting? What is on your mind at those times? /How do the thoughts make you feel?

Future: How do you see your illness in the future?

Leave the situation as it is if unable to identify any evidence of awareness.

• Explore patient perspective.

Example: What is your understanding of your illness and what the future may hold?

• Challenge any inconsistencies.

Example: "You say your illness isn't serious and yet you have recently completed a course of chemotherapy. . . ."

• Pose a hypothetical question as a means to explore goals and to identify significant issues that are important to address while the patient remains well enough.

Example: "Have you thought about what might happen if things don't go as you wish? Sometimes having a plan that prepares you for the worst makes it easier to focus on what you hope for most" [34]

• Offer an opportunity for a second opinion if the patient does not accept the futility of a treatment.

Example: "Sometimes it's useful to be able to discuss challenging issues with another experienced professional. Would you like me to arrange for a second opinion?"

Discussing life expectancy

"How long have I got to live?" is a common question posed by patients who have been made aware of a serious diagnosis. There is no clear consensus about how to respond. Prognosis might be expressed in terms such as days as opposed to weeks or months; a rough range; the proba-

bility of surviving long enough to reach key events such as birth of a grandchild; or a statistical approximation, for example, 20% survival. There is, however, agreement that exact timeframes should not be given, unless perhaps in the very terminal stages of illness when discussing whether family should be sent for, but there is value in being able to describe the difficulties of predicting survival timeframes. Evidence suggests that words and numbers are preferable to the use of graphs and pie charts when discussing prognosis although this should not be assumed and it remains important to identify individual preferences with patients [35,36].

Although a difficult issue to broach, evidence shows that the majority of patients do actually want to have full disclosure in relation to their illness and prognosis. However, a small number, about 2% of patients, do not want information [37]. Key to answering any "difficult" question is establishment of the meaning of the question, working out if the patient really does want an answer and to understand what has led to them asking the question at this time.

Responding to questions about life expectancy

• Acknowledge the significance or enormity of a "difficult" question. This is important in conveying empathy.

Example: "That must be a difficult question for you to ask."

• Explore the patient's perspective.

Example: "I'm happy to talk about this with you but I wonder what has led you to ask that question at this time?"

(It is useful to repeat this question following the patient response to elicit any other reasons the patient may have for asking.)

Before we talk about that, I wonder if you could help me to understand how things have been for you recently and if you have noticed any changes?

• Avoid giving an exact timeframe and describe the challenges associated with predicting survival if appropriate.

Example: "It's very difficult to predict with accuracy how long somebody may have to live but I might be able to guess in terms of days, weeks, months or years. Would that be useful to you?"

• Explore the impact of disclosure on the patient.

Example: "I imagine it's hard to hear that. How has it left you feeling?"

• Offer continued support.

Example: "No matter what lies ahead, I/the team will be there to support you."

When language is not shared

Where a common language is not shared between the CP and patient, effective communication becomes reliant on the facilitation of a third party such as an interpreter or bilingual advocate. The introduction of a third person is not without challenge; it has been shown that the use of an interpreter can result in a significant reduction and revision of speech with consequences for linguistic features such as content, meaning, reinforcement/validation, repetition, and affect. Additionally, the "three-way" relationship created through use of an interpreter limits rapport building, which is key in promoting an open, honest, and trusting relationship. Undoubtedly, what is said and heard by patients and CPs is significantly affected by the presence of an interpreter—the use of untrained interpreters increases the challenge and introduces the possibilities of misdiagnosis and misunderstanding through misinterpretation [38].

Using "lay" interpreters

It is not uncommon for friends and relatives of the patient, or bilingual colleagues to be recruited to the role of interpreter. This may be due to a lack of available professional interpreting services or maybe because of a lack of awareness of their existence. While some patients may prefer a familiar figure to act as interpreter, it should not be assumed that this is always the case, and CPs should be aware of some of the issues that may arise as a result of using lay interpreters. Table 6.3 shows the possible consequences for the patient and the lay interpreter.

Working with a professional interpreter

In light of the above, wherever possible a professional interpreter should be used as they possess a good awareness of cultural sensitivity and knowledge of medical and colloquial terminology together with an understanding of the need for confidentiality and sensitivity [40].

Table 6.3 Possible consequences of use of a lay interpreter.

Impact on patient	Impact on lay interpreter
Important information may be omitted as a result of having to communicate potentially embarrassing information through a particular family member, for example, a female patient explaining gynaecological problems through her son	Information passed on may be "censored" as a result of embarrassment at having to transmit intimate details
May be attempts to hide sensitive information from family member interpreting in order to protect them	Unfamiliarity of medical concepts or terminology may create problems in expressing information
Concerned that their family status may be affected as a result of younger members or in-laws finding out what is wrong with them	May not appreciate the significance of expressing the information accurately and completely
Concern that their family member may keep information from them	The wrong information may be passed on, crucial elements could be missed out or new information added
Fear that confidentiality is at risk if somebody from his or her community acts an interpreter	May not appreciate the need to be impartial or for the need for confidentiality
	May not have the confidence to say when they do not understand or if they need something to be repeated
	Tendency to use the third person rather than direct address, which may make the patient feel disempowered and may limit the development of rapport between the patient and the CP

Source: Adapted from Kai J (ed.). *PROCEED: Professionals Responding to Ethnic Diversity and Cancer*. London: Cancer Research UK, 2005 [39].

While the presence, even of a professional interpreter, increases the difficulty of achieving effective communication, it is not impossible and guidelines exist [39,41] to support the goal of this mode of communication as defined by Lubrano et al. [41]:

"collaboration" with the interpreter to achieve an optimal interaction with the patient which:

- privileges the CP—patient dialogue;
- promotes shared understanding; and
- is sensitive to cultural differences.

Seating arrangement

Commonly the patient, CP, and interpreter position themselves in a triangular arrangement. In this position, it is difficult for the patient and CP to address each other directly as attention can be diverted to the interpreter. Additionally the triangular arrangement can set up a situation where the interpreter and patient are conversing for long periods of time to the exclusion of the CP. To overcome these issues, a parallel seating arrangement is advocated [41] as illustrated in Figure 6.2. The rationale for this seating that seeks to prioritise the CP–patient relationship should be explained to the patient who might not be aware of its purpose.

Table 6.4 highlights the key tasks required to promote effective communication when working with an interpreter. Clarity is essential to the consultation, and therefore, both the pre- and postmeeting with the interpreter

Table 6.4 How to work well with an interpreter.

Action	Tasks
Arrange a preconsultation meeting with the interpreter to explain the content and expectations of the consultation	Allow sufficient time for a preconsultation meeting with the interpreter
	Identify way in which you will work together
	Enquire if interpreter is aware of any cultural issues that may affect consultation, for example, family avoidance of the word "cancer"
	Check that the interpreter and the patient speak same language and same dialect
	Ask the interpreter to teach you how to explain the patients name correctly
Establish the CP, patient, interpreter relationship	Arrange seating before consultation (see above).
	Allow time for the interpreter to introduce himself or herself to the patient and to explain the interpretation process including the confidential nature of the process
	Check that the interpreter is acceptable to the patient
	Address the patient directly; avoid looking at the interpreter
Promote effective communication throughout the consultation	Plan ahead what you are going to say
	Use straightforward language and avoid jargon
	Actively listen to the patient and the interpreter
	Allow enough time for the consultation: perhaps double the time for a patient with whom you share the same language
	Avoid colloquial expressions or metaphors, which may be difficult to translate
	Pause frequently
	Encourage the interpreter to interrupt/intervene as necessary throughout the consultation in order to check accuracy
	Check that patient has understood everything and if he/she wants to ask any questions
Review consultation with interpreter	Hold a postconsultation discussion with the interpreter
	Provide opportunity for the interpreter to highlight any possible culturally sensitive issues identified through consultation

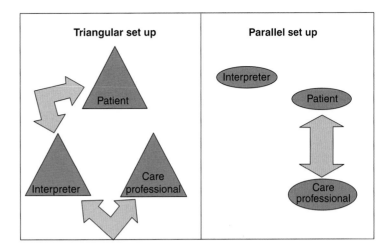

Figure 6.2 Recommended seating plan. (Adapted from Lubrano et al. [41].)

are an important part of the process. While this may seem time consuming, such meetings can help to avoid misunderstanding and can therefore save time in the long run.

Conclusion

Effective communication skills are essential to good palliative care, promoting greater patient choice and involvement, increasing patient and carer satisfaction and positively impacting on the motivation and satisfaction of the CP.

Communication skills can be developed and are not the sole domain of the "naturally gifted." However, knowledge of the skills alone is insufficient; the facilitative skills outlined in this chapter should be used with purpose. Any consultation should be structured and facilitative skills used in a meaningful way with the intention to create an open, honest, and sensitive dialogue that encourages patient disclosure and enables the CP to gain insight into the patient's situation, associated concerns and wishes and to form an agreed plan with ongoing rapport and trust.

References

1. Kai J, Beavan J, Faull C, et al. Professional uncertainty and disempowerment responding to ethnic diversity in health care: a qualitative study. *PLoS Med* 2007; 4: e323. doi:10.1371/journal.pmed.0040323.
2. Stewart MA. Effective physician-patient communication and health outcomes: a review. *Canadian Medical Association Journal* 1996; 152: 1423–1433.
3. National Audit Office. *Department of Health: Tackling Cancer—Improving the Patient Journey.* London: The National Audit Office, 2005.
4. Butow PN, Brown RF, Cogar S, et al. Oncologists' reactions to cancer patients' verbal cues. *Psychooncology* 2002; 11: 47–58.
5. Fallowfield L and Jenkins V. Effective communication skills are the key to good cancer care. *Eur J Cancer* 1999; 35: 1592–1597.
6. Taylor C, Graham J, Potts HWW, et al. Changes in mental health of UK hospital consultants since the mid-1990s. *Lancet* 2005; 366: 742–744.
7. Wilkinson S, Perry R, Blanchard K, et al. Effectiveness of a three-day communication skills course in changing nurses' communication skills with cancer/palliative care patients: a randomised controlled trial. *Palliat Med* 2008; 22(4): 365–375.
8. Maguire P. Improving communication with cancer patients. *Eur J Cancer* 1999; 35: 2058–2065.
9. Omdahl BL and O'Donnell C. Emotional contagion, empathic concern and communicative responsiveness as variables affecting nurses' stress and occupational commitment. *J Adv Nurs* 1999; 29: 1351–1359.
10. Zimmermann C, del Piccolo L and Mazzi MA. Patient cues and medical interviewing in general practice: examples of the application of sequential analysis. *Epidemiol Psichiatr Soc* 2003; 12: 115–123.
11. Silverman JD, Kurtz SM and Draper J. *Skills for Communicating with Patients,* 2nd edition. Oxford: Radcliffe Medical Press, 2005.
12. Tschuden V. *Counselling Skills for Nurses,* 3rd edition. London: Balliere Tindall, 1991.
13. Eide H, Quera V, Graugaard P, et al. Physician-patient dialogue surrounding patients' expression of concern: applying sequence analysis to RIAS. *Soc Sci Med* 2004; 59: 145–155.

14. Del Piccolo L, Goss C and Bergvik S. The fourth meeting of the Verona Network on Sequence Analysis "consensus finding on the appropriateness of provider responses to patient cues and concerns". *Pat Edu Couns* 2006; 61: 473–475.

15. Levinson W, Gorawara-Bhat R and Lamb J. A study of patient clues and physician responses in primary care and surgical settings. *JAMA* 2000; 284: 1021–1027.

16. Heritage J, Robinson JD, Elliott MN, et al. Reducing patients' unmet concerns in primary care: the difference one word can make. *J Gen Intern Med* 2007; 22: 1429–1433.

17. Dowsett SM, Saul JL, Butow PN, et al. Communication styles in the cancer consultation: preferences for a patient-centred approach. *Psychooncology* 2000; 9: 147–156.

18. Buckman R. Breaking bad news: why is it still so difficult? *BMJ* 1984; 288: 1597–1599.

19. Buckman R. Breaking bad news: the S-P-I-K-E-S strategy. *Community Oncol* 2005; 2: 138–142.

20. Ptacek JT, Ptacek JJ and Ellison NM. " I'm sorry to tell you. . . ." Physician's reports of breaking bad news. *J Behav Med* 2001; 24: 205–217.

21. Fallowfield L and Jenkins V. Effective communication skills are key to good cancer care. *Eur J Cancer* 1999; 35(11): 1592–1999.

22. Cartwright CM and Parker MH. Advance care planning and end of life decision making. *Aust Fam Physician* 2004; 33: 815–819.

23. Burgess TA, Brooksbank M and Beilby JJ. Talking to patients about death and dying. *Aust Fam Physician* 2004; 33: 85–86.

24. Bloomer M, Tan H and Lee S. End of life care: the importance of advance care planning. *Aust Fam Physician* 2010; 39: 734–737.

25. Clark K and Philips J. End of life care: the importance of culture and ethnicity. *Aust Fam Physician* 2010; 39: 210–213.

26. Clayton JM, Hancock KM, Butow PN, et al. Clinical practice guidelines for communication prognosis and end of life issues with adults in the advanced stages of a life limiting illness and their caregivers. *Med J Aust* 2007; 186: S76–S108.

27. http://oxforddictionaries.com/definition/collusion.

28. Kemp C. Cultural issues in palliative care. *Semin Oncol Nurs* 2005; 21(1): 4–52.

29. Chaturvedi SK, Loiselle CG and Chandra PS. Communication with relatives and collusion in palliative care: a cross-cultural perspective. *Indian J Palliat Care* [serial online] 2009; 15: 2–9. Available at: http://www.jpalliativecare.com/text.asp?2009/15/1/2/53485(accessed on September 17, 2011).

30. The AM, Hak T, Koλter G, et al. Collusion in doctor-patient communication about imminent death: an ethnographic study. *BMJ* 2000; 321: 1376–1381.

31. Pitorak EF. Learning to have difficult conversations leads to increased hospice referrals. *Home Healthc Nurse* 2003; 21: 629–632.

32. Clayton JM, Butow PN and Tattersall MHN. The needs of terminally ill cancer patients versus those of caregivers for information regarding prognosis and end of life issues. *Cancer* 2005; 103: 1957–1964.

33. Rousseau P. The art of oncology: when the tumour is not the target. Death denial. *J Clin Oncol* 2000; 18: 3998–3999.

34. Tulsky JA. Beyond advance directives: importance of communication skills at the end of life. *JAMA* 2005; 294: 359–365.

35. Clayton JM, Butow PN and Tattersall MHN. When and how to initiate discussion about prognosis and end of life issues. *J Pain Manage* 2005; 30: 132–144.

36. Clayton J, Butow P, Arnold R, et al. Discussing life expectancy with terminally ill cancer patients and their carers: a qualitative study. *Support Cancer Care* 2005; 13: 733–742.

37. Jenkins V, Fallowfield L and Saul J. Information needs of patients with cancer: results from a large study in UK cancer centres. *Br J Cancer* 2001; 84: 48–51.

38. Aranguri C, Davidson B and Ramirez R. Patterns of communication through interpreters: a detailed sociolinguistic analysis. *J Gen Intern Med* 2006; 21: 623–629.

39. Kai J (ed.). *PROCEED: Professionals Responding to Ethnic Diversity and Cancer.* London: Cancer Research UK, 2005.

40. Romero CM. Curbside consultation. Using medical interpreters. *Am Fam Physician* 2004; 69: 2720–2722.

41. Lubrano di Ciccone B, Brown RF, Gueguen JA, et al. Interviewing patients using interpreters in an oncology setting: initial evaluation of a communication skills module. *Ann Oncol* 2009; 21: 27–32.

7 Adapting to Death, Dying, and Bereavement

Christina Faull[1], Sue Taplin[2]

[1]University Hospitals of Leicester and LOROS, The Leicestershire and Rutland Hospice, Leicester, UK
[2]LOROS The Leicestershire and Rutland Hospice, Leicester, UK

Introduction

The fear of death and the loss of a loved one are two of the most monumental emotional challenges of human existence. This fear and ensuing anxiety is usually suppressed and is only exposed when the reality of a possible death is confronted. Fear of death stems from two main sources: the thought of our nonexistence [1,2] and the fear of the unknown, of what, if anything, lies beyond death [2,3]. Palliative care has recognised the powerful impact of this on patients living with the certainty of dying and on families in their loss and bereavement and is concerned with helping people to cope and adapt.

This chapter discusses what people may experience when confronted with the possibility of their own death or that of a "significant other" (usually someone who is loved but it may be someone with whom the individual has a deep but less positive connection). It will consider the positive consequences and the pitfalls and limitations of bereavement support and the role of health professionals in supporting the dying and people who have been bereaved.

Fear of death in society

The fear we, as humans, may have of death has interested artists and scientists alike. Philosophers have considered death in terms of fear of extinction and insignificance [1,2,4]; psychologists have devised models that explain death-related emotion [5]; and sociologists have observed how death anxiety can bind groups (e.g., societies, reli-

gions, armies) [6]. Freud claimed that social life was formed and preserved out of fear of death. In industrialised and technological societies, death and dying have been removed from the family home into institutions, with care provided by professionals. This has resulted in a lack of familiarity with the dying process, which may contribute further to a fear of death and dying within society.

In day-to-day life, individuals usually contain such fears. "Death anxiety," a term used to conceptualise the apprehension generated by death awareness [7,8], can be provoked when confronted with the reality of death and may be hugely influential on behaviour. The factors that underpin and fuel death anxiety are outlined in Table 7.1.

People differ in how they respond to the prospect of death. In caring for people who are dying and people who have been bereaved, it is useful to try to understand the different factors that influence this behaviour. Although personal factors are very important (e.g., gender, nature of disease and treatment, coping mechanisms, social support, personality), these partly relate to what is known as the "death system" in a society. This phenomenon varies between societies and depends on the following four factors [12]:

1. Exposure to death—prior experience of death of a significant other has a strong influence on the approach to subsequent deaths, including our own.
2. Life expectancy—society holds an estimate for what is considered a reasonable life span, based on observations of the community in which one lives.
3. Perceived control over the forces of nature—beliefs about one's ability to influence destiny (fate vs. control) will affect perceptions of death.

Handbook of Palliative Care, Third Edition. Edited by Christina Faull, Sharon de Caestecker, Alex Nicholson and Fraser Black.
© 2012 by John Wiley and Sons, Inc. Published 2012 by John Wiley & Sons, Inc.

Table 7.1 Factors that induce fear of death.

Drivers of death anxiety affecting males and females (Nayatanga [9])	Factors affecting the general public (Diggory and Ruthman [10])	Death fears as advocated by (Chonnon [11])
• Dependency • Pain in dying process • Isolation • Indignity of dying process • Afterlife concerns • Leaving loved ones • Fate of the body • Rejection • Separation	Grief of relatives and friends End of all plans and projects Dying process being painful One can no longer have experiences Can no longer care for dependents Fear of what happens if there is life after death Fear of what happens to one's body	Fear of what happens after death Fear of the act of dying (e.g., pain, loss of control, and rejection) Fear of ceasing to be

4. Perception of what it means to be human—"meaning" in this context relates to various belief systems that can be defined as a person's "spirituality." The clarity and conviction with which a society holds these views will influence how death is considered in that society.

Each death will be influenced to varying degrees by a combination of personal factors within a particular cultural death system. For instance, an older Indian widow who views illness from a religious perspective will respond differently from the young Western atheist who has never experienced death and believes in his or her own ability to control life events.

Holistic needs assessment and identification of emotional distress

A basis for exploring and understanding the impact of a terminal illness on a patient or those close to them is to assess people's well-being and distress in the key domains of physical, emotional, social, and spiritual so-called holistic assessment. Guidance from the National Institute for Clinical Excellence in the United Kingdom recommends that holistic assessment should be an ongoing process throughout the course of illness [13]. For cancer patients, a structured assessment is needed at key transition points:
- Around the time of diagnosis
- Commencement of treatment
- Completion of the primary treatment plan
- Each new episode of disease
- The point of recognition of incurability
- The beginning of end of life
- The point at which dying is diagnosed.

Box 7.1 Key transition points in chronic obstructive pulmonary disease (COPD) [15]

- Diagnosis.
- Retirement on medical grounds.
- Starting long-term oxygen therapy.
- Hospital admission for an exacerbation of COPD.
- A positive answer to the "surprise" question (would you be surprised if this patient died in the next 12 months?).

Similar transition points are now being clearly identified for patients with other diseases (Box 7.1) [14,15].

There is much guidance available on the process of undertaking the holistic assessment and a range of tools available to support this [16–18]. An example of a tool to assess emotional well-being and distress is the *Emotions Thermometer* (Figure 7.1), which has been validated as a screening tool in cancer and cardiovascular disease (CVD) [19].

Personal spirituality

Spirituality is concerned with how individuals understand the purpose and meaning of their existence within the universe. For some, but by no means all, there may be a strong religious component to this aspect of their life. These differences are readily seen in pluralistic Western societies such as the United Kingdom and may have a profound effect on how individuals view death and dying. There may be increased questioning and searching for

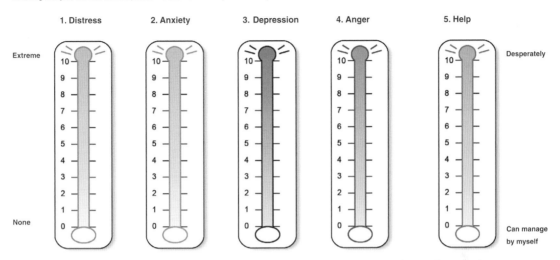

Figure 7.1 The emotions thermometer. A screening tool for emotional distress. (Reproduced from Reference 19.)

meaning, an awakening of the spiritual dimension, toward the end of life [20].

Death poses a challenge to these personally held belief systems. Some individuals possess a set of beliefs that adequately answer this challenge, but others can suffer as they strive to attain an inner peace. A patient's individual spirituality can never be assumed. Professionals must remain aware of this when considering the spiritual needs of patients. Spiritual health can be encouraged in several ways:

• By eliminating the distraction caused by physical suffering.

• By encouraging the expression of repressed emotion but with caution not to dismantle constructive adaptive processes.

• By assisting patients to attain spiritual "peace," either by personal reflection or with the help of an adviser (professional or lay).

• By respecting the individual and their culture in all interactions.

The spiritual component of well-being is an important part of the philosophy of palliative care and is recognized as one of the four tenets of holistic assessment [13,21]. One specialist palliative care group has developed a standard for the assessment, delivery, and evaluation of spiritual care, which includes three levels:

1. Routine assessment (for all patients).

2. Multidisciplinary assessment (which can be particularly sensitive to spiritual issues).

3. Specialist assessment (which may be, e.g., that undertaken by a chaplain) [22].

Such standards provide a framework for practitioners to address what is often a neglected area of palliative care. This is explored further in Chapter 24, *Spirituality in Palliative Care.*

Adapting to the stark reality of dying

There are many studies that give us insight into the challenges for people when faced with dying, and there is also a richness of personal accounts, especially those about cancer [23]. Michele Petrone, an artist who has now died from lymphoma, shared his journey in pictures and thoughts and thus gave us an insight into how the physical and the emotional are intertwined:

My journey has two intertwined threads—elements which mirror each other as exactly as the two chains of the double helix. One is the medical history. The physical injury, the illness, the happening, the happened, the inevitable and the unavoidable. The parallel thread is my emotional response. The disbelief, the grief, the doubt, the flung out, the anger, the banter, the bargaining, the accepting, the clenching of teeth, the sick to the teeth, the pain, the no-gain. Why me? Why me now? I'm living, I'm dying. I want to live and escape it. I want to die to escape it. I'm trapped and that's that. Get me out of it. I hate it. I hate this illness, what its done to me. It took away my love, my love of life, my freedom—my freedom to love. It threatened my life. I want my life back. This is not me. But it happens and this for me is more than no good. And even if it makes me stronger, why should I have to go through it—I don't want to go through it [24].

Psychosocial theories

Various psychological models have been developed, which provide insight into patients' responses to their impending death. The most well-known work is that of Kubler-Ross [25], who described a five-stage model of dying: denial, anger, bargaining, depression, and acceptance. The stage theory has been seen as too mechanistic an approach when measured against the actual experience of people working with dying patients, which suggests that people who are dying may experience feelings of calm, fear, hope, depression, anger, sadness, and withdrawal and that some but not all will gain acceptance, some reaching it very early. In addition, the reactions of an individual are dependent on their personal characteristics. For instance, some may use predominantly problem-focused coping mechanisms (e.g., searching the Internet for new treatments) and others predominantly emotion-focused coping mechanisms (e.g., drinking too much to dull the effect of emotional crisis). Other authors have proposed different models that also contribute to our understanding [12,26–31]. The main advantage of these theories is that they allow us to make sense of people's behaviour more constructively and support them more effectively. Parkes sums this up succinctly:

> It is not enough for us to stay close and open our hearts to another person's suffering: valuable as this sympathy may be, we must have some way for stepping aside from the maze of emotion and sensation if we are to make sense of it [32].

However, these models have their limitations. They should only be used to assist in our understanding of patients and help us support them and their carers, thus enabling the carer especially not to be overwhelmed by the emotions observed. Too rigid an application of such models may prevent the individual needs of patients and carers being assessed and met.

A time for personal growth?

Knowing that you are dying soon may be very distressing for the individual and for those around them. However, some patients do see the time before dying as very spe-

cial and use it to achieve amazing goals and as a time of personal growth. Patrick Joyce is an optimist with motor neurone disease who has reflected on this subject:

I met a man the other day.
I met a man the other day, an old friend from years before. Amongst the rocks and dinosaurs I was, when he suddenly appeared. A great bear of a man, towering above me in my chair, a man in the full flood of his life—confident, secure, complete. Twenty years and more have gone since I saw him last, and five minutes of him I had before he had to go, but as he talked, and smiled and laughed, I saw before me there, the boy I used to know. It was odd really, as he talked, the boy with the wooden sword appeared, with his cheeky grin, bike and pet frog. And as he talked he aged and grew, and became the man that now I sat before. Twenty eight years of him that I didn't share, twenty eight years of life, of love, experience—years I didn't know. I saw a man confident amongst the collections in his museum, doing good work and knowing it. I wondered what he saw as he looked back at me. He didn't see a man in his prime, those days are gone. Did he see the twilight? A man marking his days till the end? Did he feel pity? A sadness for the boy he once knew. . . . What if the twenty eight years had been seventy eight? What if we had met in our shared twilight? There would have been no sadness then, just joy in a rich life lived and childhood shared. And so there should be none now. It is a privilege to be in the twilight at forty, bittersweet with the missing years to come and the slow death that awaits me, but a privilege nonetheless. I've had a very rich life, and in the three years since getting MND I've had time to reflect, and learnt to value this time I've been given, learnt to be thankful for my life and the chance to look back on it, from its certain end. Do not pity me, I have something you do not. Clarity [33].

The Household Guide to Dying [34], while being a work of fiction, does nonetheless capture something very poignant about the journey of terminal cancer and the need to find resolution and meaning in life's works. Bingley et al. [23] have identified the very positive value for individuals about writing about the experience of living and dying with cancer. Others have their personal "bucket list" [35] and a few, such as Jane Tomlinson [36], have made quite miraculous achievements. For some, spiritual growth is an explicit and significant component of the dying trajectory [37].

Particular problems in adapting to dying

The extent of the distress experienced by patients depends on a wide variety of factors. In many cases, the psychosocial needs of the patient and carers are met, with honest information provided sensitively. However, in more complex instances, the debilitating effects of the adaptive process require more intense professional support. Physical symptoms can be influenced by the emotional state of patients. The concepts such as "total pain" are at the core of the philosophy of palliative care. Consequently, emotional, social, or spiritual distress can be an important component in physical suffering and therefore in its management [38].

There is an array of emotional responses that can occur when facing death, which can be difficult for patients to bear. These can include anger, anxiety, guilt, and depression. As patients grapple with all these emotions and the changing nature of their illness, feelings of isolation can also occur. This alienation can compound the many other losses that may be experienced at this time.

Not surprisingly, the enormity of the adaptive process can be overwhelming and result in psychiatric morbidity resulting in high prevalence of depression and anxiety and an increased risk of suicidal behaviour [39].

Some patients use techniques such as "positive reappraisal" and "cognitive avoidance strategies" [40]. To the professional observer, some of these strategies may seem like distortions or misinterpretations of the facts, but to the patient they can insure against emotional overload. It is important not to dismantle individual adaptive processes, but some may need to be challenged if the consequences to the patient or the carer are significant (e.g., incurring debt to explore treatments which are not evidence-based).

The debilitating effect of the emotional consequences of a terminal illness can compound the physical deterioration to produce significant social costs. Social losses are closely related to quality-of-life issues and include such things as employment, recreation, and relationships both within and outside of the family.

The demands of caring for a terminally ill patient should not be ignored by professionals. Indeed, in some cases the multidisciplinary team (MDT) focus is more appropriately directed not so much at the patient but at the patient's family and friends. The need for constant nursing care at home can be physically draining and can occasionally result in illness or injury to the carer. In addition, family and friends are subjected to a series of actual and potential losses that require considerable emotional strength. Examples of these challenges include the following:
- Loss of a certain future.
- Loss of role within the family and the outside world.
- Concerns about the burden of caring.

- Issues about sexuality.
- Loss of financial security.

In many cases these questions provoke emotions in carers that are similar to those experienced by the person who is dying. Such emotional strain can result in significant levels of sleeplessness, anxiety, and weight loss.

The social consequences of caring for a terminally ill person can be far-reaching. The time and energy required can impinge on employment, recreation, and relationships. Although society may recognise this in terms of respect for altruism, the economic burden can be considerable and only partially compensated for by statutory government allowances.

The MDT has an important role in recognising the potential dangers of caring for a loved one and should endeavour to intervene to prevent problems.

Managing the adaptation process

Assessing the emotional needs of dying patients and significant others requires an empathic attitude complemented by adept communication skills and familiarity with the issues surrounding the subject. To get an accurate picture of the patient, it may be necessary to meet on a number of occasions and incorporate the opinions of all members of the MDT. Hospice day care can play a particular role in this.

Symptom control: Unremitting physical symptoms can be "soul destroying," therefore symptom management is a key requirement of the adaptation process. This may then facilitate the management of emotional needs.

Communication: Skills in communication are pivotal to effective and sensitive care (see Chapter 6, *Communication skills in palliative care*).

Counselling and therapy: Counselling is concerned with enabling individuals to find solutions to emotional challenges by using particular techniques [41]. This approach can be especially helpful in unusually difficult situations. Such interventions can be made either through one-to-one work or as part of group work and may require the support of a trained professional.

Maintaining hope: Patients require hope to be sustained. This can be achieved either by setting achievable goals or sometimes by the use of intermittent or persistent denial. What is usually important is that the hope should reflect or be based on the reality of the situation; otherwise the goals may not be achieved.

Drugs: Appropriate use of psychotropic medicines (antidepressants, anxiolytics, or antipsychotics) is occasionally useful in palliative medicine. In some cases, it is difficult to differentiate between clinical psychiatric morbidity, which may respond to pharmacological inter-vention, and the normal emotions of dying. In cases of psychiatric morbidity, a referral for specialist assess-ment is important and trial of medication is a reasonable approach.

Complementary therapies: These can be helpful in relieving physical and emotional distress (see Chapter 23, *Complementary approaches to palliative cancer care*).

Hospice day care support and peer support groups including those for carers have a very important role in helping people adapt to what is happening to them.

Emotional crises

This subject cannot be discussed in sufficient depth here, but the reader is referred to Stedford [42], Vachon [40], Panke & Ferrell [43], and Lloyd-Williams [44].

Emotional crises do not arise without a trigger and/or premorbid factors of vulnerability. Various risk factors have been identified:

• Strong dependency issues, for example, hostility, ambivalence.
• Other stresses within the family, for example, relation-ship problems, poor housing, debts.
• Illness and bereavement history—previous experiences of death and loss are important both in the quantity and in the quality of experience and coping mechanisms that may or may not have been developed in previous times of distress.
• Psychiatric history.

Understanding these factors for the patient and fam-ily will help in the management of distress. Vulnerable patients and families should be identified in order to try to prevent crises and target support usually through proac-tive referral to additional support such as a specialist pal-liative care nurse.

Management of emotional crises

It is important to have a team approach, with more than one professional available to a family in acute distress, although one professional should take the lead role and act as the patient's key worker during the episode of care. The distress needs to be acknowledged and space must be given for the patient and/or family to regain control. To facilitate this, the cause of the distress should be explored. The "cues" to this may need to be "picked up" from the patient. Once the background and the triggers have been understood, a plan can be negotiated. Many crises arise because the patient and/or family feel trapped, with no control and with no choices and options. Any physical and practical input required should be provided in order to

reduce concerns and facilitate a sense of control over the situation. Discussing options that they themselves have not considered can diminish distress. Follow-up is essen-tial to review the situation, to devise a plan, which can be modified when necessary, and to explore any unresolved issues. A sense of security for the patient and family and also trust in the professional team are important thera-peutic components.

Adapting to bereavement

Many people possess sufficient inner resources to move through bereavement. Social networks are the main source of support for most people, and many report that they do not need formal bereavement support services. Need for formal bereavement support is associated with the avail-ability of social support and nature of the death. For some people the emotional challenge can be exacting and a risk to health. Bereavement is associated with excess risk of mortality, increased use of health service, and subsequent worse mental and physical health [45]. This observation has encouraged some health workers to develop patterns of care for the bereaved, most noticeably within the hos-pice movement [46] and voluntary sector.

Bereavement support is a fundamental aspect of pal-liative care and end-of-life care. All care staff need to understand the reactions of loss and grief, so that they may provide appropriate support to families. All those who are recently bereaved need to be provided with prac-tical information including insight into typical emotions and experiences and clear signposting to accessing sup-port services if they are needed. Bereavement should not be over medicalised, but there must be provision of spe-cialised services for those who are struggling [45].

Psychological theories on bereavement

It might be tempting to view bereavement as a variant of depression and anxiety, but doing so would ignore the separate literature that enables us to understand more clearly the processes and emotions involved.

Freud's influential work [47] described grief as a period of time where the reality of a death is repeatedly tested until attachment is withdrawn from the deceased. Although complete withdrawal is advocated by Freud, in reality individuals find means of coping with their loss by, for example, finding an inner place to "shelve" their attach-ment or memories while attending to other business. From observations made of bereaved people, Lindemann [48] describes five subgroups of grief symptoms: somatic distress, preoccupation with images of the deceased, guilt, hostility, and activity that appears restless and meaningless.

Bowlby, building on his psychoanalytical theories on attachment and loss, developed a four-stage model for bereavement [49]. It is important to apply this model flexibly and to recognise that individuals move back and forth between stages. The phases are described as:

1. Phase of numbing
2. Phase of yearning and searching
3. Phase of disorganisation and despair
4. Phase of reorganisation.

The suggestion from Bowlby's theory is that only where there is an attachment bond will loss be experienced. It is also correct to suggest that the deeper or stronger the bond is, the more intense the loss that is felt.

William Worden formulated a task-based approach to bereavement [50]. He described grief as a process, not a state, and suggested that people need to work through their reactions to grief in order to make a complete adjustment. According to Worden's "tasks of bereavement," grief is considered to consist of four overlapping tasks, requiring the person who has experienced bereavement to work through the emotional pain of their loss, while at the same time adjusting to changes in their circumstances, roles, status, and identity. The tasks are said to be completed when the bereaved person has integrated the loss into their life and "let go" of the emotional attachments to the deceased, thus allowing them to invest in the present and the future [51].

Stroebe and Schut [52] developed their ideas as a challenge to the dominant emotion—focus of previous theories of grief and proposed the Dual Process Model of Coping with Grief. This theory describes a process where the person who has been bereaved may oscillate between two orientations, loss and restoration (see Figure 7.2). Individuals oscillate as they grapple with the emotional consequences of their loss and the adjustment to the changed day-to-day reality of their lives.

Drawing from empirical and anthropological observations, Walter [53] has proposed that people who have been bereaved need to talk about the person who has died in order to construct a "durable" biography that is meaningful, reflecting both positive and negative aspects of the relationship that they had with them and that they can integrate into their ongoing lives. This allows the creation of a new identity that includes the persistent and usually unobtrusive memory of the deceased. This contrasts with models that suggested a task of bereavement was to forge a life without such integration of the person that had died.

A similar important development in grief theory has been provided by the work of Klass et al. [54] who also suggested that the purpose of grieving was not to break the bonds with the person who has died, but rather to maintain a continuing, healthy attachment to the individual, which can be seen as compatible with other new and continuing relationships.

A contemporary model of grief explores and identifies the spectrum of diverse reactions which are triggered by loss. This model, the Range of Response to Loss (RRL) [55,56] proposes that core grief reactions occur in immediate response to loss and fall within a range from "**overwhelmed**," where emotions dominate and may be disabling to "**controlled**" where emotions are avoided. A second range of responses occurs as people begin to actively engage in coping with the consequences of their loss. Initially bereavement is likely to generate a sense of "**vulnerability**" in most people as they experience the powerlessness of loss. Vulnerability may persist where there is **limited personal capacity** to deal with loss and change, for example, difficulty in dealing with stress, physical, or emotional problems, etc. where there are other **circumstantial stresses**, for example, ongoing caring responsibilities, financial/employment/housing problems, etc., or **limited social support**. As personal inner resources gain strength "**resilience**" becomes more evident. Qualities of flexibility, courage, perseverance, hope, finding meaning, setting new life goals, and making good use of social support, contribute to a growing capacity to accept the loss and effectively manage its consequences. The two dimensions of grief response in the RRL model—core grief and coping response—have been used diagrammatically as a matrix and used as the basis for assessing bereavement need in palliative care contexts [57,58].

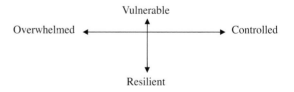

It is important to remember when thinking of the losses associated with the dying process that patients, their families, and professionals will all be managing some aspect of their own grief, and this will influence the triadic relationship between them and thus the quality of care provided [58].

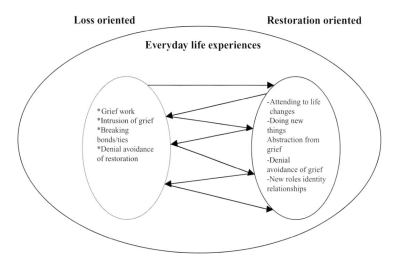

Loss oriented   **Restoration oriented**

Figure 7.2 A dual process model of coping with grief [52].

While theories and models can guide us, we have to accept the individuality of each bereaved person. Grief creates chaos in the world of the bereaved person, and people will try and bring some order to their own chaos in their own time.

Consequences of bereavement

There has been considerable research into the adverse health consequences of bereavement [59,60]. Studies have attempted to confirm the lay theory that patients can die of a "broken heart." In fact this has been very hard to prove, but it is probably true that people who have been bereaved are at greater risk of death themselves, although this risk remains low in absolute terms. Other work has examined the psychiatric morbidity following bereavement. This research has been difficult to perform, but it seems to suggest that the bereaved are at risk of the following complications:

• Depression
• Anxiety
• Alcohol abuse
• Increased use of prescribed drugs
• Suicidal tendencies and behaviour.

Complicated bereavement

The boundary between the normal emotions of grief and those exaggerated responses that would constitute complicated grief has been the subject of considerable debate. For severe psychiatric disease, the notion of "abnormality" is straightforward (like suicidal activity, alcohol abuse). However, for less severe affective disorders such as depression, anxiety, it could be said that the symptoms fall within the normal range of grief responses. Various

authors have proposed means to differentiate the normal from the abnormal or the more helpfully termed "complicated" grief. Duration of extreme or unhelpful emotional responses has been suggested as a useful, if arbitrary, discriminator. Unfortunately, no consensus appears to have been agreed upon and times ranging from 2 to over 12 months have been suggested [59,60].

Other research has concerned itself with describing symptoms that combine to produce particular bereavement syndromes (Table 7.2). It is hoped that in defining new conditions in this way, clinicians will be able to develop care for those bereaved individuals who present with particular problems [61].

Table 7.2 Examples of complicated bereavement reactions.

Absent
Individuals show no evidence of the emotions of grief developing, despite the reality of the death. This can appear as an automatic reaction or the result of active blocking

Delayed
This initially presents in a similar way to absent grief. However, this avoidance is always a conscious effort and the full emotions of grief are eventually expressed after a particular trigger. This may be seen in more compulsively self-reliant individuals

Chronic
In this instance, the normal emotions of grief persist without any diminution over time. It is postulated that this is most often seen in relationships that were particularly dependent

---

Box 7.2 Risk factors for pathological bereavement

- Younger age
- Poor social support
- Sudden death
- Previous poor physical health
- Previous mental illness
- Poor coping strategies
- Multiple losses
- Stigmatised death
- Economic difficulties
- Previous unresolved grief

Assessment of bereavement needs

As in other aspects of palliative care, accurate assessment is a necessary part of management. This could be performed by any member of the MDT and is best achieved by someone with the following attributes:

- Good communication skills to facilitate expression of emotion.
- An ability to screen for psychiatric disease (e.g., depression, anxiety, suicidal intent).
- Familiarity with events surrounding death.
- An understanding of the social background.
- An awareness of risk factors of pathological grief (see Box 7.2).

The routine use of risk assessment tools is of some value. The ability to accurately appraise a person's level of vulnerability should target help to those most in need and those most likely to benefit. But there is a concern about the ability of such tools to accurately predict the need for support. They are most useful if combined with informal assessment. Melliar-Smith describes the development and practical use of a risk assessment tool for bereavement, which is adaptable to various palliative care settings [62]. Linked with the RRL model is the Adult Attitude to Grief (AAG) scale, a nine-item self-report measure, used to explore the way grief is experienced by individuals. The scale has been modified for use prebereavement, with young people and for losses other than bereavement. Research is currently being undertaken to validate the use of the AAG scale to calculate the level of vulnerability manifest in grieving people.

Other needs should also be considered when assessing people who have been bereaved. These include social needs, that is, the social consequences of a bereavement that may need attention, and in some circumstances, there are also physical needs; for example, where a death results

---

Box 7.3 Elements of the three-component model of bereavement support [13]

Component 1:	Grief is normal after bereavement and most people manage without professional intervention.
	All bereaved people should be offered information about the experience of bereavement and how to access other forms of support, for example, leaflet.
Component 2:	Some people may require a more formal opportunity to review and reflect on their loss experience.
	Volunteer bereavement support workers, self-help groups, faith groups, and community groups provide much of the support at this level.
Component 3:	A minority of people will require specialist interventions.
	This will involve mental health services, psychological support services, specialist counselling/psychotherapy services, specialist palliative care services, and general bereavement services.

---

in unmet nursing needs in the bereaved person, for example, in the case of an elderly couple.

Management of bereavement needs

Although there are known adverse health consequences of bereavement, many bereaved individuals adapt to their loss with minimal assistance from health-care professionals. Indeed, there are potential dangers in overmedicating grief. For instance, bereavement can promote emotional growth within individuals and families. However, accurate assessment of risk remains the key component of appropriate bereavement management [63].

The Supportive and Palliative Care Guidelines for England and Wales outline a three-component model of bereavement support, which it recommends should be implemented in each Cancer Network (Box 7.3) [13].

Bereavement services

As a result of the assessment, it may be necessary to provide some emotional support. This could involve brief intervention by the professional making the assessment or by using the array of bereavement services available. The services listed below do not include the very important help provided by religious advisers, but focus more on the work of health professionals and allied workers. Besides the bereavement services, various communities have developed social groups designed to overcome loneliness.

Written information

For those with low risk, providing written information may be all that is needed. This could range from pamphlets on where to get help should problems arise, to practical guides on what to do after a death and self-help books that normalise the bereavement process. Story books can be particularly helpful when explaining death to children (see www.bbc.co.uk/radio4/gfi/bestbits/bereavement.shtml, e.g., Badgers Parting Gifts by Susan Varley and Waterbugs and Dragonflies by Doris Stickney).

Primary care team

The involvement of family physicians in bereavement support promotes continuity of care. This could include such things as a bereavement visit, brief emotional support, referral to practice counsellor, use of psychotropic drugs, or the involvement of other services. The key worker may have an ongoing supportive role for some time and should assess the need for referral to other agencies.

Specialist palliative care services

The hospice movement has seen bereavement care as integral to its service and has adopted a proactive approach. In some instances, these teams are considered as specialists within this field. They can provide an array of services, including one-to-one support, telephone contact, written information, anniversary letters, social activities, group work, and memorial services [46]. In general, trained volunteers who are supervised by hospice staff perform this work.

Voluntary services

In the United Kingdom the main voluntary service is CRUSE Bereavement Care. This national organisation takes referrals from any source and can provide one-to-one or group work. It is staffed by trained volunteers and functions with a system of formal supervision. They prefer to take self-referrals and are contactable by phone. The experience of some volunteers makes them able to tackle complex bereavement reactions. Other organisations can provide support for parents who have lost a child (e.g., Compassionate Friends).

Hospital-based services

Most hospitals in the United Kingdom have bereavement officers to assist with certain aspects of the arrangements following the death of an in-patient. Some departments provide other aspects of support for particular bereavements:
- Some emergency departments have a role following sudden deaths brought to them.
- Midwives or maternity units may provide support to their patients who suffer loss.
- Intensive care units may have well-developed bereavement support pathways.

In addition, psychiatric teams are involved in the more damaging bereavement reactions, particularly those resulting in major psychiatric illness.

Funeral directors

Some funeral directors are beginning to consider bereavement support as part of their service.

Bereavement counselling/therapy

Supporting the bereaved involves the application of the communication skills outlined in Chapter 6 in this book (e.g., active listening, empathy, clarification). Specialist authors have gone further and formulated approaches that provide greater guidance on bereavement counselling, either as general principles or in particular situations. Generally these have been based on the concept of "grief work," of which Worden's book has been the most influential [50]. He suggests that it is helpful to separate counselling (helping people facilitate normal grief) from therapy (specialist techniques that help with complicated grief). Central to his approach is the need for the bereaved to work through the four "tasks of mourning" (see Table 7.3).

This model has recently been criticised for not allowing denial as a valid coping mechanism for some people, lacking evidence of effectiveness, and for inconsistencies in

Table 7.3 Worden's four tasks of mourning [50].

Task 1	To accept the reality of the loss
Task 2	To work through the pain of grief
Task 3	To adjust to the environment in which the deceased is missing
Task 4	To emotionally relocate the deceased and move on with life

regards to cross-cultural or historical perspectives. While this theoretical controversy continues, readers may find some of Worden's suggestions helpful.

Summary

Death, dying, and bereavement often challenge the fundamental values and meaning of the human experience. Such a threat has the potential to provoke considerable distress and has therefore interested health professionals. This has considerable implications for the work of healthcare professionals. Likewise, guidelines for palliative care and end-of-life care specify the need for bereavement care and specific services [13,21].

It is important while providing care that we do not lose sight of the individual patient involved and the individuality of each experience of dying, death, and bereavement. This chapter has detailed some of the literature on this subject with an aim to improve understanding of the process involved and the role of professionals in providing care as well as the recognition of grief and bereavement as a normal and expected part of the human experience.

References

1. Heidegger M. *Being and Time*. New York: Harper & Row, 1927.
2. Tomer A, Eliason G and Wong PTP. *Existential and Spiritual Issues in Death Attitudes*. Mahwah: Lawrence Erlbaum Associates, 2008.
3. Parkes CM. Bereavement as a psychosocial transition: process adaptation and change. In: Dickinson D and Johnson M (eds), *Death, Dying and Bereavement*. London: Sage, 1978.
4. Christian JL. *Philosophy: An Introduction to the Art of Wondering*, 11th edition. Boston: Wadsworth, 2012.
5. Kastenbaum R and Aisenberg R. *The Psychology of Death*, 3rd edition. New York: Springer Publishing Company, 2000.
6. Kellehear A (ed.). *The Study of Dying: From Autonomy to Transformation*. Cambridge: Cambridge University Press, 2009.
7. Neimeyer RA. *Death Anxiety Handbook*. Washington DC: Taylor and Francis, 2004.
8. Abdel-Khalek AM. Death anxiety in clinical and non-clinical groups. *Death Studies* 2005; 29: 251–259.
9. Nyatanga B. *Why is it so Difficult to Die?* 2nd edition. Wiltshire: Quay Books, 2001.
10. Diggory J and Rothman D. Values destroyed by death. *J Abnorm Soc Psychol* 1961; 63(1): 205–210.
11. Chonon J. *Death and the Modern Man*. New York, NY: Macmillan, 1974.
12. Pattison EM. The living-dying process. In: Garfield CA (ed.), *Psychosocial Care of the Dying Patient*. New York, NY: McGraw-Hill, 1978.
13. National Institute for Clinical Excellence. *Improving Outcomes for Palliative and Supportive Care*. London: NICE, 2004.
14. Boyd K and Murray SA. Recognizing and managing key transitions in end of life care. *BMJ* 2010; 341: c4863.
15. Pinnock H, Kendall M, Murray SA, et al. Living and dying with severe chronic obstructive pulmonary disease: multiperspective longitudinal qualitative study. *BMJ* 2011; 342: d142.
16. Richardson A, Tebbit P, Sitzia J, et al. *Common Assessment of Supportive and Palliative Care Needs for Adults with Cancer: Assessment Guidance*. London: Department of Health, 2007.
17. Holistic needs assessment for people with cancer: a practical guide for healthcare professionals. National cancer action Team. Available at: http://www.ncat.nhs.uk/our-work/living-with-beyond-cancer/holistic-needs-assessment (accessed on November 4, 2011).
18. *NCCN Clinical Practice Guidelines for supportive care. Distress Management V.1.2011* Available at: http://www.nccn.org/professionals/physician_gls/PDF/distress.pdf (accessed on March 25, 2007).
19. Mitchell AJ, Baker-Glenn EA, Granger L, et al. Can the distress thermometer be improved by additional mood domains? Part I. Initial validation of the Emotion Thermometers tool. *Psychooncology* 2010; 19: 125–133.
20. Kaufman W. *Existentialism, Religion and Death: Thirteen Essays*. New York: New American Library, 1976.
21. Department of Health. *End of Life Care Strategy*. London: Department of Health, 2008.
22. Hunt J, Cobb M, Keeley VL, et al. The quality of spiritual care-developing a standard. *Int J Palliat Nurs* 2003; 9(5): 208–215.
23. Bingley AF, et al. Making sense of dying: a review of narratives written since 1950 by people facing death from cancer and other diseases. *Palliat Med* 2006; 20: 183.
24. Petrone M. *The emotional cancer journey*. Available at: http://www.mapfoundation.org/exhib.suff/forward.html (accessed on April 2, 2011).
25. Kubler-Ross E. *On Death and Dying*, 40th anniversary edition. Abingdon: Routledge, 2009.
26. Glaser BG and Strauss AL. *Awareness of Dying*. Chicago, IL: Adeline, 1965.
27. Timmermans S. Dying awareness: the theory of awareness revisited. *Sociol Health Ill* 1994; 16: 322–337.
28. Glaser BG and Strauss AL. *Time for Dying*. Chicago, IL: Adeline, 1968.
29. Greer S. Psychological response to cancer and survival. *Pyschol Med* 1991; 21: 43–49.
30. Copp G. Patients' and nurses' constructions of death and dying in a hospice setting. *J Cancer Nurisng* 1997; 1: 2–15.

31. Noyes R and Clancy J. The dying role: its relevance to improved patient care. In: Corr CA and Corr D (eds), *Hospice Care—Principles and Practice*. London: Faber & Faber, 1983.

32. Parkes CM. Bereavement as a psychosocial transition: process adaptation and change. In: Dickinson D and Johnson M (eds), *Death, Dying and Bereavement*. London: Sage, 1993.

33. Joyce P. Patrick the incurable optimist. Patricks Blog February 1, 2011. Available at: http://patricktheoptimist .org/?m=201102 (accessed on June 8, 2011).

34. Adelaide D. *The Household Guide to Dying*. Hammersmith: Harper, 2009

35. The Bucket List. Warner Brothers, 2007

36. Wainwright M. Jane Tomlinson: obituary. *The Guardian*, September 5, 2007, p. 38

37. Rinpoche S. *The Tibetan Book of Living and Dying*. London: Rider & CO, 2008

38. Clark D. Total pain: the work of Cicely Saunders and the hospice movement. *Am Pain Soc Bull* 2000; 10: 4.

39. Robson A, Scrutton F, Wilkinson L, et al. The risk of suicide in cancer patients: a review of the literature. *Psychooncology* 2010; 19: 1250–1258.

40. Vachon MLS. The emotional problems of the patient in palliative medicine. In: Hanks G, Cherny NI, Christakis NA, Fallon M, Kaasa S, Russell K and Portenoy RK (eds), *The Oxford Textbook of Palliative Medicine*, 4th edition. Oxford: Oxford University Press, 2010.

41. Davy J and Ellis S. *Counseling Skills in Palliative Care*. Buckingham: Open University Press, 2000.

42. Stedford A. *Facing Death*, 2nd edition. Oxford: Sobell Publications, 1994.

43. Panke JT and Ferrell BR. The family perspective. In: Hanks G, Cherny NI, Christakis NA, Fallon M, Kaasa S, Russell K and Portenoy RK (eds), *The Oxford Textbook of Palliative Medicine*, 4th edition. Oxford: Oxford University Press, 2010.

44. Lloyd-Williams M. *Psychosocial Issues in Palliative Care*, 2nd edition. Oxford: Oxford University Press, 2008.

45. Arthur T, et al. *Bereavement Care Services: A Synthesis of the Literature*. London: DH, 2010.

46. Payne S and Relf M. The assessment of need for bereavement follow up in palliative and hospice care. *Palliat Med* 1994; 8: 291–297.

47. Freud S. Mourning and melancholia. In: *Collected Papers Vol IV*. London: Hogarth Press, 1925.

48. Lindemann E. Symptomatology and the management of acute grief. *Am J Psych* 1944; 101: 141–148.

49. Bowlby J. *Loss: Sadness and Depression (Attachment and Loss)*, Vol. 3. New York, NY: Basic Books, 1980.

50. Worden JW. *Grief Counselling and Grief Therapy*. London: Routledge, 1992.

51. Dent A. Supporting the bereaved: theory and practice. *Healthc Counsell Psychother J* 2005; 5: 16–19.

52. Stroebe M and Schut, H. The dual process model of coping with bereavement: rationale and description. *Death Studies* 1999; 23: 197–224.

53. Walter T. A new model for grief: bereavement and biography. *Mortality* 1996; 1: 7–25.

54. Klass D, Silverman PR and Nickman, SL (eds). *Continuing Bonds: New Understandings of Grief*. Washington, DC: Taylor and Francis, 1996.

55. Machin L. Exploring a Framework for Understanding the Range of Response to Loss: A Study of Clients Receiving Bereavement Counselling. Unpublished PhD Thesis. Keele University, 2001.

56. Machin L. *Working with Loss and Grief*. London: Sage, 2009.

57. Relf M, Machin L and Archer N. *Guidance for Bereavement Needs Assessment in Palliative Care*. London: Help the Hospices, 2008.

58. Machin L Loss responses at the end of life; a conceptual reflection. *End of Life Care* 2010; 4(1): 46–52.

59. Woof WR and Carter YH. The grieving adult and the general practitioner; a literature review in two parts (part 1). *Br J Gen Pract* 1997; 47: 443–448.

60. Woof WR and Carter YH. The grieving adult and the general practitioners: a literature review in two parts (part 2). *Br J Gen Pract* 1997; 47: 509–514.

61. Middleton W, Moylan A, Raphael B, et al An international perspective on bereavement and related concepts. *Aus NZ J Psych* 1993; 27: 457–463.

62. Melliar-Smith C. The risk assessment of bereavement in a palliative care setting. *Int J Palliat Nurs* 2002; 8(6): 281–287.

63. Parkes CM. Bereavement counselling—does it work? *BMJ* 1980; 281: 3–10.

Acknowledgments. We acknowledge the work of Brian Nyatanga and Richard Woof for the previous editions of this chapter and Linda Machin for her contribution concerning the RRL model.

8 Advance Care Planning

Richard Wong

University Hospital of Leicester NHS Trust, Leicester, UK

Introduction

In our modern society, socioeconomic and medical advances have contributed to increases in life expectancy but have also changed the nature of death and dying and an increasing proportion of people are living with progressive disease burden and dependency. Advance care planning (ACP) is a process, whereby within this context, individuals can discuss and prepare for their care in the event of future decisional incapacity, usually with input from health-care or other professionals [1]. It has become associated predominantly with the refusal of specific medical technologies (e.g., not wishing to have assisted ventilation) in advance of a loss of capacity. To limit its remit to such narrow practice however, would be to underestimate the scope and potential of ACP and also to misunderstand the key principles of the process.

A medical model of ACP, where medical information alone is given and medical decisions alone are made, lacks sufficient utility for individuals and their families. ACP should additionally include exploring an individual's general understanding of what end-of-life events may entail and what their hopes or fears may be for this time, giving them an opportunity to discover more information about their condition(s), reflect on their concerns and look at their life values in the context of all of this.

The ACP process supports a holistic practice of multidirectional communication between patients, those in close relationship to them and those professionally involved in care for them.

> The important principle is that patient involvement in any decision-making process is maximised, be it when they lose capacity or when they still have it.

For the majority of people, planning for the end-of-life scenario (which pertains to the "final *phase*" of a person's life and can last weeks, months, or even longer, as opposed to just the terminal few *days* of life) is not something at the forefront of their consciousness. Even if it was, most people would know very little about the anticipated natural history of their own decline and dying, what care could or could not be provided in different health-care settings, the mechanisms of various medical interventions, benefits, and success rates of such things as cardiopulmonary resuscitation (CPR) and the implications of dying in a nursing home, a hospice, an acute hospital bed, or an intensive care unit. Therefore, through a process of ACP, professionals can be a support and resource to individuals, informing and empowering them with a degree of choice over health-care matters.

Three notable drivers to the evolution of ACP are:

1. **Medical progress** may have contributed to populations living longer and generally in better health, but there is a feeling that new medical technologies have also blurred the distinction between saving life and prolonging suffering.

2. **Autonomy** for the individual has become a much-vaunted societal value. In the medical context, this has shifted decision making from paternalistic to self-determined with an emphasis on patient information, patient choice, and informed decision making. The complex nature of "informed consent," especially in relation to modern medical management, requires a significant input from health professionals to guide and counsel patients through such processes. In practice, the much desired individual autonomy is rarely "patient-exclusive" but is in effect a "relational autonomy," reflecting the decisions made in relation to the social, cultural, medical, and health context of the individual [2].

3. **Trust**, a key component of the doctor–patient relationship, has arguably seen some degree of erosion due to various stressors. Health-care organisations and professionals

Handbook of Palliative Care, Third Edition. Edited by Christina Faull, Sharon de Caestecker, Alex Nicholson and Fraser Black.
© 2012 by John Wiley and Sons, Inc. Published 2012 by John Wiley & Sons, Inc.

may come under suspicion from the general public over standards of care, fuelled by high-profile media coverage of medical negligence cases, medical misconduct, and unlawful practice. On the contrary, health professionals may also develop wariness for their patients, particularly related to anxiety over medico-legal litigation that may perversely drive patient care in nonbeneficial or even deleterious directions.

The legislation and guidance surrounding ACP differs between countries and jurisdictions within countries. This chapter draws specifically on the legal framework for ACP in England and Wales [3] to illustrate and discuss principles, which are generally applicable.

Terminology and definitions

There are three possible ways of formally stating an individual's position:
1. **Advance Statements** indicate an individual's preferences for care; they are not legally binding. In the United States, this may be known as a values history.
2. **Refusals of Treatment** that may be legally binding. In England and Wales, the advance decision to refuse treatment (ADRT) is a legally binding record of informed consent for withholding or withdrawal of certain treatments, including life-sustaining measures, under particular health scenarios. For the withholding or withdrawal of life-sustaining measures, the records must be in writing and signed by both the individual and a witness and include the term *"even if my life is at risk."*
3. **Proxies for health-care decisions** may be appointed. Such surrogate decision makers are known in England and Wales as Lasting Powers of Attorney for Health and Welfare. Elsewhere these may be known as Welfare Powers of Attorney (Scotland); Durable Powers of Attorney for Health care (Australia, Canada, and United States), or Representatives (Canada). These appointments may pertain to decision making for health and welfare and/or financial matters. Where appointments are made for health and welfare decisions, there will usually be a requirement to assign specific decision-making rights over life-sustaining measures.

The rationale and evidence for ACP

ACP will not be desirable or beneficial to everyone facing declining health but nonetheless should always be considered by the care team. Yet it is not unusual for health-care professionals to overestimate the prognosis or underes-timate the planning needed as an illness progresses. For the practitioner, discomfort may be felt at the prospect of raising end-of-life care issues and particularly planning for end-of-life care with patients [4]. Intuitively it may seem an unpalatable proposition to make, but surveys actually suggest the contrary; that although most people have not discussed how they would like to die, they would actually want to be told if they were dying [5].

Does ACP confer benefits to the individual?

The main intention of ACP is to increase an individual's control and planning over their future (and particularly end-of-life) care, maximising the chance for empowerment in situations that are often chaotic and subject to medical paternalism. Most studies have originated from North American or Australia with a paucity of data relating to the effectiveness of ACP in the United Kingdom. Geographical differences in health and social care infrastructure and public acceptance of such processes, as well as methodological variations between studies, make it difficult to understand the direct impact of ACP but some general observations can be made:

• Importantly, documentation of ACP per se does not necessarily lead to a reduction in medical over-intervention during the end-of-life period, particularly if the records lack adequate clarity and detail on specifying the type of care and treatment or if they had not been communicated with others [6].

• The most consistent demonstration of benefit from ACP has come from its inception in long-term care facilities with nursing, or in residential facilities that were well supported by regular specialist (geriatrician) medical input. In this setting, it has been shown to reduce rates of acute hospitalisation and use of hospital-bed days [7,8]. More recently, the practice of undertaking ACP in a hospital environment has also been shown to improve concordance with an individual's prior wishes [9].

• A key benefit of ACP seems to be its ability to improve communication, an opportunity to reflect with patients on their current health, ongoing medical conditions, and future concerns. This has been shown to give patients a sense of empowerment over their care and also a sense of hope, by acting as a therapeutic and preparatory step to the future end-of-life period [10].

• Contrary to initial concerns, ACP discussions have been shown to be acceptable to patients from a wide variety of health and age backgrounds, promoting increased satisfaction with overall care largely through the aforementioned effects of enhanced communication [7–9,11,12].

Does ACP benefit caregivers and carers?

Although it seeks primarily to deliver benefits to the individual, advantages may arise for other parties involved in care for the individual, typically the health and social care professionals (CPs) and also family and close friends. Once a patient has lost decisional capacity, the presence of an Advance Statement, or something similar, might guide health professionals in determining with greater certainty, the "best interests" of a patient in a given situation. Similarly for caregivers, family, and friends, there is the potential benefit of being prepared for the situation due to prior anticipation of events and planning of care.

The indications are that guidance for health-care professionals and confidence in their decision making can be enhanced by the presence of an ACP under the appropriate circumstances. There are however provisos for this:

• The detail and specificity within the plan will determine the degree of direction that is given and the confidence of the professional in interpreting this [6,13].
• The practical application of ACP also requires investment in education and training to improve the interpretation of these documents by health-care professionals [13].

Where informal caregivers and family members are concerned, there is consensus that ACP can alleviate anxiety, depression, and reduce bereavement stress following the loss of a loved one [14]. This stressful period is sometimes exacerbated by the decision-making burden that is often incumbent upon family or significant carers in the end-of-life situation. Such burdens may be ameliorated by the opportunity to improve all round communication between patients, their informal carers, and medical professionals, particularly as these are areas of discussion that sometimes go unexplored or are perceived as taboo, even between those in close relationships.

Content of an ACP discussion

Each ACP conversation will be tailored to the individual. For many people, an important aspect is the opening up of conversations with their loved ones or those with a significant relationship. This might include discussing any deeply held values and beliefs and subjects that are often taboo, even in close, intimate relationships, such as thoughts about death and the value of life. Similarly, in conjunction with their physician, nurse, or other mem-

bers of their care team, it is an opportunity to reflect on their illness/condition and to voice any fears, concerns, or uncertainties. Some of this will involve expanding an understanding of the illness, particularly looking at its natural history; it might even entail an appreciation of prognosis. Possible treatments and management strategies might also be included in these discussions.

Even small conversations can build toward the jigsaw of care planning, especially if they are communicated (such as through referral letters to specialists, shared case manager annotations/letters or hospital discharge letters). It is impossible to anticipate all potential events and possible treatments, but after discussion with health-care professionals, someone who has gone through the ACP process should have a good idea of what *key* life-sustaining interventions entail: what CPR does and how well it works, what is involved in artificial feeding, and (if an appropriate potential event) what happens in an intensive care unit. Finally, a skilled discussion will attempt to weave this information within the context of the patient's beliefs, values, culture, and experience, arriving at an idea of what constitutes "best interests" for that patient. The key issues often encountered in such ACP discussions are summarised in Box 8.1.

Undertaking ACP discussions

ACP is a process and will often involve multiple discussions between patients and care providers. The response to introducing the discussion is subject to wide variations between cultural groups and individuals. Indeed, ACP is not for everyone and the conversations should never be forced. Nonetheless, opportunity should be given, and it should be entered into the understanding that it will often take time and should not be hurried. As an approximate guide, one study showed these discussions could take an average of 60 min altogether spread over two to three separate meetings [9]. In reality this is an organic process with the discussions frequently being informed by piecemeal conversations between patient and CP that take place along the patient journey.

People need time to understand, reflect, and discuss the elements of ACP, and then a number of conversations may be needed to help someone understand the practical implications of their choices. It is helpful to conceptualise discussions as progressing through stages of *considering*, *discussing*, and *planning* end-of-life care [15]. If there are barriers to progress, one might recognise or attempt to identify an individual's stage in this process

Box 8.1 Key components of ACP discussions

With support from health-care professionals, the person making an ACP may do the following:

- Attain a fuller understanding of their condition(s), possibly including prognosis, providing the health-care professional has explored and assessed their desire to understand the current health situation.
- Discuss and develop an awareness of the disease trajectory of their condition(s) (e.g., cancer may result in progressive loss of appetite and weight. Dementia may progress to not only worsen intellectual function but also decline physical attributes such as mobility, continence, and swallowing). Through this there may be an anticipation of certain key problems.
- Consider the need for further assessments and investigations, exploring any benefits versus potential detrimental effects or disadvantages to well-being (physical or mental).
- Explore their feelings on health-care management (both current and future), appraising the various options for care and treatment of their particular condition(s).
- Learn about possible medical treatments for the very ill and their implications, through structured discussions with the health-care team and other resources (e.g., artificial ventilation, nutritional support, hydration, and CPR).
- Consider what makes their life meaningful and under what circumstances the burdens of treatment would outweigh any benefits that the treatment offers.
- Contemplate how treatment choices would reflect their values, culture, beliefs, and goals. From this they may decide whether they would want future management to focus on comfort care rather than life-sustaining or prolonging measures and at what stage of the illness such a strategy should be implemented. Related to this, the health-care professional can help elaborate options for alternative care, for example, hospice-at-home, community palliative care, and intermediate care teams.
- Choose someone to act as a substitute decision maker if the time comes when they cannot make their own medical decisions. Opportunity should be given to discuss these choices with those closest to them and in particular with those who might be called upon to make health-care decisions for them in the event of incapacity.
- Make a record of the conversations in the form of an ACP. This should be circulated to the medical records and relevant care providers.
- Agree to a process for periodic review and updating of the ACP.

Box 8.2 Key requirements for ACP discussions

- The patient has adequate mental capacity for discussions.
- A mood disorder has been excluded.
- The patient's comfort has been optimised (mental and physical).
- Any sensory impairment has been optimised.
- The practitioner has good communication skills.
- The practitioner exhibits sensitivity (to verbal and nonverbal cues).
- Adequate time is provided for unhurried discussions.

and understand the impediments to progression. Postponing or ceasing discussions may certainly be entirely appropriate in this context. Undue focus should not be given to the completion of formal documents per se, which are not necessarily associated with improvements in patient–physician communication or other outcomes [6]. On the contrary, there is a suggestion that the mere act of having these conversations and of stimulating a change in culture toward end-of-life care could lead to genuine changes in the care approach for such individuals at a time of future decline [8]. The important ingredients for ACP conversations are summarised in Box 8.2.

Who should undertake ACP?

The generic requirements for ACP are good communication skills, sensitivity, and responsiveness to patient cues (verbal and nonverbal). Consequently, ACP discussions may be carried out not only by doctors but also by other CPs such as specialist nurses and social workers. Circumstances may dictate who is best placed to coordinate any ACP discussions, and in some cases, there is also a role for unqualified care workers, the voluntary sector and independent advocacy services to participate in discussions. Occasionally discussions take place solely within a family or social network. This is usually assisted by written or "online" materials to facilitate such discussion, planning, and self-determination.

Ideally, an ACP facilitator should possess knowledge relating to the condition(s) suffered by a patient, so that questions regarding the natural history of the illness and prognosis can be met with informed answers. In turn, this is important for shaping patient choice and preferences for care. In practice, given the increasing complexity of medical diagnostics and treatments, the whole process may involve discussions with a range of professionals to benefit from the knowledge offered by each group, with the facilitator acting as a lynchpin in coordinating these inputs.

When and where should ACP be undertaken?

Given the sensitive nature of ACP and its associated conversations, it is unsurprising that health professionals might desire or expect their patients to be the initiators of such discussions. Although patient initiation of such dialogue does occur, it is not the norm. The concept of ACP is alien to most lay people, and patients largely expect such conversations to be introduced by their physician. Indeed, the indications are that patients are actually open to discussions at an earlier stage of their illness than clinicians anticipate [16].

The timing of ACP discussions can be prompted by a number of clinical triggers that are summarised in Box 8.3. Thus as well as direct patient initiation, there may be clinical prognostic indicators of advanced disease for a number of medical conditions; guidance on applying these may be obtained from resources such as the Gold Standards Framework (GSF) [17] or the National Health Service (NHS) Lothian guidelines shown in Chapter 1, *The context and principles of palliative care*. Such indicators allow for a structured assessment of prognosis in a number of categories of chronic disease (cancer, heart failure [HF], chronic obstructive pulmonary disease [COPD], renal failure, motor neurone disease [MND], Parkinson's disease [PD], stroke, dementia, and frailty) according to physical, functional and investigational parameters. Although these tools might point to a particular condition being in an *advanced* stage or suggest that an individual might possibly be in their final year of life, it should

be emphasised to individuals that prognostication is an inherently difficult and often inaccurate process.

A professional's intuition regarding prognosis can sometimes be a more operational form of determining the appropriate timing for ACP discussions, when the practitioner "would not be surprised" if survival did not extend beyond the next 6–12 months [17]. Consistent with this, it was shown in a hospice setting that unqualified nursing assistants were accurate at predicting prognosis in this fashion, probably because they often had a close relationship with patients and a more intimate understanding of the impact of illness on them [18]. Especially in the non-cancer groups of conditions, there is a practical benefit of changing thinking toward this more instinctive, and anticipatory thinking, rather than purely predicting the likely timescale.

Ensuring the individual is comfortable, both physically and emotionally, is a key priority before commencing ACP discussions. For in-patients, physical comfort is more likely to be compromised and the chances of having just received distressing information regarding an illness are also higher, making them less ready to absorb and digest further information on matters such as ACP. Decisional capacity (see Box 8.4) may be similarly influenced by the effects of physical and/or mental stress as either may affect retention of information or drive the decision-making process in an uncharacteristic direction.

Box 8.3 Triggers to initiate discussions on end-of-life care and planning

1. *The surprise question*: "Would you be surprised if this patient were to die in the next 6–12 months?"—An intuitive question integrating comorbidity, likely illness trajectory, social and other factors.
2. *Patient choice/need*: The patient with advanced disease makes a choice for comfort care only, not "curative" or active treatment, for example, refusing renal transplant or dialysis.
3. *Clinical indicators*: Specific indicators of advanced disease for each of the three main end-of-life patient groups—cancer, organ failure, frail elderly/dementia (see Gold Standards Framework, Prognostic Indicator Guidance [14]).

Box 8.4 Mental capacity

As the intention of ACP is to provide guidance on care following loss of decisional capacity, it is implicit that the validity of ACP rests on an individual possessing adequate capacity to decide on these issues.

The decisions contemplated in ACP potentially carry great bearing on matters of life and death and consequently should result in extra care being taken over assessment of capacity before such discussions. It should not be assumed that someone with cognitive deficits is automatically incompetent to engage in ACP as capacity is decision-specific and might be present for certain decisions but not others. An individual will be deemed to have capacity if they:
- are able to understand the information given to them;
- are able to retain that information;
- are able to use and weigh the information to formulate a decision; and
- are able to communicate back that decision.

Adapted from GSF [14].

The location of the discussion per se is not the main issue but rather the fact that the timing of these discussions should not happen too close to an acute illness or new diagnosis, when patients are unwell or coming to terms with a condition, or if the person has just had a significant change in circumstances (e.g., moving into a new care home setting). There are, however, sometimes potential benefits of being in the surroundings of the acute hospital. An accessible clinician–patient relationship and an environmental context of death and illness (open awareness) may support the promotion of end-of-life discussions [19].

Preliminary arrangements before commencing ACP

In line with the aim of ensuring patient comfort (physical and mental) for ACP discussions, attention to the following areas should help enhance the process:

1. *Optimising the environment*

Every effort should be made to optimise the setting for conversations, giving consideration to privacy, comfort, adequate time for the discussions and measures to ensure that interruptions are minimised.

2. *Consider ancillary services*

Other agencies may be helpful in supporting ACP discussions, such as a professional interpretation service. These may require organising ahead of time. There should not be a dependence on family members for interpreting if at all possible. They may not understand medical terms precisely enough and consequently pass along inaccurate information to the patient. Secondly, their own views and the emotion of the situation may colour their translation of the discussion.

3. *Ensure the discussion group has the right composition and balance*

Some people will be comfortable meeting with several people at once (e.g., nurse, social worker, chaplaincy, and physician), while others may prefer to meet one-on-one with each professional, finding being faced with a team of people overwhelming. Similarly, some people may want to face their discussions alone while others may want to have one or more family members or perhaps a close friend to accompany them. Although one might advocate for having the whole team present for the discussion in order to facilitate questions and answers more efficiently, the decision in these matters should ultimately be given to the person who is the subject of the discussions.

In the context of facilitators, cultural considerations are particularly important, as people from some cultural backgrounds may be uncomfortable talking about their care with professionals of the opposite sex or may have more confidence talking to certain professional groups. The ultimate aim is to ensure as comfortable a relationship with the facilitator(s) as possible.

4. *Prior preparation on the person's medical problems, management options, and prognosis*

It is important to have an idea about what will be discussed and how the conversations will be opened. Usually a key component is a clear narrative on the patient's condition in addition to a professional view on the future management of any related health problems. To maximise sensitivity, it is preferable not to have to rely on continuous glancing at medical records; hence, preparation is important. Moreover, if there are anticipated topics of discussion that are beyond the knowledge of the facilitator(s), then every effort should be made to research and gain a specialist opinion on these areas beforehand, realising there may still be a need to refer for specialist advice later.

Initiating the discussions

Initiating ACP discussions presents certain challenges. Although understanding the illness and discussing it may engender empowerment and hope for the future, trepidation may accompany these discussions due to connotations that this is synonymous with "giving up." Forethought should be given on how to open conversations. A particular communication challenge is that it might be necessary to prompt the individual into contemplation of potential future uncertainty. The thrust of the discourse becomes one of "hoping for the best but preparing for the worst." The following are some suggestions of opening statements that may be helpful:

- For stable individuals but with advanced disease:

  Despite your medical problems, you are not doing too badly at the moment. Perhaps now is a good time to think a bit about the future in case things change with regard to your health. We could discuss any concerns you have about your health or related matters and if appropriate, get some idea about any particular wishes you have for your health care in the future. Is this something you would be interested in discussing?

- For people without significant illness but who are getting frailer:

  You never know what can happen in life. Have you thought what may happen if an accident or illness left you without the ability to decide things for yourself? Do you think it is a good idea to let people know certain things you would want? Would you want someone else to make decisions for you?

  Have you ever thought about the future? Do you have any worries about the future?

- For an individual with medical issues that are progressing, these questions can be applied specifically once an outline has been given of the condition's natural history along with key anticipated events.

> We've discussed what may be going to happen over the next months. Would you like to talk about what is important to you in the future as things change? Things you might not want to happen perhaps? Where you would want to be cared for?

Communication strategies and pitfalls of the discussion

Ambiguous or carelessly phrased questions can result in misunderstandings and subsequent block to the progress and effectiveness of discussions. As an example, when exploring a person's feelings on end-of-life care, it is best to avoid asking whether they "wish for everything to be done" in a certain situation. If the professional opinion is for management to be palliative, then rather than asking for a decision from the patient concerning an intervention that is clinically futile, it would be better that the medical position is stated in a gentle and sensitive fashion to the patient, along with the rationale; *informing not asking* is the key here (see resuscitation decisions below). An assurance can then be made in terms of "*doing everything to control discomfort and manage symptoms.*"

Discussions about withdrawing or not instituting artificial hydration or nutrition have a tendency to induce feelings of guilt, particularly among family members, as if they were abandoning them and allowing them to "starve to death." In these situations, clarity on the distinction between treatments (e.g., intravenous (IV) hydration and artificial nutrition) and basic care (e.g., the offer of food and fluids via the natural route) may help the discussion process. It is also useful to describe how the physiology of hunger is altered in many disease states (such as cancer, dementia, and progressive organ failure), with diminishing or absent appetite and the potential adverse effects of such interventions in these circumstances (see Chapter 21, *Terminal care and dying*). Similarly it can be explained that at the end of life, there is often no systemic discomfort from dehydration, with the main symptoms relating to a dry mouth (which can be palliated effectively by conservative means such as mouth care, use of ice cubes and artificial saliva/oral lubricants) and that without artificial hydration/nutrition, the result is typically a gradual slip into a coma rather than any form of suffering.

Health professionals should be aware of the trap of interpreting a patient's statement out of context. Thus an individual who states "I would not want to go on a life support machine" may be indicating this in terms of management after a catastrophic intracerebral event rather than a pneumonia, for which intensive management may be appropriate at a particular time and may result in an extension of quality of life.

Potentially ambiguous statements such as "avoiding of life-sustaining measures" will need to be clarified, as the type of treatment fulfilling this concept will vary according to clinical circumstances. Whereas it may be entirely reasonable to have IV antibiotics or fluids that may be life-sustaining in the situation of a superimposed acute, reversible illness, these options may be ineffective and declined if the cause of deteriorating health was felt to be from the progression of an underlying chronic disease state.

Measures to assist patient and professional through ACP discussions

Guiding individuals through ACP can be a technically and emotionally complex activity for health-care professionals. A number of written tools exist to support this, consisting mainly of structured questionnaires that prompt discussion and documentation. An evaluation in a hospital setting of one such tool (which was accompanied by explanatory notes and could be left in the patient's care for them to read alone or with others) was found to be associated with high rates of end-of-life care discussions between patients and medical staff and between patients and "those close to them." It was also rated by patients as being highly informative, helpful, and reassuring with little evidence that it caused any emotional upset [19].

Video decision support tools are a relatively new addition to the arena of ACP and have been used in dementia and cancer. They seem to improve communication and decision making for patients by helping them to visualise future health states. Although the number of studies is limited, they have been shown to significantly alter choices for end-of-life care, with individuals more likely to choose conservative care as opposed to active management. The choices are more likely to be stable over time, and importantly, the tools appear to be highly acceptable to patients without evidence of significant detriment to morale or emotion [20].

Recording the advance care plan

There is no set format for recording the outcome of ACP discussions. Structured tools may allow both for facilitation of the discussions and a means to record the

Table 8.1 Downloadable tools for facilitation and documentation of ACP discussions.

ACP tool	Web address
"Thinking Ahead"	www.goldstandardsframework.nhs.uk/ACP/ACPandGSF
"Preferred Priorities of Care"	www.endoflifecareforadults.nhs.uk/tools/core-tools/preferredprioritiesforcare
"Let Me Decide"	www.planningwhatiwant.com.au/Documents/c let me decide.pdf
"Expression of Healthcare Preferences"	old.rcplondon.ac.uk/clinical-standards/organisation/Guidelines/concise-guidelines/Documents/Expression-of-Health-Care-Preferences-Hammersmith-tool-form.pdf
"Physicians Orders for Life Sustaining Treatment"	www.ohsu.edu/polst/

output. A number of these tools exist in downloadable form (Table 8.1).

However professionals or patients will differ in their preference for the use of structured tools or for having more of a free rein in documenting discussion outcomes; indeed, a different approach may be used at different times. Some of the benefits and disadvantages of these two methods are described in Table 8.2.

All the structured ACP tools differ quite substantially in their content, layout, and approach, and care is needed in selecting a format that best suits the needs of the individual. Some formats may be too generic in their questions, resulting in outputs that are not sufficiently informative to guide care, while the converse is that some formats are so detailed they can be overwhelming in their decision-making requirements and come across as too mechanical

Table 8.2 Merits of structured tools to record ACP outcomes versus free documentation.

	Benefits	Disadvantages
Structured tools	Relatively simple for the CP to access and use and therefore helpful when one is less experienced with ACP discussions	The tools that focus on specific treatments in different scenarios may be viewed as restrictive in their coverage and unable to inform on situations outside of their precise remit
	Allows for a standardised format that may be appropriate in certain care settings, for example, as a format within a care home	May not allow for sufficient documentation of detail with regard to patient wishes leading to ambiguity of preferences
	Simultaneously acts as a prompt and provides a structure to the discussion process	Utilisation of a fixed format during a sensitive discussion process might appear to make the conversations stilted and less responsive to patient needs and cues
Free documentation	Allows for a more fluid approach to the planning process, responding instead to patient cues	Requires the facilitator(s) to be reasonably experienced in the ACP process
	Gives potential for documentation of patient preferences to be made with greater clarity and detail and tailored to patient needs	Lack of standardisation may result in varying quality of documents and variability of interpretation
	Conversations may be less likely to come across as rigid and planned	Certain topics of discussion may be missed

for such a sensitive subject. The more specific medical care plans may give patients a feeling of greater control over future care, albeit with concerns that they provide less guidance on routine decisions compared to critical treatments, and cannot inform on situations outside of their specific remit.

When drafting freehand documentation of ACP discussions, key elements can be enlisted from the structured ACP that exist. One of these is to record patient preferences within the two following categories:

1. The patient's values

For example, "If you were dying, how important would it be for you to avoid pain and suffering, even if it means that you might not live as long?"

2. Consideration of specific treatments

For example, "If I am aware but have brain damage that makes me unable to recognise people, speak meaningfully, or live independently, and I do not have a terminal illness, then I would not want artificial ventilation."

One of the advantages of a freely documented ACP is that it may allow the individual to "get the best out of both worlds," through an individually tailored plan that elaborates a strong expression of values and positive preferences (i.e., a clearly worded Advance Statement), combined where desired with a directive for refusal of specific treatments such as artificial ventilation, nasogastric (NG)/percutaneous endoscopic gastrostomy (PEG) feeding and CPR under specific circumstances.

Guidance on writing an ADRT is given in Box 8.5. Legal assistance can be sought for their formulation if there is a lot of uncertainty, difficulty in being clear and specific, or likely family or professional controversy.

Sometimes, patients express their desire for refusal of treatment only in a verbal fashion. A written, dated entry should be made (preferably somewhere in the medical record) by the medical professional who witnessed the verbal declaration. Verbal ADRTs can be legally recognised in the United Kingdom if the same validating criteria apply: the individual must not have an active mental health disorder, must have capacity for the decision, and must give adequate detail on specific treatments to be withheld under specific circumstances. Verbal ADRTs do not, however, legally apply to the withholding of life-sustaining treatments in the United Kingdom; these require a formally written ADRT (Box 8.5).

In summary, a tailored written output may include information on any of the following areas:
- Feedback to the individual and their carer or next-of-kin regarding the medical condition of the individual and their prognosis in more detail.

Box 8.5 Formatting an ADRT in the context of the mental capacity act for England and Wales [3]

When drafting an ADRT, the following points should be observed:
- It should be in writing. If the person is unable to write, someone else must write it down for them such as a family member or CP.
- Details of the person making the ADRT should be included: full name, date of birth, home address, name, and address of general practitioner (GP).
- It should state the date it was composed and the dates of any subsequent revision.
- There should be an introductory statement indicating that the ADRT is to come into force only if the person subsequently lacks capacity to make treatment decisions.
- It must specify the particular treatment that is to be refused and the scenarios in which the ADRT will apply.
- The signature of the individual making the ADRT must be evident. If they are unable to sign, they can direct someone else to sign on their behalf in their presence.
- The above signing must be witnessed with the witness themselves signing in the presence of the person making the ADRT.
- If the ADRT incorporates the refusal of life-sustaining treatment, then the following must be ensured additionally: An inclusion of a clear, written statement that the ADRT is to apply to a specific treatment "even if life is at risk."

- An anticipation of the disease "trajectory," including key potential problems.
- A statement of preferences for future health-care related to anticipated events.
- A statement on the values of the individual with regard to life, illness, and death.
- Preferences specifically for care at the very end of life, particularly in terms of where this is managed.
- A confirmation of discussions on resuscitation/CPR status and preferences for life-sustaining treatments that may translate into the initiation of a separate ADRT (either drafted with legal advice or utilising an available proforma).

At the end of any written document, even if it is just for an Advance Statement of preferences, it is desirable to get a signed endorsement signifying agreement with the discussions and plans.

Once complete, it is vital to ensure that the documents are circulated to all relevant personnel. A suggested

Box 8.6 Distribution list for ACP documents

- Individual
- Relatives/next-of-kin (if appropriate)
- Primary care practitioner
- Hospital medical records
- Out-of-hours services
- Social worker/key worker
- Care home records
- Solicitor (optional)

distribution list is given in Box 8.6. It is also preferable that any recorded documents are reviewed from time to time to allow for changes in patient preferences. This could be set at an arbitrarily agreed periodicity, such as annually, with a suggestion to further review such records following a change of individual circumstances. This takes into account phenomenon such as "response shift" [21] whereby an individual may adapt to a state of functional decline or ill health and come to view that state as being actually acceptable to remain in, contrasting perhaps with earlier negative views of that functional state made from a condition of relative health. However, it is not just changes in health status that may prompt a review of the ACP. A change in domestic circumstances, such as a new relationship or birth of a new child/grandchild, may imbue an individual with a new sense of purpose and outlook and fundamental reconsideration of the benefits and burdens of treatments.

Patients are generally encouraged to share their ACP with those close to them, including family members, an act which will increase the likelihood of any ACP or ADRT being brought to professional attention at the relevant time. However, this is not obligatory and professionals have to respect nondisclosure of such discussions and plans to family if indicated by the patient. In such cases, a clear recording of this position should be made on the ACP, preferably at the beginning, stipulating anyone who is not to be informed of its existence.

Appointing health-care proxies

If a patient losses capacity for decision making about their health, in some jurisdictions or countries this decision-making passes, by law, to a temporary substitute decision maker. The list of who can be the substitute decision makers is defined by law in priority order. If the patient would

want a different order of priority or the substitute to be someone not on the defined list, then they can appoint representatives.

In the United Kingdom the "next of kin," while enshrined legally for some responsibilities, has no legal responsibility or power for health decisions. Some people may wish to appoint such a proxy decision maker. This is called a lasting power of attorney (LPA) for health and welfare. The uptake of appointing an LPA seems to be less than uptake for making Advance Statements and ADRTs. Factors influencing this include: awareness of this facility, educational level, cognitive function, and whether the individual has close family members to them. LPA decision-making rights can be given to one or more individuals, jointly or severally. Authority of the attorney with respect to decisions on life-sustaining measures (e.g., artificial ventilation, CPR) needs to be specifically stated. Appointment of an LPA can be made with or without formal legal assistance, but registration of the LPA must be made with the Office of the Public Guardian and requires a fee.

In practice, even with no formal appointment of a health-care proxy, most people in a significant relationship with the individual generally come forward and discuss perceived best interests for that individual at times of need, with these pieces of information often sufficient to inform the necessary medical judgements.

What to do when individuals lack capacity for discussions

For those individuals without an ACP who have cognitive impairment and/or lack capacity to inform ACP discussions, there may still be a place for planning future care issues. This may be instigated by those in a significant relationship with the individual or by their physicians. Owing to patient incapacity, this process can no longer be termed ACP and ADRTs cannot be created. Instead, the outcomes of such planning could be termed simply as care plans or plans of treatment. This is not too dissimilar to the discussions that take place when physicians counsel a patient's next-of-kin on an escalation plan for care in times of serious illness. Box 8.7 indicates the appropriate steps that might be taken to plan care in such instances.

The aspects of health information, anticipation of events, and establishment of patient values and preferences are still important in care planning for the patient without capacity, but there will be clearly a much greater

Box 8.7 Care planning for the individual who lacks capacity for ACP discussions

1. It is important to assess firstly whether the person might regain capacity (e.g., after receiving medical treatment). If so it may be that the care planning discussions can be delayed. Even if capacity appears irreversibly impaired, effort should be made to maximise that individual's participation where practically feasible.

2. If the decision concerns life-sustaining treatment, it must not be motivated by a desire to bring about the person's death.

3. Any legally appointed health-care proxies present should guide the subsequent process as much as possible.

4. If no such proxy exists, attempt to identify all relevant participants who can inform discussions (family, informal carers, paid carers). Ensure all key participants are included in subsequent discussions, trying to keep those who know the patient best in the center of decision making.

5. Establish rapport with each participant, ascertaining their relationship with the patient and how each of them is responding to the patient's present condition.

6. Endeavour to achieve a consensus about the patient's clinical condition with the key participants, ensuring a shared understanding of diagnoses and trajectories of illnesses (and with the patient too, where this is still possible). Discussing prognosis and anticipating future clinical events may also be explored in this light.

7. Attempt, where possible, to elicit values and preferences of the patient based on information from the invited participants. For example, the patient might have previously expressed their thoughts on certain clinical procedures (e.g., CPR, dialysis) or given an idea of their values (e.g., "don't keep me going artificially in such a condition").

8. In considering how to manage key anticipated events, clarify the difference to the participants between substituted judgements (trying to put themselves in the patient's "shoes") and what they themselves perceive to be the best interests of the patient. Discuss positive and negative aspects of hospitalisation, medical treatment, artificial nutrition, and hydration in this context.

9. The facilitator's role must remain active during all of this, helping to interpret any known or inferred patient values in the context of the clinical situation, thereby providing a professional observation upon which the participants can build. Ultimately there will be some need to establish a level of professional-led advocacy and make recommendations to support the interests of the individual in a range of situations. Attention should be given to ensure these recommendations are understood and receive consensus support from other participants. The recommendations may be recorded as statements of mutually held beliefs pertaining to the individual's care (e.g., most appropriate place for death, mutually held thoughts on avoiding particular treatments/interventions).

10. After such a discussion, if the patient did have prior expressed or inferred values, it may be helpful to re-assert what these are and check that the discussions have indeed given due respect to them.

11. In summing up, it is helpful to hold up the values of "survival" and "end-of-life comfort measures" equally, especially if decisions are made not to pursue active lines of investigation or treatment. This will help reassure all participants of the active attention to patient comfort and dignity that will occur.

12. Where consensus between physicians and care-giving participants is not attained, discussions may be postponed, with care being managed expectantly until such time as renewal of discussions may be appropriate. However, throughout the discussion process, there may well be opportunities to respond to the feelings of the invited participants, to support them and to explore their own feelings toward the process that may help with understanding some of the differences of opinion.

---

reliance on other informants to gain such information and plan care accordingly. When decisions are required further down the line, the UK General Medical Council (GMC) guidance on end-of-life care states that the doctor may also explore which options these informants might see as providing overall benefit for the patient, but must not give them the impression they are being asked to make the decision. Doctors must take the views of those consulted into account in considering which option would be least restrictive of the patient's future choices and in making the final decision about which option is of overall benefit to the patient [22].

"Do not resuscitate" discussions

During ACP, the issue of CPR will naturally become a focus for many discussions, although it should be only one of the issues covered when discussing extent of treatment and preferences for care. It is important to acknowledge how emotive this subject is to the layperson and therefore to offer great clarity in discussions on the nature of the CPR intervention, outlining its potential to benefit as well as cause harm and its actual success rates as opposed to perceived success rates; with respect to this, the lack of efficacy of CPR in various advanced disease states may need to be emphasised [23]. The phrase "allow natural death" (AND) instead of do not resuscitate (DNR) may rationalise and align with the clinical intent of care and lessen the initial "blow" of discussing DNR status, but the nature of "AND" will ultimately need to be clarified in order that the patient and family are not misled with regard to their care. Whether framing such conversations in terms of "DNR" or "AND," it is often an idea to combine these declarations with a defined level of ongoing support. Thus a patient's health management could be given as follows:

- "DNR"/"AND" with ongoing measures to ensure comfort care and relief of symptoms.
- "DNR"/"AND" with continued basic medical support (consisting of IV hydration, antibiotics) explaining the aim is to "nudge" the patient through the illness where possible, but that if this fails, they will be allowed to pass "peacefully" without further intervention.

In general, any approach to discussions on CPR will vary according to three commonly encountered clinical circumstances [24]. Box 8.8 outlines an algorithm for this whole process:

1. For an **active or relatively healthy individual** (for whom cardiopulmonary arrest would be unexpected and cause of death would be uncertain), there should not be any proactive discussion of CPR as it is not relevant to their care, and it would be expected that they undergo CPR in the event of unexpected cardiopulmonary arrest. If there is a strong desire from the individual to elicit a DNR order (due to their perceptions/values on the intervention), then the reasons for this should be explored sensitively, ensuring the person has capacity to make this decision and that they have been given a full knowledge of the facts with access to clear information on their condition and treatment and about CPR itself.

2. In **individuals with a chronic or terminal illness where CPR may be deemed to have an unrealistic chance of success** or likely to cause more harm than benefit on balance of reasoning, any decision to withhold it would be made on medical grounds, and an individual cannot demand it. Nevertheless, an explanation of this approach with the individual or next-of-kin might enhance the whole communication aspect of care and should still be considered. In such situations, it is advisable to "set the argument" before an individual as opposed to raising the question with them, which as previously mentioned will effectively be a futile question and may actually result in distress to the individual.

3. For **individuals with chronic illness where the chance of CPR succeeding is possible**, albeit with concerns over potential drawbacks from the procedure (e.g., in terms of functional decline from cerebral hypoxia), it is important to share the facts and the decision-making process with the patient/next-of-kin, providing they have adequate mental capacity to do so, as their own views and values will be central in shaping any subsequent conclusion.

Concerns with ACP

Does ACP bias care against an individual?

There is potential to misinterpret ACP as generically equivalent to a mandate for "comfort care only" [13]. In the clinical setting, this may lead to a denial of potentially appropriate active and life-saving treatment. Safeguarding against this requires attention to detail in the formulation of any care plans, particularly in the area of specifying DNR status and in clarifying which procedures are to be avoided under what particular circumstances. ACP may also be phrased in such a way as to express treatments in a graduated fashion, with initial management being very active, particularly where there is some clinical uncertainty, with a licence to withdraw measures once a more accurate prognosis is known.

Can ACP decisions be overruled?

If a clinician, when encountering a patient lacking decision-making capacity, is confronted by the possible existence of an ACP, they should make every effort to obtain the plan before the initiation of care and review the content to see whether it falls within the charter of an Advance Statement or a Refusal of Treatment. An Advance Statement specifying preferences for care carries no legal mandate, and it may not always be possible or appropriate to adhere to each and every preference. An example would be where a desire was stated for terminal care to be administered at home, and this was earnestly attempted, but the individual required admission for problematic symptom control or because of extreme family stress. Preferences made within an Advance Statement therefore should be seen as allowing an individual to have aspirations for care, yet allow for flexibility of subsequent management.

Where a refusal of treatment has legal standing however (such as an ADRT in England and Wales), contravention may potentially result in legal action. Yet a number of scenarios exist where even a Refusal of Treatment drawn up by an individual may be overruled once they reach a state of decisional incapacity. Such cases may be justified if the following criteria are met:

1. If a surrogate decision maker is appointed with powers to make decisions covered in the Refusal of Treatment,

Box 8.8 An example of an approach to CPR decision making

Taken from the Unified principles for adult do not attempt CPR for the Eastmidlands, UK 2011 with permission

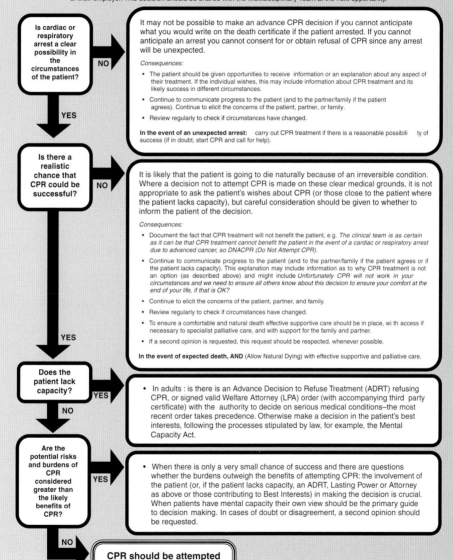

MAKING A DO NOT ATTEMPT CARDIOPULMONARY RESUSCITATION (DNACPR) DECISION FRAMEWORK

Health-care Professional Completing This DNA-CPR Form

This will vary according to circumstances and local arrangements. In general, this should be the most senior health-care professional immediately available. Whether in the acute hospitals or the community setting, this will be a senior experienced, doctor or nurse, who has undertaken appropriate training and education in communication and resuscitation decision making, according to the requirements of their employer. This decision should be shared with the Multidisciplinary Team at the next opportunity.

Is cardiac or respiratory arrest a clear possibility in the circumstances of the patient? — NO →

It may not be possible to make an advance CPR decision if you cannot anticipate what you would write on the death certificate if the patient arrested. If you cannot anticipate an arrest you cannot consent for or obtain refusal of CPR since any arrest will be unexpected.

Consequences:

- The patient should be given opportunities to receive information or an explanation about any aspect of their treatment. If the individual wishes, this may include information about CPR treatment and its likely success in different circumstances.
- Continue to communicate progress to the patient (and to the partner/family if the patient agrees). Continue to elicit the concerns of the patient, partner, or family.
- Review regularly to check if circumstances have changed.

In the event of an unexpected arrest: carry out CPR treatment if there is a reasonable possibili ty of success (if in doubt, start CPR and call for help).

↓ YES

Is there a realistic chance that CPR could be successful? — NO →

It is likely that the patient is going to die naturally because of an irreversible condition. Where a decision not to attempt CPR is made on these clear medical grounds, it is not appropriate to ask the patient's wishes about CPR (or those close to the patient where the patient lacks capacity), but careful consideration should be given to whether to inform the patient of the decision.

Consequences:

- Document the fact that CPR treatment will not benefit the patient, e.g. *The clinical team is as certain as it can be that CPR treatment cannot benefit the patient in the event of a cardiac or respiratory arrest due to advanced cancer, so DNACPR (Do Not Attempt CPR).*
- Continue to communicate progress to the patient (and to the partner/family if the patient agrees or if the patient lacks capacity). This explanation may include information as to why CPR treatment is not an option (as described above) and might include *Unfortunately CPR will not work in your circumstances and we need to ensure all others know about this decision to ensure your comfort at the end of your life, if that is OK?*
- Continue to elicit the concerns of the patient, partner, and family.
- Review regularly to check if circumstances have changed.
- To ensure a comfortable and natural death effective supportive care should be in place, wi th access if necessary to specialist palliative care, and with support for the family and partner.
- If a second opinion is requested, this request should be respected, whenever possible.

In the event of expected death, AND (Allow Natural Dying) with effective supportive and palliative care.

↓ YES

Does the patient lack capacity? — YES →

- In adults : is there an Advance Decision to Refuse Treatment (ADRT) refusing CPR, or signed valid Welfare Attorney (LPA) order (with accompanying third party certificate) with the authority to decide on serious medical conditions–the most recent order takes precedence. Otherwise make a decision in the patient's best interests, following the processes stipulated by law, for example, the Mental Capacity Act.

↓ NO

Are the potential risks and burdens of CPR considered greater than the likely benefits of CPR? — YES →

- When there is only a very small chance of success and there are questions whether the burdens outweigh the benefits of attempting CPR: the involvement of the patient (or, if the patient lacks capacity, an ADRT, Lasting Power or Attorney as above or those contributing to Best Interests) in making the decision is crucial. When patients have mental capacity their own view should be the primary guide to decision making. In cases of doubt or disagreement, a second opinion should be requested.

↓ NO →

CPR should be attempted

v49 Adapted from: 2007 BMA/RC/RCN Joint Statement on CPR; Regnard C and Randall F. *Clinical Medicine*, 2005; 5: 354–360; and *A Guide to Symptom Relief in Palliative Care*, sixth ed Radcliffe medical Press, 2010.

Case Study 8.1

You are a GP visiting an elderly man in a care home at the request of his daughter. He has Alzheimer's disease and COPD and his daughter has requested that he has a formal decision about resuscitation in place (DNR form). You establish that the man himself has no mental capacity to make such decisions. He knows his own name, but otherwise communication is limited. He uses a frame to mobilise but can manage only a short distance due to breathlessness and has started to deteriorate in the last few months with loss of weight and some difficulty in swallowing his food and drink.

You agree to fill in the DNR form but feel that he is declining and likely to end up in hospital soon. When you mention this to his daughter, she says that she wants him to go into hospital "only if absolutely necessary."

Was the daughter's original request for DNR documentation appropriate? How might you proceed to discuss future care for this man?

Discussion

This man appears to have advanced comorbidities of dementia and COPD. In terms of a decision on CPR, there is a reasonable probability that this man may suffer a cardiopulmonary arrest given his advanced age and COPD alone. However, the chances of success with CPR would be low in the presence of these advanced conditions, and it would be a medical decision not to administer the CPR on those grounds (see Box 8.8). Although this could still be put before the patient, it is likely this man lacks capacity to understand such issues; hence, it would be unhelpful in this case. His daughter seems to be in agreement with it; moreover, she actually initiated the request.

In this situation, the man has no ability to participate in ACP discussions. However, as a professional you have identified that there is potential for him to suffer adversity with respect to future health decline and its management. His daughter also seems to have some appreciation of this fact;

hence, the issue would be to see if a general escalation of care policy could be derived for him. It would be important to establish the other relevant parties who might represent his interests and to confirm the issue of DNR status with these people as well. An arrangement should be made to meet with these people with the purposes of outlining your concerns on his ongoing decline, the possibility of hospitalisation in the near future and considering a plan of treatment for him with regard to perceived best interests. This might include exploring anticipated events (e.g., falls, exacerbations of COPD, loss of mobility, loss of swallowing ability altogether, delirium), looking at what acute hospital services might have to offer in respect of some of these problems and noting any problems from previous encounters with the acute hospital environment.

After a series of discussions, with agreement from the relevant participants, a care plan might be formulated, which should be noted as carrying no legal significance. It would not be able to specify an ADRT (the DNR issue is considered separately), but it could state any known values and preferences of the elderly man or any concerns with hospitalisation, perhaps borne out of past experiences. These might subsequently be sufficient to guide health-care professionals (GP, secondary care doctors) in their decision making. The care plan might typically suggest that this man is given limited care only, consisting of a trial of appropriate medications so long as they could be administered orally and subcutaneous (SC) fluid drips, if appropriate, on a short-term basis (with support from relevant community teams such as intermediate care or community palliative care teams), but excluding invasive procedures and IV access. It might outline the conditions for which hospitalisation might be deemed appropriate such as if the man was to be in severe pain or distress that could not be relieved in the community setting. As he is still currently mobile, it might also suggest hospitalisation following a fall with a suspicion of a fracture, since repair/management of the latter might be an appropriate palliative procedure.

then the decisions of this proxy decision maker take precedence once the individual loses capacity.

2. The validity of a Refusal of Treatment may be questioned in the following circumstances:

- An individual acting in a manner suggestive of a change of view subsequent to making the Refusal of Treatment.
- Concerns about capacity at the time the Refusal of Treatment was devised.
- Changes in circumstances that may not have

been anticipated by the person and might have affected their decision (e.g., a recent therapy that radically changes the outlook for their particular condition).

In general where there is doubt regarding the presence, validity or applicability of a Refusal of Treatment, clinicians may continue management decisions according to the principle of "beneficence" until clarity is gained; they are required only to demonstrate that this belief was a reasonable one at the time.

Conclusions

ACP is an important component of holistic end-of-life care and could be considered earlier in the stage of an illness than is generally appreciated. Initiation should come from the professional side with a range of health and social CPs being able to assist with the process. Adequate time for discussion and reflection is required as an individual explores the nature of their condition(s), their values on life, and through this the implications of how they would prefer to be cared for should they eventually lose capacity to engage with the health-care profession. Communication features strongly in this process, with the discussions being arguably more important than the written output per se. Viewing ACP as a method solely to effect prior patient wishes and reduce over-intervention at the end of life may be too simplistic an expectation. Even though this may be achievable, particularly for residents of long-term care establishments, there are other potential benefits from the process, including the opening up of communication channels between patients, their families and their health-care professionals, better preparation of patients for the end-of-life situation and reducing carer strain and bereavement stress. The positive aspect of using patient values and preferences to guide and inform CPs, and expressed largely through the medium of Advance Statements, should be emphasised rather than to focus too singularly on the withholding of specific therapies that can be made through a vehicle such as a Refusal of Treatment. This chapter has not attempted to discuss the specifics of the diversity of legislation surrounding ACP across the world, and it is vital that practitioners familiarise themselves with that of their own country.

References

1. Conroy S, Fade P, Fraser A, et al. Advance care planning: concise evidence-based guidelines. In Turner-Stokes L (ed), *Concise Guidance to Good Practice Series*. London: RCP, 2009.
2. Simon J and Murray A. Facilitated advance care planning: what is the patient experience? *J Palliat Care* 2008; 24(4): 256–264.
3. Mental Capacity Act. 2005. C.9. Available at: http://www.legislation.gov.uk/ukpga/2005/9/contents.
4. Munday D, Petrova M and Dale J. Exploring preferences for place of death with terminally ill patients: qualitative study of experiences of general practitioners and community nurses in England. *BMJ* 2009; 339: b2391.
5. ICM/Endemol/BBC Poll. *Survey of General Public*. 2005.
6. Teno J, Lynn J, Wenger N, et al. Advance directives for seriously ill hospitalized patients: effectiveness with the patient self-determination act and the SUPPORT intervention. SUPPORT Investigators. Study to Understand Prognoses and Preferences for Outcomes and Risks of Treatment. *J Am Geriatr Soc* 1997; 45(4): 500–507.
7. Molloy D, Guyatt GH, Russo R, et al. Systematic implementation of an advance directive program in nursing homes. A randomized controlled trial. *JAMA* 2000; 283(11): 1437–1444.
8. Caplan GA, Meller A, Squires B, et al. Advance care planning and hospital in the nursing home. *Age Ageing* 2006; 35(6): 581–585.
9. Detering KM, Hancock AD, Reade MC, et al. The impact of advance care planning on end of life care in elderly patients: randomised controlled trial. *BMJ* 2010; 340: c1345.
10. Davison SN and Simpson C. Hope and advance care planning in patients with end stage renal disease: qualitative interview study. *BMJ* 2006; 333: 886–890.
11. Tierney WM, Dexter PR, Gramelspacher GP, et al. The effect of discussions about advance directives on patients' satisfaction with primary care. *J Gen Intern Med* 2001; 16(1): 32–40.
12. Barnes K, Jones l, Tookman A, et al. Acceptability of an advance care planning interview schedule: a focus group study. *Palliat Med* 2007; 21: 23–28.
13. Mirarchi FL, Kala S, Hunter D, et al. TRIAD II: do living wills have an impact on pre-hospital lifesaving care? *J Emerg Med* 2009; 36(2): 105–115.
14. Rabow MW, Hauser JM and Adams J. Supporting family caregivers at the end of life: "they don't know what they don't know". *JAMA* 2004; 291(4): 483–491.
15. Rizzo VM, Engelhardt J, Tobin D, et al. Use of the stages of change transtheoretical model in end-of-life planning conversations. *J Palliat Med* 2010; 13(3): 267–271.
16. Johnston SC, Pfeifer MP and McNutt R. The discussion about advance directives. Patient and physician opinions regarding when and how it should be conducted. End of Life Study Group. *Arch Intern Med* 1995; 155(10): 1025–1030.
17. www.goldstandardsframework.nhs.uk/Resources/Gold Standards Framework/PDF Documents/Prognostic IndicatorGuidancePaper.pdf.
18. Oxenham D and Cornbleet MA. Accuracy of prediction of survival by different professional groups in a hospice. *Palliat Med* 1998; 12(2): 117–118.
19. Schiff R, Shaw R, Raja N, et al. Advance end-of-life healthcare planning in an acute NHS hospital setting; development and evaluation of the Expression of Healthcare Preferences (EHP) document. *Age and Ageing* 2009; 38(1): 81–85.
20. Volandes AE, Paasche-Orlow MK, Barry MJ, et al. Video decision support tool for advance care planning in dementia: randomised controlled. *BMJ* 2009; 28(338): b2159. doi: 10.1136/bmj.b2159.

21. Schwartz C. Decision making at the end of life: shifting sands. *J R Soc Med* 2005; 98(7): 297–298.

22. General Medical Council. *Treatment and Care Towards the End of Life: Good Practice in Decision Making.* London: GMC, 2010.

23. Larkin GL, Copes WS, Nathanson BH, et al. Pre-resuscitation factors associated with mortality in 49,130 cases of in-hospital cardiac arrest: a report from the National Registry for Cardiopulmonary Resuscitation. *Resuscitation* 2010; 81(3): 302–311.

24. Decisions relating to Cardiopulmonary Resuscitation. A Joint Statement from the British Medical Association, the Resuscitation Council (UK), and the Royal College of Nursing, 2007.

9 Pain and Its Management

Alex Nicholson

South Tees Hospitals NHS Foundation Trust, Middlesbrough, UK

Introduction

Pain is a common problem for palliative care patients whatever their diagnosis. This chapter provides an overview of a huge topic with a very extensive international literature. First the extent of pain as a problem is described, and this is followed by definitions and terminology including the concept of "total pain." Next the biology of pain is reviewed with consideration of its different clinical subtypes. Pain management requires consistent clinical assessment and guidance on this and possible tools are discussed. The majority of the chapter is concerned with treatment approaches, offering general principles including the framework for pharmacotherapy that is provided by the World Health Organisation (WHO) analgesic ladder. This is followed by more detail on the use of non-opioid, opioid, and adjuvant analgesics and concludes with a brief overview of interventional and other pain treatment modalities.

A note on terminology: in this chapter, reference will be made to formulations of opioids that have a prolonged duration of effect. The term "modified release (MR)" should be taken to mean the same as "extended release" or "sustained release." Opioid formulations that have not been adapted to deliver over a prolonged period of time are referred to as "normal release (NR)," which means the same as "immediate release."

The problem of pain in palliative care

In a recent Canadian study [1] of cancer palliative care patients, 70% of patients reported pain. Half of these patients rated pain as "little" or "mild," but half had moderate to severe pain, which they considered to be an important ongoing problem. The group of patients with the worst pain tended to be younger, have poorer general condition and a shorter survival. Their pain was also associated with a higher rate of other distressing symptoms including nausea, weakness, drowsiness, and anxiety. The same study reported that the concept of "suffering" was most strongly linked to physical problems [2], reminding us that pain must never be assessed in isolation but considered as part of the whole clinical picture.

Data on patients with any diagnosis (cancer and non-cancer) are similar. A study [3] examining pain during the last two years of life revealed a prevalence of 30% two years before death rising to 47% in the last month of life. The prevalence rates (shown in brackets) were similar whatever the terminal diagnosis: cancer (45%), heart disease (48%), frailty (50%), sudden death (42%). This study sought patient reported data although, due to functional decline and comorbidities, the proxy reporting rate rose from 16% at 2 years premortem to 33% in the last month of life.

Pain is also perceived by informal carers to be a significant problem. Two studies gathering information from carers after the death of the patient demonstrate this. The study to understand prognoses and preferences for outcomes and risks of treatments (SUPPORT) [4] looked at dying patients with malignant and nonmalignant disease and revealed that 40% of carers perceived the patient to have had severe pain for some or all the time during the last 3 days of life. In the Regional Care of the Dying Study [5], which included only cancer patients, 88% patients were thought to have had pain of any severity at some time in the last year of life and 66% to have had pain in the last week.

Handbook of Palliative Care, Third Edition. Edited by Christina Faull, Sharon de Caestecker, Alex Nicholson and Fraser Black.
© 2012 by John Wiley and Sons, Inc. Published 2012 by John Wiley & Sons, Inc.

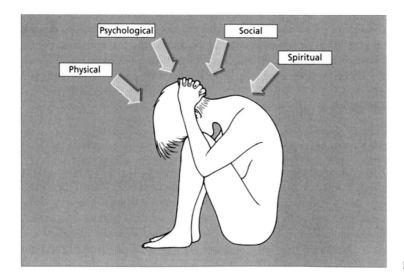

Figure 9.1 The concept of "total pain".

Definition of pain and the concept of "total pain"

Pain has been defined [6] as "an unpleasant sensory and emotional experience associated with actual or potential tissue damage, or described in terms of such damage." Pain is therefore highly subjective since it can only be identified and quantified by the person reporting it. This has given rise to a pragmatic definition "pain is what the patient says hurts," which is widely used. However, it is important to remember that patients with limited or no communication still experience pain even though they cannot report it. Observation of behaviour and physical signs that may be associated with pain will provide additional information but correlation between observer- and patient-reported pain may be poor. Whether communication is normal or impaired, one individual's response to a given painful stimulus will differ from another's.

The subjective nature of pain, individual variability in response to it, and an appreciation that the experience of pain is influenced by a multitude of other factors, has given rise to the concept of "total pain."

"Total pain" was a term used by the late Dame Cicely Saunders in the 1960s to capture the fact that the pain experience is influenced by physical, emotional, social, and spiritual factors [7]. Many of these factors encompass some form of loss. All the dimensions are important in a person's suffering. To achieve successful pain management, it is essential to consider a holistic, multifaceted assessment. Lack of attention to aspects other than the physical is often the reason why a pain syndrome appears refractory to treatment. Figure 9.1 provides a simple depiction of this concept. Table 9.1 classifies the problems that a patient in pain may encounter according to the relevant domain of "total" pain.

Terminology

Certain descriptive terms are used to define different types of pain experience [6]. While pain is notoriously difficult for patients to frame in words, it is useful for clinicians to have means of classifying the symptoms, particularly when discussing a case with a colleague. However, unless there is a shared understanding of the meaning of the term being used, it may be safer (and simpler) to restrict the discussion to descriptors used by the patient. Correct and consistent use of terminology is also important when designing and interpreting research studies although such considerations are beyond the scope of this handbook. The glossary below is included for practical, clinical purposes, and for interest. Different *types* of pain are considered separately.

Allodynia: Pain perceived in response to a stimulus that does not normally cause pain such as touch, light pressure, or moderate temperature. This term applies equally whether the skin is known to be damaged or sensitised (e.g., in the early period after radiotherapy) or appears normal on examination.

Table 9.1 The dimensions of total pain.

Physical	Psychological
"Traditional" pain	Anxiety/fear of worsening pain
Impaired mobility	Equating "pain" with "dying"
Requirement for analgesia	Equating pain relief (especially morphine) with dying
Other physical symptoms	Sense of inevitability of future severe pain
	Reminder of ill health/limitations/sick role
	Anger, despair and hopelessness
Social	**Spiritual**
Inability to work	Loss of sense of purpose
Loss of role as earner, practical person, or carer for another person	Loss of role(s) and identity
Restricted social activities and contacts	Change to expected life narrative or journey
Loss of income	Feeling of being punished
Changes to housing to accommodate functional changes	Altered relationship with/feelings about a "higher authority" in whatever form

Dysaesthesia: An unpleasant abnormal sensation that is either spontaneous or provoked. It is the "unpleasant" character that distinguishes this from paresthesia (see below), although such distinctions are, naturally, subjective and individual. Determining whether the sensation has a recognisable precipitating factor (rather than being entirely spontaneous and unpredictable) may be relevant in planning management.

Hyperalgesia: An exaggerated pain response to a stimulus that would normally be expected to be painful. Note the distinction from allodynia in which a nonpainful stimulus is perceived as pain whereas in hyperalgesia "pain" is felt as "super-pain."

Hyperesthesia: An increased sensitivity to *any* stimulus. Heat is felt to be "extra hot" but not as a pain, so there is no change in the resulting sensation.

Hyperpathia: A pain syndrome where there is an abnormally painful reaction to whatever trigger is involved (provoked or spontaneous, painful or nonpainful stimulus). It is often rather "explosive" in character, possibly delayed, poorly localised and with radiation to other areas and after sensations. Hyperpathia may be associated with any of the phenomena listed above.

Paresthesia: An abnormal sensation, either provoked or spontaneous, but which is not unpleasant (and therefore not truly a "pain").

The biology of pain: neuroanatomy and neurophysiology of nociception and analgesia

Nociception is the detection of noxious stimuli by specialised nerve endings known as nociceptors. Activation of nociceptors by mechanical, thermal, or chemical stimuli leads to the perception of so-called nociceptive pain. An understanding of the physiology that underlies this will allow improved pain assessment and management. A simplified schema of the neuroanatomy of pain and site of action of various analgesics is shown in Figure 9.2.

Nerve fibres are classified as A, B or C fibres, with alpha (α), beta (β), gamma (γ), and delta (δ) subcategories. A-β, A-δ, and C are sensory nerve fibres and therefore have a role in pain perception. A-δ nociceptors respond to pricking, squeezing, or pinching and lead to the "fast," sharp pain of an injury. "Polymodal" C fibres respond to many noxious stimuli to produce "slow," throbbing, more diffuse pain. All these nociceptive afferent fibres synapse with neurones within the dorsal horn of the spinal cord and project through interneurones to the thalamus and cortex. A-β and other sensory afferent nerve fibres also synapse with these dorsal horn neurones and may inhibit the transmission of the painful stimulus to the thalamus and cortex. This is known as "gate control" and is the mechanism of action of physical treatment with transcutaneous electrical nerve stimulator (TENS).

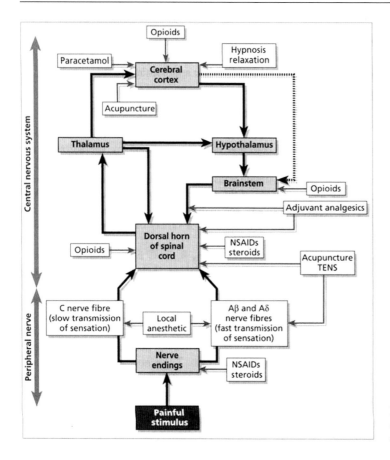

Figure 9.2 A schema of the neuroanatomy of pain and the sites of action of different analgesic modalities.

Normal activation of nociceptive pathways (i.e., a noxious stimulus triggers nociceptor firing) is known as nociceptive pain. *Abnormal* activation of nociceptive pathways is manifest as neuropathic pain. Descending inhibitory neural pathways from the brain to the spinal cord modulate incoming nociceptive information. The major neurotransmitters involved in these descending inhibitory pathways are serotonin and noradrenaline. This is the probable site of action of many adjuvant analgesics.

Opioid receptors

Four opioid receptors have been identified: Mu (μ), Delta (δ), Kappa (κ), and ORL-1 (opioid-receptor-like). These are distributed widely throughout the body predominantly, but not exclusively, in the central nervous system (CNS) and peripheral nervous system. Receptors in the peripheral nervous system are activated by inflammation resulting from injury or other tissue damage. The clinically relevant actions are shown in Box 9.1. Morphine, fentanyl, hydromorphone,

methadone, and oxycodone are strong agonists at the μ-opioid receptor. Oxycodone is also a strong agonist at the κ-opioid receptor, mediating analgesia. μ, δ, and κ receptors are all antagonised by naloxone.

Box 9.1 Opioid receptors

Opioid receptor subtype	Effect of agonist
μ	Analgesia, respiratory depression, reduced gastrointestinal (GI) motility, hypotension
κ	Analgesia, sedation, psychomimetic effects; some respiratory depression
δ	Analgesia, respiratory depression

Pain types and syndromes

Many different types and syndromes of pain are recognised, and this is clinically relevant when determining an appropriate management plan. Classification and subclassification of pain types is of considerable academic interest but also supports a practical clinical approach. Table 9.2 offers a classification of different pains linked to clinical scenarios and gives an indication of the relative role of opioids and coanalgesics (adjuvant analgesics) in their treatment. Opioid responsiveness is not an "all or nothing" phenomenon but rather a spectrum, and it is recognised that some pains may be opioid "partially-responsive." Neuropathic pain used to be regarded as opioid "poorly-responsive," but this notion has been challenged in the past decade. The classification is discussed more in the text that follows the table.

Table 9.2 Pain classification related to likely analgesic response.

Classification/type of pain	Temporal characteristics	Example	Opioid response	Coanalgesic or other modality
Nociceptive somatic	Constant	Bone metastasis	Partial	Nonsteroidal anti-inflammatory drug Paracetamol/acetaminophen Radiotherapy, Bisphosphonates
		Cutaneous metastasis	Partial	Topical anti-inflammatory or tricyclic
Nociceptive somatic	Episodic	Bone pain due to incipient pathological fracture or vertebral collapse	Partial but may not cover movement-related pain. Muscle spasm may also be involved	Surgical stabilization Nerve block Radiotherapy
Nociceptive visceral	Constant	Liver capsular pain	Partial	Corticosteroid
Nociceptive visceral	Episodic	Partially obstructing bowel tumour	Partial response but may exacerbate constipation element	Anticholinergic
		Radiation induced cystitis	Poor response	Anticholinergic
Neuropathic	Constant	Central poststroke pain	Partial response	Tricyclic Antiepileptic
		Chemotherapy induced painful peripheral neuropathy		
		Post-herpetic neuralgia		
Neuropathic	Episodic	Lancinating pain due to brachial plexopathy	Poor response	Tricyclic or other antidepressant Antiepileptic Benzodiazepine

Pain may be distinguished by the underlying pathophysiology into nociceptive and neuropathic pain. While this classification seems attractive as a way of fitting the presenting clinical picture into some sort of framework, it is rather a simplification of what is actually a much more complex situation.

Nociceptive pain

This is pain associated with tissue damage due to trauma, pathology, or other insult to an organ (visceral nociceptive pain) or body part (somatic nociceptive pain). The pain continues due to ongoing activation of nociceptors by the insult. Nociceptive pains tend to respond to simple and/or opioid analgesics, but may require interventional techniques.

Visceral pain is usually perceived to be rather vague or diffuse—that is, not well localised—but severity, location, associations, and other characteristics will depend on the organ involved. Pain arising from damage to luminal organs such as obstruction to the gut or urinary tract will have episodic, colicky features. Damage to a parenchymal organ, such as bulky metastatic disease within the liver, pathology within the lung or in the retroperitoneal structures, causes a more constant, dull, aching feeling. Involvement of peritoneum or pleura will enhance the localisation. Visceral pain may be "referred" to other areas—for example, pathology causing irritation of the diaphragm may cause pain to be felt in the shoulder.

Somatic pain is usually well localised and described in terms such as "aching," "burning," "throbbing," or "sharp."

Neuropathic pain

Neuropathic pain arises either from injury or pathology involving the peripheral nervous system or CNS or from the development of abnormal sensory perception or transmission [8].

Peripheral neuropathic pain complicates cancer or its treatment in 40% patients and includes brachial or lumbosacral plexopathies (caused directly by tumour infiltration or indirectly following radiotherapy), paraneoplastic sensory neuropathies, chemotherapy-induced peripheral neuropathies, and postsurgical pain. Peripheral neuropathic pain is also a complication of many nonmalignant diseases including peripheral vascular disease, multiple sclerosis (MS), diabetes mellitus, and human immunodeficiency virus/acquired immunodeficiency syndrome (HIV/AIDS).

Central neuropathic pain may also be due to primary or secondary malignant disease in the brain or spinal cord, but commoner causes are stroke, MS, and spinal cord injury.

Clinically neuropathic pain is suspected when there is pain associated with sensory loss or with motor or autonomic dysfunction. Clues may also arise from the characteristics of the pain (e.g., unprovoked episodes of pain like an "electric shock"), from its distribution (which may implicate an underlying neuropathy or plexopathy) or as a result of investigations that identify a lesion in a relevant neurological area.

Neuropathic pains may be less responsive to standard and opioid analgesics, sometimes being described as opioid-poorly, or opioid-partially, responsive. Their successful treatment often requires use of adjuvant or coanalgesics or interventional methods.

Pain may also be differentiated by its temporal characteristics. The main distinction here is between "background" pain and "breakthrough" pain. Some explanation around these is important.

Background pain

This is also known as "baseline" or "basal" pain and refers to the more constant element of pain in the patient's history, lasting for more than 12 h per day.

Breakthrough pain

Breakthrough pain is a concept, which, although commonly referred to in pain and palliative care literature, guidelines, teaching and clinical practice, is not universally recognised in all health-care settings. An early definition was "a transitory exacerbation of pain that occurs on a background of otherwise stable pain in a patient receiving chronic opioid therapy" [9]. In this reference, the focus was on cancer patients, but in clinical practice, it is clear that this phenomenon occurs also in noncancer patients and in those not using opioid analgesia. Other terms used to refer to breakthrough pain include "episodic pain," "pain flare," and "transient pain" [10].

The clinical relevance of understanding the nature of "breakthrough pain" is in order to establish an appropriate management plan, and the subclassification proposed by Davies [11] is helpful in guiding this. He suggests three different categories based on the clinical context. Bear in mind that more than one "breakthrough pain" may be present in an individual patient:

1. Paroxysmal pain occurring wholly unexpectedly (also called "spontaneous" or "idiopathic" pain).

2. Incident pain (also called "precipitated" pain) that is related to specific events and further grouped into the following:

  i Volitional pain provoked by a voluntary action such as reaching for an item, changing position, standing, walking. The term "movement-related" pain is also applied depending on the situation.

 ii Nonvolitional pain caused by an involuntary action such as coughing.

 iii Defaecation-related pain might fit either of the above categories. It is voluntary, and can usually be controlled, but cannot be prevented indefinitely.

 iv Procedural pain related to an intervention such as a wound dressing change.

3. End-of-dose failure is a term applied when a predictable exacerbation of pain occurs toward the end of the interval between doses of either NR or MR analgesia.

Spiritual and cultural aspects of pain

Spiritual pain is a concept recognised as one of the dimensions that contributes to the notion of "total pain" described earlier. The holistic ethos of palliative care practice seeks to ensure that this dimension is not overlooked. While not easy to define clearly, the literature emphasises that "spiritual" encompasses issues that are greater than simply religious considerations. Perceptions of spiritual pain and existential distress may be used to frame the concept of suffering [12] and recognise a two-way interaction between physical symptoms and existential experience. Suffering in turn has been described as "a state of distress brought about by a real or perceived threat to accomplish or fulfil previously held hopes or expectations for the life plan or narrative" [13].

 The myriad ways in which pain (and other physical symptoms) is felt, interpreted, and reported or expressed by patients may also vary due to the individual's characteristics including factors such as gender, culture, social and economic status, ethnicity, and others [14]. Thus, individuals may be observed to be highly demonstrative, calmly stoical, or quietly passive and may perceive their symptom to be a challenge to be overcome, an affront to be endured with dignity or a punishment for mistakes known or unknown.

Assessment of pain

Successful management of any symptom depends on an initial careful evaluation. Since pain is subjective, the main assessment must be a careful history taken from the patient (see Box 9.2). Observation of behaviour, including the consistency of this with the elicited history, appropriate examination and relevant investigations are important but secondary elements. When managing a patient with impairment of communication, cognition, or conscious-

---

Box 9.2 Key aspects of assessment

Careful initial assessment is very important and should include clear documentation of findings.

 This allows the assessing clinician, and others, to compare progress in management against the early features.

 Many pains change with time, and frequent reassessment is necessary, especially during and after interventions.

 Multiple sites and/or types of pain are common. EACH pain should be assessed, documented, managed, and reviewed.

 Charts may be used to record site and radiation of pains and associated clinical findings.

 Pain scores or scales, though subjective, may allow the patient to rate the severity of the pain.

 Each pain should be assessed for the following:
- Site, severity, radiation, and characteristics of its timing/frequency/variation.
- Quality using descriptive terms (e.g., burning, tingling, throbbing, etc.).
- Exacerbating and relieving factors including the effects of drug and nondrug interventions.
- Associated symptoms and features.

 Patient's understanding, fears and concerns, previous experience of pain and expectations of treatment, and other aspects relevant to social, psychological, and spiritual should be determined.

 Clinical examination should be performed to assist in determining the likely type and cause.

 Relevant investigation, appropriate to the patient's condition, should be considered. This might include biochemistry (which may influence drug choice) and X-rays/scans.

---

ness, a narrative from the carer who knows the patient well combined with careful behavioural observation are crucial.

 Throughout assessment, it is important to remember two points:

1. Multiple pains are common—for example, in cancer patients, one-third will have one pain, one-third will have two, and one-third will have three or more pains.

2. Multiple causes may be involved—some of the pains may not relate to the presenting pathology or diagnosis. Not all pain in a cancer patient is a cancer pain, and the same principle applies in other diagnoses.

Assessment tools

Pain assessment instruments exist in various forms.

 The simplest are single-dimension scales using words (verbal rating scale [VRS]), numbers (numerical rating scale [NRS]), lines (visual analogue scale [VAS]), or images to prompt a rating by the patient from "no pain" to "worst imaginable pain." In a patient with intact cognition and communication, these can contribute an objective element to the pain assessment process, and this can be useful when trying to assess the impact of pain relief by medication or other intervention.

Many tools exist to measure pain and its impact on the patient. The Edmonton Symptom Assessment System has been developed by the regional palliative care programme in Edmonton, Alberta, Canada (www.palliative.org) and provides a screening tool by means of NRS for pain and other symptoms including tiredness, nausea, appetite, breathlessness, depression, and anxiety among others. A body map is also incorporated to record sites of pain. Although many of these tools tend to be used more in clinical research rather than in routine clinical practice, there is considerable value in a formal, systematic assessment.

Figure 9.3 shows the short form of the Brief Pain Inventory (BPI) [15] (reproduced with permission from the Pain Research Group at the MD Anderson Cancer Center, Texas). The BPI incorporates many elements including a body chart, NRS of pain intensity, relieving/exacerbating factors and pain medications, a scale to record relief from medication, patient's perceptions of cause of pain and scales of the impact of the pain on domains of daily life such as mood, working, relationships, and sleep. The BPI has been translated into nearly 50 languages and linguistically validated in these and has undergone psychometric evaluation in almost half of them.

Detection, evaluation, and monitoring of pain in patients with cognitive and communication impairment, for example, dementia [16], is more complex. Chapter 17 explores this area in more detail.

In patients with mild impairment and preserved communication, the unidimensional scales may be useful. Evaluation in patients without communication requires observational methods. All these require some training of the user, some more than others, and some are better applied by someone who knows the patient's normal behavioural patterns well. The validity and reliability of these tools is subject to ongoing research. A useful overview of this area is provided by Herr and Ersek [17].

Assessment of pain in children may involve picture representations as they draw their bodies, perhaps adding colour to depict intensity of pain, or the use of visual images such as the face pain scales. Pain assessment in children is discussed further in Chapter 15.

Assessment tools and scales have also been developed to evaluate neuropathic pains. In the neuropathic pain

---

Box 9.3 General principles to support pain management

- Clear communication, information sharing, and explanations.
- Consider modification of underlying disease/pathology.
- Raise the pain threshold.
- Modify the environment and provide assistance with activities of daily living.
- Modify pain perception.
- Interrupt pain pathway.

---

scale [18], the intensity of 11 aspects of pain are recorded including intensity and timing, and also more qualitative features such as itching or burning. The Leeds Assessment of Neuropathic Symptoms and Signs (LANSS) pain scale [19] was developed to support clinicians in making a distinction between nociceptive and neuropathic pain and can also be used to measure and monitor treatment effects. This tool has been validated in a number of different cancer and noncancer pain models and includes seven elements. Five are symptom measures and two record examination findings—assessment for allodynia and pin-prick testing.

Management of pain

General principles
Following assessment, a specific treatment plan is agreed. The following framework is recommended in all cases to assist in formulating a management plan (see Box 9.3).

Communication
First discuss the results and conclusions of assessment using language and terminology appropriate to the patient, and a communication approach that checks understanding and facilitates further questions at intervals. Next outline the management plan including purpose, dose, and side effects of medication proposed. Realistic objectives must then be agreed with the patient. For a person with constant severe pain, the first goal may be to achieve freedom from pain at night to allow sleep, the next to achieve freedom from pain when resting by day, and the final goal might be relief of pain allowing activity. Lastly agree and confirm review arrangements and responsibilities in terms of who will provide guidance or advice in the intervening time, both by day and by night, should further problems arise.

STUDY ID #:_____ DO NOT WRITE ABOVE THIS LINE HOSPITAL #: _____

Brief Pain Inventory (Short Form)

Date:____ / ____ / ____   Time:_____

Name:_____ _____ _____
              Last   First   Middle Initial

1.   Throughout our lives, most of us have had pain from time to time (such as minor headaches, sprains, and toothaches). Have you had pain other than these every-day kinds of pain today?

                1.   Yes   2.   No

2.   On the diagram, shade in the areas where you feel pain. Put an X on the area that hurts the most.

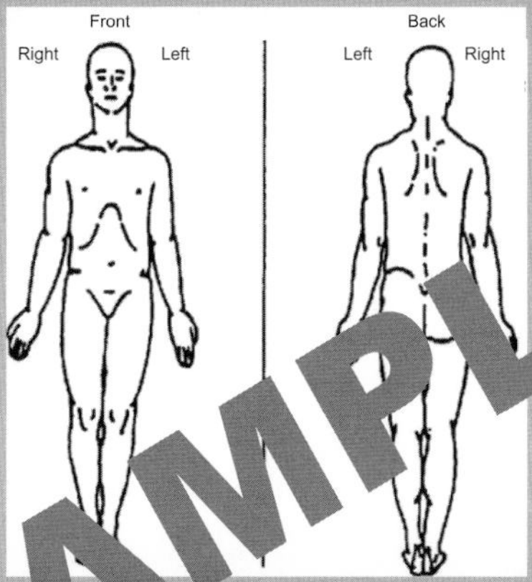

Front   Back

Right   Left   Left   Right

SAMPLE

3.   Please rate your pain by circling the one number that best describes your pain at its worst in the last 24 hours.

      0   1   2   3   4   5   6   7   8   9   10
      No   Pain as bad as
      Pain   you can imagine

4.   Please rate your pain by circling the one number that best describes your pain at its least in the last 24 hours.

      0   1   2   3   4   5   6   7   8   9   10
      No   Pain as bad as
      Pain   you can imagine

5.   Please rate your pain by circling the one number that best describes your pain on the average.

      0   1   2   3   4   5   6   7   8   9   10
      No   Pain as bad as
      Pain   you can imagine

6.   Please rate your pain by circling the one number that tells how much pain you have right now.

      0   1   2   3   4   5   6   7   8   9   10
      No   Pain as bad as
      Pain   you can imagine

Page 1 of 2

Figure 9.3 Brief pain inventory (short form).

STUDY ID #:_ _ _ _ _ _ _ _   DO NOT WRITE ABOVE THIS LINE   HOSPITAL #: _ _ _ _ _ _ _ _

Date:_ _ _ _ / _ _ _ _ / _ _ _ _   Time:_ _ _ _ _ _ _ _
Name:_ _ _ _ _ _ _ _ _ _ _ _ _ _ _   _ _ _ _ _ _ _ _ _ _ _ _ _ _ _   _ _ _ _ _ _ _ _ _ _ _ _
            Last   First   Middle Initial

7.   What treatments or medications are you receiving for your pain?

8.   In the last 24 hours, how much relief have pain treatments or medications provided? Please circle the one percentage that most shows how much relief you have received.

0%	10%	20%	30%	40%	50%	60%	70%	80%	90%	100%
No Relief										Complete Relief

9.   Circle the one number that describes how, during the past 24 hours, pain has interfered with your:

A.   General Activity

0	1	2	3	4	5	6	7	8	9	10
Does not Interfere										Completely Interferes

B.   Mood

0	1	2	3	4	5	6	7	8	9	10
Does not Interfere										Completely Interferes

C.   Walking Ability

0	1			5	6	7	8	9	10
Does not Interfere									Completely Interferes

D.   Normal ... (includes both work outside the home and housework)

0	1	2	3	4	5	6	7	8	9	10
Does not Interfere										Completely Interferes

E.   Relations with other people

0	1	2	3	4	5	6	7	8	9	10
Does not Interfere										Completely Interferes

F.   Sleep

0	1	2	3	4	5	6	7	8	9	10
Does not Interfere										Completely Interferes

G.   Enjoyment of life

0	1	2	3	4	5	6	7	8	9	10
Does not Interfere										Completely Interferes

Page 2 of 2

Figure 9.3 (*Continued*)

Consider modification of underlying cause or disease process

In many situations where a patient is being managed with a palliative care focus, it will be because no further disease modifying therapy is deemed beneficial or tolerable, or patient choice has excluded it. However, new situations arise where the risk/benefit balance changes. In cancer patients for example it will be appropriate to consider whether palliative chemotherapy might reduce symptoms caused by a bulky mass, or palliative radiotherapy relieve pain from a bony metastasis, or orthopaedic surgery permit stabilisation of a painful bony lesion.

Raise the pain threshold

The patient's ability to tolerate pain will be affected by many factors. Any of the nonphysical dimensions of the total pain model may have a bearing on pain tolerance and complement other aspects of the management plan. A tired, depressed, anxious patient who feels abandoned and unsupported and is distressed by their inability to work or provide in other ways for their family has many reasons to have a worse experience of pain. In some cases, there are elements of total pain that require high levels of specialist intervention. Where psychological and spiritual factors are predominant and more complex than can be supported by the usual clinical team members or specialist palliative care colleagues, referral to a clinical psychologist or chaplain or other spiritual care provider can be extremely beneficial.

Modify environment and support activities of daily living

The pain assessment is likely to have identified factors that provoke or exacerbate the pain. This information should be used by members of the multi-professional team to determine how the occupational therapist and physiotherapist can support the patient and to highlight social or nursing care needs that must be met.

Modify pain perception

Prescribed drug intervention is one of the main aspects of this principle. Additionally some patients benefit from acupuncture and other complementary therapies (CTs). Specific pharmacotherapies are described in more detail in the following text, and the role of CTs is discussed in Chapter 23.

Interrupt pain pathways

Interventional techniques including nerve blocks, epidural or intrathecal analgesia, joint injections, ablative techniques, or neurosurgical interventions have a role in some cases, especially where pain is refractory to drug treatment alone. The timing of these interventions must be individualised: too early and there is a risk of subjecting a patient to a procedure that might not be necessary; too late and the patient's general condition may have deteriorated, so that the intervention can no longer safely be performed.

Pharmacotherapeutic intervention

It is not practicable to provide a fully comprehensive account here of every analgesic available. The purpose of this text is not to replace the excellent regional, national, and international guidelines and formularies to which clinicians will have access but to provide an overview of options with some practical information. Prescribers must consult formularies for more specific detail about doses, adverse effects, and interactions and for guidance on locally available products and formulations. Prescribers are responsible for the safety of the prescriptions that they issue, and if uncertain should always consult the manufacturers published product information and seek specialist advice.

The *Palliative Care Formulary*, with its fourth edition published in the United Kingdom in 2011, provides detailed authoritative guidance on prescribing in palliative care practice (www.palliativedrugs.com) and versions have been produced specifically for the United States and for Canada that are accessible through the same website.

To assist clinical decision making and a logical approach to treatment decisions, analgesics may be broadly classified into three groups:

1. Non-opioid analgesics—this includes paracetamol (acetaminophen), aspirin (acetylsalicylic acid) and nonsteroidal anti-inflammatory drugs (NSAIDs).
2. Opioids—this group is further divided into "weak opioids" (sometimes referred to as "opioids for mild-moderate pain") and "strong opioids" (also referred to as "opioids for moderate-severe pain"). Examples of opioids from the different groups are given in Table 9.3, and the role of different opioid drugs is discussed later in the chapter. Box 9.4 outlines briefly the distinction between the terms "opiate" and "opioid."
3. Adjuvant analgesics, sometimes called "coanalgesics"— a group that comprises drugs whose primary purpose or design was not as analgesics but which have analgesic effects in particular clinical situations.

The WHO analgesic ladder

In 1986 an expert committee brought together by the Cancer and Palliative Care Unit of the WHO met to consider how to tackle the worldwide problem of cancer pain. The committee proposed a three-step framework to guide

Table 9.3 Classification of opioids by potency.

Opioids for mild-to-moderate pain	Opioids for moderate-to-severe pain
Codeine	Morphine
Dihydrocodeine	Diamorphine
Tramadol	Oxycodone
Buprenorphine	Fentanyl
	Methadone
	Hydromorphone
	Alfentanil

Box 9.4 Terminology of opioids

Opiate: the term referring to a naturally occurring drug derived from juice of the opium poppy (*Papaver somniferum*), that is, morphine and codeine.

Opioid: the term for a broader class including all drugs with "opiate-like" actions, which exert their effects on opioid receptors and whose effects are antagonised by naloxone. The group includes the opiates and other naturally occurring drugs and all the other synthetic and semi-synthetic drugs with these characteristics.

cancer pain management based on the fundamental principle that pain intensity, rather than a etiology, should direct clinical decision making [20]. This framework became known as the WHO analgesic ladder and continues to be recognised as a guiding principle in cancer pain management and one that has been extrapolated to non-cancer pain treatment. It incorporates the non-opioid, opioid, and adjuvant analgesics and should be applied in a way that also integrates other treatment modalities (such as radiotherapy, surgery, interventional analgesia, and others). Two further key guiding principles are also recognised to achieve simple, tolerable, and effective relief. First, pain relief should be given by mouth unless there is a particular reason to choose an alternative nonoral route (Box 9.9 suggests reasons why a change of route may be necessary). Second, patients with persistent pain should be prescribed, and be encouraged to take, pain relief on a regular basis ("by the clock") rather than in a random manner or only "as required."

A further important component of pain management is use of "rescue" or "breakthrough" analgesia. A simple representation of a pain management plan is shown in Figure 9.4.

Figure 9.5 outlines the WHO ladder.

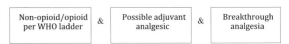

Figure 9.4 Three components of pain management.

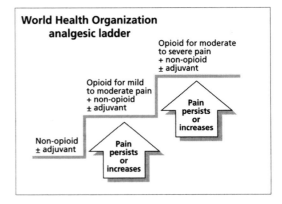

Figure 9.5 The WHO analgesic ladder.

Applying the principles of the WHO ladder in clinical practice

Box 9.5 summarises the treatment elements at each step of the WHO ladder reinforcing the principle that a

Box 9.5 Three steps in the WHO analgesic ladder

Step 1
Paracetamol (acetaminophen) and/or NSAID +/- adjuvant

Step 2
Paracetamol (acetaminophen) and/or NSAID + opioid for mild/moderate pain +/- adjuvant
  Examples of opioid for mild/moderate pain are codeine, dihydrocodeine or tramadol.
  (for rescue analgesia, use low-dose step 3 opioid, for example morphine 5 mg or equivalent)

Step 3
Paracetamol (acetaminophen) and/or NSAID + opioid for severe pain +/- adjuvant
  Examples of opioid for severe pain are morphine, diamorphine, oxycodone, fentanyl or hydromorphone.
  (for rescue analgesic, use 1/6th daily dose of regular opioid)

non-opioid should be tried first, with or without an adjuvant. Next a weak opioid may be added. If this does not provide adequate pain relief, the weak opioid is replaced with a strong opioid. Note that an adjuvant analgesic may be started, and continued, at any step.

Step 1: Initial treatment involves a non-opioid analgesic, typically paracetamol (acetaminophen), and effectiveness judged after 48 h. Depending on the degree of pain relief reported by the patient, paracetamol alone may be sufficient or an adjuvant may be added depending on the type of pain (see Table 9.2). Assessing the effectiveness of an adjuvant will take longer than 48 h and may need as long as a couple of weeks. If paracetamol provides limited or no useful pain relief, an NSAID may be substituted assuming there are no contraindication (e.g., peptic ulcer disease, cardiac failure, renal failure).

Sometimes a combination of paracetamol and NSAID may be appropriate. This is a clinical decision to be negotiated with the individual patient. The number of tablets that the patient is being asked to take may affect what is acceptable.

Step 2: If pain is not fully controlled after 48 h of simple analgesia or if pain remains distressing whilst adjuvant analgesics are being introduced and titrated, the treatment plan moves to step 2. An opioid for mild-to-moderate pain (e.g., codeine–see Table 9.3) is prescribed and administered regularly. Simple analgesics are continued if the patient believes they have provided partial relief. Any adjuvant analgesic that has been started previously should be continued.

In some countries, it is common practice to prescribe compound formulations comprising a non-opioid and "weak" opioid, and many preparations exist which combine different doses of opioid with paracetamol (acetaminophen). Advantages of this approach include fewer tablets for the patient to swallow, but disadvantages include higher cost and limitations on titration caused by a ceiling dose of one of the components.

Step 3: If the pain remains uncontrolled after a further 2–3 days on step 2 opioids, you should move to step 3. Do not switch between weak opioids as their relative potencies are broadly similar, and there is limited opportunity for upward dose titration. Oral morphine is the first choice strong opioid at step 3. An algorithm for morphine initiation and titration is shown in Figure 9.6 (strong opioid alternatives to morphine are discussed later). As in step 2, adjuvant analgesics and effective simple analgesics should also be continued. If adjuvants are not currently included in the management plan, this should be considered as should other interventions for pain relief.

When complex, multifactorial or multiple pains are being treated, it is quite normal for the management plan to include several components.

The step-wise model of the WHO analgesic ladder provides a logical framework for pain management. However, in a severe pain crisis, strong opioids may be appropriate from the outset. This would constitute a palliative care emergency and specialist advice is recommended. The management of acute severe pain is discussed toward the end of this chapter.

Three steps, or two?

The distinction between "weak opioid" and "strong opioid" is somewhat arbitrary, based more on traditional practice than pharmacological considerations. High doses of codeine have similar potency to low doses of morphine, and, again depending on the dose prescribed, the analgesic effect of tramadol bridges the step 2/step 3 divide. There have been discussions about a two-step approach [21], and some clinicians practise this. The most recent review of available evidence [22] on whether a "two step" WHO analgesic ladder might be proposed concluded that there were insufficient data to recommend abandoning the three-step approach for cancer patients with mild-to-moderate pain. Furthermore, given the nonavailability of strong opioids in many parts of the world (for political, cultural, and economic reasons) retaining step 2 in the three-step analgesic ladder approach remains true to the WHO's ambition to bring relief to the greatest number of patients with pain. Using low-dose strong opioid combined with a non-opioid as the second step is not, however, "wrong."

Breakthrough analgesia

The staged approach described above supports the management of persistent or background pain. Breakthrough pain, discussed earlier, must also be managed in an anticipatory fashion. This will not only relieve suffering by ensuring prompt access to additional pain relief but also increase the patient/carer sense of empowerment and control and aim to reduce "predictably unpredictable" demands on health-care resources, especially for parts of the day or week when routine services are unavailable, and only emergency cover is in place.

The drug choice for rescue analgesia will depend on the step in the WHO ladder being applied to the patient's care. At step 1, regular paracetamol (acetaminophen) may be backed up by an NSAID or weak opioid, or both. If paracetamol and an NSAID are already being used regularly, then a weak opioid alone would be prescribed. At

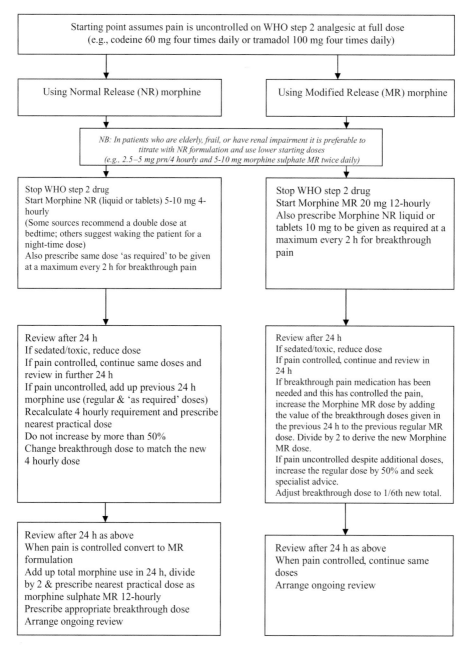

Starting point assumes pain is uncontrolled on WHO step 2 analgesic at full dose
(e.g., codeine 60 mg four times daily or tramadol 100 mg four times daily)

Using Normal Release (NR) morphine

Using Modified Release (MR) morphine

NB: In patients who are elderly, frail, or have renal impairment it is preferable to titrate with NR formulation and use lower starting doses (e.g., 2.5–5 mg prn/4 hourly and 5-10 mg morphine sulphate MR twice daily)

Stop WHO step 2 drug
Start Morphine NR (liquid or tablets) 5-10 mg 4-hourly
(Some sources recommend a double dose at bedtime; others suggest waking the patient for a night-time dose)
Also prescribe same dose 'as required' to be given at a maximum every 2 h for breakthrough pain

Stop WHO step 2 drug
Start Morphine MR 20 mg 12-hourly
Also prescribe Morphine NR liquid or tablets 10 mg to be given as required at a maximum every 2 h for breakthrough pain

Review after 24 h
If sedated/toxic, reduce dose
If pain controlled, continue same doses and review in further 24 h
If pain uncontrolled, add up previous 24 h morphine use (regular & 'as required' doses)
Recalculate 4 hourly requirement and prescribe nearest practical dose
Do not increase by more than 50%
Change breakthrough dose to match the new 4 hourly dose

Review after 24 h
If sedated/toxic, reduce dose
If pain controlled, continue and review in 24 h
If breakthrough pain medication has been needed and this has controlled the pain, increase the Morphine MR dose by adding the value of the breakthrough doses given in the previous 24 h to the previous regular MR dose. Divide by 2 to derive the new Morphine MR dose.
If pain uncontrolled despite additional doses, increase the regular dose by 50% and seek specialist advice.
Adjust breakthrough dose to 1/6th new total.

Review after 24 h as above
When pain is controlled convert to MR formulation
Add up total morphine use in 24 h, divide by 2 & prescribe nearest practical dose as morphine sulphate MR 12-hourly
Prescribe appropriate breakthrough dose
Arrange ongoing review

Review after 24 h as above
When pain controlled, continue same doses
Arrange ongoing review

Figure 9.6 Initiation and titration of morphine sulphate using either normal release (NR) or modified release (MR) formulations.

step 2, to back up the regular weak opioid, a small dose of a strong opioid is appropriate. At step 3, normal practice would be to ensure access to a dose of the same strong opioid being given routinely, but calculated as a fraction of the total daily dose of that opioid. This is covered more in opioid titration later in the chapter.

Non-opioids

Paracetamol (acetaminophen)
Paracetamol is a synthetic analgesic that acts in the CNS to inhibit cyclo-oxygenase involved in the prostaglandin (PG) cascade. This inhibitory effect is thought to be

different from the mechanism by which NSAIDs act. Paracetamol is also antipyretic. Metabolism is age- and dose-dependent and occurs primarily in the liver with conversion to glucuronide and sulphate metabolites. Available routes of administration are oral, rectal, and intravenous (IV). The recommended maximum daily dose of 4 g is drawn from evidence that higher doses are associated with a risk of acute hepatic failure. This risk is increased in chronic alcohol abuse, old age, anorexia, malnourished states and when enzyme inducing drugs are coadministered. Paracetamol should be used cautiously in renal failure and in patients taking warfarin and avoided in liver failure. The 5HT3 antagonist anti-emetics have been reported to block the analgesic effects of paracetamol.

Nonsteroidal anti-inflammatory drugs

The NSAIDs comprise a group of drugs with anti-inflammatory activity, mediated by inhibition of cyclo-oxygenase in the arachidonic acid cascade, which results in reduction in PG synthesis. PGs are inflammatory mediators with peripheral and central effects. Peripherally increased sensitivity to noxious stimuli is induced in peripheral nerve endings by PGs resulting in increased response and pain. Centrally higher levels of PGs cause sensitisation of neurones in the dorsal horn of the spinal cord resulting in further amplification of the pain signal. The antiinflammatory actions of NSAIDs provide most of their analgesic effects. These drugs are antipyretic agents and may have beneficial effects in preventing development and growth of tumours and in down-regulating cytokines involved in the anorexia-cachexia syndrome.

It is essential to balance the advantages and disadvantages of this group of drugs carefully in every clinical scenario because they are associated with significant side effects. Adverse effects of NSAIDs are described by site in Table 9.4. Table 9.5 categorises NSAIDs by their risk of causing GI adverse effects. Decisions on the use of NSAIDs should be made with a full understanding of the adverse effects. The choice of particular NSAID, dose and duration of treatment will be guided by information in locally agreed guidelines and formularies. Box 9.6 lists factors that increase the risk of GI toxicity from NSAIDs.

Opioids

Opioids for mild-to-moderate pain

The opioids used on the second step of the WHO ladder include codeine, dihydrocodeine, tramadol, and buprenorphine. Typical doses, available formulations, and

---

> ### Box 9.6 Risk factors that amplify the GI toxicity of NSAIDs
>
> *NB: Risk is compounded if multiple factors apply, as is common in palliative care patients:*
> - Increased age.
> - Helicobacter pylori infection.
> - Previous peptic ulcer disease, dyspepsia, upper GI haemorrhage (either proven endoscopically or clinically highly suspected).
> - Concurrent medication, especially aspirin, corticosteroids, selective serotonin reuptake inhibitors (SSRIs).
> - Concurrent anticoagulation.
> - Other comorbidities: malignancy, cardiac, renal, liver disease.

---

other considerations are outlined in Table 9.6. It is useful to have an understanding of the approximate relative potency of these drugs when compared with "strong" opioids. This matters in clinical practice when a switch is made from one drug to another. For example, codeine is deemed 1/10th as potent as oral morphine. Thus a patient taking the maximum typical dose of codeine (60 mg four times daily) can be thought of as taking approximately 24 mg morphine. If a switch is made from codeine to morphine because pain appears opioid responsive but is inadequately controlled, the starting dose must reflect the "opioid value" that has already been trialled. The initial daily morphine dose should be 30 mg or more (prescribed in an appropriate formulation) if an improvement in pain control is to be achieved.

A further clinical caution must be added regarding switching from codeine to morphine. Codeine has little direct analgesic effect. The majority is due to its transformation to morphine, which is dependent on a cytochrome enzyme (CYP2D6). There is genetic variation in expression of this enzyme; hence, some patients do not transform codeine to morphine, and these patients will have very little analgesic benefit from codeine. Consequently when these patients are switched to morphine, there is a risk that the initial dose recommended is too potent. Intolerance (resulting in sedation, confusion, cognitive impairment, or myoclonic jerks) will require a dose reduction. Provided the clinical effects of any morphine rescue doses given to the patient before the switch have been taken into consideration when determining the morphine dose at the time of the switch, it is unlikely that harm will occur. However, the possibility of a greater than expected

Table 9.4 Adverse effects of NSAIDs.

Site or system involved	Adverse effects	Notes
Gastrointestinal tract	Gastro-duodenal inflammation, ulceration, bleeding, and perforation Pain, nausea, vomiting Lower GI bleeding	Common NSAIDs differ in risk profile (see Table 9.5) Risk amplified by other factors (see Box 9.6) Concurrent prescription of GI protection [23] (esp. proton pump inhibitor (PPI)) indicated for majority of palliative patients
Renal system	Water and sodium retention, oedema Hyperkalaemia Antagonism of diuretics and anti-hypertensives Acute renal failure especially if elderly, dehydrated, and/or arteriopathic (e.g., if renal artery stenosis present)	Risk of renal failure is real but uncommon (less than 1% patients treated). Rehydration before use reduces risk Myeloma and renal failure are contraindications
Cardiovascular system	Increased risk of thrombotic events (myocardial infarction and stroke) Fluid retention precipitating or exacerbating congestive cardiac failure	Contraindicated in severe heart failure (HF) Thrombotic risk greater with COX-2 inhibitors—these should be avoided in patients with ischaemic heart disease and cerebrovascular disease Minimise risk by using lowest dose for shortest time Adding aspirin to counter the increased thrombotic risk of COX-2 negates the reduced GI toxicity benefit and is not recommended
Respiratory system	Bronchospasm Exacerbation of known asthma Rhinitis	Contraindicated if known previous sensitivity Avoid if known severe asthma, chronic rhinitis, nasal polyps Use cautiously under close supervision in asthmatic patients aged >40 years (other options preferable)

Table 9.5 Relative gastrointestinal toxicity of different NSAIDs.

Low risk	Medium risk	High risk
COX-2 inhibitors	Flurbiprofen	Aspirin
Diclofenac	Indometacin	Ketorolac
Ibuprofen	Ketoprofen	
Meloxicam	Naproxen	
Nabumetone	Piroxicam	

morphine dose effect should be considered and discussed when the patient is counselled about the opioid change.

Opioids for moderate-to-severe pain

Morphine is a naturally occurring opioid derived from the opium poppy and has been used to treat pain for more than two centuries. It is the strong opioid analgesic recommended as first choice in the original WHO declaration on Cancer Pain Relief in 1986 and was further endorsed in 2001 [25]. The most recent review of this guidance was published in 2011 [26] and

Table 9.6 Opioids for mild-to-moderate pain (where paracetamol is stated this also implies acetaminophen).

Drug	Dose range and formulations	Potency relative to morphine [24]	Notes
Codeine	30–60 mg four times daily Tablets, oral syrup, and solution (injection not recommended in palliative care) Compound preparations with paracetamol and aspirin exist	Codeine 30 mg ~ Morphine 3 mg (see notes on transformation above)	Often used as an antitussive agent Metabolised to morphine Metabolites accumulate in renal failure
Dihydrocodeine	30–60 mg four times daily Tablets and oral solution modified release tablets exist Injection not commonly used in palliative care Compound preparations with paracetamol exist	Dihydrocodeine 30 mg ~ Morphine 3 mg Similar potency to codeine when given orally but twice as potent as codeine when injected	Unlike codeine, dihydrocodeine is not a pro-drug; hence, its therapeutic effect is not limited by CYP2D6 inhibition Toxic in renal failure due to accumulation of glucuronide metabolite
Tramadol	50–100 mg four times daily Modified and normal release tablets and capsules Oro-dispersible tablets Injection Compound preparations with paracetamol exist	Trial evidence suggests 1/5th as potent as morphine by mouth (Tramadol 50 mg ~ Morphine 10 mg) but clinical experience suggests 1/10th Studies suggest a range of relative potencies to morphine by injection; in clinical practice 1/10th is applied	Less constipating than codeine/DHC but causes more nausea/vomiting Non-opioid properties (through noradrenaline and serotonin) responsible for efficacy and adverse effects Preferred weak opioid in renal failure as converted by liver to inactive metabolites that are renally excreted
Buprenorphine	Sublingual tablets, transdermal patches, injection	SL buprenorphine ~80 times as potent as oral morphine Transdermal buprenorphine 100 times as potent as oral morphine (35 mcg/h Buprenorphine patch ~ 84 mg oral morphine per day) (recommended in practice by PCF4)	Patches not suitable for unstable pain requiring rapid titration. Highly lipid-soluble facilitating transdermal use. Low strength TD formulations provide an option for less severe pain or for patients sensitive to other strong opioids. Suitable in renal failure. Toxicity not reversed by standard doses of naloxone (higher doses needed)

morphine remains first choice. However, the authors acknowledge that there is insufficient good quality comparative evidence for the superiority of morphine over other strong opioids, and state that morphine, oxycodone, and hydromorphone offer similar profiles of efficacy and side effects.

Morphine is well absorbed from the upper GI tract after oral administration and acts through central and peripheral opioid receptors. The peripheral nerve opioid receptors involved in pain pathways are activated in the presence of inflammation. Metabolism occurs by glucuronidation in the liver, with the main metabolites being morphine-3-glucuronide (M3G) and morphine-6-glucuronide (M6G). Metabolism is not significantly affected by liver impairment unless liver function is sufficiently impaired to extend the prothrombin time, in which case the half-life of morphine will be extended. The metabolite M6G binds to opioid receptors and is predominantly responsible for both therapeutic (analgesic) and adverse (nausea, vomiting, sedation, respiratory depression) effects. The peripheral actions of morphine on smooth muscle result in delayed gastric emptying and constipation. Morphine metabolites are excreted by the kidneys. Renal impairment therefore results in accumulation of M6G, and a risk of toxicity unless dose and frequency are adjusted. Pre-existing or new onset renal impairment/renal failure is one indication for a switch to an alternative strong opioid.

Opioid initiation and titration

An expert working group of the European Association for Palliative Care (EAPC) published guidelines on the use of morphine in cancer pain in 1996, and these were reviewed, revised, and republished in 2001 [25] and 2012 [27]. These guidelines were based on review of the available scientific evidence but mostly on expert consensus and recommended the use of NR morphine preparations for initiation and during early dose titration. This approach has long been considered as the classical method of opioid titration. In the most recent review of this topic, published in 2011 [28], the research evidence base for this recommendation is acknowledged to remain limited and the guidance remains essentially based on expert opinion and consensus.

The original justification for titration with NR formulations was based on pharmacological considerations. Since the plasma half-life of morphine is 2–4 h and a steady state will be achieved within 4–5 half-lives, a dose regime may be evaluated clinically within approximately 24 h. However, it is recognised that for practical reasons (includ-

---

> **Box 9.7 Practical points when starting oral strong opioids**
>
> 1. Ensure patients have been given very clear oral and written instructions and that their understanding has been confirmed.
> 2. MR opioids should be prescribed by time interval (i.e., stating "12-hourly") rather than the less precise instruction "twice daily."
> 3. Clarify with the patient that the regular prescription should still be taken even if a dose of breakthrough medication has just been used.
> 4. Ensure that a regular laxative has been prescribed and that bowel habit is monitored as well as pain control.
> 5. Ensure that patients have a supply of anti-emetic for regular or as required use for at least the first week on a strong opioid.
> 6. Monitor closely for efficacy, adverse effects, and toxicity.

ing reduced concordance—it is not easy to remember to take prescribed medication 5–6 times each day—and the nursing time required to dispense controlled drugs (CDs) every 4 h in busy health-care settings) titration using MR formulations may be an option. This was examined in a study of hospitalised cancer patients who were randomised to titration using normal or MR morphine for their pain [29]. Outcomes suggested titration using a MR formulation was acceptable. The time to achieve pain control was 1.7 days for the MR group and 2.1 days for the NR group. In addition, the NR group reported more tiredness. Other studies undertaken on cancer outpatients with pain report similar findings. Titration with NR preparations is highly recommended in frail elderly patients, patients with renal impairment, and patients in whom the previous analgesic intake is not known. Doses, adjustments, effects, and tolerability must be monitored very closely in these groups. Expert consensus recommends that individual dose increases during a titration schedule should not exceed 33–50% in any 24-h period [30].

The algorithm in Figure 9.6 offers an approach to WHO pain ladder step 3 opioid dose titration using either NR or MR formulations of morphine sulphate. Box 9.7 lists points to consider when starting strong opioids and Box 9.8 summarises guidance points on opioid titration.

Opioid breakthrough or "rescue" doses

All patients whose pain is managed with an opioid should also be prescribed a dose of NR opioid as a "rescue" or

---

Box 9.8 Important considerations when titrating opioids

1. The total regular daily dose given should not be increased by more than 33–50% every 24 h.
2. It is not recommended to titrate with transdermal preparations when there is unstable pain or in opioid naïve patients without specialist advice.
3. Always adjust the breakthrough dose if the regular dose is changed (*up or down*).
4. Do not use two or more MR opioid formulations at the same time.
5. If pain control deteriorates, a whole reassessment of pain is necessary.
6. If an intervention takes place that may change the pain burden, the opioid dose may require reduction to avoid intolerance and adverse effects.

"breakthrough pain" treatment to be given as needed. The drug given should be the same as the regular opioid. When a patient is being treated with a fentanyl patch options include a NR oral formulation of morphine, oxycodone or hydromorphone, or a transmucosal form of fentanyl.

Guidance on the rescue dose follows the EAPC 2001 recommendations suggesting that this should be approximately 1/6th of the total 24-h opioid dose. Other work has suggested that the appropriate rescue dose lies somewhere between 5% and 15% of the 24-h regular daily dose [31], and a further publication identified no specific relationship between the regular and an effective rescue dose [32].

The practical clinical approach is to use the 1/6th "rule" as a starting point and tailor the particular dose to a specific patient following careful clinical review of efficacy and tolerability.

The frequency at which the rescue dose may be given depends on the time to peak onset of action. Orally administered NR opioids such as morphine and oxycodone have an onset of action after 20–30 min with a peak effect after 60–120 min. Parenterally administered opioids (typically by the subcutaneous (SC) route in palliative care practice) have onset of action after 10 min with a peak after 30–60 min. Allowing repeat rescue doses after 2 h if given orally and after 1 h if given parenterally provides a safe framework for practice. Clinical judgement, with specialist advice where needed, should determine the dose and frequency, especially in the context of severe pain.

Opioid switching

There are several indications for a switch from morphine to an alternative strong opioid including efficacy, tolerability, patient factors and preferences. Before making a switch, it is important to consider whether the switch is really necessary. If there is uncertainty, or if staff are unfamiliar with making an opioid switch, specialist advice should be sought.

Pharmacogenomics and opioid analgesia [33]

The genetic diversity of humans and the impact of this on response to pain treatment is an active and expanding area of medical research. The clinical consequences of this work and its translation into "bedside" practice will become evident in the future. However, one area of research suggests that there may be genetic polymorphism in the μ-opioid receptor. This may explain why patients' responses to opioids vary in efficacy, dose requirements, tolerability, and presence and severity of adverse effects. It is exciting to imagine the potential impact that some future pharmacogenetic testing process might have on opioid analgesic selection. Until then, morphine remains the first choice.

Opioid alternatives to oral morphine

In general, morphine is no less and no more effective an analgesic than the alternative strong opioids. Differences lie in the side effect profiles of each drug. For example, fewer patients report constipation when being treated with fentanyl than with morphine [34]. Others report less sedation with oxycodone treatment than with morphine, and this means they are better able to tolerate the dose increases that are needed to control their pain. However, a significant proportion of cancer patients with pain can be treated effectively with morphine and do not require an alternative, and this is why it has been emphasised several times that morphine remains the first-choice strong opioid analgesic. The particular characteristics, formulations, and potential routes of administration of alternative opioids are what make opioid switches a recognised part of clinical practice in palliative care. Specific properties or factors will determine what change is made. This chapter does not explore these in significant detail but provides an overview of some of the alternatives and associated indications (Table 9.7).

The information presented in Tables 9.8 and 9.9 give indications of relative potencies. It is absolutely essential that this information be applied with clinical wisdom and with guidance from experienced clinical colleagues. The

Table 9.7 Opioid alternatives to morphine.

Opioid	Formulations	Characteristics/comments
Oxycodone	Normal release liquid and capsules, MR tablets, injection	Similar properties to morphine
Hydromorphone	Normal release and MR capsules, injection	Suitable option for patients with renal impairment
Fentanyl	Transdermal patches, transmucosal lozenges, buccal and sublingual tablets, nasal spray, injection	Potency often underestimated. Less constipating than morphine. Patches not suitable for unstable pain requiring rapid titration. Novel formulations permit options for rapid absorption, but this requires close supervision in initial titration. Suitable in renal failure
Diamorphine	Tablets, injection	Not widely used outside United Kingdom. Oral form rarely used. No intrinsic advantage over parenteral morphine but more soluble and thus commonly used by infusion, especially when high doses are needed. Compatible with many drugs in SC infusion
Methadone	Tablets, oral solution, injection	Non-opioid receptor actions potentiate analgesic action. Highly variable pharmacokinetics and pharmacodynamics between individuals; hence, switching from other opioids and titration should be managed by specialists [35]

stated dose "equivalence" should be considered as a guide and not as an absolute protocol. Factors that influence the effective dose after a switch include:
• the reason for the switch (e.g., inefficacy vs. intolerance);

• the dose, choice, and duration of the previous opioid including the degree of cross-tolerance that has developed; and
• metabolic and genetic characteristics of the individual patient.

Table 9.8 Opioid dose conversion ratios—oral morphine to other opioids.

Opioid dose ratio	Example of converted prescriptions
Switching between oral formulations	
Morphine : Oxycodone = 1.5 : 1	Morphine 15 mg = Oxycodone 10 mg
Morphine : Hydromorphone = 5 : 1	Morphine 30 mg = Hydromorphone 6 mg
Switching from oral to transdermal formulations	
Morphine PO : Fentanyl TD = 100 : 1	Morphine MR 60 mg/24 h = Fentanyl TD patch 25 mcg/h
Morphine PO : Buprenorphine TD = 100 : 1	Morphine MR 60 mg/24 h = Buprenorphine 25 mcg/h (in practice a 20 mcg/h patch would be used)

These figures are a guide. Please note that this table follows the PCF4 clinical recommendations rather than the manufacturers' stated ratios (see Chapter 15 in PCF4).

Table 9.9 Opioid dose conversion ratios—oral (PO) opioids to SC infusion.

Opioid dose ratio	Example of converted prescription
Morphine PO : Morphine SC = 2 : 1	Morphine MR 30 mg PO 12 hourly = Morphine 30 mg/24 h through SC infusion
Morphine PO : Diamorphine SC = 3 : 1	Morphine MR 30 mg PO 12 hourly = Diamorphine 20 mg/24 h through SC infusion
Morphine PO : Oxycodone SC = 2 : 1	Morphine MR 30 mg PO 12 hourly = Oxycodone 30 mg/24 h through SC infusion
Morphine PO : Hydromorphone SC = 10–15 : 1	Morphine MR 30 mg PO 12 hourly = Hydromorphone 4 mg/24 h through SC infusion
Oxycodone PO : Oxycodone SC = 1.5 : 1	Oxycodone MR 20 mg PO 12 hourly = Oxycodone 25 mg/24 h through SC infusion
Hydromorphone PO : Hydromorphone SC = 2 : 1	Hydromorphone CR 8 mg PO 12 hourly = Hydromorphone 8 mg/24 h through SC infusion

These figures are a guide. Please note that this table follows the PCF4 clinical recommendations rather than the manufacturers' stated ratios (see Chapter 15 in PCF4 listed in further reading).

For these reasons, whenever a switch is made from one opioid to another, it is recommended to calculate the "equivalent" dose and then apply a relative dose reduction. Provided a NR formulation is also provided for rescue use to treat breakthrough pain, further titration can be achieved. For more detail on switching between opioids, including less common dose conversions not included here, the reader is advised to consult the *Palliative Care Formulary*, 4th edition (PCF 4e) (see Further Reading) (www.palliativedrugs.com).

Transdermal opioids

Two opioids are currently marketed in transdermal formulation as patches, fentanyl and buprenorphine. These offer a useful mode of delivery, but it is important that their particular characteristics are understood. Problems arise when transdermal opioids are prescribed by those unfamiliar with their use or when insufficient information is given to patients.

The use of transdermal patches may be considered for patients with stable, opioid-responsive pain as an alternative to morphine or other opioid analgesic for one or more of the reasons indicated in Box 9.9. With particu-lar reference to fentanyl, this may be because the patient is unable to tolerate morphine (i.e., a patient who has intolerable side effects, including constipation), unable to take oral medication (e.g., dysphagia) or is requesting an alternative method of drug delivery.

Patches are also indicated where the problem is poor concordance and pain control might be improved by reliable administration. This might be useful in patients with cognitive impairment or those who for any reason find regular self-medication difficult. Transdermal patches are not suitable for acute pain, where rapid dose titration is required.

Starting transdermal patches

The following description is a general guide to using transdermal patches, but readers are referred to the manufacturer's guidance for further details. It takes 24–48 h to reach a steady state of analgesia using transdermal patches; hence, NR rescue opioid analgesia may be required until the steady state is reached.

Converting from oral opioids:
- Calculate the appropriate patch strength using the opioid dose conversion guidelines (Table 9.6).

> ## Box 9.9 Clinical issues to consider before making an opioid switch
>
> 1. Persistent pain. Review whether the pain appears opioid-responsive and consider adjustment of the non-opioid or adjuvant opioid analgesic regime.
> 2. Adverse effects. Consider whether morphine dose may be reduced or the adverse effects may be treated more effectively, for example, with an appropriate antiemetic or laxative regime. Morphine toxicity may occur due to renal or liver impairment that requires dose adjustment. Measures to improve renal function must be considered, for example, by treating dehydration, stopping nephrotoxic drugs, or surgical/radiological intervention to correct renal failure due to obstruction if this is clinically appropriate.
> 3. Problems with oral route. The route may need to be changed if there is failure of absorption due to gastric stasis, gastric outlet obstruction, or small intestinal obstruction. Other factors resulting in difficulty with oral administration include dysphagia or odynophagia caused by neurological dysfunction, oropharyngeal infection, or the consequences of head, neck, and oesophageal cancer or their treatments.
> 4. Patient choice and concordance. It is always important to review the patient's understanding of the management plan, to address their concerns and review their expectations.

- Apply patch and continue oral medication for the next 12 h (i.e., give last dose of 12-hourly morphine or three further doses of 4-hourly morphine).
- Ensure analgesic breakthrough doses are available.
- Patients should be warned that they may experience more breakthrough pain than usual in the first 1–3 days.

The dose of the patch should not be changed within two days of the first application or of any change in dose. Adequate analgesia should be achieved using breakthrough medication as needed. Subsequent dose changes should be made according to the patient's requirement for breakthrough analgesics or follow the "33–50%" rule discussed in opioid titration earlier in this chapter. The patch dose that is closest to the calculated dose should be prescribed.

Practicalities when using transdermal patches

Fentanyl transdermal patches are designed to give 72 h of analgesia. They should be replaced at the same time every 3 days, although the site of application should be varied with each patch change. In a small number of patients

analgesia decreases on the third day and patches need to be changed every 48 h. Buprenorphine patches are marketed in different formulations, some designed for 7-day use and others to last 96 h—in practice the latter is to enable changes twice a week on a set day. The steady state is maintained provided the appropriate change interval is observed. The patches should be stuck to a flat, clean, dry area of hairless skin, usually on the trunk or back or on the upper outer arm. Men may need to cut, not shave, body hair, but the skin integrity must be preserved. The patches should not be cut.

Patients are able to shower with the patches in place, but hot baths and directly applied heat will rapidly increase absorption, as will raised body temperature from pyrexia. Used patches should be folded sticky side together, and disposed of safely or returned to a pharmacist.

In 10% of patients a physical and/or depressive opioid withdrawal syndrome occurs on changing from morphine to transdermal fentanyl. This is short lived (usually a few days) and easily treated by the use of normal-release morphine when symptoms occur.

Discontinuing transdermal patches

Once a patient is established on transdermal patches, they should be continued, with dose titration if necessary, unless there is a significant reason to change. Change may be clinically indicated if the pain has become unstable or if the pain has improved so much due to other treatments that the analgesic is to be reduced or even withdrawn.

The dose of the new opioid that is equivalent to the existing fentanyl transdermal patch dose should be calculated using dose conversion charts. It is advisable to make a dose reduction (~25%) when switching between opioids because there may be incomplete cross tolerance (the patient responds more to a new opioid than to an equivalent dose of one used longer term). This is especially important if the opioid switch has been made due to opioid toxicity. It is advisable to seek specialist advice in these situations in order to discuss appropriate dose reduction for the clinical situation. Guidance on timing when switching between different routes of administration is given below.

Switching between different routes of administration

Changing between different *routes* of administration also requires careful consideration. The time to peak effect differs between opioid formulations (NR or MR) and routes (oral, transdermal, and continuous SC infusion). Box 9.10 provides a summary for guidance and this

Box 9.10 Switching between different routes of opioid administration

Oral to continuous SC infusion (e.g., through syringe driver)
  From NR opioid: start SC infusion immediately.
  From 12-hourly MR opioid: start SC infusion 8 h after the last oral dose.

SC infusion to oral
  When switching to either NR or MR opioid, stop the SC infusion at the same time as giving the first oral dose.

Oral to patch
  From NR opioid: apply patch when convenient and use oral NR opioid only as required.
  From 12-hourly MR opioid: apply patch at same time as last dose of MR oral opioid.
  From once daily MR opioid: apply patch 12 h after last dose of MR opioid.
  Breakthrough/rescue doses may be needed whilst transdermal absorption is established.

Patch to oral
  Remove patch 6 h before giving first dose of oral MR opioid.
  For first 24 h give HALF the calculated equivalent dose since the transdermal fentanyl will take time to be cleared from plasma and SC reservoir.
  After 24 h increase to the calculated equivalent dose if clinically indicated by pain.

Patch to SC infusion
  This does not apply to patients in the last days of life when recommended practice is to continue the patch and add a SC infusion—see Chapter 21.
  In other situations where a change from patch is required, remove patch and start SC infusion 6 h later. For the first 24 h use HALF the calculated opioid equivalent dose. After 24 h adjust according to symptoms.

SC infusion to patch
  Apply patch. Continue SC infusion for a further 6 h then discontinue.

Normal release (NR), modified release (MR).

Adapted from North of England Cancer Network Palliative Care Guidelines with permission.

information should be observed whenever a change is made between an opioid administered by one route and another.

Opioid adverse effects

Opioid adverse effects should be discussed with patients when the decision to commence opioids is made. Adverse effects occur with both weak and strong opioids and should be anticipated at both step 2 and step 3 of the WHO ladder.

Common adverse effects include mild sedation, constipation, nausea, and vomiting. Other well-recognised side effects are dry mouth, itching, sweating, myoclonic jerks, and occasionally hypotension. Hallucinations, confusion, and vivid dreams may necessitate a dose reduction or a change to an alternative opioid; alternatively they can be managed with a small dose of haloperidol (1.5–3 mg) at night:

• Constipation is common (95%) and persists during opioid treatment. It should be anticipated and prevented with a combination of softening and stimulant laxatives and reviewed every 2–3 days to achieve a bowel habit acceptable to the patient.

• Nausea and vomiting are common (nausea 30–60%; vomiting 10%) at the initiation of opioid therapy, but patients usually become tolerant to these effects within one week. An antiemetic (either haloperidol 1.5 mg nocte or metoclopramide 10 mg tds) should be available—ideally prescribed regularly for the first week—then withdrawn if possible to avoid polypharmacy.

• Sedation is usually mild but affects the majority of patients during the first few days of treatment and after further dose adjustments. Tolerance usually develops to this, and the patient can be reassured but advised not to drive or operate other machinery during initiation and dose titration until doses are stable and/or they feel unimpaired. It is a matter of judgement. If sedation is severe or persists, opioid dose reduction may be necessary and the possibility of using adjuvant analgesics considered.

In some cases, adverse effects persist or are so troublesome that an opioid switch is indicated.

Fears and concerns related to use of morphine and other opioids

Despite the availability of education and clinical guidelines, and increasing clinical experience, some professionals and patients continue to have fears about the use of strong opioids, particularly morphine (see Box 9.11). For some there are concerns about the potential for opioids to be used as "recreational" drugs of abuse or supplies diverted to this. These concerns are compounded by excessively tight restrictions on use, and even nonavailability, of opioid analgesia in some parts of the world. Fears are worsened by rare but notorious events such as the arrest in 1998 of the British General Practitioner Dr Harold Shipman who was convicted for murdering his patients with morphine.

Box 9.11 Fears about opioids

Professional	Patient
Patient addiction/dependence	Addiction/dependence
	Social stigma
Respiratory depression	Adverse effects
Excess sedation/confusion/ cognitive impairment	Morphine = imminent death
Seen to be expediting death	Pain will become resistant to analgesia so "nothing left when pain severe later"
Diversion of patient supply to illegal use	

Extensive clinical experience of using morphine (and other opioids) within a defined framework according to consensus guidelines demonstrates that these fears are unjustified [36] and largely unfounded. However, these fears are common, and failure to address them in discussions with the patient about a pain management plan may lead to reservations on the part of the patient, anxieties that are unresolved, poor concordance, and ultimately poor pain management. Three particular areas of concern are discussed further:

• Addiction—this does not occur when opioids are used for the management of pain. If the cause of the pain is removed (e.g., by a nerve block or radiotherapy), then opioids can generally be reduced or withdrawn with no psychological problems. There may be a degree of physical dependence, with a physical withdrawal syndrome apparent upon withdrawal of the drug. However, with withdrawal of opioid in staged decrements this is easily managed.

• Respiratory depression—this is a clinical possibility and may occur in opioid-naive patients given an inappropriately large dose of an opioid for acute pain, or in other situations due to a drug error or accumulation of morphine metabolites in renal failure. However with careful judicious titration and in chronic use, tolerance to the respiratory depressant effects occurs rapidly and provided the dose is titrated against the patient's pain, morphine can be used safely, even in patients with chronic lung disease.

• Tolerance—anxieties about developing "resistance" (tolerance) to the effects of opioids are not uncommon. Some patients express the view: "If I take it now, it won't work later, when I really need it." Explanations that a changing analgesic requirement is usually due to a change in pain due to altered burden of disease rather than to

tolerance are necessary. Increasing experience of the use of opioids in both cancer- and noncancer-related pain confirms that tolerance is rare. Specialist advice should be sought about a patient who appears to have tolerance to the effects of opioids.

Adjuvant analgesics or coanalgesics

An important aspect of the WHO pain ladder is the recognition that some sorts of pain respond only partially, or even poorly, to simple and opioid analgesics. Examples of such pains include neuropathic pain, muscle spasm, intestinal colic, ano-rectal pain and bladder spasms. It is therefore important to appreciate that other drugs can be used alongside an existing analgesic regime, and the roles of these drugs are the following:

• To enhance the effect of concurrent simple and opioid analgesics.
• To permit dose reduction of opioid analgesic in order to improve tolerability and reduce adverse effects.
• To treat pains that fail to respond to simple and/or opioid analgesics.

Table 9.10 summarises some of the drug groups, indications, examples, and dose ranges.

Adjuvant analgesics used in the treatment of neuropathic pain

Neuropathic pain is common in palliative care, and several drugs from a number of different classes are used in its treatment. The classes include antidepressants, antiepileptics, N-methyl-D-aspartate (NMDA) receptor antagonists, and others. Deciding which specific drug from which class to choose in a particular clinical situation is difficult. A traditional view that a "burning" pain be treated with a tricyclic antidepressant (TCA) and a "shooting" pain with an antiepileptic drug has no evidence base to support it.

Antidepressants [37]

Drugs developed as antidepressants have been in use for many years as treatments for neuropathic pain, especially the TCAs such as amitriptyline and imipramine. TCAs act on multiple receptor sites (including noradrenaline, serotonin, histamine, and acetylcholine) and ion channels (sodium and calcium). The nonlinear nature of their pharmacokinetics means that dose adjustments do not result in a predictable change in the magnitude of the response in the same patient (a small dose increase may result in a large effect in terms of useful and adverse effects), and these drugs are also noted for showing considerable variability

Table 9.10 Examples of adjuvant analgesic drugs used in palliative care (detail on doses, adverse effects, contraindications, and interactions should be obtained from a suitable formulary, e.g., PCF 4).

Group	Indication	Example(s) with maximum dose range
Antidepressants	Neuropathic pain	Duloxetine 60–120 mg/day
		Amitriptyline 10–100 mg nocte
		Mirtazapine 15–45 mg nocte
Antiepileptics	Neuropathic pain	Gabapentin 100 mg tds – 900 mg qds
		Pregabalin 25 mg bd – 300 mg bd
		Sodium valproate 200 mg – 1500 mg/day
Corticosteroids	Neuropathic pain	Dexamethasone 8–12 mg daily initially reducing every few days to stop
	Liver capsular pain	
Bisphosphonates	Bone pain (e.g., in myeloma and breast cancer)	Zoledronic acid 4 mg in 100 ml 0.9% saline infused over 30 min given monthly
Benzodiazepines	Muscle relaxant	Diazepam 2–10 mg daily
		Midazolam 2.5–5 mg SC per dose
	Neuropathic pain	Clonazepam 0.5 mg nocte – 4 mg daily
Muscle relaxants	Muscle spasm	Baclofen 5 mg bd – 20 mg tds
Anticholinergics	Bowel or bladder spasm	Oxybutinin 5–10 mg tds
	Anorectal pain	Hyoscine butylbromide 60–120 mg/24 h SC infusion
Ketamine (for use under specialist supervision only)	Neuropathic pain	Starting dose: 10–25 mg orally four times daily or 50–100 mg/24 h by SC infusion
		Usual maximum dose: 50–100 mg orally four times daily or 500 mg/24 h by SC infusion

of effect between patients. The commonest side effects are caused by the anticholinergic properties and include dry mouth, sedation, blurred vision, hypotension, constipation, and urinary hesitancy. These are noted especially in the elderly, in whom there is an increased risk of falls, and when combined with opioids (as is often the case when treating cancer-related neuropathic pain). Doses that have analgesic action are generally lower than those needed for antidepressant effects. Newer antidepressants with more receptor selectivity (SSRIs—such as fluoxetine, and serotonin noradrenaline reuptake inhibitors—SNRIs—such as venlafaxine) are associated with fewer side effects, but the relative efficacy of these newer drugs compared with TCAs is unclear.

Trial evidence to support the use of these drugs is drawn from studies involving neuropathic pain conditions such as diabetic neuropathy and post-herpetic neuralgia. These pain syndromes make good study models because of their stability over time but are not truly representative of many neuropathic pain patients, especially in cancer neuropathic pain, where the condition is changing. Therefore, the direct applicability of the study findings is limited and clinicians need to bear this in mind when making treatment recommendations.

Antiepileptics [38]

Antiepileptics have been used for many years especially in neuropathic pain conditions such as trigeminal neuralgia. The pharmacological actions vary between drugs, but potential mechanisms include actions on sodium and calcium channels, involvement of serotonin and effects on pathways involving gamma-amino-butyric acid (GABA). Adverse effects common to all include drowsiness and fatigue. As for TCAs, these will be exacerbated by the simultaneous use of opioids and other medication. More serious effects that require monitoring are changes to liver enzymes and impaired bone marrow function.

NMDA receptor antagonists [39]

The NMDA receptor situated in the dorsal horn of the spinal cord controls an ion channel that is closed in the nonactivated state and blocked by magnesium. Activation opens the channel allowing sodium and calcium to flow into the neurone resulting in excitation out of proportion to the original stimulus. This is the phenomenon known as "wind up," and it is believed to be responsible for the component of chronic neuropathic pain that causes limited response to opioid analgesia and some of the particularly unpleasant clinical features. Drugs that block the NMDA receptor include ketamine and methadone. Ketamine is an anaesthetic agent that, in addition to NMDA receptor antagonism, acts on opioid and muscarinic anticholinergic receptors, sodium and potassium channels, and serotonin and dopamine uptake. Its analgesic effects are associated with a high incidence of significant adverse effects, especially on cognitive and higher cerebral function (such as confusion, hallucinations, dysphoria, and sedation) and the cardiovascular system (causing tachycardia and hypertension). Up to half of patients treated may suffer side effects.

As well as opioid receptor effects, methadone is thought to cause analgesia through NMDA receptor antagonism giving a potential role in management of neuropathic pain. The pharmacokinetics and pharmacodynamics of methadone, and its interactions, make this a complex drug to initiate and titrate.

Ketamine and methadone are drugs to be used only with specialist initiation and guidance.

Other adjuvant analgesics [40]

Other drugs and formulations are used to manage neuropathic pain. Topical agents may have a role in well-localised and small areas of peripheral neuropathic pain. Capsaicin cream (its active ingredient is derived from the chilli pepper) acts by reducing substance P release in nerve endings and reducing the number and density of peripheral nerve receptors. These actions take time to occur and capsaicin is highly irritant and these two factors may reduce patient concordance or the acceptability of the treatment. Doxepin is a TCA formulated as a cream for topical application, acting through the mechanisms described for TCAs earlier. The local anaesthetic agent, lidocaine, has been incorporated into a medicated plaster for transdermal administration and can be applied to areas of superficial pain.

Some specialist centres have experience in the use of antiarrythmics (such as mexiletine) and in administration of local anaesthetics (such as lidocaine) and anticonvulsants (such as phenytoin) through infusion. These options really are the remit of the "super-specialist" and are mentioned in order to give an overview of the whole range of options assuming appropriate patient selection, consent, and supervision.

Choosing and combining adjuvant analgesics in neuropathic pain

In some cases, addition of a single agent is sufficient to improve the pain management, but in other situations there may be a need for complex combinations. The key message here is to develop experience and confidence in initiating and titrating two of these drugs, for example, one antidepressant and one antiepileptic, and to seek specialist advice at an early stage if there is limited benefit or adverse effects. The role of the specialist here is to guide choices and combinations, and to take responsibility for monitoring and supervision in partnership with the generalist. This is essential for drugs such as methadone or ketamine.

The trial evidence to support one agent over another both within and between drug groups is very limited.

A practical approach is to choose either a TCA or one of the antiepileptic drugs with a more favourable side effects profile (such as gabapentin or pregabalin) based on patient characteristics. After dose adjustment and review, it may be appropriate—depending on clinical assessment of efficacy and tolerability—either to change to, or to add, the second adjuvant. If the pain remains refractory to these measures, or if there are side effects or complications that mean the drugs are not tolerated, specialist advice should be obtained.

Following a detailed review of studies of adjuvant analgesics for peripheral neuropathic pain, Finnerup [41] derived the "numbers needed to treat" (NNT) for a range of drugs. NNT is a calculation to determine how many patients must be treated with drug "X" in order to have one patient respond, where "response" is taken to be a 50% reduction in pain score. Although attractive as an aid to decision making on choice of drug, using only the NNT does not consider the weight of evidence (i.e., how many subjects were included in the studies from which the recommendation is derived) nor the tolerability (sometimes referred to as "numbers needed to harm").

Interventional analgesia

Some patients present extremely challenging pain scenarios. There may be pain refractory to a range of drug and nondrug interventions or persistent problems with intolerance to medications used. Individual nerve blocks and nerve plexus blocks present an option to control some pains. Other pains require epidural or intrathecal analgesia. A patient whose pain may require such intervention should be under the care of specialist palliative care services who can liaise with interventional pain specialists to review the whole clinical situation and recommend an appropriate interventional management plan.

Acute severe pain

Sudden onset new pain, or rapidly escalating existing pain, is a palliative care emergency and must be recognised and treated as such. Possible causes of acute severe pain are listed in Box 9.12.

The principles of pain assessment and management described earlier in this chapter are entirely relevant but the choice of drug, route of administration, and rate of review and dose titration will need to be adapted to the severity of the situation. There are situations in managing acute severe pain when it will be appropriate, guided by

---

Box 9.12 Causes of acute severe pain

Fracture, for example, pathological fracture through a bony metastasis.

Acute nerve compression, for example, vertebral collapse and nerve root compression or spinal cord compression.

Haemorrhage, for example, bleeding into a liver metastasis, intra-abdominal/pelvic cavity, retroperitoneum, joint capsule.

Perforation of GI tract.

Infarction/ischaemia, for example, myocardial infarction, mesenteric infarction, pulmonary embolism, critical limb ischaemia.

Obstruction of hollow viscus, for example, bowel obstruction with colic, ureteric colic, or bladder outlet obstruction cause by clot from renal/renal pelvic tumour.

---

the clinical situation and dependent on careful communication with the patient and family/carers, to accept a different balance of benefit and adverse effects in order to secure relief from the crisis. For example, sedation may be acceptable to the patient provided that pain is brought under control, or the risks associated with use of parenteral NSAIDs may be justified in the aim to relieve acute, severe distress.

Emergency admission will usually be necessary and, depending on the underlying cause, surgical or anaesthetic intervention may be appropriate.

The analgesic options for immediate use are outlined in Table 9.11. Parenteral administration is recommended and, provided the patient is not severely shocked or hemodynamically compromised, the SC route allows ready access and reliable absorption without the need to find and secure venous access (an important consideration in frail patients or those whose veins have become fragile following chemotherapy).

Nondrug interventions

The management of pain has many dimensions, and two important elements of pain management should be re-emphasised in the final part of this chapter:
1. The importance of modifying the underlying pathology where possible.
2. The concept of "total pain" and the need to address its holistic dimensions.

Pain is a demanding symptom to manage. It is essential to recognise its multiple facets and to appreciate the role of the extended multiprofessional team, including surgeons, oncologists, physiotherapists, occupational therapists, psychologists, complementary therapists, and others. Interventions that go beyond the use of drugs are listed in Box 9.13. Having an appreciation of these not only ensures that the patient gains the breadth of opinions necessary to benefit but also provides partnership and support to the patient's primary clinician. It is rare that a single practitioner has all the solutions to the pain problems presented by a palliative care patient.

Conclusion

Pain is a common and multidimensional experience for palliative care patients. Successful management depends on understanding the underlying mechanisms and conducting a systematic assessment. A wide array

Table 9.11 Analgesia for acute severe pain.

Drug group/example	Dose guidance	Comments
Opioid, for example, morphine injection	Already on regular morphine: 1/6th of the parenteral morphine daily dose equivalent Opioid-naïve: 10 mg morphine	For somatic, visceral, and bone pain Under close observation dose may be repeated every 30 min
NSAID, for example, ketorolac	15–30 mg SC	May be repeated after 4 h. For somatic, bone, and visceral pain. Possibly for nerve pain Maximum daily dose 90 mg Only licensed in United Kingdom for use by injection for 2 days
Benzodiazepine, for example, midazolam	5 mg SC If already taking benzodiazepines may tolerate/require higher doses	Indicated for nerve pain, muscle spasm, severe fear/anxiety related to uncontrolled pain Often used with other drugs
Anticholinergic antispasmodic, for example, hyoscine butylbromide	20 mg SC	Repeated hourly if effective. Primarily for colic associated with bowel obstruction. May relieve bladder spasm

of drugs is available for therapeutic intervention, and the WHO analgesic ladder provides a framework for the judicious introduction of non-opioid, opioid, and adjuvant analgesics. The variety of opioids and their different formulations and the numerous drugs that are used as adjuvant analgesics can be overwhelming, and it would be unrealistic for every practitioner to have a detailed knowledge of all of these. Familiarity and experience with a small personal formulary provides a sound basis to a safe therapeutic approach. Specialist referral can then be made, or discussions undertaken, to consider the role of other agents, opioid switching, interventional techniques, and non-drug interventions including physical therapies, surgery, and radiotherapy.

Box 9.13 Examples of nondrug interventions

Medical/surgical specialists may provide:
Radiotherapy.
Orthopaedic and spinal surgery including kyphoplasty.
Allied health professionals may provide:
Physiotherapy.
Occupational therapy (OT), rehabilitation, and goal setting.
TENS.
Massage, hydrotherapy, and other physical therapies.
Acupuncture.
Clinical psychology and cognitive behavioural interventions.
CTs.
Music therapy.
Please note that this list is not exhaustive!

References

1. Wilson KG, Chochinov HM, Allard P, et al. Prevalence and correlates of pain in the Canadian national palliative care survey. *Pain Res Manag* 2009; 14(5): 365–370.
2. Wilson KG, Chochinov HM, McPherson CJ, et al. Suffering with advanced cancer. *J Clin Oncol* 2007; 25(13): 1691–1697.
3. Smith AK, Cenzer IS, Knight SJ, et al. The epidemiology of pain during the last two years of life. *Ann Intern Med* 2010; 153(9): 563–569.
4. Lynn J, Teno JM, Phillips RS, et al. Perceptions by family members of the dying experience of older and seriously ill patients. SUPPORT investigators. Study to understand prognoses and preferences for outcomes and risks of treatment. *Ann Intern Med* 1997; 126(2): 97–106.

5. Addington-Hall J and McCarthy M. Dying from cancer: results of a national population-based investigation. *Palliat Med* 1995; 9(4): 295–305.

6. Merskey H and Bogdum N (eds.). Part III: Pain terms, a current list with definitions and notes on usage. In: *Classification of Chronic Pain*, 2nd edition. IASP task force on taxonomy. Seattle: IASP Press, 1994.

7. Saunders C. The symptomatic treatment of incurable malignant disease. *Prescriber's Journal* 1964; 4: 68–73. Cited in: Clark D. An annotated bibliography of the publications of Cicely Saunders – 1: 1958–1967. *Palliative Medicine* 1998; 12 (3): 181–193.

8. Finnerup NB and Jensen TS. Neuropathic pain. Section 10.1.3. In: Hanks G, Cherny NI, Christakis NA, et al. (eds), *The Oxford Textbook of Palliative Medicine*, 4th edition. Oxford: Oxford University Press, 2010.

9. Portenoy RK and Hagen NA. Breakthrough pain: definition, prevalence and characteristics. *Pain* 1990; 41(3): 273–281.

10. Colleau SM. The significance of breakthrough pain in cancer. *Cancer Pain Release* 1999; 12(4) Available at: www.whocancerpain.wisc.edu/?q=node/219.

11. Davies AN. Current thinking in cancer breakthrough pain management. *Eur J Palliat Care* 2005; 12(Suppl): 4–6.

12. Strang S and Strang P. Questions posed to hospital chaplains by palliative care patients. *J Palliat Med* 2002; 5(6): 857–864.

13. Cassell EJ. *The Nature of Suffering and the Goals of Medicine*. New York: Oxford University Press, 1991.

14. Koffman J and Crawley L. Ethnic and cultural aspects of palliative medicine. Section 3.7. In: Hanks G, Cherny NI, Christakis NA, et al. (eds), *The Oxford Textbook of Palliative Medicine*, 4th edition. Oxford: Oxford University Press, 2010.

15. Daut RL, Cleeland CS and Flanery RC. Development of the Wisconsin brief pain questionnaire to assess pain in cancer and other diseases. *Pain* 1983; 19(2): 197–210.

16. Scherder E, Oosterman J, Swaab D, et al. Recent developments in pain in dementia. *BMJ* 2005; 330(7489): 461–464.

17. Herr K and Ersek M. Measurement of pain and other symptoms in the cognitively impaired. Section 7.9. In: Hanks G, Cherny NI, Christakis NA, et al. (eds), *The Oxford Textbook of Palliative Medicine*, 4th edition. Oxford: Oxford University Press, 2010.

18. Galer BS and Jensen MP. Development and preliminary validation of a pain measure specific to neuropathic pain: the neuropathic pain scale. *Neurology* 1997; 48(2): 332–338.

19. Bennett M. The LANSS pain scale: the leeds assessment of neuropathic symptoms and signs. *Pain* 2001; 92(1–2): 147–157.

20. WHO (World Health Organization). *Cancer Pain Relief*. Geneva: WHO, 1986.

21. Maltoni M, Scarpi E, Modonesi C, et al. A validation study of the WHO analgesic ladder: a two-step vs. three-step strategy. *Support Care Cancer* 2005; 13(11): 888–894.

22. Tassinari D, Drudi F, Rosati M, et al. The second step of the analgesic ladder and oral tramadol in the treatment of mild to moderate cancer pain: a systematic review. *Palliat Med* 2011; 25(5): 410–423.

23. Rostom A, Dube C, Wells G, et al. Prevention of NSAID-induced gastroduodenal ulcers. *Cochrane Database Syst Rev* 2002; (4), CD002296. (Edited and republished with no change in conclusion, Issue 5, 2011).

24. Twycross R and Wilcock A (eds.). *Palliative Care Formulary*, 4th edition. Nottingham: Palliativedrugs.com Ltd, 2011.

25. Hanks GW, de Conno F, Chenry N, et al. Morphine and alternative opioids in cancer pain: the EAPC recommendations. *Br J Cancer* 2001; 84(5): 587–593.

26. Caraceni A, Pigni A and Brunelli C. Is oral morphine still the first choice opioid for moderate to severe cancer pain? A systematic review within the European palliative care research collaborative guidelines project. *Palliat Med* 2011; 25(5): 402–409.

27. Caraceni A, Hanks G, Kaasa S, et al. Use of opioid analgesics in the treatment of cancer pain: evidence-based recommendations from EAPC. *Lancet Oncology* 2012; 13(2): e58–86.

28. Klepstad P, Kaasa S and Borchgrevink PC. Starting step III opioids for moderate to severe pain in cancer patients: dose titration: a systematic review. *Palliat Med* 2011; 25(5): 424–430.

29. Klepstad P, Kaasa S, Jystad A, et al. Normal release or sustained release morphine for dose finding during start of morphine to cancer patients: a randomized double blind trial. *Pain* 2003; 101(1–2): 193–198.

30. Analgesics. Starting a patient on PO morphine. Box 5.J. In: Twycross R and Wilcock A. (Editors-in-chief). *Palliative Care Formulary*, 4th edition. Nottingham: Palliativedrugs.com Ltd, 2011, p 364.

31. Cherny N and Portenoy RK. Cancer pain management: current strategy. *Cancer* 1993; 72(11 Suppl): 3393–3415.

32. Coluzzi PH, Schwartzenburg L, Conroy Jr JD et al. Breakthrough cancer pain: a randomized trial comparing oral transmucosal fentanyl citrate and morphine sulphate immediate release. *Pain* 2001; 91(1–2): 123–130.

33. Fallon M, Cherny NI and Hanks G. Opioid analgesic therapy. Section 10.1.6. In: Hanks G, Cherny NI, Christakis NA, et al. (eds), *The Oxford Textbook of Palliative Medicine*, 4th edition. Oxford: Oxford University Press, 2010.

34. Tassinari D, Sartori S, Tamburini E, et al. Adverse effects of transdermal opiates treating moderate-severe cancer pain in comparison to long-acting morphine: a meta-analysis and systematic review of the literature. *J Palliat Med* 2008; 11(3): 492–501.

35. Nicholson AB. Methadone for cancer pain. *Cochrane Database Syst Rev* 2007; (4): CD003971. doi:10.1002/14651858.CD003971.pub3.

36. McQuay H. Opioids in pain management. *Lancet* 1999; 353(9171): 2229–2232.

37. Saarto T and Wiffen P. Antidpressants for neuropathic pain. *Cochrane Database Syst Rev* 2007; (4): CD005454. doi:10.1001/14651858. CD005454.pub2.

38. McQuay HJ and Wiffen P. Antidepressants and antiepileptics for neuropathic pain. Chapter 9. In: Bennet M (ed.), *Neuropathic Pain*. Oxford Pain Management Library. Oxford: Oxford University Press, 2006.

39. Fallon MT and Fergus C. Ketamine and other NMDA receptor antagonists. Chapter 11. In: Bennet M (ed.), *Neuropathic Pain*. Oxford Pain Management Library. Oxford: Oxford University Press, 2006.

40. McCleane G. Local anaesthetics and other pharmacological approaches. Chapter 10. In: Bennet M (ed.), *Neuropathic Pain*. Oxford Pain Management Library. Oxford: Oxford University Press, 2006.

41. Finnerup NB, Otto M, McQuay HJ, et al. Algorithm for neuropathic pain treatment: an evidence based proposal. *Pain* 2005; 118(3): 289–305.

Further reading

Hanks G, Cherny NI, Christakis NA, et al. (eds.). Section 10.1. *The management of Pain. Oxford Textbook of Palliative Medicine.* 4th edition. Oxford: Oxford University Press, 2010.

Twycross R and Wilcock A (eds.). *Palliative Care Formulary*, 4th edition. Nottingham: Palliativedrugs.com Ltd, 2011.

10 The Management of Gastrointestinal Symptoms and Advanced Liver Disease

Andrew Chilton[1], Christina Faull[2], Wendy Prentice[3], Monica Compton[1]

[1] Kettering General Hospital Foundation Trust, Kettering, UK
[2] University Hospitals of Leicester and LOROS, The Leicestershire and Rutland Hospice, Leicester, UK
[3] King's College Hospital NHS Foundation Trust, Cicely Saunders Institute, London, UK

Introduction

Patients with advanced disease, of whatever nature, commonly have symptoms related to the gastrointestinal (GI) tract. All such patients should be specifically asked about dry and sore mouth problems, eating, nausea, and constipation. Unrelenting nausea can be more disabling than pain, and effective management requires a logical, systematic, and persistent approach. Constipation is often neglected and can be prevented for most patients. Cancer may obstruct the GI tract causing well-defined syndromes and the options for palliation of these symptoms are described in detail in this chapter.

Eating and defecating can be a major point of reference for patients and their carers about their health, and their dysfunction may carry enormous significance about sustaining life and the approach of death. The importance of this in caring for patients should never be underestimated.

The palliative care needs of patients with advanced liver disease are now more recognised [1,2]. Given the dramatic and often highly symptomatic complications of end-stage liver disease, many of these patients spend the last months of their lives in acute hospitals where many of them will also die. A small number of patients access specialist palliative care services, and further work is needed to support this increasing number of patients to receive appropriate palliative care delivered according to need and if possible in a place of their choosing.

Cachexia, anorexia, and nutrition

Cachexia and anorexia are commonly experienced symptoms of advanced malignant and nonmalignant disease, and up to 10% of patients with cancer in the community will have a body mass index of less than 20 m^2/kg. The associated distress can be marked especially in terms of body image and quality of life. Cachexia has been found to be associated with a shorter prognosis for many diseases including cancer [3], chronic obstructive airways disease [4], heart failure (HF) [5], liver disease [6], and the "wasting disease" acquired immunodeficiency syndrome (AIDS) [7].

Detailed discussion of pathophysiology is beyond the scope of this book but might include the following:
- Unresolved nausea.
- Mechanical effects of tumours and ascites.
- Cytokines (e.g., tumour necrosis factor) causing increased basal metabolic rate; increased hepatogluconogenesis, using protein as substrate; increased glucose intolerance; altered lipid metabolism; and anorexia.
- Adverse effect of medications.
- Jaundice and obstructed biliary system.
- Poor oral hygiene.
- Psychological factors including low mood and anxiety.
- Unresolved pain.

Management requires active involvement of the multidisciplinary team (MDT), and best outcomes are gained by using a range of approaches that aim to ameliorate the

Handbook of Palliative Care, Third Edition. Edited by Christina Faull, Sharon de Caestecker, Alex Nicholson and Fraser Black.
© 2012 by John Wiley and Sons, Inc. Published 2012 by John Wiley & Sons, Inc.

underlying cause and address symptoms directly. Patients and carers need to be fully involved in decision-making and goal-setting. It is often the carer's job to prepare meals, and this sustaining role is of vital importance to them. Before embarking on enteral nutritional support, clear goals and plans need to be thought through and discussed with the patient.

Enteral tube feeding is considered to be a medical treatment in UK law. Initiation, stopping and withdrawal are medical decisions; however, these need to be made in concert with the patient [8]. If the patient is not competent to make decisions, then it is incumbent on the doctor to make these decisions in the "best interests" of the patient in consultation with those who know the patient best, the wider multiprofessional team and taking into consideration any previously expressed wishes. In some countries, there is legal provision for an individual to nominate another individual to be involved in health-care decisions for them, if they are to lose the capacity in the future [9].

Drugs to increase appetite and weight gain

The following drugs have been shown to have some effect on the symptoms in cancer patients [10]. They should initially be used on a trial basis, with treatment being continued only if benefit is confirmed.

Steroids

Dexamethasone 2–4 mg (or equivalent dose of an alternative steroid) is useful for increasing appetite and energy but not weight gain. The side effects of these drugs can limit their use (e.g., diabetes, psychological effects, immunosuppression, fluid retention, and proximal muscle weakness).

Progesterones

Megestrol acetate 160 mg daily (increased up to 800 mg if required), and medroxyprogesterone acetate 480–960 mg daily, can improve appetite and weight in cancer and perhaps also AIDS patients. These drugs are usually well tolerated but can cause mild oedema, impotence, and vaginal bleeding. Unlike steroids their effect is not immediate but may occur within 2 weeks and is generally more sustained [11].

In cardiac cachexia, both angiotensin-converting enzyme (ACE) inhibitor and beta blockers can reduce weight loss.

Nutritional support

Nutritional support has benefits for nonterminal patients in terms of quality of life and other outcomes. For exam-

ple, it increases patient tolerance of chemotherapy, in alcoholic cirrhosis may influence prognosis and nutritional supplements benefit people during acute exacerbations of illness [12]. In advanced disease previously advised dietary restrictions, such as reducing salt to assist in managing ascites, should be regularly reviewed as they can exacerbate a reduced intake and outweigh the benefits.

The causes of insufficient nutritional intake in advanced disease are multifactorial and can place emotional strain on both the patient and the carer. In most situations, patients are unable to meet requirements in both the macro and the micronutrients. Improvements can be made concentrating on energy and protein sources in the diet with a multivitamin mineral tablet to provide micronutrients. The key message to the patient is to think differently about his/her diet, there is no such thing as "bad" food. Cream and chocolate provide a beneficial source of energy. Additionally, the following advice can be helpful:

• Eat when and what is enjoyable. Little and often can assist in reducing nausea.
• Make foods interesting and if possible plan ahead.
• Have snacks freely available around the house or when going out to maximise when the patient has an appetite and/or nausea is reduced.
• Use a small plate (it gives the impression of finishing a complete meal. Some patients feel defeated when seeing large portions, reducing intake further).
• Softer foods that reduce chewing can sometimes be better tolerated.
• Readymade meals reduce energy expenditure for fatigued patients.
• Encourage the family and carer to create a rota system for supplying hot meals (can be frozen and used later).
• Provide emotional support to the patient and carer to ensure meal/food related tension and anxiety are reduced.
• Make use of aperitifs.

When attempts at diet manipulation do not improve, commercially prepared supplements may be helpful in some situations [13]. Patients undergoing treatments or having episodic illness seem to benefit the most with supplements. There are many types of supplements varying in composition and presentation, such as milk and juice-based drinks (sweet and savoury flavour), puddings, prethickened drinks, and powders made into drinks. They are available on prescription in the United Kingdom and are therefore free to most patients. Nutritional companies are continually introducing new products with varying nutrient formulations.

The most appropriate type and quantity of supplement should be determined based on the patient's food preferences, medical condition, nutritional requirements, and nutrient deficit [14]. If there is not a clear understanding of the specific composition when selecting the supplement, the patient's diet will be further imbalanced negating any potential improvement. Regular reviews are essential to ensure tolerance and effectiveness. Nutritional supplements can leave an unpleasant after-taste, are rich in texture and can lead to a monotonous diet; therefore, it is unlikely the patient is able to sustain this as an effective long-term option. Supplements should be used for short periods of time transitioning back to food as the patient's intake improves. Dietitians provide more detailed advice on nutritional needs of patients and are an excellent source of information on dietary supplementation. The Royal College of Physicians and the British Society of Gastroenterology have published an excellent resource to guide decision making for patients with oral feeding difficulties toward the end of life and is recommended to the reader [15].

As the patient deteriorates further, the main aim of nutritional intervention shifts to the emotional support since there is little clinical benefit from nutritional supplements, and supplements can have a deleterious effect on the GI system and mouth care. The carer may feel they are providing the best for the patient by offering nutritional supplements; however, they should be reassured that sips of soup and favourite drinks are equally beneficial, if not superior, to the quality of the patient's death.

For some patients, the inability to meet nutrition and hydration requirements or ability to administer medications orally will severely impact on the quality of life, necessitating the decision to proceed with enteral nutrition. If the patient has a functional GI tract, the patient should be referred to the Nutrition Team or Gastroenterologist in secondary care to conduct an assessment, present the most appropriate plan of care and to assist in coordinating community support with the Community Home Enteral Nutrition Team. Enteral feeding tube options available to the patient are nasogastric (NG) tube or gastrostomy tube.

Nasogastric tube

An NG feeding tube is generally 5–8 French gauge, placed in the nostril and fed down into the stomach. Professionals, who have competency to pass NG tubes, typically insert them at the bedside. They are generally indicated for short term and dependent on the material of the tube can be left in-situ up to 6 weeks before requiring replacement. Indications are:

- Patients undergoing chemotherapy/radiotherapy.
- Preparation for surgery in severely malnourished patients [14].
- Postsurgery complications impeding oral nutrition.
- As a trial to assess effectiveness and tolerability (e.g., patients with motor neurone disease) before commencing more permanent feeding options if appropriate.

There are many practical difficulties in using the NG tube in the community; most importantly is the risk of tube displacement into the lungs. The risk is minimised by checking the pH of aspirated tube contents (should be less than 5.5 unless taking a proton pump inhibitor [PPI]) before each administration of feed, water, and medication. In secondary care an X-ray is conducted if the pH cannot confirm position; however, this is not practical in primary care. The safest option for the patient without confirmation is to withhold the feed and consider having a new tube placed [14]. There may be limited professionals in the community with competency to pass NG tubes, requiring the patient to have it passed in secondary care. The arduous process limits the feasibility of this option.

Percutaneous endoscopic gastrostomy tube

Fixed placement of a tube through the abdominal wall into the stomach is useful for patients who require long-term interventional nutrition (months to years) or those undergoing treatment for head and neck cancer. The procedure is well tolerated even by quite sick patients and is generally done under benzodiazepine sedation (Figure 10.1). It may be placed endoscopically (the majority), radiologically, or by a mini laparotomy. It is a day case procedure endoscopically, but patients may remain in hospital while learning about the enteral feeding apparatus and techniques. Around 6% of people will die within 30 days (around 40% of endoscopic deaths), and robust consideration of risks by the MDT is needed to assure selection of appropriate patients [17].

Box 10.1 outlines the indications and contraindications and Box 10.2 describes the possible complications of PEG.

Jejunal tube feeding

Some patients have considerable problems with enteral feeding into the stomach with symptoms of reflux, hiccup, aspiration, nausea, and vomiting. If prokinetic agents (e.g., metoclopramide) do not resolve this, then jejunal placement of the NG or PEG tube (usually endoscopically)

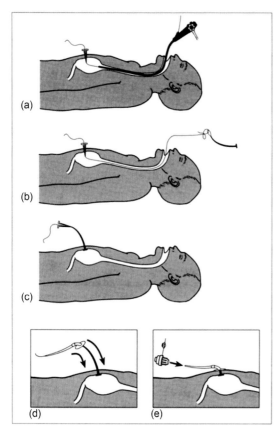

Figure 10.1 Positioning a PEG tube. (a) Gastric puncture with a sheathed needle and introduction of a string or metal wire through the sheath after the removal of the needle. While grasping the string or the metal wire, the endoscope is removed. (b) The loop of the gastrostomy tube is knotted at the string projecting from the mouth and by pulling at the abdominal end of the string the gastrostomy tube passes through the oesophagus and stomach and finally pierces the abdominal wall. (c) The retention disc of the gastrostomy tube is apposed against the gastric wall. (d) The outer retention disc, and (e) the feeding adaptor are put in place. (Reproduced from Reference 16.)

may alleviate symptoms. However, patients with jejunal feeding tubes will be unlikely to tolerate bolus feeds since there is no longer the gastric reservoir and therefore will be more practically constrained by the time required for feed to be given.

Daily care for patients requiring enteral feeding
Risk can be minimised with good daily care and the Community Home Enteral Nutrition team can be a valuable resource for the patient and carer providing training and support.

Box 10.1 Factors to assess before PEG insertion

Indications	Contraindications
	Ileus
Oropharyngeal disease	Blood coagulation disorder
Oesophageal obstruction- but may be technically problematic	Poor wound healing
	Ascites
Neurogenic dysphagia with risk of aspiration	Sepsis
Neurological injury and neurodegenerative disease	Tumour infiltration of stomach
	Respiratory insufficiency on lying flat (radiologically inserted gastrostomy [RIG] may be possible)
Major oral surgery	
Preradiotherapy	

If it is impossible to site a gastrostomy endoscopically, it may be possible radiologically with ultrasound guidance (RIG)

Flushing before and after each administration with either freshly drawn tap water or cooled boiled water will reduce the risk of the tube becoming blocked with feed and/or medication residue. Any medicine administered through the enteral feeding tube must be in the liquid form or a dissolvable preparation. The community

Box 10.2 Complications of PEG

Major	Minor
Perforation with peritonitis	Wound infection/stomal leak
Haemorrhage	Regurgitation and aspiration (consider jejunal placement)
Haematoma	
Death	Ileus, abdominal bloating, diarrhoea
	Tube migration/extubation
	Anorexia

pharmacist or prescribing advisors supporting the general practitioner (GP) can provide advice. If the tube does become blocked, the Home Enteral Nutrition team may be contacted to provide support. Techniques available are:

- Inspect the tube to see if the blockage is visible. Wrap a warm flannel around the tube and once cooler massage the tube at the blockage. With a 50-ml syringe **gently** attempt to aspirate alternating with flushing warm water. If this is not successful, rest and repeat in 30 min.
- Carbonated water and pancreatic enzymes dissolved in water may be useful to unblock tubes. Pancreatic enzymes will only help if the blockage is caused by feed. Clogg Zapper® (CorPack Medsystems) is a powder containing pancreatic enzymes marketed for breaking up feed-related blockages in enteral feeding tubes [18].
- Do not force-flush a tube.
- If all attempts fail, seek specialist advice or replacement.

Many patients do not feel it is necessary to continue with mouth care if not eating and drinking orally. Daily oral, dental, and pharyngeal hygiene will help to minimize incidence of oral thrush, tooth decay, and halitosis. Evidence suggests oropharyngeal microorganisms can migrate into the respiratory tract causing infections [19,20].

PEG care

To minimise the risk of infections the puncture site (stoma) requires daily cleaning with warm soapy water. Discharge can be common and is not always indicative of an infection. Dressings may assist in managing the discharge however should be balanced with the risk of infections caused from ideal breeding conditions. The Home Enteral Nutrition team and/or District Nurse can support the patient and provide advice.

Trouble shooting

The tube can be displaced regardless of the type of fixation device used. In the United Kingdom, National Patient Safety Agency (NPSA) put out a Rapid Response Alert in 2010, recommending that in the first 72 h.

> If there is pain on feeding, prolonged or severe pain postprocedure, or fresh bleeding, or external leakage of gastric contents, stop feed/medication delivery immediately, obtain senior advice urgently and consider CT scan, contrast study, or surgical review [21].

If late displacement occurs (i.e., once the tract is mature), the stoma tract can potentially close within hours. Some Home Enteral Nutrition teams have staff competent in changing balloon gastrostomies and may be available for immediate support, or the patient should be instructed to go to hospital as soon as possible bringing spare tubes if available. If indicated a urinary Foley catheter can be inserted to maintain the integrity of the tract.

Gastroesophageal reflux is common and can be treated with a PPI. Positional change and avoidance of overnight continuous feeding is also helpful. Aspiration occurs frequently in both NG and PEG feeding and may present with pneumonia. Patient position, type of feed and prokinetic medication may be useful. Jejunal feeding may benefit patients with persistent problems.

Nausea, bloating, and cramps occur frequently. Diarrhoea occurs in approximately 30% of patients and can present a significant challenge. These problems can be addressed by alteration of feed type and mode of feeding. Close liaison with the Community Home Enteral Nutrition team is essential.

Parenteral nutrition

If the gut is functional use it! Parenteral nutrition (PN) is not physiological and is fraught with pitfalls. PN is never an emergency. Electrolytes and micronutrients must be corrected to prevent the re-feeding syndrome in malnourished patients.

In the United Kingdom, most home PN is given for intestinal failure due to the short bowel syndrome. In parts of Europe and the United States however, the bulk of home PN is provided for malignant disease. There is, however, no convincing evidence that PN enhances either quality of life or survival in patients with *advanced* malignancy. Patients with advanced cancer who currently receive PN in the United Kingdom have usually either been commenced on it before diagnosis or before potentially curative treatment and have continued on it. PN may occasionally be used in cancer patients who have intestinal failure (complete bowel obstruction) with no other disease spread. For patients with cachexia due to advanced nonmalignant disease, the place of PN is equally uncertain. This is an area of practice that is likely to continue to challenge us all in the coming years.

Care for patients with oral feeding difficulties should have their needs carefully assessed by the MDT. As far as possible the oral route should be preserved by detailed assessment and modification of food and liquid to facilitate maintenance of oral nutrition.

Mouth care

Mouth care is very important. Studies have shown that in the elderly aspiration pneumonia is related to poor oral hygiene [19,20]. The aim of oral hygiene is to keep the lips and oral mucosa clean, soft, and intact and the basis for this is daily tooth brushing, dental flossing, and consideration of a mouth wash (one teaspoonful of sodium bicarbonate per large cup of water). Commercial mouthwashes may cause pain in patients with stomatitis since they contain alcohol, lemon, and glycerine.

Oral complications including a dry mouth (xerostomia) are common and a major problem for many patients with advanced disease [22]. Saliva helps us to chew, talk, and swallow. It protects against infection and begins digestion of food. Normally about 1–1.5 L of saliva containing amylase and bicarbonate are produced daily. A reduction in this is most commonly a side effect of drugs (e.g., opioids, antihistamines, anticholinergics, diuretics, beta blockers, and anticonvulsants) but dehydration, anxiety, and mouth breathing also result in a dry mouth. Patients who have had radiotherapy to the head and neck may have considerable problems with dry mouth, altered anatomy, and function leading to debris accumulation and pain. Dentures in patients who have lost weight can become ill-fitting and cause soreness and abrasions.

As well as keeping the lips and mucosa moist, clean and intact patients may need extra mouth care in order to:
- prevent infection;
- alleviate pain and discomfort thus enabling greater oral intake;
- prevent halitosis;
- enhance taste and appetite;
- facilitate speech; and
- minimise psychological distress.

Key point in mouth care

The *frequency* of mouth care is of greater importance than what is used to clean it.

Painful mouth

Mouth ulcers can be helped by choline salicylate gel (bonjela) or, if persistent, corticosteroid in the form of hydrocortisone oromucosal tablet (e.g., corlan pellets 2.5 mg) dissolves slowly in contact with the ulcer up to four times a day. The bioadherent gel, *Gelclair*, can also sooth and promote healing.

A sore mouth, from whatever cause, may be helped by sucking anaesthetic lozenges or using local anaesthetic mouthwashes or sprays. Severe pain may require opioid analgesia often by subcutaneous (SC) rather than oral administration.

Management of xerostomia

Table 10.1 outlines the measures that may help patients with dry mouths. Sialogogues increase the production of saliva, and chewing gum (sugar free) has been shown to be helpful and liked by patients with advanced cancer who are able to produce some saliva [23]. Most salivary substitutes provide relief for only a short time, and those that contain mucin improve symptoms more than those that don't. However, the mucin is derived from pigs and may therefore not be suitable for some patients. Salivary substitutes that have a low pH may cause demineralisation of teeth.

A few additional tips: Salivary substitutes should be applied or sprayed beneath the tongue and between the buccal mucosa and the teeth (i.e., mimic the pooling of saliva) and not in the back of the throat, the mouth should be moistened with water before spraying; lemon and glycerine swabs and mouthwashes containing glycol should not be used due to adverse effects of irritation and rebound drying effects; moist cotton swabs (e.g., Moistir) or sponge swabs on sticks dipped in water may help very frail patients.

Cholinergic agonist agents such as pilocarpine have been shown to increase saliva production postirradiation.

Table 10.1 A summary of approaches to the management of a dry mouth.

General measures	Cleanliness/tongue coating	Salivary substitutes	Increased salivary secretion
Sips of water	Pineapple	Carboxymethycellulose	Chewing gum Pilocarpine 5 mg tds with or after food
Ice poles Brushing with soft toothbrush Moistened sponges on stick Mild bicarbonate mouth wash	Effervescent vitamin C	Mucin	

It is very useful in patients with postradiotherapy xerostomia in head and neck cancer (start with 5 mg tds with meals. However, it is often poorly tolerated, usually because of sweating or GI side effects. It is contraindicated in obstructive airways disease and asthma.

Prevention and management of oral infections

Thrush

Attention to the care of the oral cavity, teeth, and dentures will help minimise infection. Patients on steroids, antibiotics, or those who have diabetes are at particular risk. Thrush is the commonest infection. Candida prefers an acid environment and sodium bicarbonate mouthwashes repeated regularly (2 hourly), coupled with gentle brushing of the teeth (or cleaning dentures) twice per day is effective prevention [23].

Established thrush is treated with nystatin or miconazole topically. Patients should be instructed to keep the gel or suspension in contact with as much of the oral mucosa as possible, for as long as possible. Ice lollipops made with diluted nystatin are soothing and engender a long duration of mucosal contact. Miconazole acts both topically and systemically. If the patient is severely affected, has symptoms suggestive of oesophageal infection, or is taking antibiotics and/or steroids a systemic antifungal is indicated; for example, fluconazole 50 mg od for 7–14 days, or itraconazole 100 mg o.d for 10–15 days. To avoid reinfection, dentures must be cleaned in Sterident or Milton with or without nystatin. If oral thrush persists then mouth swabs should be taken to evaluate further.

Herpes simplex

Herpes simplex infections present as very painful, vesicular, and ulcerating lesions. Oral acyclovir 200 mg five times daily, or valacyclovir 500 mg bd for 5 days is indicated.

Oesophageal problems

Swallowing may be difficult for patients with oesophageal cancer for several common reasons:
- Oesophageal compressive and/or obstructive lesions
- Functional dysphagia
- Odynophagia (painful swallowing)
- Oro-Oesophageal thrush.

In addition, patients may experience copious thick, tenacious mucus, which may cause coughing.

Treatment options include surgery (not for disease with metastatic spread), external beam and endoluminal radiotherapy, chemotherapy, endoscopic recanalisation, and expanding metal stents. Endoscopic interventions are discussed below. General symptom control is vital whatever the cause of obstruction or possibility of intervention.

Pain should be managed by the standard titration of analgesics as per the World Health Organisation (WHO) analgesic ladder. Strong (nonoral) opioids, such as SC diamorphine/morphine or transdermal fentanyl, may be required to control background pain. Sucralfate will coat ulcerated tumour and may reduce bleeding and pain.

In total obstruction of the oesophagus, coping with saliva and secretions can be distressing for the patient. The following may be helpful:
- Hyoscine hydrobromide (Kwells), 1–2, tablets sublingually qds.
- Hyoscine hydrobromide SC 1.2–2.4 mg/24 h.
- Hyoscine butylbromide SC 40–120 mg/24 h (less sedating than hydrobromide).
- Glycopyrronium bromide SC 0.6–1.2 mg/24 h (less sedating than hyoscine hydrobromide).

Nebulized water or saline may help reduce the tenacity of mucus secreted by the cancer, and nebulised local anaesthetic (5 ml of 0.25% bupivacaine) may be helpful in very advanced disease if the pharynx is dysfunctional and swallowing of saliva or mucus results in aspiration with distressing bouts of coughing.

Endoluminal recanalisation

Exophytic growth of tumours into a lumen will lead to obstruction. Endoscopic procedures that recanalise the oesophagus may offer alternatives or additional options to endolimunial stenting (see below) for dysphagia:
- *Argon plasma coagulator (APC)*: This is a safe and effective method. APC provides predictable penetration of normal and abnormal mucosa. The equipment is relatively cheap and has multiple other applications. The main drawback is that it may take a number of sessions to achieve the desired outcome.
- *Laser (YAG)*: Not widely available and has statutory restriction on its use. Very "powerful" with limited room for error.
- *Injection of absolute alcohol*: Cheap with good results if injected into exophytic tumour. It usually requires multiple sessions and can give rise to mediastinal discomfort at the time of injection. Will cause ulceration of the normal mucosa if injected into it.
- *Dilatation*: Useful for constrictive rather than exophytic tumours. Dilatation can be done with bougies over a guide

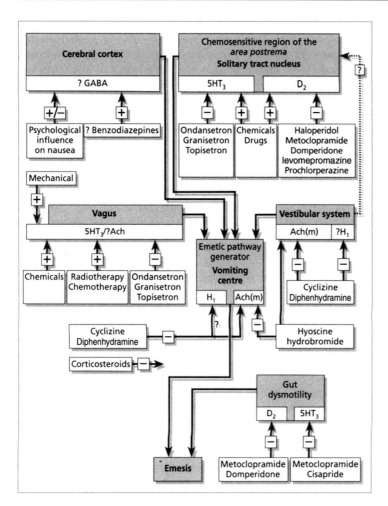

Figure 10.2 A schema of the pathways of emesis (nausea and vomiting), important neurotransmitters, and site of action of antiemetics. The neurokinin receptor and antagonist is not shown as this is an area of specialist only prescription in oncology. Receptor types—GABA; H, histamine; D, dopamine; Ach(m), acetylcholine muscarinic; 5HT, serotonin (5-hydroxytryptophan). Subscript denotes receptor subtype: + denotes agonist or enhancing stimulus; − denotes antagonist or blocking stimulus; ? denotes limited evidence for effect through this mechanism.

wire or balloons under direct vision. Balloon dilation of the oesophagus, pylorus, duodenum, and colon can be undertaken. The perforation rate is 1–5%.

A combination of the above modalities focused on the nature of the individual clinical problem should be employed.

Nausea and vomiting

Nausea and/or vomiting are common in advanced disease and can be a major cause of poor quality of life. The prevalence in patients with advanced cancer is up to 70% and up to 50% in those with advanced nonmalignant disease [24]. The symptoms may be more distressing than pain.

Five components are the key to management:
1. Careful assessment of the patient to try and identify possible avoidable and reversible aetiologies.
2. Knowledge of common syndromes.
3. Reversal of the reversible (where appropriate).
4. An understanding of the mechanism of action of antiemetic drugs (Figure 10.2).
5. Consideration of the route of administration of antiemetic and other drugs. Since nausea can cause gastric stasis, the SC or rectal routes may be needed even when there is no vomiting.

Figure 10.3 outlines the management. An aetiological-based approach to management generally underpins most guidelines although an empirical-based approach may be as effective [24,25]. Generally the first-line choice of antiemetic is one of metoclopramide, haloperidol, or

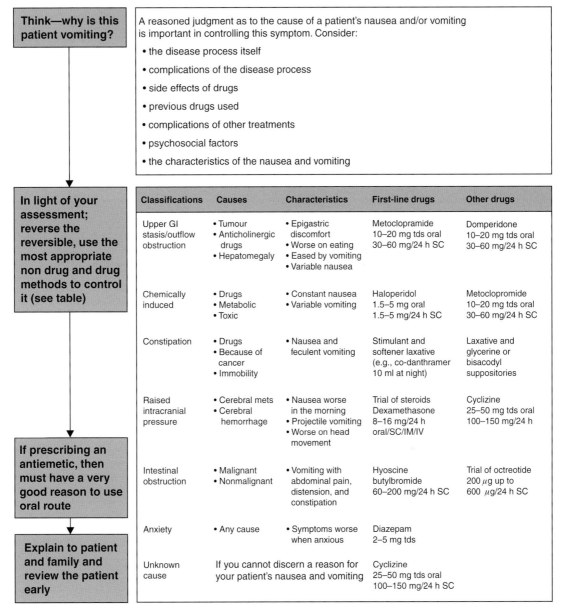

Flowchart (left column):

- **Think—why is this patient vomiting?**
- **In light of your assessment; reverse the reversible, use the most appropriate non drug and drug methods to control it (see table)**
- **If prescribing an antiemetic, then must have a very good reason to use oral route**
- **Explain to patient and family and review the patient early**

A reasoned judgment as to the cause of a patient's nausea and/or vomiting is important in controlling this symptom. Consider:

- the disease process itself
- complications of the disease process
- side effects of drugs
- previous drugs used
- complications of other treatments
- psychosocial factors
- the characteristics of the nausea and vomiting

Classifications	Causes	Characteristics	First-line drugs	Other drugs
Upper GI stasis/outflow obstruction	• Tumour • Anticholinergic drugs • Hepatomegaly	• Epigastric discomfort • Worse on eating • Eased by vomiting • Variable nausea	Metoclopramide 10–20 mg tds oral 30–60 mg/24 h SC	Domperidone 10–20 mg tds oral 30–60 mg/24 h SC
Chemically induced	• Drugs • Metabolic • Toxic	• Constant nausea • Variable vomiting	Haloperidol 1.5–5 mg oral 1.5–5 mg/24 h SC	Metoclopromide 10–20 mg tds oral 30–60 mg/24 h SC
Constipation	• Drugs • Because of cancer • Immobility	• Nausea and feculent vomiting	Stimulant and softener laxative (e.g., co-danthramer 10 ml at night)	Laxative and glycerine or bisacodyl suppositories
Raised intracranial pressure	• Cerebral mets • Cerebral hemorrhage	• Nausea worse in the morning • Projectile vomiting • Worse on head movement	Trial of steroids Dexamethasone 8–16 mg/24 h oral/SC/IM/IV	Cyclizine 25–50 mg tds oral 100–150 mg/24 h
Intestinal obstruction	• Malignant • Nonmalignant	• Vomiting with abdominal pain, distension, and constipation	Hyoscine butylbromide 60–200 mg/24 h SC	Trial of octreotide 200 μg up to 600 μg/24 h SC
Anxiety	• Any cause	• Symptoms worse when anxious	Diazepam 2–5 mg tds	
Unknown cause	If you cannot discern a reason for your patient's nausea and vomiting		Cyclizine 25–50 mg tds oral 100–150 mg/24 h SC	

Figure 10.3 Summary of the approach to the management of nausea and vomiting. Add levomepromazine as a second-line agent for unknown cause of vomiting. 6 mg od oral 6.25 mg–25 mg/24 h SC. (Adapted from Faull C and Woof R. 2002. *Palliative Care: An Oxford Core Text* with permission from the publishers Oxford University Press.)

cyclizine. Control of symptoms using one antiemetic is possible in 60% of patients. However, about one-third of patients require concurrent administration of a second antiemetic. In these patients antiemetics of different mechanisms of action should be combined (e.g., cyclizine and haloperidol). A third-line choice would be a broader spectrum antiemetic, which has risks of more side effects. This is discussed further below under the section "Persistent nausea and vomiting."

Acupuncture and ginger are two commonly used complementary techniques. Other approaches such as relaxation therapy, hypnosis, or neurolinguistic programming

Table 10.2 Antiemetic prescription.

Drug	Oral dose	Subcutaneous dose	Rectal dose
Metoclopramide	10–20 mg tds	30–120 mg/24 h	
Domperidone	10–20 mg tds	–	30 mg tds
Levomepromazine	5–25 mg od	6.25–25 mg/24 h may be given once daily	
Haloperidol	1.5–5 mg od	1.5–5 mg/24 h may be given once daily	
Ondansetron	8 mg bd	–	16 mg od
Granisetron	1–2 mg od	1–2 mg/24 h	
Cyclizine	50 mg tds	50–150 mg/24 h	
Prochloperazine	3–10 mg tds	Not suitable	
Hyoscine hydrobromide	300 μg qid	0.8–2.4 mg/24 h	25 mg tds

(NLP) are invaluable for patients with a high degree of anxiety or to combat the anticipatory nausea induced by chemotherapy treatments.

Table 10.2 provides a quick view of the range of antiemetics and gives prescription guidance.

Common syndromes of nausea and vomiting and their management

Gastric stasis and outflow obstruction

This is common in patients with GI malignancy because of ascites, liver enlargement, and direct effects of tumour on the stomach. It is also common in patients with advanced congestive cardiac failure because of ascites and in patients with diabetics because of autonomic neuropathy. It is a component of the nausea induced by opiates. Nausea is of varying intensity. It may be very transient, just before vomiting and is often relieved by vomiting. The vomitus can be of considerable volume and may contain undigested food. Vomiting may be provoked by movement of the torso. A succussion splash and other features of autonomic failure may be present.

Metoclopramide or Domperidone are the drug treatments of choice. Erythromycin may be helpful in a few patients but needs to be given intravenously. Flatulence may be relieved with dimethicone.

In complete obstruction prokinetic drugs should be stopped. PPIs may be helpful in reducing acidity and volume of secretions. A NG tube (for aspiration or free drainage) may help to relieve symptoms and is tolerated well by some patients but many prefer to have intermittent vomiting and no NG tube, especially if nausea is controlled. Insertion of a gastrostomy tube (see above) for venting purposes has been found to be effective

and acceptable but is not commonly used in the United Kingdom [26].

Chemically induced nausea

A vast array of drugs cause nausea. The initiation of opioids cause nausea in up to 30% of patients but usually settles within 3–4 days although can reappear with an escalation of dose, and it persists in a small percentage of patients. Metabolic causes of nausea are common in advanced disease: renal failure, liver failure, hypercalcaemia, hyponatraemia, and ketoacidosis. Anti-dopaminergic are the drugs of choice, for example, haloperidol. $5HT_3$ antagonists are useful for highly emetogenic chemotherapy and perhaps in cases of intractable vomiting of metabolic cause, but their cost-effectiveness in other circumstances is not yet established. These drugs are also used in the postoperative period.

Raised intracranial pressure

Nausea may be worse in the morning, and the vomiting can be projectile in nature. Nausea and vomiting provoked by head movement is associated with vestibular pathway aetiology. There is usually headache, which may be worse in the morning. Neurological signs may be absent. Steroids and cyclizine are the treatments of first choice. If there are signs of vestibular pathway aetiology, hyoscine hydrobromide may be useful.

Persistent nausea and vomiting

Thirty percent of patients require the concurrent use of two antiemetics. These should be selected for different mechanisms of action that are compatible in effects. Haloperidol with cyclizine is a good choice. Both cyclizine and hyoscine hydrobromide will counteract the prokinetic effect of metoclopramide and domperidone but will not counteract the central antiemetic effect of metoclopramide.

Alternatively, low-dose levomepromazine can also be useful. It is a "broad-spectrum" antiemetic (Achm, D_2, and 5HT antagonist activity) and in low doses does not generally cause troublesome sedation or hypotension.

Corticosteroids are potent antiemetics although their mechanism of action is not fully understood. They are thought to potentiate the effects of other antiemetics but also have an entiemetic effect in their own right. Dexamethasone at 2–6 mg od is useful to add to an antiemetic regimen for patients with resistant problems.

Malignant bowel obstruction

Malignant GI obstruction occurs most commonly in patients with advanced abdominal or pelvic cancers: in 25% of patients with a primary bowel cancer; in 6% of patients with a primary ovarian cancer; and in about 40% of advanced ovarian cancer patients.

Where surgery is technically not possible, is inappropriate, or is not acceptable to the patient, medical management of malignant GI obstruction can offer good symptom control. Patients may live for surprisingly long periods of time (sometimes months) and be able to take small quantities of food and fluids as desired, usually without the need for a NG tube or parenteral fluids. Most patients can be cared for at home.

The clinical scenario may only have some of the classic features of complete bowel obstruction outlined in Box 10.3. Malignant obstruction may present acutely but more commonly is gradual in onset, intermittent, and variable in severity. Gross distension is often absent, even in lower bowel obstruction since the bowel may be

---

Box 10.3 Classical features of complete intestinal obstruction

- Large-volume vomits.
- Nausea worse before vomiting.
- Nausea relieved by vomiting.
- Nil per rectum or per stoma.
- Abdominal distension.
- Visible peristalsis.
- Increased bowel sounds, classically tinkling, but may be absent.
- Background abdominal pain.
- Colicky abdominal pain.

---

constricted at several points. Patients with lower bowel obstruction will often have infrequent, faeculent vomiting, while those with high bowel obstruction may vomit undigested food. It is always useful to determine whether colic is present or absent since this will affect the management strategy (see below).

Nonmalignant causes of obstruction or gut paresis must be considered, which may be amenable to surgical or other appropriate intervention. These include adhesions, constipation, drugs, unrelated benign conditions, metabolic abnormalities.

Investigations can be helpful and may include a biochemical profile (hypokalaemia may cause ileus, hypercalcaemia may cause pseudo-obstruction due to constipation). A plain abdominal X-ray will demonstrate constipation, but can be misleading when multiple levels of obstruction are present. A CT/MRI scan can be indicated if surgery is to be considered.

Chemotherapy may offer a palliative option for some patients with chemosensitive tumours, for example, ovarian carcinoma. Any surgical or oncological intervention should run in parallel with more immediate symptomatic treatment. Expanding stents placed endoscopically or radiologically are occasionally helpful and are discussed below.

Surgical intervention

Surgery should always be considered in malignant GI obstruction. However, it will often be inappropriate or technically impossible. Surgical intervention is unlikely to be successful in the following situations:

- Radiological or previous surgical evidence indicating that a surgical procedure will not be technically possible.
- A stiff, doughy abdomen with little abdominal distension [27].
- Diffuse intra-abdominal carcinomatosis.
- Massive ascites that re-accumulates rapidly after paracentesis.
- Poor general physical status [28].
- Previous radiotherapy to the abdomen or pelvis, in combination with any of the above.

Medical management

A NG tube and intravenous (IV) fluids are rarely necessary if the following strategy is used.

Pain

Analgesia for background pain is obtained by using a continuous SC infusion of an opioid, for example, morphine (dose: 1/2 total daily oral morphine equivalent dose

± 30–50% increment as dictated by the pain). If opioid naive, start on a morphine dose of 10 mg/24 h. Not all patients require opioid analgesia if no background pain is present and colic can be relieved by more appropriate drugs (see below).

Colic and gut motility

If colic is present avoid all drugs that could worsen this (i.e., metoclopramide, bulk-forming, osmotic, and stimulant laxatives). If colic persists, add hyoscine butylbromide SC, starting at 60 mg/24 h (up to 200 mg/24 h as needed).

If colic is absent, a trial of metoclopramide SC 30–80 mg/24 h should be cautiously instigated with close monitoring for development of colic. In the absence of colic, incomplete obstruction in the large bowel may be helped by a stool-softening laxative, such as docusate sodium 200 mg bd-qds. Corticosteroids may reduce bowel obstruction in those with advanced malignancy, particularly GI and ovarian cancer. A 5-day trial of dexamethasone 6–16 mg SC/IV should be given [29].

Nausea

The choice of antiemetic depends on whether the patient is experiencing colic. If colic is not a feature, metoclopramide is administered SC 30–80 mg/24 h (see above). If colic is present, give haloperidol (SC 3–5 mg/24 h) or cyclizine (SC 100–150 mg/24 h). A combination of haloperidol and cyclizine is sometimes necessary.

$5HT_3$ antagonist antiemetics may have a role in relief of the nausea induced by bowel distension and stimulation of the vomiting centre through vagal afferents (see above), but this is unclear. They can be given rectally or subcutaneously.

Vomiting

Reduction in the volume of GI secretions will reduce colic, nausea, pain, and the need to vomit. This can usually be adequately achieved with hyoscine butylbromide (SC 60–200 mg/24 h [30]) with or without an H_2 antagonist or PPI.

If large-volume vomiting persists despite hyoscine butylbromide, the somatostatin analogue, octreotide, will further decrease the volume of intestinal secretions in the gut lumen [31]. A trial of octreotide, given at a rate of 300 μg/24 h by SC infusion, should be performed. The dose can be titrated over 2–3 days to 600 μg/24 h; If there is no benefit at 600 μg/24 h it should be stopped. The dose should be reduced daily by 100 μg/24 h to the lowest effective dose (mean dose 300 μg/24 h) [32].

In some cases, particularly in high obstructions such as gastric outlet obstruction, these strategies are not effective. It may then be helpful to use a NG tube or consider a venting gastrostomy to allow the patient to continue to drink and eat as desired without the fear of provoking immediate vomiting. Venting gastrostomy can be performed under local anaesthetic either endoscopically or radiologically and may facilitate discharge and dying at home. In one series of 51 patients median survival was 17 days with a range of 1–190 days; 92% of patients gaining symptomatic improvement of nausea and vomiting with some restoration of diet [26].

Contraindications to the use of a venting gastrostomy are:
• The presence of significant ascites as it would precipitate peritonitis.
• Tumour infiltration of the stomach.

In an obstructed abdomen with malignant infiltration, the risk of perforating the bowel with resultant peritonitis is significant and the patient should be clear about this risk.

It is important that at least a 16–20 F bore gastrostomy tube should be used to facilitate adequate decompression.

Subcutaneous drug delivery

Patients may require the use of more than two drugs to obtain symptom control and not infrequently two SC infusions are required. Studies of the compatibility of multiple drug combinations are often not available (see Chapter 22), but clinical observation suggests the following drugs mixed in water for injection are compatible and maintain efficacy:
• Morphine/diamorphine, haloperidol, and cyclizine.
• Morphine/diamorphine, haloperidol, and hyoscine butylbromide (compatibility may depend on order of mixing).
• Morphine/diamorphine and octreotide.
• Morphine/diamorphine, haloperidol, and octreotide.

Diet and hydration

Sensitive, pre-emptive discussion of the situation is a vital part of care for the patient and family. Many patients with obstruction can eat and drink in modest amounts when symptoms are controlled. A liquid, low-residue diet may be the least problematic.

Hydration should be considered on an individual basis. Oral discomfort and dryness can largely be relieved by frequent, attentive mouth care, ice to suck, and drinks as desired and tolerated. Profound thirst is not common but some patients may benefit from parenteral fluids, for example, SC infusion of 1–2 l 0.9% saline/24 h or IV fluids. The use of parenteral fluids can impact on choices regarding place of care.

Hiccup

This is an abnormal respiratory reflex characterised by spasm of one or both sides of the diaphragm, causing sudden inspiration with associated closure of the vocal cords. The phrenic nerve, vagus nerve, thoracic sympathetic fibres, brainstem, and hypothalamus are all involved in the reflex arc. An inhibitory pathway through the pharyngeal and glosspharyngeal nerves is present. Disturbance of any of these components may cause hiccup. Identification of cause may sometimes enable a logical and successful approach to treatment.

Management
Stimulation of the pharynx may be successful in reducing hiccup. This can be achieved in various ways, including holding iced water in the oropharynx, soft palate massage, oropharyngeal, or nasopharyngeal catheter placement.

Common empirical treatments are:
• A defoaming antiflatulent before and after meals and at bedtime (e.g., Asilone 10–20 ml).
• Domperidone 10–20 mg tds; or metoclopramide 10 mg tds half an hour before meals if delayed gastric emptying.
• Nifedipine 10–20 mg bd-tds (assess effect on blood pressure).
• Midazolam 5–10 mg SC/24 h (increasing to 60 mg/24 h occasionally).
• Baclofen 5–10 mg bd-tds (higher doses can be used with caution).
• Chlorpromazine—use with care and only if simpler measures fail: 10–25 mg po tds (it has a diffuse depressant effect on the reticular formation).
• Sodium valproate—for hiccup of central origin.

In general the drugs should be started at low dose and gradually increased to avoid side effects.

Phrenic nerve stimulation or ablation is only occasionally an appropriate treatment in patients with advanced disease.

Endoluminal stents

Stenting is a widely used therapeutic intervention for palliation of GI and hepatobiliary malignant obstruction. Stents are available as expandable metal systems (covered or uncovered) or in plastic (for biliary obstruction).

Stents are usually placed through a guidewire under endoscopic and fluoroscopic guidance, although radiologists do place them under fluoroscopic guidance alone. Uncovered stents embed well in luminal tissues but may become occluded by further tumour growth. Covered stents prevent the ingress of tumour but are more prone to migration and displacement. Stenting is usually a day case procedure but depends on patient performance status and complications.

Oesophageal stents
Expandable metal stents (EMS) provide relief or improvement of dysphagia in 90% of cases and result in shorter hospital stays and fewer procedures than nonstenting options. Covered stents are particularly effective in tracheoesophageal fistula. Stents are most useful in mid-to-low oesophageal tumours. Tumours of the gastroesophageal junction respond well, but stent migration is more common and the function of the lower oesophageal sphincter is lost and can result in problematic gastroesophageal reflux (patients will need PPIs). Stenting of high oesophageal tumours can cause significant and persistent discomfort.

Complications:
• 0.5–2% mortality as a result of stent insertion [33].
• Pain/mediastinal discomfort (NB: surgical emphysema may indicate perforation).
• Bleeding.
• 3% perforation rate.
• Stent migration (more common following chemotherapy and tumour regression).
• Tumour overgrowth.
• Food blockage.

After stenting patients need to modify their diet: more liquidised/sloppy food, avoid leafy vegetables and chunks of steak, etc. Possible acute food blockage may be relieved by carbonated drinks. Total dysphagia with drooling and aspiration requires emergency review.

Tumour overgrowth can be dealt with by laser, alcohol injection, or argon (see recanalisation earlier).

Gastroduodenal stents
Pancreatic, duodenal, and gastric cancers frequently precipitate gastric outflow obstruction, and EMS are as effective in relieving this as palliative bypass surgery. Most patients gain significant clinical improvement. Where there is functional gastric-outlet obstruction due to tumour invasion of neural supply or diffuse peritoneal infiltration with bowel encasement and gut failure, improvement will not be seen.

The EMS are best placed using the combined modalities of endoscopic and fluoroscopic guidance; however, this can be achieved fluroscopically alone. Gastroduodenal stents can be inserted as an outpatient procedure. Patients with duodenal involvement frequently develop biliary obstruction, and it is advisable that the biliary obstruction is treated first. Complications are similar to those mentioned above.

Biliary stents

Patients with biliary obstruction experience nausea, anorexia, weight loss, fat malabsorption with steatorrhoea, itch, and occasionally cholangitis, although the severity of these symptoms varies between individual patients. Jaundice can also be a significant visual reinforcement affirming the disease process. The obstructed biliary tree is decompressed by endoscopic retrograde cholangiopancreatography (ERCP) or percutaneous transhepatic cholangiography (PTC). Plastic stents are subject to bacterial and biliary encrustation resulting in occlusion and usually last between 3 and 4 months. The more expensive EMS have larger diameters and longer patency than plastic stents. If patient survival is greater than 4–6 months, then metal stents appear more cost-effective with fewer endoscopic interventions and hospital admissions required.

Patients may benefit from re-stenting and recurrence of jaundice should not be assumed to be due to tumour progression.

Complications of biliary stenting (ERCP and PTC):
- Pancreatitis
- Bleeding
- Perforation
- Biliary leak and peritonitis
- Malposition
- Cholangitis.

Colorectal stents

Colorectal stents can be used as a bridge to surgery or in patients with extensive disease who are poor surgical candidates. Covered stents are also useful in assisting closure of colo-vesical and colo-vaginal fistulas. Right-sided colonic stents require endoscopic placement. Left-sided stents can be placed radiologically.

Complications:
- Perforation (devastating as it will cause a florid faecal peritonitis)
- Stent migration
- Stool occlusion
- Bleeding

- Tenesmus[1]
- Faecal incontinence[1].

Patients should be advised to consume a low residue diet and take faecal softeners.

Liver disease

Liver disease is the only major cause of death that is continuing to rise year on year, and it is now the fifth "big killer" in England and Wales after heart disease, cancer, stroke, and respiratory disease [34]. Therefore, cirrhosis and advanced chronic end-stage liver disease represent a major public health and potential palliative burden. Worldwide hepatitis B and C are the most common causes of cirrhosis. In the developed world, alcohol is the most common cause, but hepatitis C is rapidly increasing along with liver disease associated with obesity (non alcoholic steatohepatitis).

The UK incidence of cirrhosis is approximately 17 per 100,000 (prevalence 76 per 100,000) in adults over 25 years. More than 80% of liver-related deaths in the United Kingdom are due to cirrhosis secondary to alcohol [35].

Prognosis is related to the severity of the underlying disease (see Figure 10.4) and the development of disease-related complications. In stable compensated cirrhosis (Childs A) the 5-year survival is excellent; however, in decompensated cirrhosis (development of portal hypertension, ascites, portal hypertensive bleeding, encephalopathy), the 5-year survival is 50%. The model for end-stage liver disease (MELD) is a validated scoring system used to predict the survival of patients with end-stage liver disease in America and Europe [36]. The UK equivalent is UKELD, and a UKELD score of greater than 49 is the minimum criteria for entry onto the transplant waiting list.

Complications of cirrhosis

The development of complications (see Figure 10.5) associated with decompensated cirrhosis have a marked impact on survival:
- Refractory Ascites (RA).
- Spontaneous Bacterial Peritonitis (SBP).
- Hepatorenal Syndrome (HRS).
- Variceal Bleeding (VB).

---

[1] In stents placed in the lower rectum.

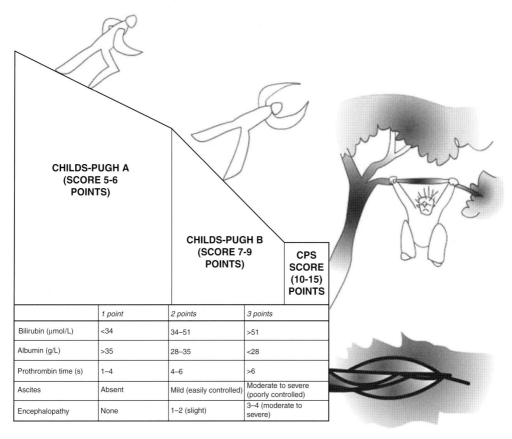

	1 point	2 points	3 points
Bilirubin (μmol/L)	<34	34–51	>51
Albumin (g/L)	>35	28–35	<28
Prothrombin time (s)	1–4	4–6	>6
Ascites	Absent	Mild (easily controlled)	Moderate to severe (poorly controlled)
Encephalopathy	None	1–2 (slight)	3–4 (moderate to severe)

Figure 10.4 The Childs-Pugh classification of cirrhosis.

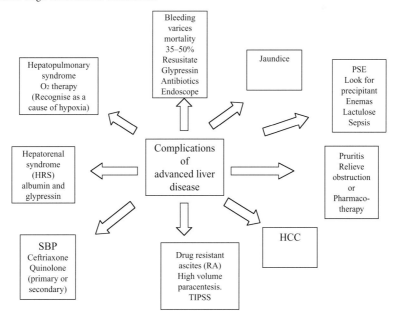

Figure 10.5 Summary of the complications that may occur in advanced liver disease. HCC, hepatocellular carcinoma; TIPSS, transjugular intrahepatic portosystemic shunt; SBP, spontaneous bacterial peritonitis; PSE, portosystemic encephalopathy.

- Hepatocellular Carcinoma (HCC).
- Portosystemic Encephalopathy (PSE).

Ascites and refractory ascites

While response to the use of diuretics in malignant ascites is variable and unpredictable, they are highly effective in ascites of decompensated liver disease. Response may be seen using spironolactone up to 400 mg/od and furosemide up to 160 mg/od Diuretics should be titrated to effect while monitoring electrolyte balance and renal function.

RA is associated with a high frequency of complications (PSE and infections). The 1-year survival is approximately 50%. Patients should have the patency of the portal vein checked (ultrasound) and development of a HCC excluded (serum alpha feto protein and imaging if appropriate).

Treatment of RA includes the following:
- *Transplantation*: By far the best treatment but not all patients will be suitable.
- *Transjugular intrahepatic portosytemic shunt (TIPSS)*: Reduces the rate of ascites recurrence and the development of HRS, has no effect on survival and is associated with a 20% incidence of encephalopathy. The ongoing management of patients with TIPSS is hospital intensive, and it is not recommended for those with severe liver failure, concomitant active infection, progressive renal failure, or severe cardiopulmonary disease.
- *Paracentesis* (see Box 10.4) [37]: The treatment of choice for most patients. Large volume paracentesis (>5 L) requires hospitalisation and concurrent administration of IV albumin; however, smaller volume paracentesis (<5 L) can be done as an outpatient, and the need for volume expansion is less clear and needs to be considered within the overall goals of care for a patient. A palliative procedure out of the hospital setting may be

---

Box 10.4 Large volume paracentesis (>5 L)

- If patient on diuretics, withhold.
- Under local anaesthetic insert suprapubic catheter into peritoneal cavity (Banano Catheter ideal).
- Give albumin 8 g/L of ascitic fluid drained.
- Drain to dryness.
- Remove catheter after 24 h to reduce chances of infection and peritonitis.
- Place stoma bag over site if ascites leakage.
Start albumin infusion before or at same time as starting paracentesis.

---

appropriate, but the risks and benefits for the patient need to be considered carefully.

Spontaneous bacterial peritonitis

SBP carries a 10–30% mortality with a 1-year survival of 38% after the first episode. It may lead to circulatory dysfunction and HRS that has a very poor survival rate. Administration of albumin with antibiotic therapy prevents HRS and improves prognosis.

There is good evidence for the administration of prophylactic quinolone antibiotics in patients with ascites due to cirrhosis for the prevention of SBP however concerns exist over the emergence of quinolone-resistant species of bacteria and antibiotic-induced complications. The suggested schedule is ciprofloxacin 250 mg od

Hepatorenal syndrome

In patients whose renal function deteriorates, HRS should be considered and urgent specialist advice sought. HRS occurs in 5–10% of cirrhotic patients with ascites and is a very sinister development with greater than 90% mortality.

Portosystemic encephalopathy

This is common and if mild is easily controlled. There are multiple causes; however, the most common are sepsis, dehydration, GI bleed, and the coadministration of sedating drugs. It is a marker of decompensation and therefore potentially reversible.

Treatment includes the following:
- Correction of the reversible (sepsis, SBP, dehydration, hypokalaemia, underlying bleeding, constipation).
- Enemas to achieve bowel clearance.
- *Laxatives*: lactulose has traditionally been used as it reduces colonic pH and nitrogen load in the gut. However, in practice it is acceptable to use alternatives that may be better tolerated.

Variceal bleeding

Varices are related to elevated portal pressure and the development of a portosystemic shunt through collateral vessels, allowing portal blood to be diverted to the systemic circulation. The size of the varix and the severity of the underlying liver disease are risk factors for bleeding. Propanolol (40 mg bd) reduces the incidence of first variceal bleeds by 50%. Alcohol causes marked increase in portal hypertension, and every effort should be made to get patients to cease drinking. Banding of varices has a role in preventing further bleeds, and if practical, should be carried out on a regular basis until the varices are obliterated.

The average mortality of a first variceal bleed is approximately 50%; however, this is closely related to the underlying severity of liver disease. Bleeding may result in severe decompensation and fatal liver injury. VB is always a frightening and dramatic occurrence.

Prescribing in liver disease

Patients with advanced liver disease are symptomatic and therefore need their symptoms to be appropriately assessed and treated. Concern exists in prescribing for patients with liver disease as there is little evidence to guide practice. The liver has a huge reserve and has to be damaged significantly before it starts to have an effect; however, this is unpredictable and each patient should therefore be assessed as an individual and closely monitored after any medication is prescribed.

Pain management in advanced liver disease

Paracetamol is safe in normal doses in patients with liver disease for short periods. Dose reduction should be considered if prolonged therapy or the patient is malnourished (<50 kg). Nonsteroidal anti-inflammatory drugs (NSAIDs) should be avoided since their salt retention and other renal effects may lead to decompensation in patients with cirrhosis.

All opioids require liver metabolism and may accumulate in liver impairment. There are also many other factors that impact on the effects of opioids, for example, underlying diagnosis and speed of deterioration, presence of ascites. There is no evidence base to inform prescribing advice and we therefore suggest:
- Use reduced doses and consider increasing the dosing interval.
- Avoid drugs with long half-lives.
- Titrate slowly against effect.
- Re-evaluate daily.

Liver transplantation issues

Liver transplant is the gold standard treatment for advanced chronic liver disease and fulminant hepatic failure with a 1 year survival of 80–90% and 5-year survival of 60–80%. However, for various reasons not all patients will be eligible for transplantation, and there is a limited pool of donor grafts available. Four people will die for every one transplanted.

For those who are not suitable for transplantation (e.g., those with alcoholic cirrhosis who cannot cease drinking or those whose performance status precludes transplanta-

tion) palliative care is the key focus of care. Even for those who are suitable for transplantation and on the waiting list, one in five will die. Appropriate symptom management and assessment of quality of life needs therefore to be considered for all those with advanced disease whether they are listed or not. This will include support for patients and their families often at a time of uncertainty and consideration of place of death when patients are removed from the transplant list because of deterioration.

Cholestatic liver disease

The key symptoms resulting from stasis of bile are pruritus and jaundice.

Pruritus

The pruritic effect is mediated through a central mechanism, a response to a rise in endogenous opioid levels. Large variations in individual response are seen and there is no correlation between plasma bilirubin concentration and intensity of pruritus. Approximately 20–25% of jaundiced patients complain of itch. There is no standard or generally accepted regimen for treatment and many different medications, with a limited evidence base, have been tried. The most effective treatment is to achieve biliary drainage, although this is not always possible and not without complications.

Drugs for pruritis include the following:
- *Antihistamine*: Sedating antihistamine has no effect on the itch but may assist in promoting sleep through their sedating effect, best avoided during the daytime.
- *Exchange resins*: Colestyramine is a bile salt binder, give 4 g bd Best taken on an empty stomach first thing in the morning and before the evening meal (can add to orange juice to improve palatability).
- *Choleuretic agents*: Ursodeoxcholic acid 250 mg tds
- *Enzyme inducers*: Rifampicin 150 mg daily or phenobarbital. Moderate to low efficacy with variable response.
- *$5HT_3$ antagonists*: Anecdotal reports of therapeutic response to IV ondansetron.
- *Selective serotonin reuptake inhibitor (SSRI) antidepressants*: Sertraline 25 mg od and titrating to effect.
- *Immunomodulating drugs*: Thalidomide 200 mg od (limited by side effects and practicalities of dispensing).
- *Opioid antagonists*: specialist guidance is required as opioid withdrawal may be provoked.

Jaundice

In cholestatic or obstructive jaundice, patients frequently feel unwell, anorexic, and nauseated. Bile is essential for digestion and absorption of fat, an essential fuel source.

They may develop symptoms of malabsorption. Active palliation through decompression of the biliary system (see endoluminal stents above) is the only effective treatment, if at all practical. The approach can be through an ERCP or PTC, either as a day case or a short stay in hospital. However, on many occasions, decompression is not practically possible and therefore active palliation of the resulting symptoms with medication needs to be aimed for.

Constipation

Constipation is a big problem for patients with advanced disease. For instance more than 50% of patients admitted to hospices in the United Kingdom complain of constipation [38]. Physical illness, immobility, poor oral intake, opioids, and many other drugs are risk factors for constipation. Constipation can be prevented in the majority of patients by prescription of appropriate laxatives and careful review.

All patients prescribed a weak or strong opioid should be advised to also take a stimulant laxative unless a contraindication exists. The dose of laxative will usually need to be increased as the dose of opioid is increased. It is not appropriate to wait until (predictable) constipation occurs before commencing laxative treatment. The vicious cycle of inappropriately treated abdominal pain and constipation should be anticipated in all patients with cancer, or others taking opioid analgesics.

Management

Management will involve removing any underlying causes if possible, prescribing an appropriate oral laxative and considering the use of per rectal/stomal measures (see Table 10.3). It should be remembered that one of the commonest reasons for failure of therapy is prescription of a laxative that the patient dislikes.

Table 10.4 shows the various types of laxative that are available. Macrogols and sodium picosulfate are probably best used as second-line laxatives for patients with established constipation resistant to other laxatives. Lactulose may cause substantial gaseous distension, especially in resistant constipation.

Rectal laxatives may be needed and include:
- *Suppositories*: glycerine (softening and mild stimulant); bisacodyl (stimulant).
- *Enemas*: arachis oil (130 ml) (softening); phosphate, sodium citrate (stimulant).

Table 10.3 Treatment of constipation.

Examination finding	Treatment
Rectum full of hard faeces	Soften with glycerin suppositories +/− arachis oil enema. Commence combined stimulant and softening oral laxative
Rectum full of soft faeces	Stimulate evacuation with bisacodyl suppository +/− stimulant enema. Commence stimulant oral laxative
Empty distended rectum	Exclude obstruction. Stimulant suppository or enema will enhance colonic contraction. Commence oral laxative

If the rectum is empty and stool is high in the colon, enemas should be administered through a rubber Foley catheter. Oil enemas should be warmed before use.

Bulk-forming laxatives have a very limited place in the management of constipation in patients with advanced disease, since they are generally troublesome to take, rely on a high oral fluid intake, and are not appropriate for the management of opioid-induced constipation. All laxative doses should be titrated according to response.

In 2008 methylnaltrexone (an opioid antagonist) was licensed for use in the United States and Europe. This is given subcutaneously and may be appropriate to consider using when standard management of constipation has failed in those patients with opioid-induced constipation. Specialist advice should be sought when considering its use in management [39]. Naloxone combined with oxycodone in an oral preparation is now available and may reduce the occurrence of constipation but has some complexity in its usage due to the ceiling dose of naloxone.

Rectal problems of advanced cancer

The presence of tumour in the rectum may lead to bleeding, faecal incontinence, and offensive discharge, in addition to pain. The quality of life may be severely impaired. Such problems occur not only in patients with primary rectal cancers but also in patients with other pelvic cancers:

Table 10.4 Laxatives and their characteristics.

Laxative type	Drugs	Starting dose	Latency of action
Stimulant	Bisacodyl Senna Sodium picosulfate	10 mg nocte 15 mg nocte 5 ml nocte	6–12 h
Softening	Docusate sodium Lactulose Macrogol	200 mg bd/tds 15 ml bd 1 sachet daily in 125 ml water	1–2 days
Combined softening and stimulant	Co-danthramer Co-danthrusate	Two capsules or 20 ml nocte. One capsule or 10 ml nocte	6–12 h

cervix, vagina, uterus, and bladder. Treatment options include:
• radiotherapy;
• palliative surgery with stoma formation;
• endoscopic injection of absolute alcohol;
• laser therapy and diathermy;
• metal stent alone or in combination with laser or alcohol; and
• pharmacological palliation.

The stool should be kept very soft to pass through the obstructive lesion. Docusate sodium is given at a dose of 200 mg at least tds but titrated to stool consistency; it can be combined with a stimulant laxative (such as in Co-danthrusate). Careful insertion of softening enemas may be useful.

Pain and tenesmus

Pain from rectal cancer may be troublesome in a number of ways; constant nociceptive, visceral and bone, which may be worsened by movement. In some cases sitting may be impossible. The pain may be present only on, or worsened by, either standing or defecation. Neuropathic pains can result from infiltration of the lumbosacral plexus. Some patients experience tenesmus: a painful sensation of rectal fullness and an urge to defecate.

The WHO ladder (see Chapter 9) will be helpful for all of these pain syndromes. Pain will be additionally helped by keeping the faeces soft. For some patients, a palliative colostomy will be the best form of pain relief.

Neuropathic pain, of which tenesmus is one type, may be helped by opioids but will probably require adjuvant analgesics such as amitriptyline 10–75 mg nocte. Tenesmus may also be helped by:

• steroids—dexamethasone 4–16 mg daily;
• calcium channel antagonists—nifedipine 10–20 mg bd-tds (smooth muscle relaxant);
• radiotherapy;
• bupivacaine enema;
• sacral epidural injection of steroid and local anaesthetic and
• intrathecal 5% phenol to posterior sacral nerve roots.

Occasionally epidural infusion of opioids and local anaesthetic may be appropriate for relief of pain at rest and on defecation, particularly if the obstructive lesion is very low in the bowel.

Rectal bleeding and discharge

While radiotherapy, alcohol injection, diathermy, or laser therapy is being planned, or if these are not possible or helpful, other measures may be needed to reduce the distress and discomfort from rectal bleeding. Enemas may be performed using various active ingredients, including: tranexamic acid (2–4 g/day made up in KY jelly) [40]; and aluminium coating through an enema (1% alum or sucralfate g in KY jelly) [41]. Distress or discomfort due to rectal discharge may be alleviated by steroid enemas and metronidazole suppositories.

Stoma care

Patients with stomas require both physical and psychological support. Good preparation before stoma formation and adequate time spent with the patient after stoma formation by a specialist (stoma care) nurse help in the transition and continued successful management. Patients vary in the time needed to adapt to and manage their stoma.

The most common physical difficulties are:
- when a bowel stoma becomes overactive, often with a more fluid faecal output;
- when constipation occurs; and
- when patients are less able to manage their own stoma care because of the effects of their treatment or their disease.

Evaluation and management of these problems will involve examination of the stoma and effluent, including a digital examination of the stoma. There must also be a review of skin protectives/adhesives and bag size, together with a review of laxatives and antidiarrhoeal agents along with all other drugs.

If a stoma is impacted, suppositories and enemas can be given as for rectal impaction; however, a stoma has no sphincter. Suppositories should be gently pushed through the stoma as far as possible and gauze held over the stoma for a few minutes. If an enema, either oil or phosphate, is used it should be administered through a medium-sized Foley catheter. This should be passed well into the stoma (identify direction of the bowel by digital examination beforehand). Inflate the balloon to 5 ml for 10 min while instilling the enema.

Control of fluid loss from an overactive ileostomy can be troublesome and specialist advice may need to be sought. Various treatments are available. The administration of opioids can reduce bowel motility; for example, loperamide 4–8 mg bd or codeine phosphate 30–60 mg qds If the patient is already taking morphine for pain relief, an increase in this may reduce bowel motility further but will also increase sedation and other central effects, and is not the preferred option unless it is also useful to improve pain control. A reduction of bowel motility and secretions may be achieved by use of anticholinergics, for example, hyoscine butylbromide SC 60–200 mg/24 h, while H_2 antagonists or PPIs can reduce gastric secretions.

Ispaghula (1–2 sachets tds) aids thickening of the motions, as does the use of isotonic and avoidance of hypotonic oral fluids. Marshmallows may also help increase stool consistency. An SC infusion of octreotide can reduce small bowel secretions (see above). However, doses required can be much greater than in treating obstruction.

The principles of management of a stoma and stoma-care equipment can also be used to contain the output from faecal fistulae and protect the skin. SC octreotide has been used to decrease the volume of fistula effluent and in some cases has aided healing.

References

1. Roth K, Lynn J, Zhong Z, et al. Dying with end stage liver disease with cirrhosis: insights from SUPPORT. Study to understand prognoses and preferences for outcomes and risks of treatment. *J Am Geriatr Soc* 2000; 48(5 Suppl): S122–S130.

2. Hansen L, Saaski A and Zucker B. End-stage liver disease: challenges and practice implications. *Nurs Clin N Am* 2010; 45: 411–426.

3. Dewys WD, Begg D, Lavin PT, et al. Prognostic effect of weight loss prior to chemotherapy in cancer patients. *Am J Med* 1980; 69: 491–496.

4. Wagner PD. Possible mechanisms underlying the development of cachexia in COPD. *Eur Resp J* 2008; 31: 492–501.

5. Anker SD, Negassa A, Coats AJ, et al. Prognostic importance of weight loss in chronic heart failure and the effect of treatment with angiotensin-converting-enzyme inhibitors: an observational study. *Lancet* 2003; 361: 1077–1083.

6. Plauth M and Schutz ET. Cachexia in liver cirrhosis. *Int J Cardiol* 2002; 85: 83–87.

7. Grunfield C. What causes wasting in AIDS? *NEJM* 1995; 333: 123–124.

8. General medical Council. *Treatment and Care Towards the End of Life: Good Practice in Decision Making.* London: GMC, 2010.

9. HM Government UK. *Mental Capacity Act.* London: The Stationary Office, 2005.

10. Bruera E and Sweeney C. Pharmacological interventions in cachexia and anorexia. In: Doyle D, Hanks GWC, Cherney N, Calman K (eds), *Oxford Textbook of Palliative Medicine,* 3rd edition. Oxford: Oxford University Press, 2003, pp. 552–560.

11. Bernstein G and Ortiz Z. Megestrol acetate for treatment of anorexia-cachexia syndrome. *Cochrane Database Syst Rev* 2005; (2): CD004310. doi: 10.1002/14651858.CD004310.pub2.

12. Stratton RJ and Elia M. A review of reviews: a new look at the evidence for oral nutritional supplements in clinical practice. *Clin Nutri Suppl* 2007; 2: 5–23.

13. Elia M (Chairman and ed.). Guidelines for detection and management of malnutrition. Maidenhead: Malnutrition Advisory Group (MAG), Standing committee of British Association of Parenteral and Enteral Nutrition (BAPEN), 2000

14. National Institute for Clinical Excellence, 2006 CG32 Guidance for Nutrition Support in Adults.

15. Royal College of Physicians. Oral feeding difficulties and dilemmas. A guide to practical care, particularly towards the end of life. Report of a working party. Royal College of Physicians, 2010.

16. Mathus-Vliegen EMH. Feeding tubes and gastrostomy. In: Tygat GNJ, Classen M, Waye JD, Nkazawa S (eds), *Practice of Therapeutic Endoscopy*. Philadelphia, PA: Saunders, 2000.

17. NCEPOD. Scoping our practice. The 2004 Report of the National Confidential Enquiry into Patient Outcome and Death. London, NCEPOD, 2004.

18. Twycross R and Wilcock A (eds.). Administering drugs via enteral feeding tubes. In: *Palliative Care Formulary*, 3rd edition. Nottingham: Palliative drugs.com Ltd, 2009, pp. 503–524.

19. Scannapieco FA. Pneumonia in nonambulatory patients: the role of oral bacteria and oral hygiene. *J Am Dent Assoc* 2010; 137: 21s–25s.

20. Bassim CW, Gibson G, Ward T, et al. Modification of the risk of mortality from pneumonia with oral hygiene care. *J Am Ger Soc* 2008; 56: 1601–1607.

21. National Patient Safety Agency. 2010 Rapid Response Alert–Early Detection of Complications after gastrostomy No.1214 NPSA/2010/RRR010.

22. Petrina Sweeney M and Bagg J. The mouth and palliative care. *Am J Hosp Palliat Med* 2000; 17: 118–124.

23. Davies A and Finlay I (eds.). *Oral Care in Advanced Disease*. Oxford: Oxford University Press, 2005, pp. 97–114.

24. Harris DG. Nausea and vomiting in advanced cancer. *Br Med Bull* 2010; 96: 175–185.

25. Ang SK, Shoemaker LK and Davis MP. Nausea and vomiting in advanced cancer. *Am J Hosp Palliat Med* 2010; 27(3): 219–225.

26. Brooksbank MA, Game PA and Ashby MA. Palliative venting gastrostomy in malignant intestinal obstruction. *Palliat Med* 2002; 16: 520–526.

27. Taylor RH. Laparotomy for obstruction with recurrent tumour. *Br J Surg* 1985; 72: 327.

28. Krebs H and Goplerud DR. Surgical management of bowel obstruction in advanced ovarian cancer. *Obstet Gynaecol* 1983; 61: 327–330.

29. Feuer DDJ and Broadley KE. Corticosteroids for the resolution of malignant bowel obstruction in advanced gynaecological and gastrointestinal cancer. *Cochrane Database Syst Rev* 2000; (1): CD001219. doi: 10.1002/14651858.CD001219.

30. DeConno F, Caraceni A, Zecca E, et al. Continuous subcutaneous infusion of hyoscine butylbromide reduces secretions in patients with gastrointestinal obstruction. *J Pain Symp Manage* 1991; 6: 484–486.

31. Ripamonti CI, Easson AM and Gerdes H. Management of malignant bowel obstruction. *Eur J Cancer* 2008; 44: 1105–1115.

32. Riley J and Fallon MT. Octreotide in terminal malignant obstruction of the gastrointestinal tract. *Eur J Palliat Care* 1994; 1: 23–25.

33. Ramirez FC, Dennert B, Zierer ST, et al. Esophageal self-expandable metallic stents-Indications, practice, techniques and complications, results of a national survey. *Gastro Intest Endosc* 1997; 45: 360–364.

34. Office for National Statistics: Health Service Quarterly, Winter 2008, no. 40; 59–60.

35. Macnaughtan J and Thomas H. Liver failure at the front door. *Clin Med* 2010; 10(1): 73–78.

36. Medici V, Rossaro L, Wegelin JA, et al. The utility of the model for end-stage liver disease score: a reliable guide for liver transplant candidacy and, for select patients, simultaneous hospice referral. *Liver Transpl* 2008; 14: 1100–1106.

37. European Association for the Study of the Liver. EASL clinical practice guidelines on the management of ascites, spontaneous bacterial peritonitis, and hepatorenal syndrome in cirrhosis. *J Hepatol* 2010; 53: 397–417.

38. Sykes NP. Constipation and diarrhoea. In: Hanks G, Cherny NI, Christakis NA, Fallon M, Kaasa S, Russell K, Portenoy RK (eds), *The Oxford Textbook of Palliative Medicine*, 4th edition. Oxford: Oxford University Press, 2010.

39. Larkin PJ, Sykes NP, Centeno C, et al. The management of constipation in palliative care: clinical practice recommendations. *Palliat Med* 2008; 22: 796–807.

40. McElligot E, Quigley C and Hanks GW. Tranexamic acic and rectal bleeding. *Lancet* 1991; 29: 37–39.

41. Regnard CFB. Control of bleeding in advanced cancer. *Lancet* 1991; 337: 974.

Further reading

Nutrition, tube feeding, and PEG

Stroud M, Duncan H and Nightingale J. Guidelines for entral feeding in adult hospital patients. *Gut* 2003; 52(Suppl VII): vii1–vii12.

Cirrhosis and its complications

Menon KV and Kamath PS. Managing the complications of cirrhosis. *Mayo Clin Proc* 2000; 75(5): 501–509.

11 The Management of Respiratory Symtpoms and Advanced COPD

Christine Jones

Palliative Medicine Physician, Victoria Hospice Society, Vancouver Island Health Authority, Victoria, Canada

Dyspnoea introduction

Dyspnoea is defined as "a subjective awareness of breathing discomfort" [1]. It is present in about 70% of patients with advanced malignancy, >90% of those with advanced chronic obstructive pulmonary disease (COPD), and in >60% of those with advanced heart disease [2]. Breathlessness is experienced by patients with renal failure, dementia, human immunodeficiency virus (HIV), and neuromuscular disease [3]. Shortness of breath affects almost 50% of all patients who receive end-of-life care, and becomes more severe in the final weeks of life [4,5].

Clinical correlates of breathlessness are fatigue, impaired sleep, anxiety, depression, and a reduced sensation of well-being [6]. It negatively impacts a patient's mobility, self-care, and social interactions. Dyspnoea intensity is an independent predictor of will to live [7]—patients sometimes say they would prefer death to the experience of breathlessness.

The perception of dyspnoea is heavily influenced by a person's previous experiences, personality, physical symptoms, and psychosocial context. Assessment and management of this symptom requires close attention to the physical, psychological, social, and existential domains [8].

Dyspnoea pathophysiology

The act of respiration is a complex neurophysiologic process under both voluntary and involuntary control (Figure 11.1). The respiratory centre in the brainstem balances incoming sensory information with motor output to the muscles of ventilation. Experiences, emotions and context are processed centrally and will influence the sensation of intensity as well as the perceived unpleasantness [9].

Sensory input

Chemoreceptors are located both peripherally and centrally. *Peripheral chemoreceptors* in the carotid body and aortic arch respond to changes in pH, pO_2, and pCO_2. The *central chemoreceptors* in the medulla respond to changes in pH and pCO_2. Acute hypercapnia is a stronger stimulus to respiration than acute hypoxia.

Pulmonary mechanoreceptors include *pulmonary stretch receptors*, activated by an increase in tension in the walls of airways; *irritant receptors*, stimulated by rapid changes in lung volume, direct mechanical stimuli, irritants, or chemicals; and *J-receptors* in the very small airways and alveolar capillaries stimulated by mechanical and chemical factors.

Chest wall mechanoreceptors include *muscle spindles* that function as stretch receptors and *tendon organs* that monitor force generation.

Motor output

The muscles of respiration include the diaphragm, intercostal muscles, and accessory muscles of respiration. Motor output is under voluntary control through the motor cortex and involuntary control through the brainstem.

Central processing

Information provided to the brainstem is fed to higher centres through the thalamus and limbic systems where previous experiences and emotions give context to the dyspnoea experience. This central processing influences respiratory muscle and behavioural responses [10].

Handbook of Palliative Care, Third Edition. Edited by Christina Faull, Sharon de Caestecker, Alex Nicholson and Fraser Black.
© 2012 by John Wiley and Sons, Inc. Published 2012 by John Wiley & Sons, Inc.

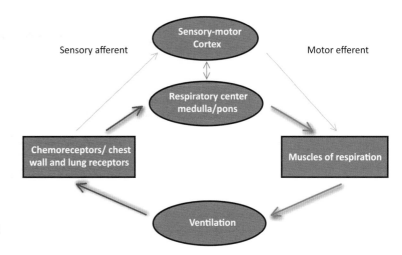

Figure 11.1 A simplified neurophysiologic diagram of the control of breathing.

Perception of breathlessness

Breathlessness results when there is a perceived mismatch between motor command from the respiratory centre and the ability of the respiratory system to respond. This mismatch has been termed *neuro-mechanical dissociation* [9–11]. For example, if chest wall and lung expansion become limited due to pleural disease or chest wall weakness, the pulmonary and chest wall receptors will not fire appropriately, and an increased sensation of dyspnoea will result.

Dyspnoea aetiology

Dyspnoea can result from any pathological process that impairs pulmonary ventilation, circulation, or gas exchange. Several causes are usually present in any one patient, particularly at the end of life [12]. Table 11.1 lists common causes of dyspnoea encountered in palliative care.

Dyspnoea assessment

All patients with life-limiting illnesses should be asked about dyspnoea, regardless of primary presenting symptom. It should be assessed in the context of a comprehensive history, physical examination, and investigations appropriate to the patient's disease trajectory and stated goals of care. History should include present and past medical history, investigations, treatments, and psychosocial history. Assessment should focus on the identification

of a possible reversible component, the pattern and severity of dyspnoea, and its effect on quality of life.

An approach to the history of dyspnoea is presented in Box 11.1 utilising the OPQRSTUV format and described fully below [14].

Onset and timing of dyspnoea

Acute and chronic dyspnoea

Chronic dyspnoea is generally due to COPD, asthma, interstitial lung disease, or myocardial dysfunction [15]. *Acute dyspnoea* usually results from an exacerbation of chronic illness, such as COPD or congestive heart failure (CHF). It may represent progression or complication of an underlying malignancy. Patients who have had dyspnoea for many years may have learned to modify their activity and lifestyle while those with acute dyspnoea may still be struggling to adjust.

Severe dyspnoea of very rapid onset is terrifying for the patient, caregiver, and professionals alike. Immediate treatment while the cause is being investigated is appropriate for some patients, while a focus on urgent symptom relief without investigation will be the priority for others. Severe dyspnoea of rapid onset in patients with advanced disease is most often caused by pulmonary embolism, pulmonary oedema, or cardiac arrhythmia [13].

Breakthrough/incident dyspnoea

Short-lived dyspnoea on a background of well-controlled breathlessness is called breakthrough or incident dyspnoea, analogous to breakthrough or incident pain. The history may be a bit misleading; background dyspnoea may be well controlled only because the patient has

Table 11.1 Common causes of dyspnoea in palliative care patients based on pathophysiology.

Defective ventilation	

Obstructed ventilation	Upper airway obstruction
	  Tumour
	  Retained secretions
	Lower airway obstruction
	  Bronchospasm
	  oedema
	  Inflammation

Restricted ventilation	Muscle weakness
	  Neuromuscular disease
	  Cachexia
	  Phrenic nerve paralysis
	Reduced compliance
	  Pulmonary fibrosis
	  Interstitial oedema
	Compression of lung tissue
	  Tumour
	  Effusion
	  Pneumothorax
	Replacement or loss of lung tissue
	  Tumour
	  Emphysema (loss)
	  Atelectesis
	  Infection/inflammation
	Reduced elasticity
	  COPD

Impaired circulation	
Reduced perfusion	Pulmonary embolism Pulmonary hypertension Cardiac failure Superior vena cava obstruction
Impaired gas exchange	
Interstitial disease	Pulmonary fibrosis Pneumonitis Oedema Emphysema (loss)
Impaired delivery/ utilisation	Anaemia Deconditioning

Source: Reproduced from Reference 13.

Box 11.1 History of dyspnoea using the OPQRSTUV approach (modified from the Fraser Health Guidelines)

Category	Possible questions
ONSET/TIMING	When does the dyspnoea occur? What is your best time of day? Are you breathless rest? Are you breathless all the time? How long have you been breathless?
PROVOKING/ PALLIATING	What makes the shortness of breath worse? Triggers may be physical, psychological, or environmental
QUALITY	What does the breathlessness feel like? Chest tightness/air hunger/ suffocation
RELATED SYMPTOMS	What other symptoms accompany the breathlessness? Pain? Anxiety? Fear? Haemoptysis? Cough? Wheeze? Congestion?
SEVERITY	How bad is the breathlessness? May use a visual analogue scale (VAS) or an numerical rating scale (NRS)
TREATMENT	Current medications and treatments Efficacy of current and past treatments? Side effects?

UNDERSTANDING/ IMPACT	Explore perception of patient and carers
	  What do they think is causing the dyspnoea
	  Effect of symptom on patient and carer?
	  Symptoms of anxiety or depression?
	  Social withdrawal?
	  Decreased activities of daily living (ADLs) or mobility?

VALUES	Goal for symptom relief
	Hope for future symptom relief
	Beliefs about symptom
	  Wonder about ongoing damage?
	  Worry about sudden death?

Source: Reproduced from Reference 14.

dramatically modified their lifestyle. Breakthrough dysp-noea is most often triggered by activity, occurs numerous times a day, and lasts for less than 10 min [6].

Provoking factors

As disease progresses, dyspnoea will be provoked at lower and lower exercise thresholds. Eventually dyspnoea may be triggered by the simple act of dressing, bathing, or, in severe cases, talking. Cool air seems to be better toler-ated than hot, humid air, and environmental pollutants such as tobacco smoke may trigger acute attacks. Anxiety or sadness may precipitate dyspnoea, and patients may avoid social outings or conversations with strong emo-tional overtones. "I can't talk about that because it will make me cry, and then I can't breathe."

Qualitative aspects of dyspnoea

Patients should be asked to describe their dyspnoea expe-rience. They may use terms such as "air hunger," "chest tightness," and "increased work of breathing" [16]. As breathlessness begins to occur at rest or takes a while to settle after activity, patients may use words that have an emotional overtone, such as "worrying," "terrifying," and "frightening" [17].

Descriptors may reflect a pathological process or dis-ease state (Table 11.2) [11,16]. However, there are multiple causes of dyspnoea at play in any one patient, particularly at the end of life, and dyspnoea is a complex qualitative experience. Descriptors may be most useful in defining the patient's unique symptom experience, and therapies can then be targeted to their distress. For example, probing into the "frightening" nature of a patient's experience may reveal that they are fearful of dying in extreme dyspnoea; this fear can be addressed through education and reas-surance. Changing the language used to discuss dyspnoea can have significant therapeutic value.

Dyspnoea severity

Dyspnoea is a subjective symptom. Physiologic assess-ments such as blood gases and oxygen saturation do not accurately reflect the patient's experience, nor do signs such as tachypnea, cyanosis, or accessory muscle use [9]. We must rely on the patient's report. Multiple assessment scales have been developed, including the Numberic Rat-ing Scale (NRS), the Visual Analogue Scale (VRS), and the modified Borg scale. Symptom inventory scales, such as the Memorial Assessment scale or the Edmonton Symp-tom Assessment Scale, incorporate ratings of dyspnoea. However, no single assessment tool incorporates all the dimensions of this complex symptom, and no one scale

Table 11.2 Common descriptors of dyspnoea in various disease states.

Disease	Description
Heart failure	Air hunger Suffocation Inspiratory difficulty
COPD	Increase effort to breathe Unsatisfying breaths Cannot get a deep breath
Acute hypercapnia or restricted thoracic motion	Air hunger
Anxiety	Can not get enough air
Acute bronchoconstriction	Chest tightness Increased effort Air hunger
Cardiovascular deconditioning	Heavy breathing
Neuromuscular disease	Increased respiratory effort
Interstitial lung disease	Inspiratory difficulty Rapid breathing

can be recommended over another at this time. NRS or VAS, in which the patients rate the symptom severity on a scale of 1–10, has the most practical value [18].

The severity of dyspnoea during different times of the day and with different types of activities should be recorded.

Related symptoms

Anxiety

All patients with dyspnoea should be asked about anxiety, although these two symptoms do not always coexist [12]. If present, there is usually significant generalised and anticipatory anxiety.

Respiratory panic attacks

Some patients become immersed in a cycle of dyspnoea causing anxiety, which in turn creates more breathlessness and panic (Figure 11.2). These respiratory panic attacks are exceedingly difficult for patients to experience and

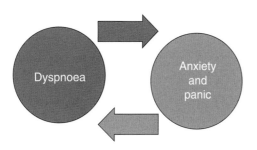

Figure 11.2 Relationship between dyspnoea and anxiety/panic.

caregivers to witness. Unless there are plans for these acute episodes, patients frequently present to the emergency department.

Cough
Coughing episodes can lead to severe, disabling incident dyspnoea. Productive sputum that is difficult to clear may temporarily obstruct the upper airways.

Symptoms clusters
Dyspnoea often presents in the context of other symptoms. In cancer patients, dyspnoea most often "clusters" with fatigue, drowsiness, nausea, and decreased appetite. Addressing dyspnoea in the context of a symptom cluster may provide superior palliation [19].

Treatment history
Previous treatments should be reviewed. Avoidance of opioids due to fear of side effects is common and generally can be resolved through education about opioid safety and appropriate prophylaxis, especially for constipation.

Some treatments may aggravate dyspnoea through the retention of fluid (steroids) or aggravation of bronchospasm (beta blockers). Dyspnoea may result from radiation pneumonitis or fibrosis, or as a side effect of some types of chemotherapy (bleomycin or carmustin).

Understanding of dyspnoea/impact of dyspnoea
Many patients fear suffocation or dying during an episode of incident dyspnoea. Education and reassurance will be necessary.

Coping strategies should be explored as some patients will push through an activity despite dyspnoea, with the knowledge that the dyspnoea will settle once they rest. Others will severely limit their activity, which could aggravate deconditioning, immobility, and dependence.

The impact of dyspnoea on the patient's ability to perform work, hobbies, household chores, and personal (ADLs) should be reviewed. The patient's world will become smaller and smaller as their activities are increasingly limited.

Relationships may be strained as a result of caregiver exhaustion and the increasing dependence of the patient [20]. Patients may become depressed or socially isolated.

Value or goal of patient and carer
Understanding patient and caregiver goals is an essential part of patient assessment. Patients may have lived for a long time with chronic dyspnoea and do not expect it to be resolved entirely. Others, particularly those who are fearful, will hope for complete resolution. Earlier in the trajectory, the focus is often dyspnoea management with concurrent improvements in mobility, alertness, and ability to perform ADLs. On the other hand, some patients nearing the end of life may be willing to compromise alertness in order to achieve relief of severely disabling and frightening dyspnoea.

Investigation
Investigation of dyspnoea will depend on the patient's underlying disease, trajectory, and goals of care. For some patients it may be important to forgo investigations and focus on symptom management. In other cases, diagnostic investigations are helpful to identify reversible causes of dyspnoea.

A chest X-ray is useful to assess the presence of infection, effusion, or progression of malignant disease. A CT scan will aid diagnosis of pulmonary embolism or interstitial lung disease. Haemoglobin helps to rule out significant anaemia. Blood gases could be measured to assess possible hypoxia or hypercapnia. In advanced disease, oxygen saturation is usually preferred.

Brain natriuretic peptide (BNP) may be measured to assess for pulmonary congestion [21].

Management of dyspnoea

Management of dyspnoea encompasses four principles:
1. Treat reversible causes if possible.
2. Palliate refractory dyspnoea and associated symptoms.
3. Enhance coping of the patient and caregivers.
4. Prepare for acute episodes.

Treat reversible causes

The underlying disease and comorbidities should be addressed, as appropriate to the patient's illness trajectory and stated goals of care. Table 11.3 lists common causes of dyspnoea in palliative care patients and possible treatments. The most common correctable causes of dyspnoea in patients with advanced malignancy are hypoxia, anaemia, and bronchospasm [12].

Symptom-targeted treatments for palliation of respiratory symptoms should occur while disease-specific therapies are being explored and continue beyond the point at which modifiable factors have been exhausted [22].

Palliate dyspnoea and associated symptoms

Nonpharmacological interventions

There is an expanding evidence base to support the use of nonpharmacological interventions, particularly in the mobile patient with COPD [23]. Systematic reviews conclude a strong level of evidence for

Table 11.3 Common causes of dyspnoea in palliative care and possible treatments.

Cause of dyspnoea	Treatment of choice
Caused by malignancy	
Airway obstruction	Radiation/steroids/stenting
Parenchymal compression or replacement	Radiation/chemotherapy
Pleural effusion	Thoracocentesis/pleurodesis
Pericardial effusion	Steroids/pericardial drainage
Lymphangitis carcinomatosis	Steroids
Related to malignancy	
Anaemia-severe	Transfusion
Cachexia and muscle weakness	None specific/minimise deconditioning
Phrenic nerve palsy	None specific
Pulmonary emboli	Anticoagulation/Caval filters
Pain	Appropriate analgesia
Ascites	Paracentesis
Superior vena cava obstruction	Steroids/radiotherapy/chemotherapy
Related to malignancy treatment	
Radiation pneumonitis/fibrosis	Steroids
Respiratory disease	
COPD	Steroids/bronchodilators
Pulmonary fibrosis	Steroids
Cardiac disease	
Cardiomyopathy	Appropriate treatment directed at cause
Pulmonary oedema	Diuretics
Neuromuscular Disease	
Amyotrophic lateral sclerosis (ALS)	Possibly, assisted ventilation
Other or nonspecific	
Hypoxia	Oxygen
Anxiety	Benzodiazepines/psychosocial support Relaxation therapies

Source: Reproduced from Reference 14.

pulmonary rehabilitation, neuromuscular stimulation, and chest wall vibration. Mobility aides and breathing techniques are supported by a moderate level of evidence [24]. However, these approaches are unevenly provided and underutilised. Other techniques such as music therapy, acupuncture/acupressure, hand-held fans, activity pacing, relaxation therapy, and psychological approaches have conflicting evidence for their use but may be very helpful in individual patients. As much of the information on nonpharmacological interventions comes from work with patients with COPD, the beneficial effect among patients with other diseases remains uncertain but therapeutic trials should be encouraged.

Pulmonary rehabilitation involves a supervised exercise programme, generally of 4 weeks duration, and may or may not include education or psychological support. Exercise training aids in the palliation of dyspnoea in many conditions, including COPD, chronic heart failure (HF), asthma, restrictive lung disease, obesity, and malignancy [11]. Exercising to greater than usual levels of breathlessness in a safe environment desensitises the patient to their dyspnoea; the patient begins to associate breathlessness with activity rather than respiratory distress [25]. For patients with COPD, rehabilitation provides relief of dyspnoea and fatigue, improves emotional functioning, and enhances patients' sense of control over their condition [26]. Unfortunately, it is provided for less than 2–4% of eligible patients. Challenges to supplying this intervention include a motivated patient population, facility support, and experienced health professionals.

Neuromuscular electrical stimulation (NMES) of the leg muscles is helpful for those patients who, due to severe dyspnoea, deconditioning, or peripheral muscle weakness, are unable to participate in an exercise programme [27]. NMES applied several times a week for 30–60 min, up to 4 weeks at a time, in patients with COPD or HF showed improved skeletal muscle function, exercise capacity, and disease-specific health status [24]. Access to this technique remains variable.

Chest wall vibration requires specialised equipment and is not widely available, but has been shown to have a significant effect on dyspnoea, perhaps by stimulating chest wall receptors [10,24].

Mobility aids have good evidence for their use, particularly in COPD, where they support the forward lean position during walking, provide support on which to rest when needed, and offer psychological reassurance.

Breathing techniques include breathing control, diaphragmatic breathing, pursed lip breathing, recovery breathing, and paced breathing [23] (see Box 11.2).

Box 11.2 Breathing techniques used for the relief of dyspnoea [23]

Technique	Description
Breathing control	Normal tidal breathing encouraging relaxation of the upper chest and shoulders
Diaphragmatic breathing	Breathing using abdominal movement; reducing the degree of chest wall movement as much as possible
Pursed lips breathing	Generation of a positive pressure against partially closed lips
Recovery breathing	Patient focuses on blowing out while gradually and deliberately increasing the length of the outbreath as their breathing recovers.
Paced breathing	Breathing to a rhythm; in time with walking or stairs

---

Positioning has little evidence to support its use, but many patients with COPD find leaning forward in a standing or sitting position helpful. This position may enhance diaphragmatic efficiency. Patients with unilateral respiratory disease will avoid lying on the unaffected side in order to maximise pulmonary expansion of functioning lung [25].

Activity pacing and planning can be provided by occupational therapists who are trained to evaluate activity, break it down to its component parts, and provide suggestions on energy conservation. Balance between activity and rest is encouraged [13].

A *hand held fan* directed at the cheeks is a commonly used and an easily applied technique to reduce breathlessness, possibly due to the stimulation of facial receptors [28]. Other methods of facial cooling may be equally effective.

Breathlessness case management clinics or *breathlessness services* may be beneficial. These services are multidisciplinary, tailored to the individual patient, and include nonpharmacological and pharmacological approaches to the relief of breathlessness, psychosocial interventions,

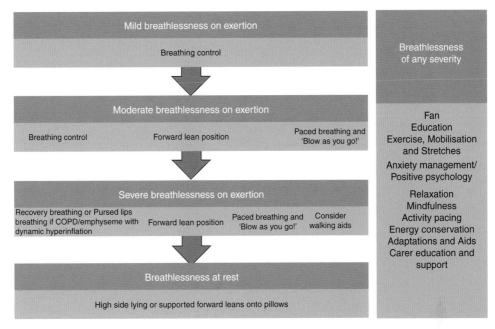

Figure 11.3 Suggested approach to the nonpharmacological management of dyspnoea. (Reproduced from Reference 23.)

and attention to end-of-life care, as appropriate. Early studies have shown benefit and results of randomised trials are pending [23].

A suggested approach to the nonpharmacological management of dyspnoea is presented in Figure 11.3 [23].

Pharmacological interventions

Opioids

Although the exact mechanism by which opioids reduce breathlessness is unclear, it is postulated that they reduce central sensitivity to hypercapnia and hypoxia, modulate the central perception of dyspnoea, and reduce oxygen consumption during exercise [24,25].

The evidence supporting the use of opioids in the palliation of dyspnoea is stronger than for any other pharmacologic agent [29]. Systematic reviews confirm the benefit of opioids for the relief of dyspnoea in both COPD and end-stage malignancy [30]. The American Thoracic Society and The American College of Chest Physicians have produced consensus statements supporting the use of opioids for the management of refractory dyspnoea in patients with advanced cardiorespiratory disease [31,32]. Clinical practice guidelines support the use of opioids for patients with advanced COPD [33].

Opioids should be started when disabling dyspnoea persists despite maximal management of the underlying condition [13]. There is no evidence to suggest one opioid as superior to another for the relief of dyspnoea, although morphine is the most extensively studied [3]. Initially, shorter acting preparations should be used and titrated to relief of dyspnoea. Once symptoms are stable, the patient could be switched to a long-acting formulation.

Box 11.3 lists suggested starting doses for patients with moderate-to-severe dyspnoea. Opioid naïve patients should be started at a low dose of morphine, usually 2.5–5 mg po q4h with breakthrough dosing available every hour. In opioid experienced patients with dyspnoea, the dose is usually increased 25–50%. The opioid dose can be titrated upwards incrementally, as required for symptom relief. Sometimes an increase of 100% is required over a period of days to obtain relief. Equal analgesic doses of other opioids may be used.

Relief of dyspnoea is determined by patient report. If the patient is unable to communicate, the clinician must assess other factors such as control of restlessness or agitation. A palliative care bowel protocol should be administered concurrently, and the prophylactic use of antiemetic medication considered.

Fear of respiratory depression and accelerated death is a significant barrier to the use of opioids for dyspnoea,

Box 11.3 Suggested opioid starting doses for patients with moderate to severe dyspnoea

---

Opioid naïve patients
Morphine 2.5–5 mg po q4h regularly.
Hydromorphone 0.5–5 mg po q4h regularly.
Oxycodone 2.5 mg po q4h.

Opioid experienced patients
Increase current opioid dose by 25–50% and titrate as for pain.
May need to increase dose incrementally by 100% or more.

Breakthrough dosing
Give $^1/_2$ of q4h po dose equivalent q1h prn.

Parenteral dosing
If used, parenteral dosing requires a dose reduction of about 1/2 (for example, 5 mg subcut = 10 mg po).

Anxiolytic (if required)
Consider Lorazepam 0.5–1 mg subling/subcut tid.

Cautions
Long-acting agents should not be used for initial titration.
In the very frail elderly, or patients with COPD, doses should be reduced.

Prevent uncomfortable side effects
When initiating, start bowel protocol and consider antiemetic.

When initiating, start bowel protocol and consider antiemetic.

particularly in patients with COPD. This fear stems primarily from experience with opioid naïve patients given large doses of opioids for acute pain. When regularly scheduled, appropriately titrated opioids are provided for the relief of dyspnoea in patients with advanced disease, clinically significant respiratory depression does not occur, even in opioid naïve patients [36–38].

Studies fail to show evidence to support the use of nebulised opioids in the relief of dyspnoea [30].

Benzodiazepines

In the past, benzodiazepines have been routinely recommended for the relief of dyspnoea; the proposed mechanism is an altered central perception of breathlessness [39]. However, a recent systematic review concluded that benzodiazepines do not provide significant relief to breathless patients with advanced cancer or COPD [40]. Notwithstanding this review, there is a widely acknowledged interplay between anxiety and dyspnoea as mutually enhancing conditions. For patients who have dyspnoea with associated anxiety or panic, benzodiazepines are likely helpful [41]. Opioids and benzodiazepines, when titrated carefully together, do not result in significant respiratory depression [41,42].

In the case of respiratory panic attacks, a combination of short-acting opioid with a benzodiazepine may be required to break the breathlessness/panic cycle.

Corticosteroids

Corticosteroids in combination with antibiotics provide relief of dyspnoea in acute exacerbations of COPD [43]. They may be beneficial in patients with lymphangitic carcinomatosis [44], superior vena cava obstruction (SVCO) [13], upper airway obstruction [45], and radiation pneumonitis or fibrosis [13]. Corticosteroids reduce peritumour oedema and decrease inflammatory infiltration of the airway and interstitium.

Phenothiazines

Although often quoted as a useful adjunct for dyspnoea, evidence for their use is sparse and of low quality [46,47]. The benefits of phenothiazines may be in their anxiolytic properties. Promethazine can only be given orally. Levomepromazine (methotrimeprazine) and chlorpromazine can be given both orally and parenterally; consequently, they may have more practical value. Both medications can cause significant sedation. If used, methotrimeprazine should be given at a starting dose of 2.5–5 mg po q8h and titrated as required.

Bronchodilators

Many patients with cancer-related dyspnoea have a history of smoking and COPD; suboptimal treatment of reversible airways obstruction is not uncommon. Bronchodilators can be very helpful in these situations.

Furosemide

Nebulised furosemide may have some benefit independent of its diuretic effect. Some studies have shown a reduction of breathlessness in healthy volunteers with experimentally induced bronchoconstriction [48]. Others suggest involvement of airway mechanoreceptors [48,49]. However, a small trial in end-stage cancer patients did not find any benefit [48]. The routine use of nebulised furosemide in the management of dyspnoea is not currently recommended.

Oxygen

Breathless patients frequently receive oxygen therapy, despite a lack of clear evidence for benefit. *Perceived* benefits include an increase in functional capacity, the belief in oxygen as a lifesaving intervention, and improved symptom control [50]. Oxygen is not without its burdens, however, as it is expensive, disrupts mobility, and impedes communication. Nasal prongs can be uncomfortable. Patients often describe barriers to access, fear of running out, and a perceived stigma when outside the home. The apparatus also represents a noisy intrusion into the home [50].

Oxygen use in hypoxic patients

For patients with COPD who are hypoxemic at rest, there is a clear role for the use of long-term oxygen therapy (>15 h/day); in this case, supplemental oxygen improves survival, quality of life, exercise tolerance, and *may* improve dyspnoea [33,51].

For hypoxic patients with advanced malignancy, oxygen therapy may provide relief of dyspnoea [52–54], although some studies fail to show benefit [55,56]. Patients may feel better with oxygen therapy [56] at the end of life, when there are multiple causes of dyspnoea, oxygenation probably plays a small role. Oxygen therapy should never be used as the *only* method to palliative breathlessness. Opioids may in fact be more helpful than oxygen for patients with end-stage malignancy, even in hypoxic patients [57].

If hypoxia exists in advanced illness, some authors suggest an N-of-1 trial where breathlessness and health-related quality of life are assessed carefully before and after supplemental oxygen is delivered. Oxygen is continued only if benefits are realised after a determined period of time [58,59]. The benefit should be reassessed as time goes on as improvement may not be maintained over the long term, and even patients who derive short-term benefits may not wish to continue oxygen due to perceived burdens of therapy.

Oxygen use in non-hypoxic patients

For patients with advanced life-limiting disease *without* hypoxia, oxygen probably does not confer benefit over medical air. Abernathy et al. studied the effect of supplemental oxygen on nonhypoxemic patients who experienced dyspnoea from various advanced conditions (64% who had COPD) [60]. Oxygen conferred no additional benefit over the administration of medical air delivered via nasal cannula. Both therapies improved dyspnoea scores about 10%, most notably in the morning. The reduction in breathlessness may be mediated through the movement of air over the nasal and facial receptors. A similar benefit may be conferred through the use of a bedside fan directing airflow toward the face [28].

Ambulatory and short burst oxygen therapy during exercise or ADLs may benefit a subset of patients who experience oxygen desaturation with activity; reported benefits include improved quality of life and exercise tolerance [61].

Enhance coping

Education

Fears of dying during an acute attack should be alleviated. Caregivers and patients should be reassured that breathlessness itself is not life-threatening and that dyspnoea is a manageable symptom. The causes of dyspnoea and known triggers should be reviewed.

The purpose of each medication should be reviewed, particularly opioids. The use of regular baseline medications should be emphasised, as well as specific circumstances in which breakthrough or pre-emptive medications should be taken. Written instructions outlining a step-by-step plan for either breakthrough, or acute severe episodes can increase confidence in the patient and caregivers ability to cope.

Regular review of medications by the medical and nursing team is important to ensure compliance.

Improving independence

Functional ability should be maximised through the use of an interdisciplinary team to assess function and to provide support. This may include a district nurse, an occupational therapist, physiotherapist, and social worker. Functional aids should be supplied to reduce dyspnoea associated with ADLs, such as raised toilet seats, grab bars, mobility aids, hospital beds, and commodes.

Improve social function

Attempts should be made to reduce feelings of personal and social isolation. This could be through palliative day programmes or pulmonary rehabilitation programmes. Support from families or patients with similar problems reduce the sense of aloneness. Respite admissions can be arranged.

Support caregivers

Most patients with advanced illness are cared for at home, with nonprofessional caregivers playing a major role in supportive care. Major stressors to caregivers that influence their ability to provide ongoing care at home include personal health problems, social isolation, negative reactions from outside, loss of personhood and acute exacerbations [20]. Breathlessness can be a particularly challenging stressor, and caregivers generally do not feel well prepared to deal with acute exacerbations. The caregivers should be supported by strategies such as provision of opportunities for respite and self-care, home-based interdisciplinary care, facilitation of patient self-care, and provision of an emergency contingency plan [20].

Prepare for acute episodes

Some centres have emergency palliative response teams that are able to attend the home in case of symptom emergencies, but this is clearly not available to all patients. Therefore, clear and detailed plans must be created and appropriate medications be made available, even at home. Plans should include detailed instructions in the use of breakthrough oral or parenteral medications along with adjuvant anxiolytics if required. Emergency contact information for on-call nursing or physician support should be made available. No patient should be made to wish for death due to breathlessness [13].

Prepare for episodic or breakthrough pain

Breakthrough or incident dyspnoea will require prn dosing of short-acting opioids (Figure 11.4). Because incident dyspnoea is often of rapid onset and short-lived (usually 10–30 min), oral opioids with an onset of action of 30–60 min may not provide acceptable, expedient relief. Subcutaneous preparations may be preferred (onset of action 15–30 min). Pre-emptive opioid dosing should be considered when the incident dyspnoea is predictable, such as prior to ADLs. Recently, the use of ultrashort-acting opioids for the relief of incident dyspnoea has been reported [34,35]. Intranasal or buccal fentanyl has a very rapid onset (10–15 min) and a shorter duration of action (about 1–3 h). The literature supporting the use of ultrashort-acting opioids is limited to case reports, and they cannot be recommended for routine use. However, therapeutic N-of-1 trials could be considered. Ultrashort-acting opioids should not be used in opioid naïve patients.

Severe, frightening dyspnoea in the final hours of life

Severe, frightening dyspnoea near the end of life should be considered a medical crisis. In these cases, the side effect of sedation may not be avoidable; patients and families should be made aware of this possible outcome. Box 11.4 details suggested medications for patients with severe, acute dyspnoea at the end of life. In this case, parenteral

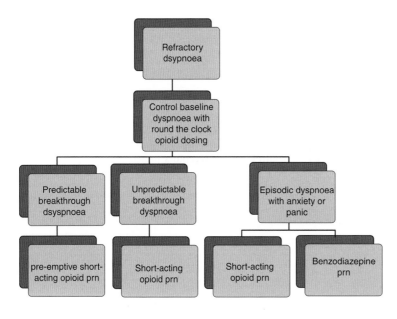

Figure 11.4 Approaches to the use of opioids for background and breakthrough/incident dyspnoea.

opioids provide expedient relief and should be offered q20 min until the symptom "breaks" or begins to subside. Once the acute episode has resolved, q4h dosing with parenteral opioids can resume, usually at doses 50–100% higher than the previous baseline opioid regime. If frequent doses of benzodiazepines were required during the crisis, they should be given regularly after the crisis, either through intermittent SC dosing, or through a continuous infusion.

Additional interventions

Noninvasive positive pressure ventilation (NIPPV)

In patients with COPD suffering an acute exacerbation and respiratory failure, NIPPV may be used to prevent acidosis and endotracheal intubation [62]. However, there is inadequate evidence to support nocturnal NPPV in stable COPD patients [63].

Box 11.4 Suggested doses for severe, frightening dyspnoea at the end of life

---

Opioid naïve patients

  Morphine 5 mg SC q20 min until dyspnoea begins to settle.

  If ineffective, double dose every third dose.

Opioid experienced patients

  Give equivalent of po q4h dose SC q20 min.

  If ineffective, double dose every third dose.

Sedative dose (if required)

  Midazolam 2.3–5 mg SC q5–15 min OR.

  Midazolam infusion 2.5–5 mg/h with 2.5–5 mg for breakthrough dosing q15 min prn.

  Lorazepam 2–4 mg SC q15 min OR.

  Methotrimiprazine 15–25 mg SC q15 min.

Ongoing dosing after crisis has settled

  Opioid: resume q4h dosing with SC opioid at an increased dose (usually 25–100% higher) with appropriate q1h breakthrough dosing.

  Sedative: if multiple dosing required, then consider ongoing, regular dosing of benzodiazepine or methotrimiprazine.

Source: Reproduced from Reference 14.

NIPPV is an intervention that must have close monitoring and consideration of the patient's goals of care (Figure 11.5). NIPPV can be successful in reducing dyspnoea and reversing respiratory failure in patients nearing the end of life from advanced cardiorespiratory disease or malignancy, but it may prolong a life with unacceptable quality. However, if respiratory failure is potentially reversible and life prolongation is consistent with the patient and family's goals of care, some providers may consider NIPPV a valid palliative care intervention [64]. The burdens must be carefully considered before embarking on this therapy and indications for discontinuation clarified.

NIPPV is also used in patients with respiratory failure due to neuromuscular and restrictive chest diseases. This is discussed in Chapter 13, *Palliative care for people with progressive neurological disorders.*

Cough in palliative care

Introduction

Cough is a cause of significant morbidity in advanced disease. Troublesome cough is associated with insomnia, exhaustion, musculoskeletal pain, and urinary incontinence [65]. It may interfere with conversation and result in social isolation. Family members may feel anxious or irritated; sleeping arrangements may be changed. Paroxysms of cough can result in significant dyspnoea.

Cough with increased mucous production is a predominant symptom in COPD [66]. Cough is the initial symptom in 65% of patients with lung cancer [65] and present in 50–90% of patients during the course of advanced malignancy.

Pathophysiology [65,67]

Like breathlessness, the cough reflex is a complex neurophysiologic process under both voluntary and involuntary control. Cough receptors present in the upper airways and pharynx are stimulated by products of inflammation, inhaled irritants, and mechanical stimuli. Afferent information is carried to the brainstem cough centre and sensory-motor cortex. Connections through the limbic system allow the higher centres to process the information, giving it context and meaning. Motor efferent activity directs the muscles of respiration to complete the cough reflex. Three phases are involved: inspiration, forced expiration against a closed glottis, and then expulsion. Cough

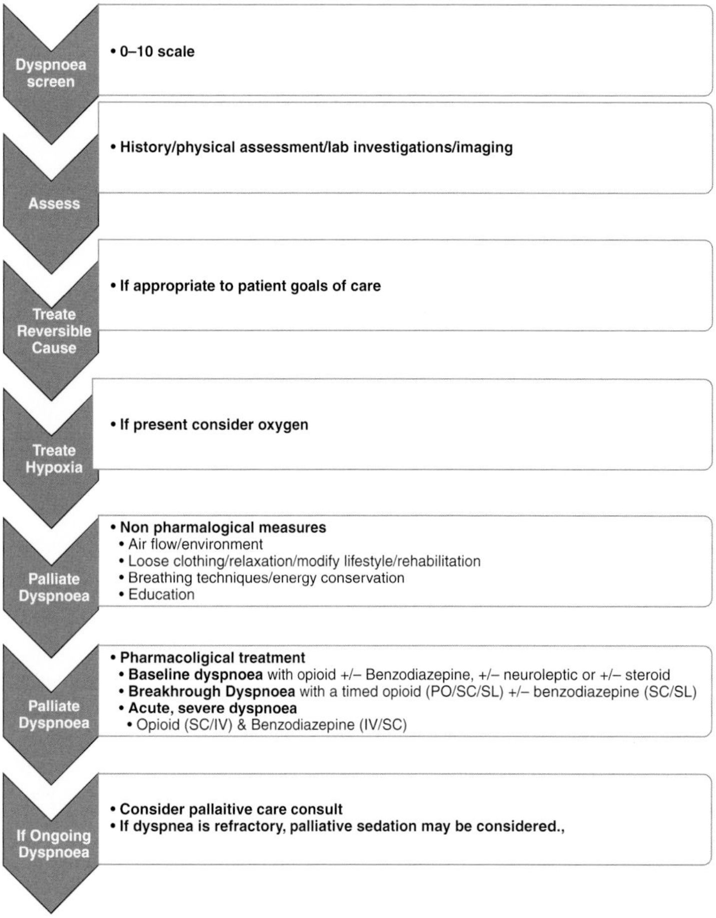

Figure 11.5 Assessment and management algorithm for dyspnoea in palliative care.

often occurs in paroxysms with a deep inspiration phase and multiple forced expiration phases.

Cough receptors are present primarily in the larger airways, are scarce in the smaller bronchioles and lung periphery. Therefore, cough is more likely to imply involvement of the airways, mediastinum, and upper respiratory tract rather than the lung periphery. Receptor sensitivity may be up-regulated by chronic stimulation, ACEIs, or acute viral infection. Central sensitisation may also occur at the level of the ganglia or brainstem.

Cough is a normal physiologic process designed to protect the airway and remove debris. It becomes pathological when abnormal in intensity, frequency, or efficacy.

Causes of cough

Chronic cough in the general population is most often caused by Gastroesophageal reflux disease (GERD),

asthma, or chronic cough syndrome (postnasal drip). Cough secondary to angiotensin-converting enzyme inhibitors (ACEIs) is less common [68]. In the palliative care population, cough generally arises from advanced cardiorespiratory disease and malignancy with its attendant complications.

While it is tempting to ascribe a troubling cough to a known cause such as malignancy, one must consider comorbid causes of chronic cough. For example, COPD is a very common comorbidity in patients with lung cancer. GERD is common in patients with advanced disease [67].

Ineffective cough can be troublesome due to an inability to clear accumulated secretions. Cough may be impaired due to pain, decreased level of consciousness, or muscle weakness. Ineffective cough is prevalent in neuromuscular diseases, central pathology (brain tumour or stroke), or in patients at the terminal stage. Such patients are also at risk for oropharygeal dysphagia and aspiration that may result in cough.

Cough is further impaired if the mucous is copious or viscous in nature. Impairment of cilia by chronic inflammation or medications will reduce cough efficacy.

Assessment of cough

Cough should be assessed in the context of an appropriate history, physical examination, and investigations according to the patient's disease trajectory and stated goals of care. History should include present and past medical history, previous investigations and treatments, as well as psychosocial history. The focus should be on identifying a possible reversible component, the presence or absence of mucous, and impact on quality of life. An approach to the history of cough is presented in Box 11.5 utilising the OPQRSTUV approach [14].

Chest X-ray or CT scans are often helpful in determining the cause of cough. Sputum can be cultured. Spirometry or barium swallow may be required.

Management of cough

Reverse what is reversible

If possible, treatment should focus on managing the underlying cause of the cough. For example, systemic chemotherapy and/or radiotherapy reduce thoracic symptoms in lung cancer [54,69]. Endobronchial treatments such as electrocautery, brachytherapy, or laser may be helpful, as may stenting of obstructive lesions [54]. Comorbidities such as GERD (GORD in United Kingdom), COPD and CHF should be optimally managed. ACEIs should be discontinued as they may sensitise cough receptors [69]. In some cases a reversible condition may be readily identified, but the goals of care in advanced disease may favour pure palliation without the burden of further investigation or invasive treatments (Table 11.4).

Education

The family and patient should be educated about the causes of cough. Common triggers such as environmental irritants, pollution, exertion, and emotion should be reviewed. If appropriate, the risk of aspiration should be discussed. Occupational therapists will assess swallowing and aspiration risk; thickened fluids may be recommended in the case of a poorly coordinated swallow. Enteral feeds can be slowed or discontinued. Many

---

Box 11.5 History of cough using the OPQRSTUV approach

ONSET/TIMING	How long has it been present?
	Which time of day does it occur (am to clear secretions, or night-time)?
	How long after a meal does it occur?
PROVOKING FACTORS	What are the triggers (laughing, eating, swallowing, bending forward, environmental)?
QUALITY	Is the cough dry or wet?
	Is it productive of sputum?
	What colour is the sputum?
	Is there blood?
RADIATION/ RELATED SYMPTOMS	Where is the cough (in throat, in chest)
	Associated pain?
	Incontinence?
	Breathlessness when coughing paroxysms?
SEVERITY	Subjective rating of mild/moderate/severe. *VAS could be used.*
TREATMENTS	What has been tried in the past?
	How effective were previous treatments?
	Is the patient on medications that will reduce lower oesophageal sphincter tone, or cause gastroparesis?
	Is patient on an ACEI?
UNDERSTANDING/ IMPACT	What do they think is causing the symptom?
	How is it affecting them (limiting conversation, eating, activity, socialisation)?
	How is it affecting their family (noise can be troublesome, anxiety provoking)?
VALUE	What are they hoping from treatment?

Table 11.4 Common causes of cough in palliative care and possible treatments.

Causes of cough	Possible treatments
Tumour related airway irritation	Radiotherapy/chemotherapy Laser treatment Steroids
Pleural effusion	Thoracocentesis/ pleurodesis; lying on the same side can decrease related cough
Superior vena cava obstruction	Steroids/radiotherapy
Post radiation pneumonitis/fibrosis	Steroids
Chemotherapy related (bleomycin)	Suppress cough/stop chemotherapy if required
End-stage weakness	Suppress cough Reduce secretions if possible Reduce aspiration risk if possible
Aspiration	Modify intake/swallowing assessment Reduce secretions
Neuromuscular disease	Reduce secretions
CHF	Conventional medications
Infection	Antibiotics
GERD	Proton pump inhibitors/H2 blockers Motility agents
Medications	Stop offending agent (ACEI)

Source: Reproduced from References 14 & 69.

patients chose to live at risk for aspiration rather than limit intake.

Nonpharmacologic treatments

Proper positioning will aid cough efficiency; furthermore, an upright posture will be helpful for a cough secondary to reflux disease or aspiration.

Humidified air delivered via nebuliser (2.5–5 ml as needed tid-qid or prn) reduces dryness and irritation of the airways and may thin viscous mucous.

Chest physiotherapy (bronchopulmonary hygiene) may be helpful for those patients with copious or difficult to clear secretions. There is not enough evidence to support or refute its use in COPD or bronchiectasis [70].

Patients can be taught to clear secretions through forced expiration (a huff). Positional drainage can be helpful in some cases, but is time consuming and may be uncomfortable [67].

Use of medications

Bronchodilators
Undiagnosed airways disease may respond to conventional bronchodilators.

Anti-inflammatory medications
Corticosteroids exert antitussive effect indirectly by reducing inflammation and oedema around a tumour, thereby limiting mechanical and chemical stimulation of the

cough receptors. Prednisone 25–50 mg once daily, or Dexamethasone 4–8 mg once daily, could be considered as a two-week trial. Corticosteroids are useful in the palliation of cough related to radiation-induced pneumonitis or fibrosis [54].

Syrups and lozenges

There are various soothing agents used to reduce irritation in the pharynx and airways. Most have high sugar content and soothe the airways by encouraging salivation and repeated swallowing. Lemon may increase the production of protective airways mucus. Menthol and peppermint may reduce the cough receptor sensitivity. However, these effects last only for a short period of time and cough syrups should be used only in mild cases of cough [71]. A recent systematic review found "some" evidence for efficacy with *citrate linctus* (simple cough syrup) in the reduction of cough related to malignancy [72].

Expectorants

Guaifenesin is an irritant mucolytic that stimulates the production of mucus that is greater in volume, but thinner in consistency and more easily expectorated [71]. *Carbocysteine* or *acetylcysteine* are chemical mucolytics that reduce the thickness of secretions. N-acetyl cysteine has been shown to be helpful in patients with chronic bronchitis [73]; it should be considered for a therapeutic trial in patients with other diagnoses, particularly in patients who develop cough or dyspnoea due to inspissated secretions.

Medications that reduce mucous clearance should be discontinued if possible (anticholinergic medications, nonsteroidal anti-inflammatory drugs [NSAIDs], aspirin, and benzodiazepines).

Antitussives (Table 11.5)

Opioids suppress the cough reflex in the brainstem, although there may be some peripheral effect.

Dextromethorphan works in mild-to-moderate cough, but is often inadequate in advanced disease. It is supplied alone, or in a mixture with guafenesin. Drug interactions should be monitored as dextromethorphan inhibits the cytochrome P450 system. It may cause serotonin syndrome if used with serotonergic drugs such as antidepressants.

Codeine is commonly used and has been found effective in several placebo-controlled trials [71]. It is supplied alone, or in combination with guaifenesin. Codeine as the "gold standard" for cough suppression is coming under question [74] as it has been found to be no more effective

Table 11.5 Antitussive medications.

Medication	Starting doses
Demulsants	
Citrus linctus	5–10 cc prn
Mucolytics	
Guafenisin	200–400 mg q4h prn
Acetylcysteine	3–5 ml nebulised tid
Carbocysteine	750 mg bid-tid
Centrally acting agents	
Dextromethorphan	10–20 mg po q4–8h
Morphine	2.5–5 mg po q4h prn
Codeine	10–20 mg po q4–6h prn
Hydrocodone	5–10 mg po q4–6h prn
Methadone linctus	2 mg at hs
Peripheral agents	
Nebulised 0.25% bupivicaine	5 ml nebulised tid
Nebulised 2% lidocaine	5 ml nebulised qid
Na cromoglycate	20 mg inhaled bid to qid
Benzonatate	100–200 mg tid
Levopropamide	75 mg po tid

than placebo for chronic cough in COPD [75] and the acute cough of viral infection [65].

Morphine has a significant and sustained benefit on refractory cough but has only been studied in small randomised trials [76]. *Hydrocodone* is as effective as codeine with fewer gastrointestinal (GI) effects. It is often sold as a combination product with the antihistamine chlorpheniramine that contributes to the product's sedative effects.

There is no good clinical evidence to support the use of one opioid antitussive over another [71]. Empiric trial is likely the best approach. Dextromethorphan, codeine, and morphine are probably all good first choices. For those patients already on an opioid, there is unlikely benefit to opioid rotation or the addition of another opioid [77]. Opioid dose should be increased by 20% and titrated to effect [77].

Peripherally acting antitussives

In refractory cases, *nebulised bupivacaine and lidocaine* have been tried [13], and these agents work by anaesthetising the sensory nerve endings involved in the cough reflex. However, they also anaesthetise the pharynx and may increase the risk of aspiration. Patients cannot eat for about 1 h after administration. A test dose should always be given under close observation, as treatment may precipitate bronchospasm. Tolerance to the antitussive effect of lidocaine is common.

There is no evidence to support the use of nebulised opioids in the treatment of breathlessness or cough [67]. Furthermore, nebulised opioids may paradoxically aggravate cough through airway irritation and histamine release causing bronchoconstriction.

Other medications

Levodropropizine, a peripherally acting agent, was found to have equivalent effect to dihydrocodeine with less somnolence, but is not widely available [78].

Sodium cromoglycate, which usually acts as a bronchodilator, has been shown to reduce cough in lung cancer without changes in lung function. Further studies are required, and its role is still being determined. It may take up to 36–48 h to become effective [79].

Benzonatate has been reported to have excellent efficacy in various types of chronic cough, including that associated with malignancy, by anaesthetising the upper airway receptors [80]. It is probably best used as an adjunct to an opioid antitussive.

Centrally acting drugs such as paroxetine, gabapentin, carbamazepine, and amitriptyline have anecdotal evidence of efficacy in the treatment of chronic cough [81].

Anticholinergic agents

If patients are having difficulty handling their secretions due to a weak swallow and cough, anticholinergic agents may be used to reduce salivary secretions [82]. Glycopyrrollate is particularly effective at reducing salivary secretions and has the benefit of not crossing the blood–brain barrier, but atropine, hyoscine, and scopolamine can also be used.

Suggested approach to cough

In approaching the palliation of cough, one must determine whether it is necessary to aid expectoration or to suppress cough. If mucous is present and the patient has a strong cough, then the focus should be on aiding expectoration. However, if the patient is suffering significant comorbidity such as exhaustion, pain, or dyspnoea, then the cough should be suppressed. If the cough is dry and troublesome, then again the main treatment should be antitussive agents. If the patient has a very weak cough that cannot be assisted, such as at the end of life, cough should be suppressed and secretions controlled.

Pleural effusions in palliative care

A pleural effusion is a pathological collection of fluid in the pleural space. Normally, there is about 20–30 ml of fluid present in the pleural space to provide lubrication for the movement of lungs, but in disease, several litres may accumulate [25].

Pathophysiology of pleural effusions

Pleural fluid is maintained by a balance between production and removal. Fluid enters the pleural space from the capillaries in the parietal pleura, the interstitium of the lung (through the visceral pleura), or through small holes in the diaphragm. There is a pressure gradient across the parietal and visceral pleura, facilitating resorption of the fluid through the interstitial spaces of the visceral pleura [13]. The remainder of the fluid is removed through the lymphatics. In disease, a pleural effusion develops if there is an excess production of fluid (from the parietal pleura, the interstitial spaces of the lung, or the peritoneal cavity) or when there is decreased fluid removal by the lymphatics [83].

Causes of pleural effusions (Table 11.6)

Pleural effusions are divided based on the biochemical and cytological analysis of the fluid. They may be transudative or exudative [83].

Transudates are caused by *systemic* factors that influence the formation and absorption of pleural fluid. For example, in CHF, excess fluid is released from the interstitium of the lungs into the pleural space and overwhelms the capacity of the lymphatic system. Similarly, effusions result when ascitic fluid moves through the holes in the

Table 11.6 Common causes of pleural effusion in palliative care.

Transudates
Congestive heart failure
Cirrhosis
Pulmonary emboli

Exudates
Malignancy
Infection
Pulmonary embolism

diaphragm into the pleural space more quickly than it can be removed.

Exudates occur when *local* factors affect fluid production and absorption, resulting in a much larger proportion of protein and LDH in the pleural fluid. For example, malignant pleural effusions result from tumour-induced angiogenesis and the production of vascular endothelial growth factor (VEGF) that increases vascular permeability and leakage of fluid [84]. The most common causes of exudative effusions are bacterial infections, malignancy, and pulmonary embolism. Of note, pulmonary embolism may result in either a transudative or exudative effusion.

In palliative care populations, pleural effusions are most often caused by malignant disease, particularly lung, breast, ovarian, and lymphoma [84]. For most patients, mean survival after diagnosis is only 3–6 months depending on the type of cancer and the response to anticancer therapies. Survival is higher with breast cancer (7–15 months) and ovarian cancer (mean 9 months) but lower with lung cancer (mean 2 months) [13,84].

Patients with pleural effusions often present with slowly progressive dyspnoea on exertion, cough, orthopnea, or chest pain. Occasionally, patients will experience severe respiratory compromise [85].

Assessment of pleural effusion

The evaluation of a pleural effusion should include:
1. How long the effusion has been present.
2. The identification of a potentially reversible cause.
3. If goals of care allow, pleural fluid should be examined to determine whether the effusion is a transudate or exudate. If this patient has a malignancy but the fluid is a transudate, then the cause may be concurrent CHF or pulmonary embolism.
4. The presence of loculation; if so, the effusion will be more difficult to drain.
5. The severity of symptoms. If asymptomatic, the effusion could be monitored.
6. Previous response to treatments, particularly thoracocentesis. If this procedure was not helpful, then repeat drainage may not be indicated.
7. Patient/family understanding and their hopes/values for management.

Clinical examination will detect effusions of greater than 500 ml; chest radiographs will detect effusions >200 ml [25]. It is sometimes difficult to distinguish tumour or lung collapse from pleural fluid and either an ultrasound or CT of the lung is required.

Management of pleural effusion

If appropriate, the underlying cause should be treated: diuretics for CHF, antibiotics for infection, or chemotherapy/radiotherapy for malignancy.

Initial symptomatic management of a malignant pleural effusion will depend on the general performance status of the patient and the severity of the symptoms. If the patient is declining, and nearing the end of life, the focus may be on the control of dyspnoea, cough, and pain without invasive procedures. However, if the patient is earlier in the trajectory, initial management is usually aspiration of the fluid through a small bore catheter (thoracocentesis). This allows for re-expansion of the lungs, rapid relief of symptoms, and diagnostic examination of the fluid. If relief of breathlessness does not occur, then other causes of breathlessness should be evaluated, such as lymphangitic carcinomatosis, thromboembolism, or atelectasis. Unfortunately, the fluid usually accumulates within 30 days [84]. Repeated drainage should be avoided, as it becomes less effective over time due to fibrosis and loculation of the fluid. Repeated procedures can be a burden for a patient who is probably declining [84].

For patients who have a longer prognosis (>8 weeks), chemical pleurodesis should be considered. This involves injecting a sclerosing agent into the pleural space via a small bore intrapleural catheter or video-assisted thoracoscopy. The sclerosing agent (usually talc or tetracycline) causes inflammation and adherence of the parietal and visceral pleura, thus obliterating the pleural space and preventing fluid reaccumulation. Pleurodesis should be offered to patients who have longer than 2–3 months to live, an effusion nonresponsive to systemic chemotherapy, and lung expansion to the chest wall after therapeutic thoracentesis [84]. This procedure can be quite painful due to pleural inflammation; adequate analgesia should be made available. Concurrent use of corticosteroids may reduce the inflammation and pain, but will also reduce the likelihood of success.

In the past number of years, insertion of tunnelled indwelling catheters has become much more common. These catheters remain in place and can be drained intermittently as required, either in hospital or at home, through sterile vacuum bottles. This reduces the burden of having to return to the hospital for repeated drainages. The tube may cause "auto-sclerosis" of the pleural space; drainage becomes less and less over time, and the drain can be removed. Relief of dyspnoea occurs in more than 90% of patients and outcome is particularly successful in patients with gynaecologic primary tumours and when there is complete re-expansion of the lung. Survival rates are unchanged compared to pleurodesis. Complications include dislodgement, loculation, and infections, but the indwelling catheters are generally very well tolerated [84].

Pleuroperitoneal shunting can be tried for patients with trapped-lung where lung re-expansion is inadequate for pleurodesis.

Haemoptysis

Haemoptysis, or the expectoration of blood, can be a frightening experience for patients and caregivers. It can range from occasional blood streaking of the sputum, to massive amounts of frank blood. Massive haemoptysis is defined as life-threatening haemorrhage of 100 to 600 ml/24 h [86].

Causes of haemoptysis

The most common causes of haemoptysis in the general population are bronchitis, bronchogenic carcinoma, and bronchiectasis [54]. Bleeding can occur due to diseases in the larger airways, lung parenchyma, pulmonary circulation, or through abnormalities of the coagulation cascade (Table 11.7).

Nonmassive haemoptysis is relatively common in patients with advanced bronchogenic carcinoma, occurring in approximately 20% of patients sometime in their course. However, massive terminal haemoptysis occurs in only 3% of patients with lung cancer and is usually preceded by smaller, progressive herald bleeds [54]. Massive

Table 11.7 Causes of haemoptysis in palliative care.

Airway disease
Malignancy
Acute or chronic bronchitis
Bronchiectasis
Airway trauma (as in bronchoscopy)

Parenchymal disease
Infection (tuberculosis/pneumonia/lung abscess)
Inflammatory or immune disorder

Pulmonary vascular disease
Pulmonary thromboembolism

Coagulopathy
Anticoagulants
Disseminated intravascular coagulopathy (DIC)
thrombocytopenia

haemoptysis is more common in patients with centrally located tumours, especially squamous cell carcinoma. In metastatic lung disease, the bleeding usually arises from erosion of small, friable vessels. The risk of haemoptysis is increased with the presence of airway inflammation (bacterial or fungal infection), thrombocytopenia, or coagulopathies. Massive haemoptysis occurs when the tumour erodes into a major vessel.

Approach to haemoptysis

The history should evaluate:
1. How long the symptom has been present. If progressive, then massive haemoptysis may be more likely.
2. Provoking features such as cough or infection, which, if suppressed, may reduce the frequency or severity of the haemoptysis. Sometimes bleeding may be triggered by investigations such as bronchoscopy.
3. Quality of the haemoptysis. Frank blood can be more worrying than blood streaked sputum.
4. Related symptoms such as dyspnoea. Evidence of bleeding elsewhere or history of coagulopathy should be sought.
5. Severity of haemoptysis, as measured by the volume of blood, and the associated distress.
6. Treatments such as previous radiotherapy, or anticoagulants that may aggravate bleeding.
7. The patient and caregiver understanding of the condition and their expectations for management. Although investigations and radiotherapy can be performed, the patient may feel too unwell to proceed.

Management of haemoptysis

If mild and not progressive, and the patient is reaching end stage, the patient and family can be reassured that this is a common symptom and probably will not progress [13]. Patients who are on anticoagulant medication for treatment or prophylaxis of thromboembolic disease should have the indications for therapy reviewed; sometimes these medications can be discontinued. Medications that interfere with platelet function such as ASA or NSAIDs should be re-evaluated.

If desired, and appropriate to the patient's goals of care, disease modifying therapy could be considered. Radiotherapy is the treatment of choice for patients with haemoptysis due to lung malignancy and is often very effective [54]. Chemotherapy could also be considered. Other options include bronchoscopy with laser ablation, endobronchial brachytherapy, or arterial embolisation. Medications that inhibit fibrinolysis appear effective in reducing blood in a number of conditions; tranexamic acid has been found to be anecdotally helpful in cystic fibrosis (CF) [87]. While there is little evidence for their use to control bleeding in palliative care, an N-of-1 trial could be considered after carefully weighing potential risks (increased clotting) with the benefits. If used, tranexamic acid could be tried at a dose of 500 mg to 1 g qid.

If the bleeding is progressing and there is concern that massive haemoptysis may occur, then preparations should be made either in the hospital or at home. If massive haemoptysis occurs it is generally very rapid, painless, and the patient is alert for only 1–2 short minutes before losing consciousness. This can be extremely frightening to witness. While it is important to educate and prepare patients and families, this must be done in a very gentle and careful way to reduce anxiety. Dark towels and face cloths should be made easily available; if bleeding starts the blood can be covered to reduce the visual impact. Blood should be gently removed from the patient's mouth and face. A calm presence, while holding the patient and offering comforting words, will hopefully reduce suffering.

If possible, medications could be made available in the home for such an emergency. If things are happening very quickly over the course of short minutes, time is better spent comforting the patient. However, if this is a slower bleed, then administration of an intravenous (IV) or SC opioid in combination with a benzodiazepine will reduce dyspnoea and anxiety. Dosages would be similar to that used in terminal dyspnoea at the end of life (Table 11.5).

Approach to advanced chronic obstructive pulmonary disease

In 2020, COPD will represent the third leading cause of death worldwide [88,89]. Patients with COPD experience symptom burden similar to patients with advanced malignancy [90]. As disease advances, breathlessness predominates (>90%); it is particularly severe in the last year of life [88]. Fatigue, social isolation, advancing disability, and high levels of anxiety and depression are commonly present [89]. Family members suffer significant caregiving burden [20]. Thankfully, there is a growing interest in providing improved symptom control and better quality of life for this group of patients and their caregivers.

The lengthy illness trajectory of COPD is best described in the context of "end-stage organ failure" characterised by declining function and progressive symptoms punctuated by acute exacerbations [91]. Patients die most commonly from respiratory failure (30%) and HF (13%), followed by pulmonary infection, pulmonary embolism, cardiac arrhythmia, and lung cancer [91].

Box 11.6 Clinical correlates suggesting a focus on a palliative approach

Severe airflow obstruction (forced expiratory volume in 1 s (FEV1) <30).
Significant weight loss.
Declining functional status.
Multiple hospital admissions.
Need for long-term oxygen therapy.
Clinician estimate of survival less than 12 months.
Patient expresses wish to die or wonders about dying process.

Source: Reproduced from Reference 91.

The patient may or may not return to their previous level of function after an acute exacerbation, despite recovery from the acute illness. Prognostic uncertainty results as clinicians are unable to predict which episode will result in recovery, and which in death. "Prognostic paralysis" follows [92], where professionals and patients may delay introduction of a palliative approach. Vital opportunities to discuss quality-of-life interventions, psychological support, and advanced directives may be missed.

Ideally, end-of-life discussions occur at any time in the trajectory, depending on patient circumstances. This may include at the time of diagnosis, during hospitalisations for acute attacks, or when the patient initiates a discussion. Information about prognosis should be shared, along with plans for management of acute exacerbations, emergencies, mechanical ventilation, and quality of life interventions. Box 11.6 highlights clinical correlates, suggesting that the clinician may wish to consider a more palliative approach to the patient with COPD.

Breathlessness has been addressed extensively in this chapter, and the basic approach applies to all patients with advanced disease, including COPD. Specific recommendations for the management of dyspnoea in patients with COPD have been reported by many working groups and parallel those presented in this chapter, including management of the underlying disease and comorbid conditions, the use of nonpharmacological interventions and psychosocial support, the addition of opioids for refractory dyspnoea, and oxygen for patients with hypoxemia [33]. COPD guidelines re-enforce the recommendation that benzodiazepines should not be used routinely, except in situations where anxiety and panic are significant. There is a lack of evidence to support the use of palliative oxygen in patients with COPD who are not hypoxic [33]. The place

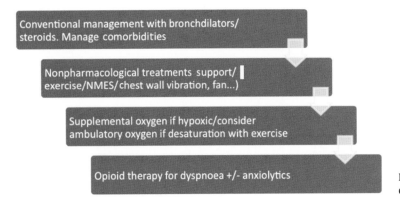

Figure 11.6 Dyspnoea "ladder" in COPD. (Reproduced from Reference 88.)

of opioids in the management of refractory dyspnoea in patients with COPD is outlined in Figure 11.6.

Recommendations on opioid dosing in COPD can vary. There is little research to guide initial dosing or ongoing titration; empiric starting doses tend to be lower for patients with advanced COPD. As a rule, the rate of opioid titration for patients with advanced disease depends on dyspnoea intensity and related distress. Patients with COPD generally have been breathless for some time and urgency is less severe. Gaining patient and caregiver confidence with opioids is of primary importance. One approach is to start with very low doses in the first week, with the expectation that symptom management may not be achieved, but patient safety and compliance will be ensured.

Some authors suggest initial starting doses of morphine as low as 0.5 mg po bid and titrated up to 1–2.5 mg po q4h while awake by the end of the first week [88]. Doses are then titrated up by 25% weekly until adequate symptom relief is achieved. Once a stable dose is achieved, an equal-analgesic switch to a long-acting opioid is recommended. Morphine is the best studied opioid in COPD and current formulations allow for very low opioid dosing strength.

Other authors have studied the use of sustained release morphine in patients with refractory dyspnoea (54% of whom had COPD) [93]. Morphine sustained release at a starting dose of 10 mg per day and titrated weekly to 20 or 30 mg per day was found to reduce dyspnoea without respiratory depression or significant side effects. Compliance may be enhanced by the use of once daily dosing.

As with all patients suffering from advanced life-limiting illness, management of patients with advanced COPD should encompass attention to the multiple physical symptoms, quality of life, functional status, psychosocial and existential domains. Where possible, care should be supplied by a multidisciplinary team comprised of physicians, nurses, occupational and physical therapists, nutritionists, respiratory therapists, counsellors, spiritual care, and volunteers.

References

1. Society, Official Statement of the American Thoracic. Dyspnea: mechanisms, assessment, and management A Consensus statement. American Thoracic Society. *Am J Respir Crit Care Med* 1999; 159: 321–340.
2. Bausewein C, Farquhar M, Booth S, et al. Measurement of breathlessness in advanced disease: a systematic review. *Resp Med* 2007; 101(3): 399–410.
3. Abernathy AP, Kamal AH, Wheeler JL, et al. Management of dyspnea within a rapid learning healthcare model. *Curr Opin Support Palliat Care* 2011; 5: 101–110.
4. Currow DC, Smith J, Davidson PM, et al. Do the trajectories of dyspnea differ in prevalence and intensity by diagnosis at the end of life: a consecutive cohort study. *J Pain Sympt Manage* 2010; 39(4): 680–690
5. Cuervo Pinna MA, Mota Vargas R, Redondo Morato MJ, et al. Dyspnea—a bad prognosis symptom at the end of life. *Am J Hosp Palliat Care* 2009; 26(2): 89–97.
6. Reddy SK, Parsons HA, Elsayem A, et al. Characteristics and correlates of dyspnea in patients with advanced cancer. *J Palliat Med* 2009; 12: 29–36.
7. Tataryn C and Chochinov HM. Predicting the trajectory of will to live in terminally ill patients. *Psychosomatics* 2002; 43: 370–377.
8. Abernethy AP and Wheeler JL. Total dyspnoea. *Curr Opin Support Palliat Care* 2008; 2: 110–113.
9. Gilman SA and Banzett RB. Physiologic changes and clinical correlates of advanced dyspnea. *Curr Opin Support Palliat Care* 2009; 3: 93–97.
10. Mahler DA. Understanding mechanisms and documenting plausibility of palliative interventions for dyspnea. *Curr Opin Support Palliat Care* 2011; 5: 71–76.

11. Williams M. Applicability and generalizability of palliative interventions for dyspnoea: one size fits all, some or none? *Curr Opin Support Palliat Care* 2011; 5: 92–100.

12. Dudgeon DJ and Lertzman M. Dyspnea in the advanced cancer patient. *J Pain Symptom Manage* 1998; 16(4): 212–219.

13. Gallager R. Dyspnea. In: *Medical Care of the Dying*. Victoria: Victoria Hospice Society Learning Centre for Palliative Care, 2006, pp. 365–375.

14. Kennedy B, McLeod B and Barwich D. *Fraser Health Hospice Palliative Care Program. Symptom Guidelines*. Dyspnea. Revised 2009.

15. Pratter, MR, Curley FJ, Dubois J, et al. Cause and evaluation of chronic dyspnea in a pulmonary disease clinic. *Arch Intern Med* 1989; 149: 2277.

16. Williams M, Catarella P, Olds T, et al. The language of breathlessness differentiates between patients with COPD and age matched adults. *Chest* 2008; 134: 489–496.

17. Horton R and Rocker. Contemporary issues in refractory dyspnoea. *Curr Opin Support Palliat Care* 2010; 4(2): 56–62.

18. Dorman S, Byrne A and Adwards A. Which measurement scales should we use to measure breathlessness in palliative care? A systematic review. *Palliat Med* 2007; 21: 177–191.

19. Cheung WY, Le LW and Zimmerman C. Symptom clusters in patients with advanced cancers. *Support Cancer Care* 2009; 17: 709–715.

20. Gysels MH and Higginson IJ. Caring for a person in advanced illness and suffering from breathlessness at home: threats and resources. *Palliat Support Care* 2009; 7(2): 153–162.

21. Maisel A, Krishnaswamy P, Nowak RM, et al. Rapid measurement of B-type nautriuretic peptide in the emergency diagnosis of heart failure. *N Engl J Med* 2002; 347: 161–167.

22. Navigante AH and Castro MA. Morphine versus midazolam as upfront therapy to control dyspnea perception in cancer patients while its underlying cause is sought or treated. *J Pain Symptom Manage* 2010; 39(5): 820–830.

23. Booth S, Moffat C, Burken J, et al. Nonpharmacological interventions for breathlessness. *Curr Opin Support Palliat Care* 2011; 5: 77–86.

24. Bausewein C, Booth S, Gysels M, et al. Non-pharmacological interventions for breathlessness in advanced stages of malignant and non-malignant diseases. *Cochrane Database Syst Rev* 2008; 16(2): CD0005623.

25. Twycross R and Wilcock A. Respiratory symptoms. In: *Symptom Management in Advanced Cancer*, 3rd edition. Radcliff Medical Press, 141–179.

26. Lacasse Y, Goldstein R, Lasserson TJ, et al. Pulmonary rehabilitation for chronic obstructive pulmonary disease. *Cochran Database Syst Rev* 2009; (1): CD003793.

27. Buckholz GT and von Gunten CF. Nonpharmacological management of dyspnea. *Curr Opin Support Palliat Care* 2009; 3: 98–102.

28. Galbraith S, Fagan P, Perkins P, et al. Does the use of a handheld fan improve chronic dyspnea? A randomized controlled, crossover trial. *J Pain Symptom Manage* 2010; 39: 831–838.

29. Abernethy AP, Wheeler JL and Currow DC. Common approaches to dyspnoea management in advanced life-limiting illness. *Curr Opin Support Palliat Care* 2010; 4: 53–55.

30. Jennings LA, Davies AN, Higgins PTJ, et al. Opioids for the palliation of breathlessness in advanced disease and terminal illness. *Cochrane Database Syst Rev* 2009; 1.

31. Lankin PN, Terrky PB, Delisser HM, et al. An Official American Thoracic Society clinical policy statement: palliative care for patients with respiratory diseases and critical illnesses. *Am J Respir Crit Care Med* 2008; 177: 912–927.

32. Mahler DA, Selecky PA, Harrod CG, et al. American college of chest physicians consensus statement on the management of dyspnea in patients with advanced lung or heart disease. *Chest* 2010; 137(3): 674–691.

33. Marciniuk DD, Goodridge D, Hernandex P, et al. Managing dyspnea in patients with advanced chronic obstructive pulmonary disease: a Canadian Thoracic Society clinical practice guideline. *Can Respir J* March/April 2011; 18(2): 1–10.

34. Guana AA, Kang SK, Trian ML, et al. Oral transmucosal fentanyl citrate for dyspnea in terminally ill patients: an observational case series. *J Palliat Med* 2008; 11(4): 643–648.

35. Benitez-Rosario MA, Martin AS and Feria M. Oral transmucosal fentanyl citrate in the management of dyspnoea crises in cancer patients. *J Pain and Symptom Manage* 2005; 30: 395–397.

36. Clemens KA, Quednau I and Klaschik E. Is there a higher risk of respiratory depression in opioid-naive palliative patients during symptomatic therapy of dyspnea with strong opioids? *J Palliat Med* 2008; 11(2): 204–216.

37. Clemens, KE and Klaschik E. Effect of hydromorphone on ventilation in palliative care patients with dyspnea. *Support Care Cancer* 2007.

38. Clemens KE and Klaschik E. Symptomatic therapy of dyspnoea with strong opioids and its effect on ventilation in palliative care patients. *J Pain Symptom Manage* 2007; 33: 473–481.

39. Thomas JR and von Gunten CF. Clinical management of dyspnoea. *Lancet Oncol* 2002; 3: 223–228.

40. Simon ST, Higginson IJ, Booth S, et al. Benzodiazepines for the relief of breathlessness in advanced malignant and non-malignant diseases in adults. *Cochrane Database Syst Rev* 2010; 20(1): CD007354.

41. Clemens KE and Klaschik E. Dyspnoea associated with anxiety-symptomatic therapy with opioids in combination with lorazepam and its effect on ventilation in palliative care patients. *Support Care Cancer* 2011; 19(12): 2027–2033

42. Navigante AH, Cerchietti LC, Castr MA, et al. Midazolam as adjunct therapy to morphine in the alleviation of sever dyspnea perception in patients with advanced cancer. *J Pain Symptom Manage* 2006; 31: 38–47.

43. Daniels JMA, Snijders D, de Graaff CS, et al. Antibiotics in addition to systemic corticosteroids for acute exacerbations of chronic obstructive pulmonary disease. *Am J Respir Crit Care Med* 2010; 181: 150–157.

44. Vaughn VM, Haymore BR, Sanchez-Rivera IJ, et al. Progressive pulmonary infiltrates in a patient with ovarian cancer. *Respir Care* 2006; 51(5): 515–518.

45. Elsayem A and Bruera E. High-dose corticosteroids for the management of dyspnea in patients with tumor obstruction of the upper airway. *Support Care Cancer* 2007; 15: 1437–1439.

46. McIver B, Walsh D and Nelson K. The use of chlorpromazine for symptom control in dying cancer patients. *J Pain Symptom Manage* 1994; 9(5): 341–345.

47. O'Neill J and Fountain A. Levomepromazine (methotrimiprazine) and the last 48 hours. *Hospital Medicine* 1999; 60(8): 564–567.

48. Currow DC and Abernethy AP. Pharmacological management of dyspnoea. *Curr Opin Support Palliat Care* 2007; 1: 96–101.

49. Currow DC, Ward AM and Abernethy AP. Advances in the pharmacological management of breathlessness. *Curr Opin Support Palliat Care* 2009; 3: 103–106.

50. Jaturapatporn D, Moran E, Obwanga C, et al. Patients' experience of oxygen therapy and dyspnea: a qualitative study in home palliative care. *Support Care Cancer* Mar 21, 2010; 18(6): 765–770.

51. Crockett AJ, Cranston JM, Moss JR, et al. Domicillary oxygen for chronic obstructive pulmonary disease. *Cochrane Library* 2000; 1.

52. Viola R, Kiteley C, Lloyd NS, et al. The management of dyspnea in cancer patients: a systematic review. *Support Care Cancer* 2008; 16: 329–337. Review of effectiveness of four drug classes: opioid, phenothiazines benzos and corticosteroids.

53. Ben-Aharon I, Gafter-Gvili A, Paul M, et al. Interventions for alleviating cancer-related dyspnea: a systematic review. *J Clin Oncol* 2008; 26(14): 2396–2404.

54. Kvale PA, Selecky PA and Prakash UBS. Palliative care in lung cancer: ACCP evidence-based clinical practice guidelines (2nd edition). *Chest* 2007; 132: 368S–403S.

55. Philip J, Gold, M, Milner A, et al. A randomized, double-blind, crossover trial of the effect of oxygen on dyspnea in patients with advanced cancer. *J Pain Symptom Manage* 2006; 32(6) : 541–550.

56. Cranston J, Crockett A and Currow D. Oxygen therapy for dyspnoea in adults. *Cochrane Database Syst Rev* 2009; 3: CD004769.

57. Clemens KE, Quednau I and Dlaschik E. Use of oxygen and opioids in the palliation of dyspnoea in hypoxic and non-hypoxic palliative care patients: a prospective study. *Support Care Cancer* 2009; 17(4): 367–377.

58. Bruera E, Schoeller T and MacEachern T. Symptomatic benefit of supplemental oxygen in hypoxemic patients with terminal caner: the use of the N of 1 randomized controlled trial. *J Pain Symptom Manage* 1992; 7: 365–368.

59. Uronis HE and Abernethy AP. Oxygen for relief of dyspnea: what is the evidence? *Curr Opin Support Palliat Care* 2008; 2: 89–94.

60. Abernethy AP, McDonald CR, Frith PA, et al. Effect of palliative oxygen versus room air in relief of breathlessness in patients with refractory dyspnea: a double-blind, randomised controlled trial. *Lancet* 2010; 376(9743): 784–793.

61. Bradley JM and O'Meill BM. Short term ambulatory oxygen for chronic obstructive pulmonary disease. *Cochrane Database Syst Rev* 2009; 1.

62. Ram FSF, Picot J, Lightowler J, et al. Non-invasive positive pressure ventilation for treatment of respiratory failure due to exacerbations of chronic obstructive pulmonary disease. *Cochrane Database of Systematic Reviews* 2009; 1.

63. Wijkstra PJP, Lacasse Y, Guyat GH, et al. Nocturnal non-invasive positive pressure ventilation for stable chronic obstructive pulmonary disease. *Cochrane Database of Systematic Reviews* 2010; 11.

64. Cuomo C, Delmastro M, Cerian P, et al. Noninvasive mechanical ventilation as a palliative treatment of acute respiratory failure in patients with end-stage solid cancer. *Palliat Med* 2004; 18: 602–610.

65. Wee B. Chronic cough. *Curr Opin Support Palliat Care* 2008; 2: 105–109.

66. Smith J and Woodcock A. Cough and its importance in COPD. *Int J COPD* 2006; 1(3): 305–314.

67. Hosneih F and Moric AH. Cough in palliative care. *Prog Palliat Care* 2008; 16(1): 91–97.

68. Pratter MR. Overview of common causes of chronic cough: ACCP evidence-based clinical practice guidelines. *Chest* 2006; 129(1 Suppl): 59S–62S.

69. Molassiotis A, Smith JA, Bennett MI, et al. Clinical expert guidelines for the management of cough in lung cancer: report of a UK task group on cough. *Cough* 2010; 6(9).

70. Jones AP and Rowe BH. Bronchopulmonary hygiene physical therapy for chronic obstructive pulmonary disease and broncheictasis. *Cochrane Database Syst Rev* 2010; 8.

71. Homsi J, Walsh D and Nelson DA. Important drugs for cough in advanced cancer. *Support Care Cancer* 2001; 9(8): 565–574.

72. Molassiotis A, Bailey C, Caress A, et al. Interventions for cough in cancer. *Cochrane Database Syst Rev* September 2010.

73. Poole PJ and Black PN. Mucolytic agents for chronic bronchitis or chronic pulmonary disease. *Cochrane Library* 2004; 1.

74. Bolser DC and Davenport PW. Codeine and cough: an ineffective gold standard. *Curr Opin Allergy Clin Immunol* 2007; 7: 32–36.

75. Smith J, Owen E, Earis J, et al. Effect of codeine on objective measurement of cough in chronic obstructive pulmonary disease. *J Allergy Clin Immunol* 2006; 117: 831–875.

76. Morice AH, Menon MS, Mulrennan SA, et al. Opiate therapy in chronic cough. *Am J Respir Crit Care Med* 2007; 175: 312–315.

77. Bonneau A. Cough in palliative care. *Can Fam Physician* June 2009; 55: 600–602.

78. Luporini G, Barni S, Marchi E, et al. Efficacy and safety of levodropropizine and dihydrocodeine on nonproductive cough in primary and metastatic lung cancer. *Eur Respir J* 1998; 12(1): 97–101.

79. Moroni M, Porta C, Gualtieri G, et al. Inhaled sodium cromoglycate to treat cough in advanced lung cancer patients. *Br J Cancer* 1996; 74(2): 309–311.

80. Charpin J and Weibel MA. Comparative evaluation of the antitussive activity of butamirate citrate linctus versus clobutinol syrup. *Respiration* 1990; 57: 800–805.

81. Chung KF. Currently available cough suppressants for chronic cough. *Lung* 2008; 186(Suppl 1): 82–87.

82. Jones C. Respiratory congest. In: Wainright W, Downing M (eds), *Medical Care of the Dying*, 4th edition. Victoria: Victoria Hospice Society, 2006, pp. 381–389.

83. Light RW. Disorders of pleura, mediastinum, and diaphragm. Isselbacher KJ et al. (eds), *Harrison's Principles of Internal Medicine*, 13th edition. s.l.: McGraw-Hill Inc, 1994, pp. 1229–1234.

84. Lombardi G, Zustovich F, Nocoletto MO, et al. Diagnosis and treatment of malignant pleural effusion. a systematic literature review and new approaches. *Am J Clin Oncol* 2010; 33(4): 420–423.

85. Hass AR. Recent advances in the palliative management of respiratory symptoms in advanced-stage oncology patients. *Am J Hosp Palliat Med* April/May 2007; 24(2): 144–151.

86. Thompson AB, Teschler H and Rennard SI. Pathogenesis, evaluation, and therapy for massive hemoptysis. *Clin Chest Med* 1992; 13(1): 69–82.

87. Graff GR. Treatment of recurrent severe hemoptysis in cystic fibrosis with tranexamic acid. *Respiration* 2001; 68(1): 91–94.

88. Rocker G, Horton R, Currow D, et al. Palliation of dyspnoea in advanced COPD: revisiting a role for opioids. *Thorax* 2009; 64: 910–915.

89. Blinderman CD, Homel P, Billings JA, et al. Symptom distress and quality of life in patients with advanced chronic obstructive pulmonary disease. *J Pain Symptom Manage* 2009; 38(1): 115–123.

90. Bausewein C, Booth S, Bysels M, et al. Understanding breathlessness: cross-sectional comparison of symptom burden and palliative care needs in chronic obstructive pulmonary disease and cancer. *J Palliat Med* 2010; 13(9): 1109–1118.

91. Seamark DA, Seamark CJ and Halpin DMG. Palliative care in chronic obstructive pulmonary disease: a review for clinicians. *J R Soc Med* 2007; 100(5): 225–233.

92. Stewart S and McMurray JJ. Palliative care for heart failure. *BMJ* 2002; 325: 915–916.

93. Currow DC, McDonald C, Oaten S, et al. Once-daily opioids for chronic dyspnea: a dose increment and pharmacovigilance study. *J Pain Symptom Manage* 2011; 42(3): 388–399.

12 Managing Complications of Cancer

Rachael Barton, Debbie Allanson

The Queen's Centre for Oncology and Haematology, Hull, UK

Introduction

Patients with advanced or metastatic cancer often experience complications caused by the cancer itself or its treatment that may have a profound effect on their functional ability and quality of life. Those with tracheostomies for head and neck cancer and patients who develop lymphoedema will require carers to have distinct knowledge and skills.

Although such complications are seen frequently within the field of oncology, they may be rare outside the speciality. It is important to identify early those who may benefit from specific treatment since a prompt referral allows the rapid palliation of symptoms and may prevent loss of function and independence. It is equally important to identify those patients who are in the terminal stage of their disease who may be helped more by symptomatic measures than by referral for investigation and treatment.

This chapter outlines the clinical problems most frequently encountered and gives management guidelines, so that the nonspecialist may have confidence in dealing with what is often a frightening situation for both patient and carer.

Spinal cord compression

This requires early recognition and prompt referral. Restoration of neurological function, especially walking, is rarely possible for those who have lost it by the time they start treatment. It is therefore essential to have a high level of suspicion in patients with known cancer and in those without a malignant diagnosis who have suspicious symptoms. Despite the development of cord compression being a poor prognostic sign, active management is indicated in all patients except those very near the end of life.

Epidemiology

Malignant spinal cord compression (MSCC) is common, affecting 3–5% of all cancer patients and in up to half of these, it is the first presentation of their cancer. 10–20% of patients with breast, lung, and prostate cancer develop MSCC and account for more than 50% of all cases. MSCC is also frequently seen in renal cell cancer, myeloma, and in lymphoma [1]. In children, MSCC is rare but may occur with Ewing's sarcoma, neuroblastoma, Hodgkin's disease, germ cell tumours, and soft tissue sarcomas.

Pathophysiology

MSCC usually results from vertebral body collapse with extension into the spinal canal or, less commonly, from the presence of a tumour deposit adjacent to or within the spinal canal. These may cause neurological dysfunction by a combination of spinal cord or cauda equina oedema, ischaemia, and ultimately infarction. Of all cases, 85–90% are due to metastases or deposits of myeloma affecting the vertebrae, while 10% result from compression from a paraspinal mass (commonly lymphoma) and a small proportion from extradural or meningeal deposits. Metastatic disease is present in more than one vertebra in >70% of patients, the commonest level being the thoracic spine, which is affected in 70% of cases and the lumbar in 20%.

Handbook of Palliative Care, Third Edition. Edited by Christina Faull, Sharon de Caestecker, Alex Nicholson and Fraser Black.
© 2012 by John Wiley and Sons, Inc. Published 2012 by John Wiley & Sons, Inc.

Prognostic factors

Ambulatory status at presentation
Of patients with MSCC, 30–40% can walk at presentation with or without help and of these, 70% will still be able to walk after treatment. In contrast, 50% of patients have complete paraplegia at presentation and few of these will regain function. Early diagnosis is therefore important before irreversible damage occurs.

Histology of the primary
Cancers that are particularly sensitive to chemotherapy and radiotherapy such as myeloma, lymphoma, small-cell lung cancer, and germ cell tumours have a more favourable prognosis for ability to walk following definitive treatment than less chemo-sensitive tumours such as non-small-cell lung cancer [2]. This assumes that the patient is fit for treatment and that it can be started promptly before irreversible damage is caused to the spinal cord. Breast and prostate cancer have a better outlook for mobility and survival than non-small-cell lung cancer or metastases of unknown primary.

Rate of neurological deterioration before presentation
A slower development of neurological deficit over days to weeks predicts for a better outcome in terms of maintaining mobility than a rapid deterioration over 24–48 h, which suggests irreversible cord damage, probably with infarction [3].

Early suspicion and clinical diagnosis
Any patient with cancer is at risk of MSCC, especially those with vertebral metastases. It is extremely difficult to exclude MSCC clinically in a patient with known cancer who complains of localised back pain and even the absence of pain cannot exclude MSCC. Patients with spinal metastases who go on to develop clinical MSCC experience pain for a median of 3 months before developing symptoms and signs giving a "window of opportunity" for diagnosis [1].

A history of increasing back pain is present in the majority. This may be localised to the vertebral column, but often a radicular pain develops, which radiates in a dermatomal distribution. The pain may be worsened by activities that raise intra-abdominal pressure, by movement, lying supine, percussion over the vertebrae, or neck and hip flexion.

The clinical picture does vary between patients and the frequency of symptoms is shown in Box 12.1 [1].

Box 12.1 The frequency of symptoms in MSCC

Symptom	% with symptom
Pain	94
Weakness or difficulty walking	85
Changes in sensation	68
Difficulty passing urine	56
Constipation	66
Faecal incontinence	5

Muscle weakness generally occurs symmetrically in the proximal leg groups while sensory loss may be in any pattern. Sphincter dysfunction occurs late except in compression of the cauda equina which usually results in a combination of the following:
- Sciatic pain
- Saddle anaesthesia
- Urine retention, constipation, or faecal incontinence
- Loss of anal tone

It is important that all health professionals recognise that new or unremitting spinal pain in a patient with known malignancy or a suspicious history with or without clinical signs in patients not known to have cancer requires urgent assessment. (Adapted from National Institute for Health and Clinical Excellence (NICE) guidelines, available at http://guidance.nice.org.uk/CG75.)

Referral guidelines
In 2008, the National Institute for Health and Clinical Excellence (NICE) published guidelines for the management of patients at risk of or with metastatic spinal cord compression that are available at http://guidance.nice.org.uk/CG75.

These set out a pathway for the identification, referral, investigation, and treatment of patients at risk of or with MSCC.

The key recommendations are:
1. Each centre treating patients with MSCC should have 24-h access to a MSCC coordinator through a single point of contact to provide advice to clinicians and coordinate the patient's pathway.
2. The MSCC coordinator will perform an initial telephone triage, advise on care of the spine, organise

admission and investigation where appropriate, and liaise with the members of the acute team to ensure timely management.

3. "At risk patients," that is, those known to have bone and especially spinal metastases and those at high risk of developing spinal metastases should be given an information leaflet explaining about spinal cord compression and the symptoms to look out for. This should include the 24-h contact details for the local MSCC coordinator.

4. The local MSCC coordinator should be contacted **urgently** (within 24 h) to discuss the care of patients with known cancer and any of the following **symptoms suggestive of spinal metastases**:

- Pain in the middle (thoracic) or upper (cervical) spine.
- Progressive lower (lumbar) spinal pain.
- Severe unremitting spinal pain.
- Spinal pain aggravated by straining (e.g., opening bowels, coughing, or sneezing).
- Localised spinal tenderness.
- Nocturnal spinal pain preventing sleep.

5. Patients without a known diagnosis of cancer who develop suspicious pain should be reviewed frequently and referred within 24 h if they develop progressive pain or other symptoms suggestive of spinal metastases (see above).

6. The local MSCC coordinator should be contacted **immediately** to discuss the care of patients with or without known cancer with symptoms suggestive of spinal metastases who have any of the following **neurological symptoms or signs suggestive of MSCC**. Such patients should be viewed as an oncological emergency:

- Neurological symptoms including radicular pain, any limb weakness, difficulty in walking, sensory loss, or bladder or bowel dysfunction.
- Neurological signs of spinal cord or cauda equina compression.

7. MRI of the whole spine should be performed in patients with suspected MSCC unless there is a specific contraindication. MRI should be done in time to allow definitive treatment to be planned within **1 week** of the suspected diagnosis in the case of pain **suggestive of spinal metastases** and within **24 h** in the case of pain suggestive of spinal metastases and neurological symptoms or signs **suggestive of MSCC**. Occasionally MRI will be required sooner than 24 h if there is a pressing clinical need for emergency surgery.

8. Patients with severe mechanical pain suggestive of spinal instability or symptoms/signs suggestive of MSCC should be nursed flat with neutral spinal alignment until bony and neurological stability are established and cautious mobilisation can begin.

9. Definitive treatment should begin before further neurological deterioration and ideally within 24 h of the diagnosis of MSCC.

10. Discharge planning and rehabilitation should begin on admission and involve the patient, their family and carers, the oncology and rehabilitation teams plus palliative care, primary care teams, and community support as required.

Treatment

Immediate management
Patients with MSCC should be prescribed dexamethasone 8 mg immediately, which should be given parenterally only when there is concern about absorption. This should be followed by dexamethasone 16 mg daily in two divided doses. Ideally the second dose should not be given after 2 pm to avoid night-time wakefulness and agitation although this should not preclude emergency administration of the first day's dose. Analgesia will often require nonsteroidal anti-inflammatories (NSAIDs), strong opioids +/− antispasmodics.

Subsequent treatment options
The multidisciplinary assessment and management of all patients is essential to ensure appropriate and timely treatment.

Surgery
Surgery should be considered when there is structural spinal instability with or without pain, particularly if progression to MSCC can be prevented. Other relative indications for surgery include malignancy of unknown primary or disease that is radioresistant. Those who are likely to benefit most from surgery are those with a relatively good prognosis and premorbid performance status with limited sites of metastatic disease. A recognised prognostic scoring system such as that described by Tokuhashi may be helpful [4,5].

Spinal decompression and stabilisation followed by radiotherapy improves the outcome in terms of maintenance of mobility and continence compared with radiotherapy alone [6].

Radiotherapy
For the majority of patients, radiotherapy is the mainstay of treatment. It will often relieve pain and may prevent deterioration but rarely restores function that has already

been lost. In general, radiotherapy is more effective when cord compression occurs without bony collapse and instability [7]. Five to ten fractions are often given, but a single fraction may suffice to relieve pain in the patient with a poor prognosis and complete paraplegia [8,9].

Chemotherapy

Chemotherapy may be indicated for chemosensitive tumours such as lymphoma, small-cell lung cancer, germ cell tumours, and myeloma and is usually followed by radiotherapy.

Rehabilitation and discharge planning

Patients with MSCC usually have a dramatic change in their functional ability; therefore, the physiotherapist and occupational therapist play a key role in rehabilitation. Patients and carers need to adapt not only to the poor prognosis and loss of mobility and bladder/bowel function but also to the loss of social status, income, and a change in body image.

Immediate needs may include the following:
- Special equipment or adaptations at home.
- An alternative place of care.
- A "package" of social and health care including respite care.
- Psychosocial support.

Outcomes

Function

Overall, 40% of patients with MSCC remain ambulant following treatment. However, 25% of patients relapse at the same site within 6 months, and 50% of those living long enough will relapse within a year. Of those who do not require a urinary catheter before treatment, 80% will remain catheter-free compared to 20% of those who require a catheter at diagnosis.

Survival

Overall median survival is 7–10 months; 10% die within 1 month and 18–30% live for more than 1 year [2]. Lung cancer carries a particularly poor prognosis, with a median survival of 2–3 months.

Place of care

Many patients with MSCC will require care in a nursing home, especially if they have other specialised care needs. If life expectancy is very short or there are particular physical, psychological, or other problems, a palliative care unit may be appropriate.

Follow-up

Patients with MSCC are at increased risk of further spinal cord compression since >70% will have other vertebral sites affected by metastatic disease. Radiotherapy is often given to such lesions although there is no evidence to support prophylactic treatment. To continue to optimise function, pain control, and quality of life, regular follow-up is vital. According to individual circumstances, this may be based in the community rather than hospital.

Superior vena cava obstruction (SVCO)

SVCO describes a syndrome characterised by obstruction to blood flow through the superior vena cava (SVC). There is a malignant cause in 88% of cases, lung cancer causing 70%, lymphoma 8%, and other malignancies 10%. In 50% of cases with an underlying malignancy, SVCO is the first manifestation of disease, and therefore, an urgent specialist referral is important to make an accurate diagnosis.

Active treatment of SVCO may give good relief from distressing symptoms and is indicated in all but the frail, terminally ill patient who may be helped more by symptomatic measures alone.

Pathophysiology

Malignant obstruction to blood flow usually results from extrinsic compression by tumour or lymph nodes although intracaval thrombus may also occur. Patients with indwelling central lines are at particular risk of thrombosis. Swelling of the face and arms results from elevation of venous pressure above the obstruction. The cyanosed appearance usually results from the delay of drainage of deoxygenated blood rather than central hypoxia, which, if present, is usually due to the effects of any underlying lung disease.

Diagnosis and early suspicion

Any patient known to have a primary lung tumour, especially right-sided, is at particular risk. The onset is usually insidious, which allows collaterals to develop, visible as engorged subcutaneous (SC) veins. Two-thirds of patients complain of breathlessness and half of facial swelling or a feeling of fullness in the head. The symptoms (see Box 12.2) may be exacerbated by bending forwards or lying down.

Management

Although symptoms are often uncomfortable, SVCO is rarely life-threatening unless oxygenation is severely

> ## Box 12.2 Symptoms and signs of SVCO
>
> *Symptoms*
> - Dyspnoea
> - Facial/arm swelling
> - Head fullness
> - Headache
> - Cough
> - Chest pain
> - Dysphagia
>
> *Physical signs*
> - Neck vein distension
> - Facial/arm swelling
> - Distension of superficial veins on chest and abdominal wall
> - Breathlessness
> - Plethora
> - Facial or conjunctival oedema
> - Central or peripheral cyanosis

compromised. Urgent telephone referral should be made to a chest physician if there is no prior diagnosis or to the oncologist if the patient has known malignant disease.

Immediate measures

If the patient with SVCO is breathless, bed rest and elevation of the bed head may be helpful although oxygen should be used only if it gives symptomatic relief. Analgesia and antitussives may help patients who have headache and cough.

The role of steroids is unproven; dexamethasone 16 mg daily in divided doses may help but should not be given "blind" if the underlying diagnosis is not known. Rarely, high-grade mediastinal lymphoma may present as SVCO, in which case steroids may induce tumour lysis, threatening renal function, and obscuring a histological diagnosis. Anticoagulants are not indicated routinely.

Subsequent treatment

The aim of the treatment is to relieve symptoms and, if possible, cure the underlying process. Patients with SVCO who are otherwise well can be treated as outpatients.

Cancers that are particularly sensitive to radiotherapy and chemotherapy will often have a rapid and dramatic response to treatment with response rates of 77% quoted for patients with small-cell lung cancer. Although non-small-cell lung cancer is less sensitive to available therapies, response rates of 60% for symptom relief are reported although there is undoubtedly some gradual improve-

ment with time as collateralisation takes place [10]. Radiotherapy is usually complete in 1–2 weeks and symptoms usually improve within 2–3 weeks.

Insertion of a stent under radiological control gives rapid and often immediate relief of symptoms, most resolving within 72 h [11]. Urgent referral for stenting should be considered for severe symptoms or for relapse following treatment with other modalities. Caution must be exercised however, with the placement of stents in patients with a good prognosis, especially those with curable disease, as fibrosis and narrowing occurring some months after stenting may require further intervention with the risk of intractable symptoms. Thrombolysis may be indicated for extensive thrombus, although this increases the chances of adverse side effects.

Outcome

The average survival of a patient diagnosed with a malignant cause of SVCO is 8 months, but the prognosis depends on the underlying histology and stage of their disease. Relapse occurs following radiotherapy and/or chemotherapy in approximately 17% of patients with lung cancer over a period of 1–16 months following treatment [10].

Follow-up

During active treatment and until toxicity has settled, care should be centred on the specialist unit providing the treatment. Following treatment, patients with incurable lung cancer may be offered infrequent hospital visits with an "SOS" option providing that appropriate community support is available. The patient, family, palliative care and primary health-care teams should all be made aware of the likely symptoms of progression of their cancer and who to contact should the need arise.

Bone metastases

Bone metastases are common, especially in cancers of the breast, prostate, lung, and kidney, and widespread bone lesions are a feature of multiple myeloma. Up to 70% of women dying of breast cancer will have bone metastases at post mortem, although many of these will have been asymptomatic. The complications of bone metastases include pain, pathological fracture, nerve compression, and hypercalcaemia.

Diagnosis and early suspicion

The cardinal feature of a bone metastasis is pain. This is commonly unrelenting, progressive, may be present at rest and may be associated with referred pain, restriction of movement, and neurological impairment.

The initial investigation should be plain X-rays of the affected area, asking for orthogonal (i.e., perpendicular) views of long bones as some metastases may be visible only on one view. At this stage it is important to rule out a pathological fracture or a bone at imminent risk of fracture (see below). Prostate cancer classically results in sclerotic metastases although lytic disease may occur, whereas myeloma causes marked lysis of the bone. Breast and lung cancer often give a mixed picture of sclerotic and lytic metastases, and renal cancer metastases are often large and vascular. Bone metastases are frequently multiple although many will not cause symptoms.

An isotope bone scan is a more sensitive investigation than a plain radiograph, assessing the whole skeleton and detecting small areas of increased isotope uptake, which may indicate a metastasis. The distinction between metastases and degenerative disease is improved by comparing the bone scan with plain radiographs. Noticeably, metastases that cause a great deal of bony lysis, for example, myeloma, may appear "cold" on a bone scan. In cases of difficulty, or if surgery is contemplated, an MRI scan of the affected area may be helpful.

Treatment

General measures

The initial priority is analgesia. Nonsteroidal anti-inflammatory druge (NSAIDs) are often useful although severe pain from bony metastases often requires strong opioids [12]. Steroids, for example, dexamethasone, 4–6 mg daily can be helpful as a short-term adjunct to other analgesics but if not helpful after a week's trial, should be discontinued. Pain may also be reduced by resting the affected area. Consultation with physiotherapists may be helpful, particularly if walking aids are required.

Systemic anticancer treatments

Consideration should be given to systemic treatments, for example, hormones for breast and prostate cancer or chemotherapy for solid tumours or haematological malignancies if the patient is fit for treatment.

Radiotherapy

For most painful bony metastases, local radiotherapy is the treatment of choice [13]. In uncomplicated bone metas-

tases, a single dose of radiotherapy, planned and delivered in one day will achieve pain relief in 60–80% of patients with a complete response in 30% [14,15].

The side effects of radiotherapy depend on the site treated and include fatigue, nausea and vomiting and looseness of the bowels. Gastrointestinal (GI) side effects are most common when the treatment field includes the abdomen and can be reduced by a $5HT_3$ antagonist plus dexamethasone 4–6 mg daily beginning on the day of radiotherapy and continuing for 3 days. Palliative radiotherapy given in this way can be repeated if the pain recurs with a good chance of a second response and little added toxicity.

Widespread, painful bony metastases are impractical to treat with many local fields. One option is "hemibody radiotherapy" in which a single dose is delivered either to the upper or to the lower half of the skeleton [16]. Toxicity can be severe, mainly comprising nausea, vomiting, and diarrhoea but a $5HT_3$ antagonist plus dexamethasone as above allows outpatient treatment in patients of good performance status who can maintain their hydration. An alternative is the use of bone-seeking radioactive isotopes, for example, ^{89}Strontium or ^{153}Samarium that are concentrated in the affected bone and deliver a local dose of radiotherapy [17]. There is little acute toxicity although there may be asymptomatic bone marrow suppression, and it is essential to ensure that patients have adequate bone marrow reserve and to check they are continent in order to deal with the radioactive urine.

Bisphosphonates

Bisphosphonates have a role in prophylaxis against bone pain, fractures, and hypercalcaemia in patients with myeloma and bony metastases from breast and prostate cancer [18–21]. There may also be a case for the treatment of other cancers although the balance of benefits against side effects is probably less favourable [22,23]. Bisphosphonates can also be used to treat patients with malignant bone pain in myeloma, breast, lung, and prostate cancer when they are usually delivered as an intravenous (IV) infusion every 4 weeks [24]. An improvement in pain is seen in 40% of patients with common solid tumours but up to 80% of those with myeloma. Oral preparations improve the convenience of treatment but are less well tolerated.

Cement injection and percutaneous ablation

Newer techniques are now being introduced for painful bony metastases which are unresponsive to conventional treatments such as radiotherapy and chemotherapy. The technique of vertebroplasty is well established, having been introduced initially for the treatment of osteoporotic vertebral fractures. A vertebra that contains a painful metastasis is injected with bone cement under sedation and radiological screening [25]. If there is loss of bony height, there is also an option to restore some of the lost height by the use of a balloon, termed a kyphoplasty [26]. Outside the spine, destruction of the bony metastasis may be achieved by the use of radiofrequency ablation (RFA) or cryotherapy with or without the subsequent injection of cement into the bone to consolidate bone structure [27]. This is particularly useful for lytic lesions of the pelvis that are not amenable to prophylactic surgical fixation although all these techniques require operator expertise and are not available in all centres.

Outcome

For bony metastases not complicated by nerve compression, fracture, or hypercalcaemia, the outlook is relatively good, and many patients will be able to reduce their analgesic requirement and/or improve their mobility. For most common solid tumours, the prognosis is better for patients with metastases in the bones alone than for patients with bone and visceral metastases.

Follow-up

Patients with bony metastases often have several sites of pain and more will usually reveal themselves with time. Close follow-up is therefore required in the community to ensure adequate analgesia and appropriate and prompt referral back to specialist services. Social services, occupational and physiotherapy services may also be needed to allow patients with reduced mobility to return safely and comfortably to their own homes.

Pathological fracture

Pathological fractures are usually associated with lytic bone metastases, particularly in weight-bearing bones. The early diagnosis and treatment of impending pathological fractures may prevent unnecessary pain and loss of function.

Impending pathological fracture

Diagnosis and early suspicion

This complication is often seen in myeloma, breast, lung, and renal cell cancer, but any primary cancer may give rise to a pathological fracture, and all patients with metastases in long bones are at risk. Pain on limb movement (func-

Table 12.1 Mirels' score for impending pathological fracture.

Variable	Score		
	1	2	3
Site	Upper limb	Lower limb	Peritrochanteric
Pain	Mild	Moderate	Functional
Lesion	Blastic	Mixed	Lytic
Size	<1/3	1/3–2/3	>2/3

tional pain) especially on bearing weight raises the possibility of a lesion at high risk of fracture. The diagnosis is usually made on plain radiograph.

Management

There is a well-established scoring system to estimate the probability of a given metastatic lesion fracturing [28] (Table 12.1). A score of eight or more indicates a high risk of fracture, and such lesions should be considered for prophylactic fixation. This can be carried out with good results in all but the most unfit patient and an orthopaedic team should be consulted in all cases. Those with an impending pathological fracture should take as little weight through the affected region as possible until definitive treatment is complete; hospital admission may be necessary to achieve this. All patients will require adequate analgesia.

Outcome

Functional outcome after surgical fixation of an impending pathological fracture is usually excellent although overall outcome will depend on the patient's general state of health and performance status.

Established fracture

Diagnosis

The sudden loss of function or mobility, especially with a sudden increase in pain, makes a pathological fracture likely. Spinal cord compression should also be considered and urgent specialist referral for investigation is indicated.

Management

An established pathological fracture in a weight-bearing long bone is treated surgically in all but the most frail patient. Those of the upper limb may be fixed surgically but in unfit patients, immobilisation, often with radiotherapy will usually provide pain relief.

Radiotherapy

Following surgical treatment of either an impending or an established fracture, postoperative radiotherapy is usually added to prevent local progression. This is given in 1–5 daily treatments beginning approximately 4 weeks after the surgery to allow for healing of the soft tissues. A pathological fracture that is not to be treated surgically is usually managed with radiotherapy alone.

Rehabilitation and discharge planning

The chances of a patient rehabilitating successfully will depend on many factors, particularly their general health and performance status. Other painful bony metastases may slow progress, especially if they occur in a limb that is required to take more weight following surgery. As for spinal cord compression, discharge planning may require the coordinated action of several teams.

Brain metastases

Metastases to the brain are a common problem in oncology, affecting 17–25% of the cancer population. They are common in lung cancer affecting 26% of patients with this disease, breast cancer (16%), renal cancer (13%), colorectal carcinoma (5%), and in melanoma (4%). In the majority of patients, the diagnosis of cerebral metastases carries a poor prognosis.

Diagnosis and early suspicion

Brain metastases frequently masquerade as a stroke or less commonly as seizures in patients not previously known to have a diagnosis of cancer, the correct diagnosis being made at CT scan. Brain metastases should be considered in all those known to have cancer presenting with any of the symptoms listed in Box 12.3.

Box 12.3 Common symptoms and signs of brain metastases

Headache
Nausea/vomiting
Focal weakness/hemiparesis
Confusion
Unsteadiness
Seizures
Visual disturbance
Dysphasia

Management

In many patients, the presence of cerebral metastases is a component of widely disseminated disease and is often associated with a poor performance status and prognosis. The focus of management for this group is general symptomatic care and consideration of psychosocial needs. For a selected group of patients with a better prognosis, active treatment may be appropriate.

General symptomatic measures

Cerebral oedema and raised intracranial pressure

Acute treatment is with steroids: dexamethasone 8 mg initially, which should be given parenterally only when there is concern about absorption, for example, in the presence of vomiting. This should be followed by dexamethasone 16 mg daily in two divided doses. Ideally the second dose should not be given after 2 pm to avoid night-time wakefulness and agitation though this should not preclude emergency administration of the first day's dose. IV mannitol may rarely be needed to reduce the intracranial pressure in a patient whose condition is worsening rapidly.

Headache

Headache usually responds to steroids, but regular paracetamol with the addition of codeine phosphate may be helpful and occasionally strong opioids may be required.

Seizures

Once the intracranial pressure is reduced, seizures may subside, but some patients require regular anticonvulsant medication. The terminally ill patient with cerebral metastases and uncontrolled fitting may require parenteral benzodiazepines, for example, midazolam by continuous SC infusion (see Chapter 22).

Nausea and vomiting

This usually responds to measures which reduce intracranial pressure, but antiemetics may be required and may need to be given parenterally at first.

Confusion, agitation, or psychosis

The introduction of steroids may reverse acute problems but occasionally sedation may be required until the steroids take effect or as part of the management of terminal agitation.

Specific treatment options

Solitary brain metastases

Surgical resection or stereotactic radiosurgery (SRS) are both used widely for the treatment of patients with an MRI-proven solitary metastasis who have limited extra-cranial disease and both a good prognosis and performance status. SRS uses finely focused beams of radiation and image guidance to treat the metastasis with a small margin to a high dose and is available in the United Kingdom in several larger radiotherapy centres. There has been no head-to-head comparison of surgery and SRS, so the choice depends on local expertise, fitness for surgery, the size and site of the metastasis and patient choice [29]. The addition of whole brain radiotherapy to either of these local treatments seems to decrease the risk of relapse in the brain but does not impact on overall survival [30].

Surgical resection may be more appropriate than SRS where there is no known primary cancer; the differential diagnosis lies between a primary brain tumour and a solitary metastasis or when the metastasis is too large for SRS. Surgery also has a role when raised intracranial pressure causes severe symptoms, especially with posterior fossa lesions.

The multidisciplinary team (MDT) is vital in the management of solitary brain metastases. Cases, which may be appropriate for surgery should be discussed at a neuro-oncology MDT meeting.

Radiotherapy

Radiotherapy to the whole brain has been a common treatment and is usually given over 2–5 days. Steroids are continued throughout the treatment but are tailed off once it is complete, at a rate determined by symptoms although it is not often possible to stop steroids completely. Good response rates have often been quoted but studies using patient-rated scales suggest that symptomatic benefit is the exception, and benefit is often outweighed by side effects (Box 12.4) [31,32]. For the patient with a poor performance status and poor prognosis, treatment with steroids and general supportive measures may be the best option.

Chemotherapy

Systemic chemotherapy is useful for some tumours which are chemosensitive, such as small-cell lung cancer and germ cell tumours and may also be useful in patients with breast cancer. Chemotherapy is usually followed by radiotherapy.

Box 12.4 Side effects of whole brain radiotherapy

Acute	Late (>6 months after completion of treatment)
Temporary alopecia	Difficulties with memory and concentration
Headache	Deterioration on neurocognitive testing
Nausea	Persistent alopecia
Redness and soreness of the skin	
Tiredness and sleepiness	

Rehabilitation and discharge planning

Many patients with brain metastases have a dramatic change in their functional ability, independence, and personality. Many of their rehabilitation needs are similar to those outlined for patients with MSCC. In addition, some patients may need speech therapy, and where appropriate, route of nutrition will need to be considered in those who have difficulty swallowing. There is a need for psychological support for both patient and carers.

Outcomes

Symptoms and quality of life

A prospective study found that 1 month following whole brain radiotherapy, 20% of patients with brain metastases reported an improvement or resolution of their neurological symptoms and a similar number were stable. The rest had progressive symptoms or had died [31]. The challenge is to identify patients who are likely to benefit from treatment, concentrating on end-of-life care and symptom control for those who are unlikely to gain from intervention.

Survival

The survival of patients with cerebral metastases is usually short. Performance status is the strongest predictor of survival although patients with non-small-cell lung cancer have a particularly poor prognosis with a median survival of 2–3 months. Box 12.5 summarises the factors influencing survival.

Box 12.5 Factors affecting survival in patients with brain metastases

Factors that improve survival	*Factors that reduce survival*
Solitary metastasis	Poor performance status
Long disease-free interval before relapse	Extracranial sites of metastatic disease
Primary site breast	Meningeal disease

Place of care

Many patients will be unable to be cared for at home because of loss of independence and need for nursing care. Changes in cognitive function in particular make care at home problematic and distressing to relatives.

Follow-up

Symptomatic progression of brain metastases is common and is often accompanied by progressive extracranial disease. Close follow-up should be arranged in the community where care is usually centred for those without further anticancer treatment options.

Surgical and interventional management of other sites of metastatic disease

Liver metastases

Liver metastases are common in colorectal cancer affecting 15–25% of patients at presentation and a further 20% at a later stage in their disease. Radical treatment of liver metastases has been shown to result in long-term survival and, in some cases, cure.

Surgery

The resectability of liver metastases largely depends on the tumour bulk, the number of metastases, and their location within the liver but each case should be considered individually. Patients must have good liver function and be fit enough to undergo major surgery; the success rate is improved if a clear resection margin can be achieved. In selected groups with optimally resectable metastases, 5- and 10-year survival rates of 30% and 20% respectively have been reported [33].

Local ablation

Liver metastases may be unresectable because of their number or location. Local ablative techniques such as RFA and cryotherapy may be directed at individual metastases to destroy tumour tissue. As an adjunct to surgery or chemotherapy, these techniques may increase survival and the NICE have issued guidelines on the use of RFA and cryotherapy in colorectal liver metastases that are available at:

www.nice.org.uk/IP248aoverview

www.nice.org.uk/guidance/IP/400/overview

Chemoembolisation describes the use of chemotherapy impregnated microscopic beads that can be introduced into the liver selectively to target inoperable metastases or primary hepatocellular carcinoma (HCC) This has been used with some success in specialist centres.

Lung metastases

Lung metastases are common, affecting 25–30% of patients dying of cancer. Rarely, resection will result in long-term survival or cure in selected patients. Cures are seen in metastatic teratoma when multiple lung metastases are resected following chemotherapy. Curative resections may also be carried out in patients with several pulmonary metastases from colorectal cancer, with 5-year survival rates of up to 50% reported in selected series [34].

Bone metastases

Renal cell carcinoma may recur as a single or a limited number of bone metastases that are usually resistant to chemotherapy and radiotherapy and may cause pathological fracture. Surgical excision and reconstruction followed by radiotherapy may be curative, and early specialist referral is mandatory.

Hypercalcaemia

Hypercalcaemia is a common metabolic complication of cancer, affecting up to 50% of patients with breast cancer and multiple myeloma. It is also common in squamous cell cancers of the lung, cervix, and head and neck and is usually, but not always, associated with widespread bone involvement (80%). The outlook is poor if the condition is untreated but prompt, active treatment may relieve symptoms rapidly with minimal toxicity. Specific therapy should be offered in all but the very frail patient at the end of their life in whom hypercalcaemia is a terminal event and who may be helped more by simple symptomatic measures.

Pathophysiology

Tumour-induced hypercalcaemia results from the action of various factors released by the immune system or from the tumour. The most common is parathyroid hormone-related protein (PTH-RP), which increases the release of calcium from bone and its GI and renal tubular absorption. Others include prostaglandins (PGs) and cytokines.

Hypercalcaemia induces vomiting and an osmotic diuresis leading to polyuria, dehydration, hypovolemia and compromised renal function, further escalating calcium levels. The action of a raised serum calcium concentration on smooth muscle and the central nervous system (CNS) leads to the characteristic symptoms of constipation, confusion, and nausea.

Diagnosis and early suspicion

The diagnosis should be considered in any patient with advanced cancer who becomes unwell. Bony metastases are often, but not always, associated. Onset is often gradual and the symptoms are nonspecific, often mimicking the general debility of a patient with advanced cancer (see Box 12.6). It should be remembered that enforced immobility, for example, following a pathological fracture or spinal cord compression will often accelerate the development of hypercalcaemia as calcium is mobilised from the bones.

Management

Serum calcium, corrected for the serum albumin should be checked along with renal function. Uncontrolled diabetes should be excluded as the clinical features are similar. For patients at home with mild symptoms suggestive of hypercalcaemia, the results of blood tests should be established within 48 h. A patient with cancer who becomes unwell with suspected hypercalcaemia should be admitted urgently for investigation and treatment.

Immediate treatment

Rehydration is the first requirement. Oral fluids are encouraged, and IV normal saline is infused at a rate determined by the clinical condition. Drugs that inhibit urinary calcium excretion or decrease renal blood flow are stopped (e.g., thiazide diuretics, NSAIDs). High-dose steroids are no longer recommended. Rehydration alone may be sufficient to relieve many of the symptoms, but analgesia may be required for the pain of bony metastases. Constipation and nausea are often severe and should be treated vigorously (see Chapter 10).

Specific treatment of hypercalcaemia

IV bisphosphonates inhibit the absorption of bone by osteoclasts and are the mainstay of treatment for malignant hypercalcaemia [35]. Several drugs are available in this class that differ in their potency: the newer, more potent formulations such as zoledronate and ibandronate have a shorter duration of infusion and provide a more prolonged normalisation of serum calcium than pamidronate or etidronate [36]. Side effects of bisphosphonate treatment include flu-like symptoms, uveitis, renal impairment, hypocalcaemia, and hypophosphatemia, most of which are well tolerated. Rarely, osteonecrosis of the jaw can occur, especially if dental extractions are carried out in a patient receiving regular bisphosphonates, and this should be avoided. The renal impairment associated with bisphosphonate treatment can largely be avoided by adjusting the dose according to the calculated creatinine clearance and ensuring adequate saline hydration for at least 12–24 h before administration. Following IV bisphosphonates, the serum calcium begins to fall rapidly reaching a nadir after 7–10 days although symptomatic improvement is usually more rapid.

Prophylactic bisphosphonate therapy either as intermittent IV infusions (usually 4 weekly) or as oral therapy has been shown to reduce the incidence of skeletal events such as symptomatic bone metastases and episodes of hypercalcaemia in patients with myeloma and metastatic breast, prostate, and other cancers (see above). Patients who have had a diagnosis of malignant hypercalcaemia are at risk of further episodes, especially if they have active cancer. Their calcium level should be monitored in the community at a frequency dictated by the rate of rise, allowing prompt outpatient intervention with IV bisphosphonates before symptoms develop.

Box 12.6 Clinical features of hypercalcaemia

General	Neurological
Thirst	Confusion
Polyuria	Psychosis
Polydipsia	Coma
Dehydration	
Weight loss	Gastrointestinal
Lethargy	Anorexia
Fatigue	Nausea/vomiting
Pruritus	Constipation
Cardiac arrhythmias	Peptic ulceration

In the event of severe hypercalcaemia causing life-threatening effects, bisphosphonates may be too slow to have a useful effect. Salmon calcitonin is effective in the rapid, short-term management of hypercalcaemia but needs to be given as regular SC injections and monitored carefully [37].

Specific treatment of the underlying cancer

With the exception of those with localised head and neck or cervical cancers, most patients will have widespread disease and cure of the underlying cancer is rarely possible. However, treatments such as chemotherapy, hormonal therapy, or radiotherapy may reduce the bulk or metabolic activity of the underlying cancer and reduce the likelihood of recurrent hypercalcaemia.

Outcome

Close follow-up in the outpatient setting or at home is vital as hypercalcaemia commonly recurs. For patients who have anticancer treatments available, the outlook is much better than for those with advanced disease resistant to treatment. In the latter case, hypercalcaemia often recurs with shorter intervals between episodes gradually becoming resistant even to the effects of bisphosphonates. At this point the patient's life expectancy is very short.

Obstructive nephropathy

Pelvic, abdominal, and retroperitoneal malignancies predispose to the development of ureteric obstruction. If left untreated, progressive disease will lead to acute or chronic renal failure, which will ultimately prove fatal. Estimates of median survival following malignant ureteric obstruction range from 3–7 months, the survival time largely depending on the patient's performance status, the presence of other sites of metastatic disease, and biochemical features of severe renal impairment [38,39].

Relief of ureteric obstruction by stent or nephrostomy is an invasive but relatively simple procedure with good resolution of symptoms in most patients. However, if renal failure is relieved in the absence of a therapeutic option for the cancer itself, the original disease process will continue to progress, causing distressing symptoms and ultimately leading to death. This gives rise to a dilemma commonly encountered in palliative care: "*is intervention and therefore prolongation of life, in the patient's best interests?*" Discussion with the patient and their informed consent are crucial, but this is often very difficult if this issue is only raised when the need for treatment has become urgent.

> **Box 12.7 Clinical features of obstructive nephropathy**
>
> - Anorexia
> - Anuria/oliguria
> - Bleeding tendency
> - Cardiac arrhythmias
> - Confusion
> - Drug toxicity
> - Hypertension
> - Myoclonic jerks
> - Nausea
> - oedema
> - Susceptibility to infection
> - Vomiting

Of patients presenting with acute renal failure secondary to bilateral ureteric obstruction, two-thirds have underlying malignant disease. For half of these it will be their first manifestation of disease. This is particularly common in cancers of the cervix, bladder, and prostate.

Diagnosis and early suspicion

Obstruction of a single kidney is often not noticed unless imaging of the abdomen takes place. Once the second kidney becomes involved, the clinical features of obstructive nephropathy become evident (Box 12.7). As with hypercalcaemia, the features are nonspecific unless anuria occurs and may mimic the general debility of a patient with advanced cancer.

Investigations

Both blood urea and creatinine are raised and often potassium. Ultrasound and/or CT scan of the renal tracts and pelvis will usually be able to confirm obstruction to renal outflow with dilation of the renal pelvis and may be able to demonstrate the cause of the obstruction.

Treatment

If appropriate, the obstruction needs to be relieved promptly before irreversible damage is caused to the kidneys. This is commonly carried out by nephrostomy or ureteric stenting [40]. Acute medical management of the associated hyperkalemia, metabolic acidosis, and fluid overload may be necessary if the deterioration in renal function has been rapid. In previously untreated carcinoma of the prostate, the rapid introduction of antiandrogens may shrink the primary tumour enough to relieve obstruction although if renal function is impaired, emergency drainage of the renal tract is usually required while the hormones take effect.

Hydration should aim to replace losses and prevent thirst while avoiding fluid overload and the distressing features of pulmonary oedema. All drugs should be used with caution in renal failure. Haloperidol given orally or by SC infusion will help control nausea, myoclonic jerks, confusion, and agitation.

Pain from hydronephrosis may require strong opioids. Many opioids accumulate in renal failure and should be used with longer dosing intervals and frequent review. Fentanyl has little renal excretion and accumulates less in renal failure than morphine (see also Chapter 19) although estimating a dose to use by transdermal patch can be difficult. If an SC infusion is appropriate, the short-acting drug alfentanil is considered to be the safest option in renal failure.

Haemorrhage

There are several reasons why a patient with cancer may haemorrhage including:
- bleeding directly from tumour or metastases;
- invasion of tumour into blood vessels;
- bleeding tendency due to thrombocytopenia, disseminated intravascular coagulopathy (DIC), uraemia, or anticoagulants; and
- bleeding from postradiotherapy telangiectasia (especially bladder and GI tract).

Conditions that increase the tendency to bleed should be dealt with whenever possible and appropriate. For example, consideration should be given to the pros and cons of stopping anticoagulation or to transfusing with platelets, etc. The management of massive, terminal haemorrhage is discussed in Chapter 21.

Radiotherapy
Palliative radiotherapy to control bleeding is usually restricted to a short course of treatment with few planning stages, a typical course lasting 1–5 days. Radiotherapy can be useful for bleeding arising from primary or metastatic cancers although it should be remembered that the affected area may already have received radiotherapy to tolerance doses. As individual cases vary, the advice of the treating oncologist should be sought. Haemoptysis often responds well to radiotherapy, which can be given in a single day in patients of poor performance status. Laser therapy may be helpful in resistant or severe cases of haemoptysis with a proximal bleeding lesion.

Vascular embolisation
Occasionally, bleeding from a vascular tumour can be reduced by embolisation of its blood supply. Advice should be sought from an interventional radiologist on the suitability of the lesion and the need for further investigation.

Symptomatic measures
Drugs that decrease the tendency to bleed may be helpful, for example, tranexamic acid or ethamsylate. Mucosal bleeding from bladder or bowel may be reduced by using 1% alum as a bladder irrigation or enema. Tranexamic acid enema (5 g in 50 ml water twice daily or 1–2 g mixed with KY jelly) may reduce bleeding from rectal tumours. The application of adrenaline-soaked swabs (1:1000), alginate dressings, and sucralfate paste (in KY jelly) may reduce superficial capillary bleeding. Oral or rectal sucralfate (1 g 2–4 times daily) may reduce bleeding from oesophageal, gastric, or rectal tumours.

Itch

Itching is a sensation that produces a desire to scratch and is a problem for many patients with cancer. It can cause profound debility as it prevents sleep and leads to painful excoriation of the skin. It is associated with various conditions:
- Blood disorders: lymphoma (itch may be the presenting feature of Hodgkin's disease); leukaemia; polycythemia rubra vera.
- Iron deficiency.
- Cholestatic jaundice (see Chapter 10).
- Uraemia.
- Allergens causing eczema and contact dermatitis.
- Drugs: opioids (histamine release); chlorpromazine (cholestasis).
- Skin infections and infestations: scabies; fungal infection.
- The presence of advanced cancer, particularly with skin involvement—directly or by metastasis.

Pathophysiology
Irritant substances in the skin such as histamine, tissue proteases, PGs, or bile acids stimulate receptors of unmyelinated nerve fibres (C fibres). It is likely that opioid and serotonin receptors are involved in the transmission of the sensation of itch [41] and in cholestasis, circulating levels of endogenous opioids are increased.

Management
There are no specific antipruritic drugs; hence, the underlying cause should always be addressed if possible.

General measures

Avoiding the following may be helpful:

- Friction from rough clothing and bed linen.
- Overheating.
- Vasodilators.
- Soap and other products that dry the skin.
- Hot or spicy food and alcohol.

Cooling and moistening the skin with moisturisers and emollients is helpful but calamine lotion may over-dry the skin.

Drug treatment

1. Oral antihistamines in the form of a sedative preparation may be useful at night, for example, chlorpheniramine with a less sedative preparation in the day, for example, loratidine although the latter may not prove as effective.

2. A trial of oral corticosteroids may be of value in some patients, particularly those with lymphoma or bile duct obstruction due to tumour or lymph nodes.

3. Systemic nonsteroidal anti-inflammatories have not been shown to have a role in cancer-related itch although they may be useful topically for the itch of cutaneous tumour infiltration.

4. Erythropoietin (EPO) is helpful for the itch of chronic uraemia.

5. Cimetidine may be helpful in itch associated with Hodgkin's disease.

6. Itch related to cholestatic jaundice may be associated with abnormal activity of endogenous opioids. This is suggested by reports of benefit seen with opioid antagonists such as low-dose naloxone or partial agonists such as buprenorphine in the management of cholestatic itch [42].

7. The $5HT_3$ antagonists such as ondansetron and granisetron have also been found to be effective for itch associated with cholestatic jaundice of advanced cancer and of nonmalignant origin.

8. The selective serotonin reuptake inhibitor (SSRI) paroxetine and the central noradrenaline and serotonin reuptake inhibitor mirtazapine have been found to be effective in cancer-related itch, mirtazapine showing activity in uraemia, lymphoma, and cholestasis without the nausea associated with paroxetine [41].

Fever and sweating

Patients with cancer may experience troublesome fever and sweating. The two are related, but sweating may occur without fever. These symptoms are generally distressing to patients and can result in fatigue, drowsiness, and confusion. The aetiology can be related directly to the tumour (neoplastic fever) or other causes, for example, infection. Both fever and sweating are more common in patients with Hodgkin's disease, leukaemia and tumours with liver metastases.

Management

Although it is inappropriate within a palliative care setting to undertake exhaustive investigations in patients with fever and sweats, it is important to consider the differential diagnoses that may aid appropriate treatment:

- Infection. Look for common foci of infection. Be especially cautious in patients who are susceptible to neutropenia (e.g., those on chemotherapy or with marrow invasion) and in those with an indwelling central line. In the presence of infection, fever may be absent in patients who are on steroids or have a markedly suppressed white cell count.
- Fever associated with advanced cancer.
- Treatment related, for example, some chemotherapy drugs produce fever (e.g., bleomycin), as can blood transfusion.
- Hormonal (e.g., thyrotoxicosis and menopause).
- Anxiety.
- Physiological (secondary to environmental conditions).

In many cases, it is necessary to resort to general measures to provide relief. Paramount among these is a high standard of nursing care, including the provision of a fan, sponging and regular washing, and encouraging the intake of oral fluids. Evidence to support the use of most drug therapies tried in generalised sweating in cancer patients is lacking but the following have been used with varying success: paracetamol; aspirin; NSAIDs; low-dose gabapentin; mirtazepine; fluoxetine, paroxetine, and thalidomide. High-dose steroids have a role in chronic lymphatic leukaemia.

Side effects of palliative oncology treatments

Severe side effects of chemotherapy and radiotherapy weigh heavily in the cost–benefit analysis of palliative interventions. It is important for the patient, the healthcare teams, and the carers to know what effects are likely, how long they may last, and what can be done to alleviate them.

Gastrointestinal system

Oral mucositis

Evidence for the efficacy of many commonly used treatments for mucositis is poor [43]. The mainstay continues to be oral hygiene measures [44]. This should include:
- frequent brushing of teeth/dentures with a soft toothbrush;
- moisturising lips;
- rinsing after each meal with saline; and
- adding sodium bicarbonate to rinse if secretions are thickened.

Patients with mucositis need analgesics, often strong opioids. Topical measures include Gelclair™ that contains polyvinylpyrrolidone and sodium hyaluronate and forms a protective barrier.

Mouthwashes often cause stinging, but the recently introduced mouthwash, Caphosol™ shows superiority over a standard regime in reducing the duration and severity of mucositis in patients undergoing bone marrow transplantation or head and neck radiotherapy [45].

Nausea and vomiting

Nausea and vomiting are worsened by anxiety about cancer, the treatment, and its side effects; hence, psychological support is vital throughout treatment.

Highly emetogenic chemotherapy

Nausea and vomiting usually occur in the first 24–72 h postchemotherapy. They can be managed by administering a $5HT_3$ antagonist plus dexamethasone intravenously prechemotherapy, followed by domperidone 10 mg po tds plus dexamethasone 4–6 mg po daily for 3 days afterwards. For severe vomiting despite the above, a trial of aprepitant is warranted but is initiated only by oncologists.

Less emetogenic chemotherapy

Where chemotherapy is less emetogenic, oral antiemetics usually suffice, for example, cyclizine 50 mg tds or domperidone 10 mg tds.

Radiotherapy

Nausea and vomiting can follow radiotherapy, especially if the stomach, small bowel, or liver is in the treatment field. The symptoms usually occur acutely after each treatment and remit once treatment is complete. Oral antiemetics usually suffice, for example, cyclizine 50 mg tds or haloperidol 1.5 mg bd although if a significant portion of the upper abdomen is within the field, $5HT_3$ antagonists plus dexamethasone as above may be required. Vomiting may be a side effect of radiotherapy to the brain, in which case it will usually respond to an increase in the dose of oral steroids with the addition of cyclizine.

Problems of the lower bowel

Diarrhoea

Diarrhoea is common with pelvic or abdominal radiotherapy. It often begins in the second week of radiotherapy and lasts 1–2 weeks after completion.

Management includes:
- dietary assessment with a reduced fibre diet for the duration of the radiotherapy;
- loperamide titrated to effect +/− codeine phosphate 30–60 mg 6 or 12 hourly (if the patient is not already receiving a strong opioid);
- attention to oral hydration; and
- barrier creams to perianal skin.

Proctitis

Proctitis is common with pelvic radiotherapy. The timing of its occurrence is the same as for diarrhoea (see above). Rectal bleeding may occur. Management involves the use of steroid foam enemas and appropriate analgesia. Warm baths may help to alleviate symptoms. Rectal bleeding occurring more than 6 months after radiotherapy is unusual but may result from telangiectasia and rarely may require surgery although this is hazardous as tissue healing is poor.

Skin

Skin reactions are common with high-dose radiotherapy. Reactions occur 1–2 weeks after the start of radiotherapy and take approximately the same time to heal. Table 12.2 details the types of skin reactions.

The skin is less commonly affected by chemotherapy although rashes are common. Discoloration, erythema, and peeling of the palms and soles are sometimes seen.

Several steps can be taken to improve the comfort of the skin and prevent further damage:
- Protect from friction, by avoiding tight clothing, elastic straps underwired bras, etc.
- Avoid strong sunlight, hot baths, wet shaving, cosmetics, deodorants, adhesive plasters, and perfumed creams.
- Wash with warm water and usual soap. Pat dry with a soft towel and air-dry if possible.
- For erythema, apply moisturising cream, for example, aqueous cream twice daily.
- For dry desquamation, increase frequency of moisturising cream to 4–5 times daily.

Table 12.2 Skin reactions to radiotherapy.

Category of skin reaction	Detail of signs and symptoms
Erythema	The area in the radiotherapy field becomes slightly inflamed and may tingle, usually occurring after 1–2 weeks of treatment
Dry desquamation	The skin becomes hot, flaky, very itchy, and uncomfortable usually occurring after 2–3 weeks
Moist desquamation	Blisters form on the epidermis that sloughs leaving a denuded, painful area of dermis that may exude serum. Moist regions with opposed skin surfaces, such as the perineum or inframammary fold, are particularly affected

- Occasionally hydrocortisone cream 1% is used, if the treated skin is itchy.
- Intrasite gel$^{®}$ is soothing for dry desquamation.
- For very itchy dry desquamation, a glycerine-based hydrogel sheet, for example, Novogel$^{®}$ is very cooling.

Moist desquamation heals best in a warm, moist environment. Dressings should be conformable, comfortable, nonadherent, must not contain metals or cause further skin damage. Intrasite gel$^{®}$ absorbs exudate and helps lift debris and can be used with mepilex$^{®}$ dressing, which is a low adherence silicone dressing.

Hair loss

Temporary hair loss is a variable feature of many chemotherapy regimes, and radiotherapy will also cause temporary alopecia if the scalp is irradiated. The psychological impact should not be underestimated, and wigs and camouflage should be discussed pretreatment.

Marrow suppression

Patients with advanced cancer may have reduced bone marrow reserve and symptomatic anaemia is common. Thrombocytopenia is less common in the absence of chemotherapy although it may occur in the presence of marrow infiltration by tumour. The platelet count may be especially low if there has been prior chemotherapy, wide field radiotherapy, or bone seeking isotopes, particularly in prostate cancer. Anaemia and thrombocytopenia may require transfusion.

Clinically significant neutropenia is uncommon without current cytotoxic chemotherapy treatment. It predisposes to overwhelming bacterial sepsis, particularly when the absolute neutrophil count is less than $1 \times 10^9/l$. Neutropenic sepsis requires urgent specialist inpatient treatment with IV antibiotics. Urgent admission to the treating oncology unit should be arranged for assessment of any patient having chemotherapy who develops symptoms or signs of sepsis, particularly sore throat, fever $> 38°C$, rigors, cough productive of purulent sputum or shock.

Lymphoedema

Lymphoedema is a progressive, chronic, incurable condition that results in the accumulation of protein-rich fluid within the interstitial tissue space. It usually affects the limbs, but it is often seen in the adjoining truncal, genital, and head and neck areas, resulting in swelling and heaviness with marked physical and psychological consequences, which may impact on quality of life, independence, function, and mobility.

There is no doubt that the earlier lymphoedema treatment is introduced, the more successful it is. However, lymphoedema is unlikely to resolve completely, particularly if there is evidence of progressive disease. As more patients spend longer in the advanced stages of cancer, the prevalence of lymphoedema will increase, and it is therefore essential that early signs of oedema are actively sought and that intervention is instigated as soon as possible. Ideally this should include an early referral to a local lymphoedema specialist.

Pathophysiology

Damage to the normal routes of lymphatic drainage commonly occurs following surgery, radiotherapy, and with tumour involvement. The patients at greatest risk of developing lymphoedema are those with melanoma and sarcoma, breast, gynaecological, urological and head and neck cancers. The risk is highest if they have undergone surgery and/or irradiation to a major group of lymph nodes causing an interruption to the lymphatic drainage routes. This leads to the remaining vessels becoming overloaded resulting in swelling and increasing the risk of an acute inflammatory episode (AIE) (also referred to as cellulitis [46]).

Clinical features

In the early stages of lymphoedema, the swollen tissues have the following features:

- soft;
- pit with pressure; and
- reduce with elevation.

If left untreated, accumulation of proteins within the tissues results in thickening and fibrosis [47] which may lead to:

- distorted limb shape
- skin folds
- skin changes (hyperkeratosis, papillomatosis)
- lymphorrhea (leakage of lymph through the skin surface)

Assessment

Early assessment and management of lymphoedema is essential in reducing both the physical and the psychological effects of this chronic condition. A holistic assessment of patients with lymphoedema is essential whether this is a new or progressive feature. This includes:

- consideration of all possible aetiologies;
- identification of any treatable precipitating factors;
- physical effects including functional impairment;
- recognition of acute complications; and
- identification of the psychological and social effects on patient and carers [48].

Skin condition

Examination of the skin for:

- dryness;
- fungal infections;
- breaks to the skin;
- AIE or cellulitis; and
- lymphorrhea.

Function and mobility

Lymphoedema can cause:

- reduction in function/mobility;
- stiffness of the joints;
- discomfort; and
- difficulties with posture and balance.

These can lead to both physical and psychosocial problems.

Pain

Lymphoedema does not cause acute pain, but some pain is reported in up to 50% of patients, most of whom take regular analgesia [49]. Most patients complain of:

- tightness of the tissues;
- aching and heaviness in the affected area;

- strain on joints/muscles due to the weight of the limb; and
- neuropathic pain.

If pain is severe, disease progression should be explored and complications considered. Infection/cellulitis, inflammation, and thrombosis may exacerbate pain.

Psychological issues

Patients' perception of body image can be affected by lymphoedema and may cause psychological distress. An insight into the individual patient's experience is important in achieving patient-centred outcomes. A patient may experience:

- reduced self-esteem;
- altered body image;
- depression/anxiety; and
- difficulty with sexual/family/social relationships [48,50].

Management

Referral to a local lymphoedema service in a timely manner is essential to achieve the best possible treatment outcome for the individual with lymphoedema, even those with advanced disease.

The aim of management includes:

- reduction of swelling;
- control; and
- palliation (comfort measures).

The use of diuretics in the treatment of lymphoedema has little benefit as there is no evidence to suggest that diuretics improve lymphatic drainage [55].

Following a holistic assessment of the patient's lymphoedema status, an individual management programme will be discussed and agreed with the patient. The choice between maintenance and intensive treatment will depend on the complexity of their lymphoedema.

Maintenance treatment

This may include a combination of:

- skin care;
- support/compression;
- exercise; and
- simple lymphatic drainage (SLD).

Intensive treatment

Intensive treatment is therapist led and is indicated for severe lymphoedema, misshapen limbs, skin folds, damaged or fragile skin, lymphorrhea, swollen digits, facial, genital, and truncal lymphoedema [51].

This may include:

- skin care;
- exercises;

- manual lymphatic drainage (MLD)/intermittent pneumatic compression (IPC) pump in lymphassist mode;
- multilayer lymphoedema bandaging (MLLB); and
- compression.

Skin care

Care of the skin is an important part of treatment for any patient with lymphoedema as this helps to reduce the risk of infection by maintaining skin integrity:
- Wash daily using a neutral soap/soap substitute.
- Dry well.
- Apply emollient twice daily.
- Observe for damage to the skin.
- Avoid injections/blood sampling and blood pressure monitoring on the affected limb.
- Treat any skin condition.

Exercise

It is important to understand the complexity of movement and its effect on lymphoedema. Exercise promotes the drainage of lymph by activating the muscle pump and also helps to maintain or improve joint mobility, posture, and function. The use of slings should be discouraged unless required to relieve pain or support flaccid limbs. It should be remembered that hosiery should always be worn during exercise, movements should be slow and controlled, and over-exertion should be discouraged as it induces vasodilation and lymph production.

Patients who are weak and debilitated and those with neurological dysfunction, such as spinal cord compression, are at particularly risk of dependent oedema [52]:
- Exercises should be tailored to the patient's need, ability, and disease status.
- The affected limb should be elevated while resting.
- Referral to a physiotherapist should be made if there is evidence of restricted movement.

Compression garments

The aim of compression garments in the long-term management of lymphoedema is to reduce/maintain the individual's swelling, but garments should only be measured and supplied by an appropriately trained practitioner [53]. Various factors must be taken into account when deciding the suitability of compression garments on the individual patient.

Contraindications:
- Arterial insufficiency <0.5ABPI for lower limbs.
- Acute cardiac failure.
- Shape distortion/skin folds.
- Lymphorrhea.

- Ulceration/fragile skin.
- Severe peripheral neuropathy.
- Infection (cellulitis in acute phase).
- DVT/PE (in acute phase).
- Patient inability to apply/remove garment.

General information for the wearing of compression garments:
- The fabric must be evenly distributed.
- It must not be too tight or too loose but should feel firm and comfortable.
- It must never be folded over at the top or bottom.
- It should be worn all day and removed at night unless advised otherwise by the lymphoedema practitioner.

Simple lymphatic drainage

SLD is a simplified version of MLD and is taught to patients and carers to carry out at home on a daily basis. Its aim is to move lymphatic fluid from the congested area to an area where it can drain more effectively. Gentle stretches of the skin against the underlying tissue help improve superficial lymphatic drainage. The use of creams and oils are not advised while carrying out SLD.

Manual lymphatic drainage

MLD is a specialised gentle massage performed by trained practitioners and is indicated as part of intensive treatment. There are several recognised techniques that follow the lymphatic pathways and are particularly useful for facial, genital, and truncal lymphoedema.

Multilayer lymphoedema bandaging

MLLB is carried out by a trained practitioner as part of intensive treatment and may also form part of long-term or palliative management. Using inelastic bandages, it is applied to the limb to form a rigid casing that produces a high working pressure, low resting pressure that produces a massaging effect while exercising. This stimulates lymphatic flow, reducing limb volume, improving limb shape and may reverse lymphorrhea [54].

Intermittent pneumatic compression pump

IPC is an electrical air compression pump that is used as part of lymphoedema treatment by practitioners who have received training at a specialist level. Its use aids lymphatic drainage, softens tissues, and helps reduce limb volume.

Cellulitis/acute inflammatory episode

Cellulitis is an acute inflammation of the skin and SC tissues caused by a bacterial infection, it is important to recognise and treat promptly episodes of cellulitis in lymphoedema patients to reduce further complications.

Clinical features may include:
- Erythema
- Pain
- Increased swelling
- Warmth
- Blisters
- Systemic upset
  Precipitating factors may include:
- Injury to the affected area
- Breaks to the skin
- Insect bites/stings
- Fungal infection.

Management

(See Consensus Document: British Lymphology Society [46])
- Commence appropriate antibiotics, to continue until cellulitis has resolved.
- Mark area of erythema.
- Bed rest/elevation of the limb.
- Appropriate analgesia.
- Removal of compression garment until able to tolerate.
- Increase fluid intake.
- Stop SLD/MLD until infection resolved.

Recurrent cellulitis

Prophylactic antibiotic treatment should be considered for patients who have two or more episodes of infection per year.

Lymphorrhea

This describes the leakage of lymph fluid through a break in the skin.

Treatment of lymphorrhea:
- Apply emollient to protect surrounding skin.
- Cover leaking area with a nonadherent, absorbent dressing to help prevent infection.
- Apply appropriate bandages (short stretch/crepes) changed frequently to avoid maceration.

Palliative phase

Reduction of swelling is often unrealistic for patients with locally recurrent advanced cancer, particularly when the trunk is congested. In these circumstances, treatment of the limb will only result in an increase of oedema centrally. The palliative phase of lymphoedema management uses modified conventional treatments to address a patient's individual needs and improve the quality of their life.

Swelling often increases as progressive tumour infiltrates into the skin and disrupts lymphatic drainage. Tissues can become very engorged, hard, and discoloured, with loss of skin integrity, and lymphorrhea. Swelling often extends beyond the root of the limb into the truncal area.

External support may be applied in the form of modified support bandaging and appropriate wound dressings for those with areas of skin breakdown, with the support of community nurses.

Airway patency and care of the patient with a tracheostomy or laryngectomy

A tracheostomy is an artificial opening from the anterior neck into the trachea. Tracheostomies are always kept patent by the use of a tube. A tracheostomy is indicated for:
- bypassing an obstructed upper airway;
- long-term ventilation; and
- facilitating suction.

A laryngectomy is surgical removal of the larynx to form an end stoma of the trachea on the anterior neck. The stoma does not usually require a tube to maintain the opening unless it has a tendency to shrink or distort. A laryngectomy is indicated for laryngeal cancer that does not respond to radiotherapy.

Types of tracheostomy tube in use

Plastic tubes with an inner tube (Shiley and Tracheotwist)

These come in various styles to include cuffs and fenestration or a combination. They need to be changed about monthly.

The cuff is used to create a seal between the trachea and the tube when ventilating a patient or to reduce excessive aspiration of secretions. Excessive pressure in the cuff (>30 mm Hg) will cause tracheal necrosis and stenosis. If a cuffed tube is in situ but the cuff is not required, it should be deflated. Cuffs should only be inflated if there is a specific rationale to do so.

Fenestrations are used to allow air into the upper airway to facilitate speech or to wean the patient before removal of the tube.

The inner tracheostomy tube facilitates cleaning of the tube and removal of secretions to prevent a build-up of crusts obstructing the tube. Inner tubes are also used to "open" and "close" the fenestration.

Metal tubes

Some patients with a long-term tracheostomy have metal tubes as they are thin walled, giving the best lumen available. Negus tubes are the most common. The inner tube may have speaking valves, and the patient usually has two sets of tubes that are changed approximately 2–3 weekly. The tubes are reusable.

Adjustable flange

This is used when an adjustable length is needed. Usually used for longer tubes but occasionally used when a short tube is needed. Tubes are flexible and armoured to prevent kinking and changed 3 monthly. Inner tubes should be replaced monthly. They come with or without cuff.

For all tube types, it is essential that a **spare tube** of the same size as the patient has and one a size smaller should be kept at the patient's bedside in case the tube is accidentally dislodged. Without this the tracheostomy would collapse and the patient asphyxiate.

Routine care for tracheostomy patients

Suction

Suction should be carried out following assessment of the patient rather than at set intervals. The patient will need suction if:

• secretions are audible and not cleared by cleaning the inner tube
• the patient is desaturating or the work of breathing is increasing
• there is any indication that the patient may have aspirated

The technique for suction is detailed in Box 12.8

Box 12.8 Suctioning of the patient with a tracheostomy

• Suction pressure should be maintained below 20 kPa.
• Using sterile gloves, the suction catheter should be gently introduced into the tracheostomy until the end is just clear of the distal end of the tube. If the patient is conscious, they will start to cough at this point.
• Suction is applied by occluding the port on the catheter with your thumb. Gently withdraw the catheter while suctioning, over a period of about 10 s.
• The suction catheters are multiholed and should not be rotated as this causes trauma.
• Disguard the suction catheter and reassess patient for continuing need for suction.
• Flush the suction tubing with water.

Inner tubes

The inner tracheostomy tube should be removed, cleaned, and replaced at least every 4 h or more frequently if the patient is very productive of secretions. Inner tubes should be cleaned under running water, using a disposable cleaning swab to dislodge any tenacious secretions and dried after cleaning. Ideally the patient should have two inner tubes used in rotation.

Cleaning the traceostomy

The tracheostomy site should be cleaned aseptically twice a day, removing all secretions from under and around the flange. Once the tract is well established and the surrounding skin has healed, the area should be cleaned using a clean technique.

Dressings and ties

The ties for the tracheostomy tube should be changed daily. One person must hold the tube in place while another changes the ties. The dressing should be changed at least daily but more if required. Precut dressings should be used to prevent lint being introduced into the tract.

Humidification

Regular saline nebulisers should be used to prevent crusting of secretions. A heat and moisture exchange (HME) device or a bib should be used to prevent the airway becoming dry between nebulisers. Any oxygen administered must be warmed and humidified. Good systemic hydration of the patient helps to prevent secretions crusting.

Cuff pressure

If a cuffed tube is being used, the cuff pressure should be monitored twice a day and maintained below 25 cm H_2O.

Spare tube

Check every day that there are spare tubes for the patient: one of the same size as the patient has and one a size smaller. The tube should be kept near the patient in case the in situ tube is accidentally dislodged.

Routine care for laryngectomy patients

Suction

Suction is carried out in the same way as for tracheostomy patients (Box 12.8). However, there is no tube in situ and the trachea is shorter; hence, the catheter is not introduced so far. The tip of the catheter usually remains visible throughout suctioning.

Tubes, studs, and ties

If the patient is using a laryngectomy tube or a stoma stud to maintain the shape of the stoma, it should be removed and cleaned at least twice a day under running water and dried before re-insertion. It is usually necessary to use lubricating gel to re-insert laryngectomy tubes. Silicone laryngectomy tubes do not have inner tubes as it is safe to remove the whole tube to clean it. Tube ties, if used, are replaced daily.

Cleaning

The skin surrounding the stoma is cleaned with tap water and a cloth. Liquid secretions can be removed from the stoma by the patient coughing and wiping them away or by suction. Crusted secretions should be removed gently from the stoma with round-ended forceps.

Humidification

An HME device should be used. This can be a bib, a disposable foam cover, or a base-plate and HME filter. Bibs can be washed and reused three times. Base-plates can be worn until they start to come away from the skin. The HME filter or foam cover is changed daily.

Nebulisers should be used regularly, and any oxygen used should be warmed and humidified.

Speaking valves

There may be a speaking valve at the back of the stoma. Care should be taken to prevent it being dislodged during cleaning. The valve can be carefully cleaned in situ, with a special brush.

Communication

Phonation can be achieved by some tracheostomy and laryngectomy patients by using finger occlusion of the airway to force air upwards into the mouth. Occasionally a patient will have an "electronic voice-box." Communication is often very frustrating and tiring for both patients and carers, and a great deal of patience is required. Nonverbal communication will be used by both tracheostomy and laryngectomy patients. This may be using body language (pointing, thumbs up, eyebrows lifted, etc.) or writing.

In tracheostomy patients, the air will pass around the outside of the tube or through the fenestration if they have one. This requires a patent airway above the tracheostomy. Some tracheostomy patients use a valve such as a Passy Muir or Voiceline valve to use "hands free" speech. In laryngectomy patients the air is passed through the speaking valve and is vibrated in the pharynx.

References

1. Levack P, Graham J, Collie D, et al. Don't wait for a sensory level–listen to the symptoms: a prospective audit of the delays in diagnosis of malignant cord compression. *Clin Oncol (R Coll Radiol)* 2002; 14(6): 472–480.

2. Rades D, Rudat V, Veninga T, et al. A score predicting posttreatment ambulatory status in patients irradiated for metastatic spinal cord compression. *Int J Radiat Oncol Biol Phys* 2008; 72(3): 905–908.

3. Rades D, Heidenreich F, Karstens JH, Final results of a prospective study of the prognostic value of the time to develop motor deficits before irradiation in metastatic spinal cord compression. *Int J Radiat Oncol Biol Phys* 2002; 53(4): 975–979.

4. Tokuhashi Y. A revised scoring system for preoperative evaluation of metastatic spine tumor prognosis. *Spine* 2005; 30(19): 2186–2191.

5. Putz C, van Middendorp JJ, Pouw MH, et al. Malignant cord compression: A critical appraisal of prognostic factors predicting functional outcome after surgical treatment. *J Craniovertebr Junction Spine* 2010; 1(2): 67–73.

6. Patchell R, Tibbs PA, Regine WF, et al. Direct decompressive surgical resection in the treatment of spinal cord compression caused by metastatic cancer: a randomised trial. *Lancet Oncol* 2005; 366(9486): 643–648.

7. Loblaw DA and Laperriere NJ. Emergency treatment of malignant extradural spinal cord compression: an evidence-based guideline. *J Clin Oncol* 1998; 16(4): 1613–1624.

8. Rades D, Stalpers LJ, Hulshof MC, et al. Comparison of 1 × 8 Gy and 10 × 3 Gy for functional outcome in patients with metastatic spinal cord compression. *Int J Radiat Oncol Biol Phys* 2005; 62(2): 514–518.

9. Rades D, Lange M, Veninga T, et al. Final results of a prospective study comparing the local control of short-course and long-course radiotherapy for metastatic spinal cord compression. *Int J Radiat Oncol Biol Phys* 2011; 79(2): 524–530.

10. Rowell NP and Gleeson FV. Steroids, radiotherapy, chemotherapy and stents for superior vena caval obstruction in carcinoma of the bronchus: a systematic review. *Clin Oncol* 2002; 14: 338–351.

11. Ganeshan A, Hon LQ, Warakaulle DR, et al. Superior vena caval stenting for SVC obstruction: current status. *Eur J Radiol* 2009; 71: 343–349.

12. McNicol ED, Strassels S, Goudas L, et al. NSAIDS or paracetamol, alone or combined with opioids, for cancer pain. *Cochrane Database Syst Rev* 2005; (2): CD005180.

13. Lutz S, Berk L, Chang E, et al. Palliative radiotherapy for bone metastases: an ASTRO evidence-based guideline. *Int J Radiat Oncol Biol Phys* 2011; 79(4): 965–976.

14. Sze WM, Shelley M, Held I, et al. Palliation of metastatic bone pain: single fraction versus multifraction radiotherapy. *Cochrane Database Syst Rev* 2002; (1): CD004721.

15. Bone Pain Trial Working Party. 8 Gy single fraction radiotherapy for the treatment of metastatic skeletal pain: randomised comparison with a multifraction schedule over 12 months of patient follow-up. *Radiother Oncol* 1999; 52: 111–121.

16. Dearnaley DP, Bayly RJ, A'Hern RP, et al. Palliation of bone metastases in prostate cancer. Hemibody irradiation or strontium-89? *Clin Oncol* 1992; 4(2): 101–107.

17. Baczyk M, Czepczynski R, Milecki P, et al. [89]Sr versus [153]Sm-EDTMP: comparison of treatment efficacy of painful bone metastases in prostate and breast carcinoma. *Nucl Med Commun* 2007; 28(4): 245–250.

18. Mhaskar R, Redzepovic J, Wheatley K, et al. Bisphosphonates in multiple myeloma. *Cochrane Database Syst Rev* 2010; (3): CD003188.

19. Pavlakis N, Schmidt RL and Stockler MR. Bisphosphonates for breast cancer. *Cochrane Database Syst Rev* 2005; (3): CD003474.

20. Yuen KK, Shelley M and Sze WM. Bisphosphonates for advanced prostate cancer. *Cochrane Database Syst Rev* 2006; (4): CD006250.

21. Saad F and Eastham J. Zoledronic acid improves clinical outcomes when administered before onset of bone pain in patients with prostate cancer. *Urology* 2010; 76: 1175–1181.

22. Aapro M, Abrahamsson PA, Body JJ, et al. Guidance on the use of bisphosphonates in solid tumours: recommendations of an international expert panel. *Ann Oncol* 2008; 19: 420–432.

23. Langer C and Hirsh V. Skeletal morbidity in lung cancer patients with bone metastases: demonstrating the need for early diagnosis and treatment with bisphosphonates. *Lung Cancer* 2010; 67: 4–11.

24. Wong R and Wiffen PJ. Bisphosphonates for the relief of pain secondary to bone metastases. *Cochrane Database Syst Rev* 2002; (2): CD002068.

25. Halpin RJ, Bendok BR and Liu JC. Minimally invasive treatments for spinal metastases: vertebroplasty, kyphoplasty, and radiofrequency ablation. *J Support Oncol* 2004; 2: 339–355.

26. Boonen S, Van Meirhaeghe J and Bastian L. Balloon kyphoplasty for the treatment of acute vertebral compression fractures: 2-year results from a randomized trial. *J Bone Miner Res* 2011; 26: 1627–1637.

27. Anselmetti GC. Osteoplasty: percutaneous bone cement injection beyond the spine. *Semin Intervent Radiol* 2010; 27: 199–208.

28. Mirels H. Metastatic disease in long bones. A proposed scoring system for diagnosing impending pathologic fractures. *Clin Orthop* 1989; 249: 256–264.

29. Fuentes R, Bonfill Cosp X and Expósito Hernandez J. Surgery versus radiosurgery for patients with a solitary brain metastasis from non-small cell lung cancer. *Cochrane Database Syst Rev* 2006; (1): CD004840.

30. Suh JH, Videtic GMM, Aref AM, et al. ACR appropriateness criteria: single brain metastasis. *Curr Probl Cancer* 2010; 34: 162–174.

31. Bezjak A, Adam A, Barton R, et al. Symptom response after palliative radiotherapy for patients with brain metastases. *Eur J Cancer* 2002; 38: 487–496.

32. Gerrard GE, Prestwich RJ and Edwards A. Investigating the palliative efficacy of whole-brain radiotherapy for patients with multiple-brain metastases and poor prognostic features. *Clin Oncol (R Coll Radiol)* 2003; 15(7): 422–428.

33. Primrose JN. Surgery for colorectal liver metastases. *Br J Cancer* 2010; 102: 1313–1318.

34. Pfannschmidt J. Surgical resection of pulmonary metastases from colorectal cancer: a systematic review of published series. *Ann Thorac Surg* 2007; 84(1): 324–338.

35. Neville-Webbe HL and Coleman RE. Bisphosphonates and RANK ligand inhibitors for the treatment and prevention of metastatic bone disease. *Eur J Cancer* 2010; 46(7): 1211–1222.

36. Major P, Lortholary A, Hon J, et al. Zoledronic acid is superior to pamidronate in the treatment of hypercalcemia of malignancy: a pooled analysis of two randomized, controlled clinical trials. *J Clin Oncol* 2001; 19(2): 558–567.

37. Kovacs CS, MacDonald SM, Chik CL, et al. Hypercalcemia of malignancy in the palliative care patient: a treatment strategy. *J Pain Symptom Manage* 1995; 10: 224–232.

38. Ishioka J, Kageyama Y, Inoue M, et al. Prognostic model for predicting survival after palliative urinary diversion for ureteral obstruction: analysis of 140 cases. *J Urol* 2008; 180(2): 618–621.

39. Kouba E, Wallen EM and Pruthi RS. Management of ureteral obstruction due to advanced malignancy: optimizing therapeutic and palliative outcomes. *J Urol* 2008; 180(2): 444–450.

40. Watkinson AF, A'Hern RP, Jones A, et al. The role of percutaneous nephrostomy in malignant urinary tract obstruction. *Clin Radiol* 1993; 47(1): 32–35.

41. Zylicz Z, Krajnik M, Sorge AA, et al. Paroxetine in the treatment of severe non-dermatological pruritus: a randomized, controlled trial. *J Pain Symptom Manage* 2003; 26(6): 1105–1112.

42. Zylicz Z, Stork N and Krajnik M. Severe pruritus of cholestasis in disseminated cancer: developing a rational treatment strategy. A case report. *J Pain Symptom Manage* 2005; 29(1): 100–103.

43. Clarkson JE, Worthington HV and Eden OB. Interventions for treating oral mucositis for patients with cancer receiving treatment. *Cochrane Database Syst Rev* 2007; (2): CD001973.

44. Shih A, Miaskowski C, Dodd MJ, et al. A research review of the current treatments for radiation-induced oral mucositis in patients with head and neck cancer. *Oncol Nurs Forum* 2002; 29(7): 1063–1080.

45. Papas AS, Clark RE, Martuscelli G, et al. A prospective, randomized trial for the prevention of mucositis in patients

undergoing hematopoietic stem cell transplantation. *Bone Marrow Transplant* 2003; 31(8): 705–712.

46. The British Lymphology Society. *Consensus Document on the management of cellulitis in lymphoedema.* Available at www.thebls.com (accessed on June 2011).

47. Linnitt N. Complex skin changes in chronic oedemas. *Br J Commun Nurs* 2007; 12(4): S10–S15.

48. Keeley V. Oedema in advanced cancer. In: Twycross R, Jenns K, Todd J (eds), *Lymphoedema.* Oxford: Radcliffe Medical Press, 2000, pp. 338–358.

49. Moffatt CJ, Franks PJ and Doherty D. Lymphoedema: an underestimated health problem. *QJM* 2003; 96: 731–738.

50. Woods M. Lymphoedema. In:Cooper J (ed.), *Stepping into Palliative Care.* Oxford: Radcliffe Medical Press, 2000, pp. 81–88.

51. Hampton S. Chronic oedema and lymphoedema of the lower limb. *Br J Commun Nurs* 2010; 15: S4–S12.

52. Hughes K. Exercise and lymphoedema. In: Twycross R, Jenns K, Todd J (eds), *Lymphoedema.* Oxford: Radcliffe Medical Press, 2000, 140–151.

53. Lay-Flurrie K. Use of compression hosiery in chronic oedema and lymphoedema. *Br J Nurs* 2011; 20(7): 418–422.

54. Linnitt N and Davies R. Fundamentals of compression in the management of lymphoedema. *Br J Nurs* 2007; 16(10): 588–592.

55. Best practice for the management of lymphoedema. In: *Lymphoedema Framework—International Consensus.* London: MEP Ltd, 2006.

Acknowledgement. We acknowledge the contribution to this chapter by Roslyn White, Macmillan Head and Neck Cancer Nurse Specialist at the University Hospitals of Leicester, UK.

13 Palliative Care for People with Progressive Neurological Disorders

David Oliver

Wisdom Hospice, Rochester, UK

Introduction

Palliative care is often appropriate for people with neurological disease from soon after the time of diagnosis, as there is no curative treatment, and at best, treatment may slow the disease progression. The involvement of palliative care with these patients and families has been stressed in the UK National Service Framework for long-term conditions [1] and the National End of Life Care Programme document "End of life care in long term neurological conditions" [2]. In the United Kingdom, it is estimated that 350,000 people need help with daily living due to a neurological disease and 850,000 people care for people with a neurological condition [1].

The aim of palliative care is to minimise the problems that may occur and maximise the abilities and opportunities for patients to live their lives as fully as possible, despite disability and disease progression. There may be specific issues for each disease, but many of the principles of care are common to all, regardless of diagnosis–motor neurone disease (MND), Parkinson's disease (PD), multiple sclerosis (MS), Huntington's disease (HD), and muscular dystrophies (MD). Although the involvement for each disease will be rare for the primary health-care team—a primary care professional (CP) such as a general practitioner (GP) may only see one patient with MND in their career—the principles of good palliative care will apply to all.

Background

Motor neuron disease

In many parts of the world, the term amyotrophic lateral sclerosis (ALS) is used to represent the condition that in the United Kingdom is referred to as MND. In the United States, clinicians may be familiar with the terminology Lou Gehrig's disease. In the United Kingdom, ALS is used to define a subgroup of patients with MND and this is explained in Table 13.1. Hereafter, the term MND will be used to refer to ALS or Lou Gehrig's disease.

MND is a progressive disease of unknown cause, although there is a familial history in up to 10% of patients—there are now several genetic associations recognised and families are often aware of the risks of MND. There is progressive loss of neurons—primarily motor neurons—but there is increasing evidence of damage to the frontal lobe of the brain and other areas. There may be loss of upper and lower motor neurons leading to a mixed pattern of weakness, wasting, spasticity, and bulbar effects, affecting speech and swallowing. The presentation is often insidious and there may be long delays in diagnosis. Cognitive change, particularly in decision making, is commonly seen and frontotemporal dementia, which may precede the symptoms of MND, is seen in 10–15% of patients. Every patient is different, and the rate of progression and areas affected vary greatly.

Handbook of Palliative Care, Third Edition. Edited by Christina Faull, Sharon de Caestecker, Alex Nicholson and Fraser Black.
© 2012 by John Wiley and Sons, Inc. Published 2012 by John Wiley & Sons, Inc.

Table 13.1 Motor neurone disease.

Motor neurone disease	Clinical findings	Prognosis
ALS; 66% of patients	Lesions of upper and lower motor neurones; with involvement of the corticospinal tracts	Median survival is 3 years
Progressive muscular atrophy (PMA); 8% of patients	Largely affects lower motor neurones in the first instance	The most, favourable prognosis, with some patients surviving more than 15 years
Progressive bulbar palsy (PBP); 26% of patients	Involvement of the brain stem motor nuclei predominates; speech and swallowing affected	Poor, 18–24 months

MND has an incidence of 1.7 per 100,000 and a prevalence of 5–6 per 100,000 [3]. Three main variants of MND are described and these are summarised in Table 13.1. The presentation may be unclear and mixed patterns are seen. The average survival is 3–5 years but 10% of patients live over 10 years [3]. In the United Kingdom, approximately 6,000 people have MND and 1,600 deaths occur every year.

The only drug treatment for MND is riluzole, which was shown in trials to increase survival and seems to slow the rate of progression [4]. In the United Kingdom, riluzole has been approved by National Institute for Health and Clinical Excellence (NICE) for patients with ALS form of MND, but should be initiated by a specialist, and monitoring of liver and haematological function is necessary.

Multiple sclerosis

MS is characterised by demyelination within the nervous system, and the symptoms and signs will depend on the area affected but include hemiparesis, hemisensory loss, internuclear ophthalmoplegia, optic neuritis, ataxia, and tremor. Bladder and bowel function can be affected and cognitive impairment is common. The classification of MS is shown in Table 13.2.

Patients may experience progressive symptoms or intermittent exacerbations, with periods of recovery between attacks. Women are more commonly affected than men, and there may be hereditary factors in the aetiology. Most patients develop the disease between 20 and 50 years of age and over time there is progressive disability. The prognosis is long with a median survival of 28 years for men and 33 years for women, but after 15 years a large number of patients are severely disabled [5].

In the United Kingdom, MS is more common than MND with a lifetime risk of 1 in 100 and a prevalence of 0.1–0.2%, and there are an estimated 100,000 people with MS and approximately 1,200 deaths every year. Steroids are used to reduce the severity and shorten the duration of relapse. There are disease-modifying treatments available that do reduce the number of relapses, namely β-interferon, glatiramer acetate, and natalizumab. These are all administered by injection or infusion and need to be carefully monitored.

Parkinson's disease

PD is a progressive disease in which there is neuronal loss from the substantia nigra, with associated inclusions in the neurons (Lewy bodies). This leads to bradykinesia (slowness of movement) with cogwheel rigidity and rest tremor. There are many other symptoms such as autonomic dysfunction and cognitive changes—including Lewy body dementia in about 20% of patients. The prognosis is very variable and with dopamine replacement therapy, the symptoms can be eased for many years. The average prognosis is 28 years [6]. In the United Kingdom, there are estimated to be 180,000 people with PD and about 7,000 deaths per year, with PD as a contributory factor.

There are parkinsonian syndromes (Parkinson's plus) that may present initially like PD but are often less responsive to treatment and progress more rapidly:
• Multiple system atrophy (MSA), with autonomic dysfunction.
• Progressive supranuclear palsy (PSP), with limited eye movement, cognitive change, and physical instability.

The prognosis is usually 2–4 years for diagnosis and there is progressive severe disability [7]. In the United

Table 13.2 Multiple sclerosis.

Multiple sclerosis type	Clinical features
Primary progressive	Gradual worsening of illness without clear exacerbations
	Usually diagnosed in people in their 40s
	Steadily worsening symptoms—rate of change varies
Relapsing remitting	85% of people diagnosed with MS
	Pattern of relapse or flare-up of symptoms (attack or exacerbation) with remissions in between
	Relapse is defined as new symptoms/return of previous symptoms for over 24 h
	Disease-modifying drugs may be helpful
Secondary progressive	65% of people with relapsing remitting disease develop this form within 15 years
	Continued deterioration over 6 months, with or without relapses
	Certain disease-modifying drugs may be helpful

Kingdom, there are estimated to be 10,000 people with PSP and 3,000 with MSA.

Huntington's disease

HD is inherited as an autosomal dominant disorder and presents usually between 30 and 50 years of age. Presentation can be as personality change, often irritability or aggression, associated with choreiform movements, bradykinesia, and slowness of speech. Depression is common and cognitive change often develops as the disease progresses, with ensuing dementia [8].

The prevalence of HD is 5–10 per 100,000 and so the estimates are that there are about 6,500 people with HD in the United Kingdom. There are no specific treatments. As it is inherited, it is possible to undertake predictive gene testing, but careful pre- and post-test counselling is essential.

Muscular dystrophies

These are a group of inherited disorders characterised by degeneration of different muscle groups. Although not strictly neurological disorders, they exhibit similar symptomatology. Duchenne muscular dystrophy (DMD) is most commonly seen in adult palliative care and is the variant that will be referred to in the remainder of this chapter. It is an X-linked recessive disorder, which means it is carried by females and is expressed in males. Thirty percent are due to spontaneous mutations.

Proximal muscle weakness is seen with patients having increasing difficulty walking and standing. This typically occurs between 4 and 5 years of age, and progresses to being wheelchair bound, usually in the teenage years.

With artificial ventilatory support, patients are now living longer into adulthood and reaching their 30s and 40s [9].

Due to its genetic nature, genetic counselling can be important for parents when making decisions about future family planning. Treatments for DMD are aimed at prevention and treatment of complications and include physiotherapy, surgery for scoliosis, and artificial ventilation for respiratory failure. With increased survival, the profile of complications in DMD is changing. By the age of 18 years, about 90% of patients will have an associated cardiomyopathy that results eventually in cardiac failure. The cardiomyopathy is incurable and treatment of heart failure (HF) is entirely supportive, using angiotensin-converting enzyme inhibitors (ACEIs) and diuretics [10]. Therapies directed at improvement in skeletal muscle function do not improve cardiac muscle function and may even worsen it. While 20% of deaths used to be from HF due to cardiomyopathy, it is thought likely this will increase as noninvasive ventilatory support prolongs life, increasing the risk of development of cardiomyopathy and its consequences [9].

Symptom management

As there are no curative treatments for these progressive neurological diseases, the primary aim of management should be symptom management and addressing other issues—physical, psychological, social, and spiritual. As outlined in Chapter 1, *The Context and Principles of Palliative Care*, good symptom management requires:

- careful history of the symptom;
- careful physical examination;

- relevant investigation; and
- discussion with the patient and family of possible options, including the advantages and disadvantages of treatment.

Pain

Pain is common in all these neurological diseases:

PD	85% [11]
MND	73% [12]
MS	34–82% [5]

Careful, systematic assessment is essential as pain may be due to a variety of causes and requires individualised management.

Musculoskeletal pain

This may occur due to altered muscle tone around joints—particularly, the shoulder—or to restricted movement. Management includes:

- careful positioning;
- physiotherapy, including passive movements, to maintain joint mobility;
- nonsteroidal anti-inflammatory drugs, although there are the risks of gastric irritation or bleeding; and
- intra-articular injections of steroid and local anaesthetic.

Muscle cramps

If muscles are spastic—due to upper motor neuron damage in MND or MS—cramp and spasm may be troublesome. Careful positioning and physiotherapy are helpful and muscle relaxant drugs may be tried:

- Baclofen 5–20 mg three or four times daily.
- Tizanidine 2–24 mg per day in three or four divided doses.
- Dantrolene 25–100 mg four times daily.
- Diazepam 5 mg at night increasing slowly.

All these drugs may cause drowsiness and may reduce mobility, as the spasticity may allow some mobility and if this is reduced walking may be more difficult.

Botulinum toxin injections can be helpful if spasticity is localised to one muscle group [13].

Skin pressure pain

If a patient is immobile and remains in one position for some time, they may experience discomfort and pain—although often they do not appreciate how much pain they are experiencing as this develops slowly over time. Good positioning and regular help in movement is essential but analgesics are often required. They should be administered according to the World Health Organisation (WHO) analgesic ladder—see Chapter 9, *Pain and Its Management*, for more detail. Opioids are often helpful and experience, particularly in MND, has shown that they can be used effectively and safely [14].

Pain specific to the condition

There may be specific pains related to the disease process itself. For instance, in MS, paroxysmal pains, similar to trigeminal neuralgia, are common and may require treatment with anticonvulsant drugs. In PD, pain may be unrelated to the disease itself, but is due to pathology that is worsened and modified due to the changes in movement and muscle tone [11].

Breathlessness and respiratory issues

Patients with neurological disease may develop problems with respiration for several reasons:

- Infection, particularly aspiration pneumonia if there are swallowing problems.
- Posture, a person who is wheelchair or bedbound may have restricted chest movement.
- Weakness of respiratory muscles—the diaphragm, intercostal muscles, and accessory muscles. This may cause breathlessness but may present as respiratory failure, particularly at night, leading to orthopnea, poor sleep due to arousals caused by hypoxia, dreams, morning headache, nonrefreshing sleep, anorexia, and a general feeling of being unwell. This is particularly problematic in MND and DMD.
- Coexistent cardiac or lung pathology, such as chronic obstructive pulmonary disease (COPD) and cardiac failure. Patients with DMD have an associated cardiomyopathy, and are at risk of arrhythmias and muscle weakness if given diuretics that reduce potassium levels.

Management

- Infection—appropriate antibiotics and physiotherapy. If there is evidence of aspiration, a full assessment of swallowing by a speech and language therapist and consideration of alternative feeding methods should be considered.
- Respiratory muscle weakness—careful positioning and raising the head of the bed may be helpful. Careful discussion of respiratory support, using noninvasive ventilation (NIV), may be appropriate. This can be very helpful in improving symptoms, although many patients find the use of the tight-fitting mask difficult and may not be able to continue to use the NIV. For patients with MND, the discussion should occur before a crisis situation and

regular monitoring and discussion of the possible symptoms is helpful [15].

With both MND and DMD although NIV may be initially helpful in alleviating symptoms, increasing dependence on NIV may occur, and it is important to discuss the issues of ventilator dependence and possible withdrawal of treatment as the disease progresses before starting NIV [15,16]. Life may be prolonged but with increasing disability, which may be less acceptable for the patient and may cause distress and strain on the family. Some patients may request invasive ventilation, with a tracheostomy, although this is rare in the United Kingdom. The importance of advance care planning (ACP) and discussions about possible advance decision to refuse treatment (ADRT) are often highly relevant in connection to respiratory support issues for these patients. Chapter 8, *Advance Care Planning*, considers ACP in detail.

Medication is helpful in alleviating the subjective experience and possible distress of breathlessness:

- Benzodiazepines, such as diazepam 2–5 mg three times daily or sublingual lorazepam 500 μg to 1 mg as needed for acute situations.
- Opioids, such as regular morphine 2.5–5 mg every 4 h. Careful titration of medication is necessary to ensure the symptoms are effectively managed, without oversedation.

Cough may be troublesome for patients with respiratory muscle weakness or where posture reduces the ability to produce a good cough. Careful physiotherapy assessment will help in ensuring the cough is as effective as possible.

If there is infection, this should be treated with appropriate antibiotics. If there is evidence of aspiration of fluid and food, consideration of alternative methods of feeding should be considered. This is covered in more detail in Chapter 10, *The Management of Gastrointestinal Symptoms and Advanced Liver Disease*. Mucolytics, such as carbocisteine 500 mg three times daily, may be helpful to relieve thick or tenacious sputum. Small doses of opioids, such as morphine elixir 2–5 mg every 4 h, may be considered.

Dysphagia

Swallowing difficulties are common in patients with neurological disorders, for example, affecting 90% of patients with MND [17]. This may be due to involvement of muscles in the chewing, handling of the bolus of food in the mouth, moving the bolus to the pharynx, or in swallowing itself. There may also be problems in eating due to arm weakness and impaired mobility, and assessment by the occupational therapist may allow aids to help with these

issues to be provided. Careful assessment by a speech and language therapist and dietitian is essential, and videofluoroscopic examination of swallowing may be helpful.

Management

Other causes of dysphagia, such as oral and oesophageal candidiasis, should be excluded and treated appropriately. Following assessment, dietary advice from the speech and language therapist and dietitian is helpful. For patients with bulbar palsy, a custard consistency is easiest to swallow and high calorific value foods should be encouraged. Initially, the patient may be able to use strategies suggested by the speech and language therapist, but as the dysphagia worsens, there will be need for education and support to be offered to carers, both family and professional, to ensure feeding is performed in the most appropriate way for the person.

If there is increasing difficulty, weight loss, and significant risk of aspiration, alternative methods of nutrition may be considered. Nacogastric (NG) feeding is rarely used, except in a crisis situation. Percutaneous endoscopic gastrostomy (PEG) or percutaneous radiological gastrostomy (PRG) may be considered—see Chapter 10, *The Management of Gastrointestinal Symptoms and Advanced Liver Disease*, for more detail. This can be a very difficult decision for patients and their families. A period of discussion, over several weeks, allows the patient to consider the issues, and it should always be stressed that the gastrostomy does not, of itself, preclude oral feeding. The tastes, pleasure, and social aspects of oral feeding remain highly important to many of these patients. Discussion about the possible withdrawal of feeding at the end of life is important, as PEG feeding may allow increasing disability to develop and lead to a poor quality of life, which may be unacceptable to the person. Consideration of an ADRT and other future care plans may be important in the context of these discussions (see Chapter 8, *Advance Care Planning*).

Drooling

If there is reduced swallowing and weakness of facial muscles, causing poor lip control, and neck weakness leading to the head falling forward, drooling of saliva may occur. This is usually due to reduced swallowing of the normal production of saliva, rather than excess production. This is often distressing to both patients and their carers, family and professionals, and affects communication and mobility and may result in social isolation due to embarrassment. It is a common symptom affecting 40% of patients with MND and 65% with PD [12,18].

Management

Careful attention to posture and explanation to the patient and family is essential and may be sufficient. For some patients, medication or other intervention may be necessary and potential options are listed below.

- Anticholinergic medication to reduce saliva production:
  - Hyoscine hydrobromide, 300 µg sublingually three times daily.
  - Hyoscine hydrobromide patches, 1-mg patch changed every 72 h.
  - Glycopyrronium bromide in its injectable formulation can be given via a PEG as 200 µg three times daily or by continuous subcutaneous (SC) infusion using a syringe driver, up to 1,200 µg over 24 h.
- Antidepressants, such as amitriptyline, have side effects of causing a dry mouth and can be helpful particularly if there is evidence of depression or anxiety.
- Botulinum toxin injections into the salivary glands have been shown to be very effective for some people [13].
- Local radiotherapy to the salivary glands can be considered, but this is obviously irreversible and the ensuing dryness can be distressing to some people.
- For some patients, the saliva can become very sticky and difficult to clear. Propranolol 10 mg three times daily, pineapple chunks, papaya tablets, or botulinum toxin can be helpful in easing the consistency or reducing the volume of saliva.

Reassessment of the symptoms is essential, as for many people the ensuing dry mouth can be distressing and careful titration of medication is necessary.

Constipation

Constipation is a common problem for people with neurological conditions due to many causes: immobility, poor diet, medication, such as opioids and anticholinergics, and the reduced abdominal muscular power needed to strain.

Management

First, the particular cause of constipation should be addressed:

- Increased roughage within the diet, including consideration of supplement feeds.
- Ensuring hydration and extra fluids—particularly in patients having enteral feeding by PEG.
- Encouraging mobility.
- Review of medication to reduce doses or discontinue those which could be causing constipation, if possible.

Second, oral aperients may be necessary:
- A combination of a stimulant laxative with a softener is helpful:
  - Co-danthramer 5–10 ml twice daily—increasing to the co-danthramer strong formulation if there is inadequate response.
  - Senna 5–10 ml or 1–2 tablets twice daily and lactulose 15–30 ml twice daily.
  - Macrogols (such as Movicol) 1–2 sachets per day.

Third, rectal measures may be necessary if sphincter control is difficult and regular suppositories or enemas may be helpful for some patients.

Insomnia

There are many causes of poor sleep—pain/discomfort, anxiety, fear of not being able to attract attention due to immobility, reduced ability to call out and be heard, cough, orthopnea/respiratory failure, cramps, and fear of incontinence, restless legs, and confusion. These will vary with disease processes, and in PD, sleep disorders are very common, often with hallucinations and confusion and may be related to medication and the development of "off periods" [18,19].

The management of poor sleep should be directed at the underlying cause and may include simple measures ranging from a call button to allow the patient to call for attention to considering medication changes in PD. Opioids can be helpful for immobile patients who develop pain that affects sleep—see Section "Pain" in this chapter and also Chapter 9, *Pain and Its Management*.

Restlessness and agitation

The causes of restlessness and agitation require careful assessment. These include infection, medication, hypoxia, as well as disease progression, particularly in PD [18,19]. Ensuring the environment is quiet and relaxed is important, as well as exclusion and treatment of reversible causes. In PD, hallucinosis and psychotic episodes are common and up to 40% of patients may experience hallucinations [19]. The cause may be medication and titration of the doses is essential. Clozapine and quetiapine are widely used in PD, and risperidone and olanzapine, often in combination with benzodiazepines, may be helpful.

Holistic care for patients with neurological conditions

In addition to management of physical symptoms, the total care of patients with progressive neurological disorders includes attention to mobility, communication, mood and cognition, the psychosocial care of the patient and wider family, and multidisciplinary team (MDT) working.

Weakness and mobility issues

Patients with progressive neurological disease will face many losses, particularly with mobility. Careful assessment by a physiotherapist and occupational therapist with specialised knowledge of neurological disease is essential. The provision of equipment to aid daily living requires sensitive communication and should be a gradual process of discussion, rather than the sudden provision of equipment that the person is not prepared to use and may not accept. Careful explanation is necessary together with forward planning, as equipment needs will change as the disease progresses. Any aids will need to be adaptable to cope with these changes.

Speech and communication

Speech may be affected by muscle weakness of the mouth and face as well as by respiratory weakness, leading to a very quiet voice. However, communication may also be affected by changes in mood, arm mobility, and cognition. Assessment of the issues may therefore be complex. Careful listening to the person is important with attention to timing and pace of the consultation and allowing them to complete what they want to say, whether this is by speech or by a communication aid. The speech and language therapist will perform an assessment and will be able to provide advice on the best way of communicating, not only for the patient but also for the lay and professional carers. The provision of communication aids can be helpful, from low-tech pads and pencils to computer systems and iPads, which can include the ability to speak the words the person has typed or entered into the system.

It is very helpful to allow patients to communicate their wishes and fears while speech is present, although this may require encouragement as these are difficult issues to discuss. It is often easier to continue these discussions later in the disease progression when communication aids are needed if they have touched upon at an earlier stage. It is important to recognise that communication is still important to the patient, as many very disabled patients will continue to have normal hearing and intellectual abilities even if they are unable to speak.

Depression

Any person with a progressive neurological disease, knowing that the progression will continue and death ensue, may have a low mood. Many will become depressed with

the prevalence estimated as 20% in MND and 40% in PD, although it may be difficult to make the diagnosis when the patient has severe communication issues and possible cognitive change [18,19].

Listening to the patient and family and providing counselling support are important. Antidepressant medication is useful and options include the following:
- Amitriptyline, particularly if there is drooling or poor sleep; suggested dose range of 25–150 mg at night.
- Citalopram 10–20 mg once daily, which has fewer side effects and may be helpful for a patient with emotional lability (in MND) or coexistent cardiac disease (in DMD).

As the disease progresses anxiety is common, often caused by fear of the disease itself and concerns about end-of-life situations and fear of the unknown. Reassurance and behavioural or cognitive therapies may be helpful either alone or supplemented by judicious use of benzodiazepines, such as temazepam (10–20 mg) or diazepam (5–10 mg) given at night.

Cognitive change

Cognitive change is now recognised in many progressive neurological diseases—up to 67% of people with MND have evidence of frontal lobe dysfunction and 10–15% have frontotemporal dementia [20]; in PD, about 30% of patients develop dementia [18]; and in MS, 40–50% show cognitive change [5]. The changes may be subtle at first and may not be recognised, except as changes in personality noticed by the family and close carers. Because there is likely to be progression to the point where the patient will lose capacity in decision making, future care planning discussions should be initiated early in the disease and sometimes even soon after diagnosis. It may be very difficult for patients and their families to cope with looking at a difficult future, but if they wish to be in a position to influence their care, and to contribute to decisions about their future management at a time when they cannot give an opinion, these issues need to be raised and support given to help all involved to cope with the issues and face these important discussions. It is important to remember that future care planning should never be forced on a patient, but the value of it can be emphasised.

Psychosocial support for the patient

It has been suggested that for patients with MND, concerns about their family are reported by almost all patients compared with physical or other health matters that are reported by about half. Interest in physician-assisted suicide or euthanasia is also apparent. Likewise, in patients with MS, the risk factors for desire for euthanasia or suicide include loneliness, concerns about (un)employment, and lack of psychosocial or spiritual support. Loss and change are common emotional challenges to these patients. It has also been shown that there can be a mismatch between symptoms noted by the professional and those that are considered most troublesome by the patient.

Assessment for psychological issues including hopelessness is therefore important and consideration should be given to early intervention from clinical psychologists with a view to interventions such as cognitive behavioural therapy and other nondrug measures, which may sustain hope, purpose, and meaning. The concepts of purpose and meaning are features within the spiritual dimension of patient care and this must also be addressed. Spiritual care is discussed in greater detail in Chapter 24, *Spirituality in Palliative Care*. Information about patient support groups is very important for these patients and should be provided at, or soon after, diagnosis. Increasingly, a key member of the team will be a specialist nurse who has developed particular expertise in the patient's neurological disorder (or a group of such conditions) and who will act as an expert resource for patient, family, lay, and professional carers alike. Often this may be a "key team" so that there is continuous support, which is not dependent on one particular person. Because concern for family wellbeing is paramount to the patient, opportunities such as respite admissions to hospice care or a care home setting, and weekly attendance at a hospice day care unit form a valuable part of a holistic management plan.

Carer support

The demands on families and close carers of people with progressive neurological disease can be profound—physically, psychologically, and emotionally. There are often multiple losses faced by both the patient and family with great changes of roles within family units. This is particularly seen when speech and communication are difficult and/or cognitive changes occur, adding increased stresses on all concerned.

There may be specific challenges for families when the disease is inherited—such as in HD and DMD. In HD, there may have been multiple deaths already within the family due to the disease. Children and siblings of patients face the dilemma as to whether they should undergo genetic testing, with the stresses of the process and the issues that may arise if they are found to be carrying the gene and will develop the disease themselves. Genetic counselling is essential before and after any testing is considered.

Following the death of the person, there may be many varying feelings, including ambivalence—sadness at the loss yet relief that the challenges of caring have ended. All involved need time to talk and members of the primary health-care team are well placed to provide the ongoing support and care.

Many of the challenges and stresses faced by families may be experienced by the professional carers as well. They may feel hopelessness and despondency at seeing the progression of the disease. The team approach, including the support and liaison with other teams, is very helpful and discussion and sharing of the feelings experienced in caring for the patient and their family is essential. Regular team meetings when the issues can be shared are helpful, and following the death a debriefing meeting allows the ambivalent feelings of team members to be expressed and shared, so that team members are not isolated.

Multidisciplinary care

As many of these diseases are relatively rare, the primary health-care team may have little experience in their management. Moreover, there is a particular need to ensure that the care involves a wide MDT in a coordinated approach. There are often specialist nurses or teams involved and the primary care team will need to work closely with them so that the care is as effective as possible and is also proactive—responding to changes that may occur and preparing for changes that are likely to occur in the future.

It is important for patients and families that the care is coordinated and it is clear as to which professional is involved and their roles. It has been suggested that patients have a nominated "key worker" who can help in liaison and coordination. Often, this may be a "key team" so that there is continuous support, which is not dependent on one particular person. The primary health-care team, when it is working well together and with other specialist teams, can provide this ongoing support.

End-of-life care

The period of end-of-life care may be more difficult to define for a person with neurological disease as there may be particular challenges:
- There is often a long duration of disease, many years in patients with PD, MS, and some patients with MND and decades in patients with DMD.
- Death may be sudden in MND and MSA.
- The course of the illness may fluctuate greatly as in PD.

• Associated neuropsychiatric problems—cognitive or behavioural—may make assessment more complex.
• Many people will die with, but not from, their neurological disease.
• Many patients fear the end of life, as they have heard of distressing deaths from neurological disease (choking, immobility, and inappropriate interventions such as ventilation), and these fears may be accentuated by the debates about assisted suicide, which often emphasise the risk of distress at the end of life.

Indicators have been suggested to help identify the end-of-life phase. These include:
• swallowing problems;
• recurring infection;
• marked decline in physical status;
• first episode of aspiration pneumonia;
• cognitive difficulties;
• weight loss; and
• significant complex symptoms [2].

The preparation for end of life would be similar to other conditions and this is discussed in more detail in Chapter 21, *Terminal Care and Dying*. There are opportunities for discussion about place of death and the person's specific wishes—although these should have been considered much earlier in the disease progression.

Management
Medication for the management of symptoms at the end of life should be continued:
• Oral medication may be possible, or could be continued via a gastrostomy.
• Transdermal patch, such as fentanyl transdermal patch for pain, may be helpful if swallowing is difficult.
• Parenteral medication may be necessary—either as SC injection every 4 h or a continuous SC infusion using a syringe driver over 24 h. Possible medications are suggested below and further guidance is given in Chapter 21, *Terminal Care and Dying*:
  ○ Morphine for pain and/or breathlessness. If morphine has been given by mouth or PEG earlier in the illness, the dose should be adjusted to take account of different potencies when administered subcutaneously.
  ○ Midazolam for sedation or anxiety. Doses of 5–10 mg every 4 h or 20–60 mg in 24 h administered by continuous SC infusion.
  ○ Levomepromazine for nausea or agitation. Doses of up to 25 mg in 24 h are used for nausea, and may be given once daily or in divided doses. For agitation, higher doses are used—up to 100 mg in 24 h may be necessary

(higher in some cases following specialist advice) and these doses are usually given by continuous SC infusion.
  ○ Glycopyrronium bromide for relief of respiratory secretions with doses of 200 μg given every 4 h or 800–1,200 μg in 24 h administered by continuous SC infusion.

Certain medication should be continued; for instance, in PD, it is important to continue dopaminergic medication, via a PEG or as patches, to reduce rigidity [22]. Care should also be taken to ensure that there are no drug interactions with existing medication, as this could lead to an increase in symptoms.

Conclusions

The palliative care of patients with progressive neurological disease requires the following:
• Coordinated care including specialist teams.
• Involvement early in the disease pathway to facilitate planning and discussion while the person can communicate and hopefully before the onset of significant cognitive impairment.
• Involvement of many disciplines working together as a team.
• Careful assessment and management of symptoms.
• Support for patients and their families considering physical, psychosocial, and spiritual dimensions.
• Proactive care with timely preparation for symptoms or problems that may occur.
• Collaboration with voluntary agencies and charities who can provide specialist advice and support.
• Good team working attitudes and mutual support.

Supportive organisations in the United Kingdom

Motor neurone disease
The Motor Neurone Disease Association (MNDA) is a national, voluntary organisation and registered charity. It has regional care development advisors who have direct contact with patients and families and also play an educational role to health-care professionals. The MNDA also runs an information service, with a wide range of publications written for both the lay public and professionals involved in the care of people with MND.

Contact: 08457 626262; www.mndassociation.org

Multiple sclerosis

The Multiple Sclerosis Society of Great Britain and Northern Ireland provides information for sufferers and professionals and local support groups.

Contact: 0808 800 8000; www.mssociety.org.uk

Multiple Sclerosis Trust: 01462 476700; www.mstrust.org.uk.

Muscular dystrophies

The Muscular Dystrophies Campaign provides useful information about current treatments, grants, and equipment and offers a support network.

Contact: 020-7720-8055; www.muscular-dystrophy.org

Huntington's disease

The Huntington's Disease Association offers news updates, information, and support for families, patients, and professionals.

Contact: 020-7223-7000; www.hda.org.uk.

Parkinson's disease

Parkinson's UK provides information and support for people with PD and their families, runs local groups, and supports research and national campaigns to influence public policy.

Contact: Helpline 0808 800 0303; www.parkinsons.org.uk

PSP Association provides support and information for people with PSP and corticobasal degeneration.

Contact: 01327 322410; www.pspeur.org

MSA Trust provides information and support to people with MSA.

Contact: 020 7940 4660; www.msatrust.org.uk

References

1. Department of Health. *National Service Framework for Long-Term Conditions*. London: Department of Health, 2005. Available at: www.dh.gov.uk/en/Publicationsandstatistics/PublicationsPolicyAndGuidance/DH_4105361 (accessed on May 5, 2012).

2. End of Life Care Programme. *End of Life Care in Neurological Conditions: A Framework for Implementation*. Available at: http://www.endoflifecareforadults.nhs.uk/news/all/neolcp-publishes-end-of-life-care-in-long-term-neurological-conditions (updated 2010, cited October 2011) (accessed on May 5, 2012).

3. Shaw C. Amyotrophic lateral sclerosis/motor neurone disease. In: Oliver D, Borasio GD, and Walsh D (eds), *Palliative Care in Amyotrophic Lateral Sclerosis: From Diagnosis to Bereavement*, 2nd edition. Oxford: Oxford University Press, 2006.

4. Bensimon G, Lacomblez L, and Meininger V. A controlled trial of riluzole in amyotrophic lateral sclerosis. *N Eng J Med* 1994; 330: 585–591.

5. Macleod AD and Formaglio F. Demyelinating disease. In: Voltz R, Borasio GD, Bernat J, Maddocks I, Oliver D, and Portenoy RK (eds), *Palliative Care in Neurology*. Oxford: Oxford University Press, 2004.

6. Royal College of Physicians Parkinson's Disease. *National Clinical Guideline for Diagnosis and Management in Primary and Secondary Care*. London: Royal College of Physicians, 2006.

7. Nath U, Ben-Shlomo Y, Thomson RG, *et al*. Clinical features and natural history of progressive supranuclear palsy: a clinical cohort study. *Neurology* 2003; 60: 910–916.

8. Roos RA. Huntington's disease: a clinical review. *Orphanet J Rare Dis* 2010; 5: 40.

9. Manzur AY, Kinali M, and Mutoni F. Update on management of Duchenne's muscular dystrophy. *Arch Dis Child* 2008; 93: 986–990.

10. Fayssoil A, Nardi O, Orlikowski D, *et al*. Cardiomyopathy in Duchenne muscular dystrophy: pathogenesis and therapeutics. *Heart Fail Rev* 2010; 15(1): 103–107.

11. Lee M, Walker RW, Hildreth TJ, *et al*. A survey of pain in idiopathic Parkinson's disease. *J Pain Symptom Manage* 2006; 32: 462–469.

12. Oliver D. The quality and care of symptom control—the effects on the terminal phase of ALS/MND. *J Neurol Sci* 1996; 139(suppl): 134–136.

13. Esquenazi A, Novak I, Sheean G, *et al*. International consensus statement for the use of botulinum toxin treatment in adults and children with neurological impairments—introduction. *Eur J Neurol* 2010; 17(suppl 2): 1–8.

14. Oliver D. Opioid medication in the palliative care of motor neurone disease. *Palliat Med* 1998; 12: 113–115.

15. Heffernan C, Jenkinson C, Holmes T, *et al*. Management of respiration in MND/ALS patients: an evidence based review. *Amyotroph Lateral Scler* 2006; 7: 5–15.

16. Oliver DJ and Turner MR. Some difficult decisions in ALS/MND. *Amyotroph Lateral Scler* 2010; 11: 339–343.

17. Heffernan C, Jenkinson C, Holmes T, *et al*. Nutritional management in MND/ALS patients: an evidence based review. *Amyotroph Lateral Scler Other Motor Neuron Disord* 2004; 5: 72–83.

18. Lee MA, Prentice WM, Hildreth AJ, *et al*. Measuring symptom load in idiopathic Parkinson's disease. *Parkinsonism Relat Disord* 2007; 13: 284–289.

19. Poewe W. Non-motor symptoms in Parkinson's disease. *Eur J Neurol* 2008; 15(Suppl 1): 14–20.

20. Goldstein L. Control of symptoms—cognitive dysfunction. In: Oliver D, Borasio GD, and Walsh D (eds), *Palliative Care in Amyotrophic Lateral Sclerosis: From Diagnosis to Bereavement*, 2nd edition. Oxford: Oxford University Press, 2006.

21. Borasio GD, Lorenzl S, Rogers A, *et al.* Palliative care in non-malignant neurological disorders. Section 12.5. In: Hanks G, Cherny NI, Christakis NA, Fallon M, Kaasa S, and Portenoy RK (eds), *Oxford Textbook of Palliative Medicine*, 4th edition. Oxford: Oxford University Press, 2010.

22. Parkinson's UK and National Council for Palliative Care. *Consensus Statement on the Management of Symptoms for People with Parkinson's and Related Conditions in the Last Few Days of Life*. London: Parkinson's UK, 2011.

Acknowledgements. The author acknowledges the previous work of Fiona Hicks and Hazel Pearse who contributed the chapter on palliative care for people with progressive neurological disorders to the second edition of this handbook.

14 Palliative Care for People with HIV Infection and AIDS

Surinder Singh[1], Nick Theobald[2]

[1]UCL Medical School, London, UK
[2]Chelsea and Westminster Hospital, London, UK

Introduction

Human immunodeficiency virus (HIV) infection and acquired immunodeficiency syndrome (AIDS) continue to cause high levels of morbidity and mortality throughout the world, the United Kingdom included. In developing countries, as many as one in three deaths can be HIV related. Most of this chapter will describe palliative care practice in the United Kingdom. We will also bring readers up to date with some of the changes that are occurring as a result of the success of antiretroviral therapy (ART).

This chapter will not cover the more specialist area of paediatric palliative care (PPC) though readers are directed to an excellent web site (http://www.chiva.org.uk) for reference.

Global epidemiology

The HIV epidemic remains a major global public health challenge, with a total of 34 million people living with HIV worldwide [1].

In 2010, an estimated 34 million people were living with HIV—a rise of over a quarter from 1999. Globally, nearly 23% of all people living with HIV are younger than 24 years, and people aged 15–24 years account for 35% of all people becoming newly infected. Sub-Saharan Africa remains the most severely affected region, accounting for 68% of all people living with HIV, 70% of new infections, and 72% of AIDS-related deaths. The epidemic, however, has not spared other regions; more than 10.8 million people are living with HIV outside sub-Saharan Africa. It continues to deepen poverty, increase hunger, slow progress on maternal and child health, and exacerbate other infectious diseases.

HIV/AIDS is the world's leading infectious killer claiming—to date—more than 25 million lives. An estimated 2 million people die every year from HIV/AIDS [2,3].

The burden of HIV in the United Kingdom is similar to other Northern European countries while in contrast southern European countries such as Spain and Portugal have experienced larger numbers among injecting drug users (IDUs). The most dramatic figures, however, emanate from Eastern Europe where the number of people living with HIV almost tripled between 2000 and 2009. An estimated 1.4 million people were living with HIV in 2009 compared to around half a million in 2000 [4]. AIDS-related deaths continue to rise in this region: an estimated 76,000 people died from AIDS-related causes in 2009 compared to 18,000 in 2001, a fourfold increase. The Russian Federation and Ukraine together account for nearly 90% of newly reported HIV infections in the Eastern Europe and central Asian region. Ukraine has the highest adult HIV prevalence in all of Europe and central Asia, at 1.1%. Annual HIV diagnoses in Ukraine have more than doubled since 2001. Between 2000 and 2009, the HIV incidence rate increased by more than 25% in five countries in the region: Armenia, Georgia, Kazakhstan, Kyrgyzstan, and Tajikistan. The epidemic in Eastern Europe is concentrated primarily among people who inject drugs, sex workers, and, to a lesser extent, men who have sex with men (MSM).

Handbook of Palliative Care, Third Edition. Edited by Christina Faull, Sharon de Caestecker, Alex Nicholson and Fraser Black.
© 2012 by John Wiley and Sons, Inc. Published 2012 by John Wiley & Sons, Inc.

HIV and AIDS in the United Kingdom

HIV continues to be one of the most important communicable diseases in the United Kingdom. In 2011, over 6,000 individuals were diagnosed with HIV for the first time [5]. It is estimated there are about 91,500 HIV-infected people alive in the United Kingdom, a quarter of whom do not know they are infected. Worryingly, half of the adults were diagnosed with HIV at a late stage of infection—that is, their CD4 count was less than 350 per mm^3 within 3 months of diagnosis (this is the stage at which antiretroviral treatment is currently recommended) [6].

These figures indicate why there is a move to encourage a wider testing policy because individuals are not seeing the benefit of treatment if started at a late stage in their disease [7]. ART has resulted in a sustained decline in HIV-associated deaths, which, with a rise in the number of new diagnoses, has resulted in a steep increase in the number of people requiring long-term treatment. London, Brighton, and Manchester are the cities in England and Edinburgh in Scotland, with the largest HIV-infected populations. Despite the obvious good news about reduced mortality, in 2010 there were 680 [8] deaths among HIV-infected persons in the United Kingdom.

Men who have sex with men

For the first time since 1998, the number of new HIV diagnoses in men who have sex with men (MSM) has surpassed new diagnoses in heterosexuals. 48% of those diagnosed in 2011 probably acquired their infection through sex between men and 47% through heterosexual contact [5]. The overall estimated prevalence of HIV infection (both diagnosed and undiagnosed) was 47 per 1,000 population (1 in 20) for MSM of all ages in the UK and 87 per 1,000 living in London (1 in 11).

Heterosexual transmission

The number of heterosexually acquired HIV infections diagnosed in the United Kingdom rose during the late 1990s and early part of the 21st century but in recent years has been falling. New diagnoses among heterosexuals infected abroad dropped from 4,160 in 2004 to 2,260 in 2010. By contrast, new diagnoses among heterosexuals who probably acquired HIV within the UK have slowly increased (from 320 in 2001 to 1,090 in 2010) and these accounted for a third of all heterosexuals newly diagnosed in 2010.

Undiagnosed HIV infection

In the UK, the estimated prevalence of HIV in 2010 was 1.5 per 1,000 population of all ages [6] and an estimated 91,500 were living with HIV (both diagnosed and undiagnosed). Approximately, a quarter (26%, 22,200) of HIV-infected people were estimated to be unaware of their infection. The percentage of people who are unaware of their HIV infection varies by "category"—thus whereas 22% of MSM do not know about their HIV, up to a third of "heterosexual" men are unaware [5,9,10].

HIV and AIDS in the Americas

North America

Canada

The number of people living with HIV (including AIDS) in Canada continues to rise, from an estimated 57,000 in 2005 to approximately 65,000 by the end of 2009 (a 14% increase). Although estimates of the number of new HIV infections are quite uncertain, it appears that the number of new infections in 2009 (estimated range between 2,300 and 4,300) was about the same as or slightly greater than the estimated range in 2005 (2,200–4,200).

Twenty-six percent of all people living with HIV are unaware of their HIV status and people with heterosexually acquired HIV infection are most likely to be diagnosed late in the course of infection [10].

The following are the most recent trends in Canada:
• Gay, bisexual, and other MSM continued to comprise the greatest proportion (44%) of new HIV infections in 2009.
• In 2008, people who inject drugs (IDU) comprised 17% of new HIV infections.
• The proportion of new infections in 2009 among male and female heterosexuals who are not from countries that have high rates of HIV was 17% and those from countries with high rates of HIV (so-called "endemic countries") was 14.1%.
• The proportion of all new infections among women was unchanged from 2005 to 2009 (26%). Aboriginal persons also continue to be overrepresented in the HIV epidemic in Canada, and comprised 12.5% of all new infections in 2009.

The United States

At the end of 2010, the estimated number of persons living with a diagnosis of HIV infection in the United States was 1.2 million. In 2010, an estimated 47,129 persons were diagnosed with HIV infection (11). Twenty percent of people living with HIV are unaware of their HIV status and people with heterosexually acquired HIV infection are most likely to be diagnosed late in the course of infection. Unprotected sex between men continues to dominate patterns of HIV transmission. New HIV infections resulting from unprotected sex between men increased by more than 50% in the United States between 1991–1993 and 2003–2006. Some racial minorities are disproportionately impacted by HIV—in the United States, African-Americans represented 14% of the population but accounted for 44% of people newly infected with HIV in 2009.

In 2009, the estimated number of HIV-related deaths was 17,774 (7.0 deaths per 100,000 population). Due to widespread access to ART, the number of AIDS-related deaths has dropped considerably, 70% lower in the United States in 2009 than in 1994.

What exactly is palliative care in the context of HIV/AIDS?

Palliative care should be a core component of comprehensive HIV/AIDS care [12,13], thus:
• access to palliative care should not be artificially restricted due to political or social constraints;
• all patients needing and wanting it should receive it, without exception;
• palliative care should be provided in accordance with the needs of the patient and World Health Organisation (WHO) standards of care;
• treatment for illnesses and conditions should not be withheld at any stage of the disease (e.g., tuberculosis (TB) treatment, ART, or substitution therapy for IDUs); and
• palliative care should be incorporated as appropriate at every stage of HIV disease, and not only when the patient is dying.

Gold standards in palliative care

Over the past few years, there has been much attention given to the care of people who enter the terminal phase of their illness irrespective of the cause (cancer, chronic diseases such as chronic obstructive pulmonary disease [COPD], heart failure [HF], or HIV infection). Three major factors play a part in this—first, the choice of where this end-of-life care should take place; second, current guidance about what is best practice; and third, the economics of health-care provision in the last few days or weeks in a person's life [14]. The Gold Standards Framework (GSF) for palliative care, now enshrined in the National Institute for Health and Clinical Excellence (NICE) guidance, is an approach to care which is critical

for those in the last few weeks or days of their lives and is being implemented in both hospitals and the community [15,16] (see Chapter 2, *Palliative Care in the Community*, for a more detailed description of the GSF).

A new paradigm?

It has been argued that in the HIV/AIDS context, the traditional "either-or" approach to care—curative or palliative—is no longer valid [17]. At first, this seems counterintuitive. After all, the success of ART has been well documented and thus the need for end-of-life care surely reduced. In many ways, it is as a result of this extended life expectancy that the need for a new palliative care has been realised. Quite simply, continued significant levels of morbidity and mortality still occur, adverse effects of ART need to be managed, the incidence of new cancers appear to be rising, and the issue of comorbidities (in an ever-increasing "older" population) are all factors that have contributed to this ethos.

Some would even argue that up to now palliative care has been neglected largely because clinicians— presumably those who are most concerned with "cure"—fail to acknowledge the complexities of dealing with patients in whom palliation of symptoms (pain control, quality of life, care of loved ones, and carers) can sit alongside curative approaches [7].

Case history—a lost opportunity?

NT was a lady of 54 years who had recently registered with a new general practitioner (GP) having moved from an address in Northeast London. Following a visit to the surgery, the practice nurse identified a previous abnormal smear and possible cervical intraepithelial neoplasia (CIN)—and NT was duly referred to the local hospital for routine colposcopy. The patient was seen by her GP two or three more times for self-limiting problems over the next year.

Two years after registration with the practice, we received notification that the patient had died in a hospital outside of London of two AIDS-related conditions—TB and toxoplasmosis.

The practice has since conducted a critical incident on this patient (and all her available notes) concluding that while it is easy to see in retrospect that NT could have been identified earlier, the practice could not identify any specific reason for testing her for HIV.

This lends some weight to the argument that all patients registering with a practice/or attending outpatients in hospital should be screened for HIV infection [7].

Issues relating to palliative care

Prognosis and the transition to palliative care

Life expectancy for patients with HIV infection in the developed world has improved significantly following the introduction of combination ART. The clinical course for any individual patient can be variable and is dependent on factors such as tolerance of drugs, adherence to complex regimes, and the development of drug resistance. For the majority of people, HIV infection can now be regarded as a chronic, manageable disease.

It is therefore more difficult than ever to determine when the emphasis of care should turn toward palliating symptoms rather than pursuing investigations and curative treatment regimens. In the majority of cases, the processes may run in parallel—with the expertise of palliative care controlling adverse symptoms while the HIV physician works to control the virus and consequences of impaired immunity.

Many patients with HIV and AIDS choose to receive much of their care from hospitals, often for reasons of familiarity, relative anonymity, and continuity of care. Unfortunately, this sometimes means that the primary care team may have very little involvement with the patient until the end of their illness, which is not ideal for all parties concerned. It is therefore important to remind patients that the GP ought to be involved at all stages of their illness. In return, there is probably more that general practice can do for the average patient or family affected by HIV infection [9,18]. There are many resources within primary care that can provide a great deal of help and support to those living with HIV and it is often the case that the patient will be attending their GP for other reasons over the course of a year (health checks, vaccination programs).

Patients with advanced disease often have multiple physical and psychosocial issues and comprehensive care for late-stage HIV disease commonly involves an increasingly complex mixture of therapies, both disease specific and palliative. This requires coordination and collaboration between acute HIV treatment centres, palliative care services, and primary care—even more reason why patients with HIV infection ought to be registered with a GP. Below are characteristics that render the care of patients with advanced HIV/AIDS a particular challenge to health-care workers:
- Up to now, predominantly younger age group (but this is changing).
- Multisystem disease.
- Polysymptomatic.
- Polypharmacy and multiple drug interactions.
- Concurrent active/palliative needs.
- Changes in prognosis following treatment advances.
- Patient involvement/knowledge/empowerment.
- Social issues of isolation, stigma, fear of breaches in confidentiality, housing problems, language and cultural barriers, religious issues, lack of family and/or support.

Stigma and confidentiality

In the context of HIV/AIDS, confidentiality is crucial. It is an integral part of patient care, as it should be in all conditions. Because HIV and AIDS remain stigmatised conditions, it is all the more important that all services, including those in palliative care, need to guard against complacency, ensure awareness, and provide training when necessary. Confidentiality is a team issue. A lapse by one member of staff means that the patient and family or caregiver is compromised. A breach of confidentiality cannot be easily rectified for an individual or family.

Some patients perceive negative attitudes toward them from doctors—perhaps GPs are perceived to be worse than most in this regard. Many patients crave anonymity and confidentiality is one of the reasons why people with HIV infection would commonly move home to be within a major conurbation like London or Manchester.

Several studies involving general practice have shown that a practice declaration—often in the form of a visible practice statement—can be important in allaying the fears of adults regarding confidentiality. The more prominently these are displayed, the better. Other features of an HIV-friendly general practice include the following:
- All members of the team are nonjudgemental and empathic to different lifestyles.
- Development and implementation of a nondiscrimination policy.
- Development and implementation of an appropriate confidentiality policy.
- The availability of routine HIV testing (including point-of-care testing).

In the specific context of palliative care, it must be remembered that the duty of confidentiality continues "beyond the grave" [19,20] (see Section "The end of life").

Eligibility for health care

The last census completed in the United Kingdom in 2001 showed that around 8% of the UK population was born abroad and in 2009, an estimated 567,000 migrants arrived in the United Kingdom [21]. A good proportion of this highly diverse group will be from sub-Saharan Africa and it is inevitable that the issue of eligibility for medical treatment and social support is raised. As the legislation in this area is subject to constant review, readers are advised to check with the appropriate authority and advocacy group. Eligibility for medical care is generally based on residence rather than nationality, but the rules are complex. A new resource specifically for clinicians throughout the National Health Service (NHS) has been launched by the Health Protection Agency [21] and is particularly useful when looking at this area.

Management of common physical symptoms

Many of the symptoms in advanced HIV infection are similar to those seen in malignant disease (Table 14.1). The principles of symptom control are identical and an understanding of the likely pathophysiology allows selection of the most appropriate management. Ideally, treatment should be holistic, tailored to the individual with frequent review of benefits, side effects, and the wishes of the patient. However, there is significantly increased risk of drug toxicities (from long-term combination antiretroviral medication) and of drug interactions.

Perhaps inevitably, some patients comment that the emphasis from HIV clinicians is on their immunological

response to treatment rather than their symptoms or quality of life [9]. Clinics have become busier as the caseload has increased, although stable patients are now seen less frequently than in the past. It is easy for patients to be taking medication prescribed by several different clinicians (HIV clinic, GP, psychiatrist, and others) without full awareness between the physicians involved—sometimes because of complicity with the mistaken belief that the patient prefers to avoid such communication for fears of confidentiality. Time spent reviewing the patient's medication can reduce toxicity, interactions, adverse effects, and overall costs.

Pain

Pain in HIV disease is common and frequently both underestimated and undermedicated, particularly in women, less educated patients, and IDUs [22,23]. Pain is more common in people who have lived with HIV for a longer time. Common pain syndromes associated with HIV infection often involve the nervous system (e.g., peripheral neuropathy), gastrointestinal (GI) tract, or the musculoskeletal system. The principles of pain control are similar to those in cancer care, based on three-step analgesic ladder of the WHO (see Chapter 9, *Pain and Its Management*, for full discussion).

Painful neuropathy

Peripheral nerve disorders are among the most common problems encountered, with a predominantly sensory polyneuropathy—generally distal and symmetrical—being most problematic. Although HIV itself can be responsible in late-stage untreated infection, in the majority of cases, treatment with nucleoside analogues (particularly stavudine and sometimes zidovudine) is the cause. Other causes (nutritional deficiencies such as vitamin B_{12}, pyridoxine, or thiamine, diabetes, hypothyroidism, syphilis, and other drugs—including vincristine, isoniazid, and dapsone) should be excluded by appropriate investigation, and diagnosis can be confirmed by nerve conduction studies that show abnormal sensory nerve amplitude and conduction velocity. Analgesia need not be delayed waiting for this to take place.

Peripheral neuropathy may present as continuous or episodic pain, sometimes associated with an exaggerated pain response to other stimulus such as touch (clothes, bedcovers, and so on). Patients generally report the nature of the pain using terms such as "burning," "stabbing," "aching," or "cramping."

Management of peripheral neuropathy (if simple analgesia has failed) sometimes starts with tricyclic agents

Table 14.1 Common physical symptoms in AIDS [12].

Symptom	Patients (%)
Pain	60
Neuropathic	22
Pressure sore	12
Visceral	10
Headaches	8
Epigastric/retrosternal	7
Joint	7
Myopathic	5
Anorectal	4
General debility	61
Anorexia	41
Nausea	21
Confusion	29
Diarrhoea	18
Dyspnoea	11

such as amitriptyline or lofepramine (which have fewer anticholinergic side effects). The dose may need to be increased gradually every 4–7 days—and the patient will need to be specifically reassured that the use of a drug that is also an antidepressant does not indicate that the physician feels that the patient is imagining the pain. If the patient fails to tolerate tricyclic antidepressant (TCAs), or pain relief is inadequate, anticonvulsants are a second choice. Both carbamazepine and phenytoin are contraindicated due to drug interactions, leaving gabapentin as the agent in most use, as it is generally well tolerated and has no interactions with antiretrovirals. Careful dose titration is the general approach, because some patients will have tolerability problems. A starting dose of 300 mg of gabapentin once daily can be increased up to 2,400 mg in gradual increments of 300 mg. Some palliative care physicians may take the daily dose up to 3,600 mg.

Individual responses are variable in terms of agents, doses, and serum levels. You should be open with your patient about the "trial and error" nature of the approach and be prepared to monitor them regularly for benefits and side effects. The most common reasons for failure to achieve adequate pain control include early termination of treatment because of side effects from increasing the dose too quickly, starting at too high a dose, or failure to reach a sufficient dose for that individual.

Some patients may benefit from a combination of tricyclic agents and anticonvulsants. In resistant peripheral neuropathy, specialist advice should be sought. Sometimes antiarrhythmics such as mexiletine are considered. Topical agents including capsaicin and lidocaine can be of benefit in a few cases, and many physicians also advocate acupuncture.

Finally, opioids are now used more often in the management of peripheral neuropathy than in the past, despite concerns about their use in patients who may live with the condition for many years. Methadone in particular, due to its wide range of receptor affinities, appears to be more effective than other opioids, and at relatively low doses (5 mg twice daily is often sufficient).

If adequate relief from the symptoms can be obtained with relative ease, and the precipitating factor seems to have been a nucleoside agent, ART may be continued without change. However, if the neuropathy is severe, disabling, not amenable to palliation, or any combination of these, a change in ART is desirable.

GI tract pain

Odynophagia (pain on swallowing) may be caused by infection (e.g., *Candida* or *Cytomegalovirus* [CMV]) or by malignancy (e.g., lymphoma). Abdominal pain may be caused by infection (such as CMV or *Mycobacterium avium intracellulare* [MAI]) or by malignancy. Antiretroviral drugs can cause pancreatitis and constipation is generally drug induced. Anorectal pain may be due to infection (herpes simplex or abscess), anal fissure, or anal carcinoma. In all of these cases, investigation is essential to establish a cause.

Nausea and vomiting

It is important to establish an underlying cause and treat appropriately. A rational approach to antiemetics should always be used, according to the emetic stimulus. A single agent is usually effective if this policy is followed, but if a second antiemetic is necessary, it should be chosen for its different mode of action. Drug-induced nausea is common, and many physicians will routinely prescribe antiemetics to patients on the initiation of ART. Other commonly prescribed drugs that may cause nausea include co-trimoxazole and dapsone, both in use as prophylaxis against *Pneumocystis carinii* pneumonia (PCP).

Case study

"Tom" is a 32-year-old, single man living alone in a flat in west London. Nigerian-born, his family has never fully accepted his homosexuality and relations with his parents are strained. He started on a social work degree but mental health problems have interrupted his studies. He has been HIV positive for 8 years and although he has tried combination antiretroviral drugs on several occasions, the side effects have been unpleasant and he is unable to tolerate them now. He has made a decision not to try any others and has made this clear in an advance decision (living will). As a result, he is extremely immunocompromised and his weight has gone down from 90 to 63 kg.

He is reliant on his primary care team to support him at home; his analgesia (methadone) and the specific treatment for his disabling neuropathy (gabapentin) are all provided by his GP in close liaison with the local HIV clinic. His GP is also prescribing co-trimoxazole and azithromycin, which Tom takes as primary prophylaxis to prevent opportunistic infections (OIs) such as PCP and *M. avium* complex (MAC) or MAI. He is supported by his local community nurse specialist who visits him weekly, and he has spent periods in the local hospice for respite care. His HIV clinic has encouraged a close relationship with his primary care team in anticipation of his request to die at home if possible.

If the nausea and/or vomiting are associated with gastric stasis, a prokinetic drug (such as metoclopramide or domperidone) is most likely to be effective. Cyclizine is more likely to be effective if there is raised intracranial pressure, or vestibular problems, due to its action on the vomiting centre. Haloperidol is the drug of choice for most chemical causes of vomiting (drug induced, renal failure) as it acts principally on the chemoreceptor trigger zone (area postrema), it is also useful for its long half-life, and it is generally given at bedtime. Finally, levomepromazine reportedly has a broad spectrum of action and may be useful if there are several possible causes, or if other agents have failed.

Very occasionally, agents such as nabilone or ondansetron are used, but under specialist supervision.

Diarrhoea

Diarrhea is common. Whereas the cause for the majority of patients with diarrhoea in the early days of the epidemic was chronic infections such as cryptosporidium or microsporidium, for most patients nowadays, the antiretrovirals—especially the protease inhibitors (PIs)—are the responsible cause. Nevertheless, investigations should always be undertaken to exclude infection, inflammatory bowel disease, pancreatic insufficiency, and/or malignancy in any case of altered bowel habit. Symptomatic treatment is crucial in improving quality of life, controlling hydration and weight loss, and improving adherence to antiretrovirals. Loperamide is effective for most patients; the dose should be flexible and titrated by the patient and physician in partnership. Doses of up to a maximum of 32 mg daily can be used (although this represents 16 tablets/capsules). It is more effective, and has fewer side effects than codeine or co-phenotrope.

Codeine phosphate is useful in those cases where loperamide is not successful, and where pain is an additional factor (at doses of 30–60 mg every 4–6 h). Very few patients require oral morphine, but this may be used if the first two choices do not succeed. Finally, subcutaneous (SC) octreotide can be useful, but under expert guidance.

Other specific HIV-related problems

Oral problems

Mouth ulcers and oral candidiasis may cause significant difficulty in eating for some patients. Topical steroids (triamcinolone in orabase or hydrocortisone pellets) may help relieve the painful ulcers, but beware of the possibility that an underlying herpetic infection or malignancy may be present. For some patients with candidiasis, treatment with antiseptic mouthwash and topical nystatin/amphotericin (2–3 hourly) may be sufficient. Others may need a course of oral fluconazole. Gingivitis is also a problem for the immunocompromised, and regular dental supervision is recommended. Hairy oral leukoplakia is a condition caused by Epstein–Barr virus, which results in adherent white lesions, usually on the lateral border of the tongue.

Respiratory problems

PCP remains one of the most common presentations of previously undiagnosed HIV-related immunosuppression. Due to the often insidious onset, early diagnosis can be difficult. A dry, nonproductive cough with significant dyspnoea on exertion is the classic presentation. Unfortunately, late presentation of PCP is still sometimes fatal. Pneumothorax is a known complication. Co-trimoxazole (or alternative) is effective prophylaxis and should be continued in all patients with a CD4 lymphocyte count less than 200.

Mycobacterium TB is very common in this group of patients, and the emergence of multidrug-resistant TB (MDR-TB) has highlighted the importance of good infection control and the need for optimal adherence to a medication regime. Continued bacterial surveillance and resistance monitoring are also essential. TB should always be considered in any respiratory illness with cough, and the patient needs to be isolated until diagnosis is excluded (generally by smear examination of sputum). Any procedures that induce cough should only be undertaken in properly ventilated sealed areas to prevent spread of infection to others. Directly observed therapy helps compliance—particularly in those with chaotic lifestyles, visual impairment, or cognitive difficulties.

Kaposi's sarcoma (KS) can cause extensive pulmonary (and GI) lesions and if it has advanced to this stage, it carries a very poor prognosis. External skin lesions would also be present.

Ophthalmic problems

Sight-threatening retinitis caused by CMV is seen only in the severely immunocompromised, and is relatively uncommon nowadays in the developed world. Significant disability can follow because the damage to the retina is irreversible—and the patient may be at risk of sudden retinal detachment affecting the remaining sight.

Ophthalmic herpes zoster (with dendriform keratitis) and herpes simplex keratitis can also cause serious problems, and advice from an experienced ophthalmologist should be sought at a relatively low threshold.

Dermatological problems

Dry skin is very common in HIV infection, and topical emollients (used liberally) are the recommended management. Yeast and fungal infections are also commonly seen and generally managed with topical combination steroid/antifungal preparations. Psoriasis can be more extensive and more aggressive.

Herpes simplex is likely to be more severe, and recurrences more frequent. Oral aciclovir may be given regularly (400 mg twice daily) as prophylaxis. Herpes zoster is also likely to be seen more often than in the immunocompetent and may affect more than one dermatome. Molluscum contagiosum is caused by a poxvirus and presents as small umbilicated vesicles.

Scabies can be a problem as immunocompromised individuals may often be heavily infected before showing significant signs. Norwegian scabies in particular may be a problem in the institutional setting.

Tumours

KS is caused by infection with the herpesvirus KS–HV or HHV-8 and appears as nodular, purplish lesions commonly affecting the face, trunk or limbs. Antiretroviral treatment is generally extremely effective; as the immune system is restored, the lesions regress. Sometimes chemotherapy and/or local radiotherapy may also be necessary.

Non-Hodgkin's lymphoma is seen significantly more common in those with HIV infection, and is treated with systemic chemotherapy. Prognosis is variable, but in general much better than in the past. However, primary cerebral lymphoma is usually associated with an extremely poor prognosis.

Nervous system

HIV-related brain impairment (once known as "AIDS dementia") is reported more commonly in recent years in the USA but not in the UK. The reasons for this are unclear. Progressive multifocal leukoencephalopathy (PML) is a rapidly progressive condition with extensive cerebral demyelination associated with the reactivation of infection with the JC virus, which carries a very poor prognosis.

Issues relating to medication and HIV/AIDS in palliative care

Antiretroviral therapy

In 1987, zidovudine (also known as AZT) was the first antiretroviral agent shown to improve survival in patients with AIDS. Now, there are a wide range of antiretroviral agents (see Table 14.2) licensed for prescription in the United Kingdom: These include nucleoside/nucleotide reverse transcriptase inhibitors (nRTIs), PIs, non-nucleoside reverse transcriptase inhibitors (nnRTIs), entry inhibitors, and integrase inhibitors. Clear benefit of combination ART is now well established and even in late-stage disease they can achieve both immunological and clinical benefit with dramatic decline in HIV viral load. Significant benefit in terms of morbidity and mortality is demonstrated as well as in the immune markers.

Nevertheless, there will always be a small number of people who are diagnosed very late in the course of their HIV infection, or who cannot tolerate the drugs, or who have significant drug resistance, or who do not wish to take them (or any combination of these factors).

Table 14.2 Antiretroviral drugs.

Nucleoside reverse transcriptase inhibitors	Protease inhibitors	Non-nucleoside reverse transcriptase inhibitors
Abacavir (ABC)	Darunavir	Efavirenz
Emtricitabine (FTC)	Fosamprenavir	Nevirapine
Didanosine (ddI)	Indinavir	Etravirine
Lamivudine (3TC)	Lopinavir	Rilpivirine
Stavudine (d4T)	Nelfinavir	
Zidovudine (AZT)	Ritonavir	
Zalcitabine (ddC)	Saquinavir	
	Tipranavir	
Nucleotide reverse transcriptase inhibitor	**Entry Inhibitors**	**Integrase inhibitors**
Tenofovir	Maraviroc Enfurvitide	Raltegravir

Toxicity of antiretroviral agents

Long-term use of antiretroviral medication is associated with a number of abnormalities related to lipid metabolism, fat distribution, and mitochondrial function. For peripheral neuropathy, see earlier. Other problems include:

- hypercholesterolemia;
- hypertriglyceridemia;
- insulin resistance and type II diabetes;
- body fat loss (face, buttocks, legs);
- body fat accumulation (abdominal, breast, buffalo hump); and
- renal toxicity;
- osteopenia/osteoporosis.

Metabolic sequelae may be treated with nutritional advice/support, exercise programs, lipid-regulating agents, and diabetic agents, as appropriate. For SC fat loss, management is often supportive—but the body changes can lead to significant psychological consequences if severe. Injections of polylactic acid are available at many centres to provide bulk to the facial area where fat loss is most prominent and visible.

Immune reconstitution inflammatory syndrome

Immune reconstitution inflammatory syndrome (IRIS) is seen after initiation of successful ART in people with relatively advanced immunosuppression. As the immune system begins to recover, it responds to a previously acquired OI with an overwhelming inflammatory response that paradoxically makes the symptoms or signs worse. Two IRIS scenarios are common: one when an occult OI activates as the immune response is improving and the other when a previously diagnosed OI appears to relapse despite a previous successful response to microbiological treatment. Although the symptoms/signs may sometimes be dangerous, they do at least indicate that the improved immune response gives the individual a better chance to overcome the infection. The best treatment is not always fully known—it may be appropriate to sit tight and await spontaneous resolution or in some situations appropriate antibacterial or antiviral agents should be prescribed. In some cases, corticosteroids are indicated.

Infections most commonly associated with IRIS include *Mycobacterium* TB, CMV, herpes zoster, PCP, and MAC or MAI. HIV-positive patients are more at risk for IRIS if they are starting combination ART for the first time.

Corticosteroids

Practitioners are often reluctant to prescribe steroids to patients with HIV because of fears that this will accelerate the disease and predispose to OIs. However, the benefits of steroids in certain situations are clearly established and they may also be helpful in palliating nonspecific symptoms by:

- lifting mood;
- reducing fatigue;
- improving anorexia resistant to anabolic steroids;
- acting as an adjuvant antiemetic for nausea or vomiting;
- promoting weight gain with improved body image;
- modulating fever associated with HIV *per se*, lymphoma, or MAC infection;
- reducing the oedema and pain from visceral KS; and
- acting as an adjuvant to analgesia for patients with painful neuropathy or myopathy.

Short courses at a higher dose probably give more benefit than prolonged low-dose treatment. Patients need to be aware of the potential side effects and offered an initial trial of treatment.

Opioid medication

There is often concern about prescribing opioids for pain when treating patients with a current or previous history of drug abuse, and pain may be undertreated for this reason. In all stages of HIV, control of pain must be a priority. Additionally, patients who have been on maintenance methadone for many years are sometimes fearful of changing to an alternative opioid. For such a patient in pain, the choices are:

1. to continue same dose of methadone and add morphine or some other opioid as an analgesic; or
2. to increase dose of methadone: using it for both "maintenance" and analgesia.

There is little evidence about the comparative efficacy of these methods, but probably the first is the most satisfactory. Although the GP may be prescribing both methadone maintenance and opioid analgesia, it is important that the patient is clear about the difference between the two.

Methadone equivalence with other opioids can be difficult to calculate owing to the comparatively longer half-life and broad-spectrum receptor affinity. Therefore, a single 5-mg dose may be equivalent to 7.5 mg of morphine, but when given repeatedly, it may be 5–10 times more potent, gram for gram, than morphine [24]. It is strongly recommended that specialist palliative care advice is sought when there is to be a combination of methadone and other opioids to manage pain in this context.

The use of the additional opioid for analgesia should be fully discussed and clear guidelines, boundaries, and a plan for review unambiguously drawn up with the patients and their carers and other professionals involved in the patient's care to prevent abuse. Many of these patients exhibit remarkable opioid tolerance and sometimes pain control may be achieved and maintained only with what may appear to be an alarmingly high opioid dose. Appropriate antiemetic and laxative agents should always be prescribed and, if needed, sedative agents.

Finally, some drug users come from families where substance abuse is common, and times of stress, such as a relative dying, may precipitate excesses of drugs and/or alcohol with unpredictable behaviour during visits. Setting clear guidelines on visiting—both in the home and in the hospital/hospice—and giving frequent and clear explanations about the patient's treatment plans and condition are crucial to avoid unpleasant confrontations around the dying patient.

Drug interactions

The antiretroviral drugs affect hepatic metabolism of many other drugs (either through inhibition or induction of the CYP3A/cytochrome P450 pathway). For full up-to-date information, the reader is referred to the web site of University of Liverpool (http://www.hiv-druginteractions.org/) or the British National Formulary. Some important interactions concern nevirapine and methadone (reduction in methadone levels can lead to withdrawal syndrome in some patients), and drugs such as fluconazole, itraconazole, ergotamine derivatives, phenytoin, phenobarbital, and carbamazepine—all of which are contraindicated with various antiretrovirals. Finally, there are potential interactions with herbal remedies (including St. John's wort and *Echinacea*) that can affect the potency of antiretroviral drugs.

Complementary therapy

Acupuncture, aromatherapy, reflexology, and massage can all be beneficial for specific symptoms, as well as the general well-being of a person living with symptomatic HIV infection. Many involve hands-on therapy with human contact that is much valued by the client—and the consultation time is often longer than that of the traditional services.

The end of life

In many cities, certain undertakers have established a good reputation for sensitivity in handling HIV-related deaths. Patient support/advocacy groups or local HIV units should be able to give advice on this, for example, Terrence Higgins Trust [25]. A good undertaker can advise on issues such as type of funeral or cremation service as well as more complex problems such as the transport of body to another country [26].

Death certification

In many countries, death certification continues to be a contentious issue largely for the reasons that a death certificate is a public document. At the same time, the law requires doctors to provide factual information, where available, about the cause of death. Add to this the fact that a doctor's duty of confidentiality to the patient continues beyond his or her death and it can be seen that the certifying doctor has dual responsibilities. The General Medical Council (GMC) in the United Kingdom is aware of this and, as a result, has issued guidance on how doctors can manage this sometimes difficult dilemma [19,20]. Anticipation is the key. Talking to and discussing this with a senior or more experienced colleague are strategies that can be adopted to try and ensure the best is done for the patient. It must also be remembered that such documentation is also critical for HIV/AIDS statistics and ultimately public health—so it is everyone's duty to provide this whenever possible [27].

Where people die?

Since the early 1990s, the improved prognosis of people with HIV/AIDS has led, perhaps inevitably, to a more aggressive approach to treatment of those who become symptomatic and ill. Although the proportion of those who die in hospice has not changed significantly, fewer deaths occur at home, with more occurring in acute hospital settings. Generally, outside of HIV/AIDS, and especially noticeable over the past generation, the proportion of home deaths in England and Wales fell from 31% to 18%, though the exact reason for this is unclear. It may well be due to a combination of factors including increased anxiety (by patient or carers) as death draws near and a lack of enhanced community support [28]. For those who require social care and nursing support, Appendix A is a brief guide for practitioners who are unused to providing care for patients with HIV.

Bereavement

Carers, family, friends, and professionals may be at risk of difficult and abnormal grief in relation to deaths from HIV and AIDS. Table 14.3 gives a synopsis of risk factors associated with abnormal or a protracted bereavement

Table 14.3 Risk factors for difficult bereavement in AIDS-related deaths.

Multiple loss experiences
History of alcohol and drug abuse
Bereaved may also be ill
Denial of status as a lover/partner
Social isolation
Stigma of the disease
Stigma of their lifestyle
Undisclosed diagnosis
Family rejection
Anger
Powerlessness

process [9]. Chapter 7, *Adapting to Death, Dying, and Bereavement*, discusses in detail the identification of risk factors and the prevention of problems.

Conclusion

Defining palliative care for people living with HIV and AIDS will always be a challenge as the advances in ART bring an increase in life expectancy. Within the HIV/AIDS context, associated drug toxicities and other problems connected with chronic illness render this as difficult a problem as any encountered in clinical practice. The arguments about defining palliative care in any patient, with any condition(s) continues unabated [28–30]. The recent focus on the GSF for end-of-life care adds impetus to this debate especially for patients with HIV infection or AIDS [15].

Many have called for a systems approach to meaningful end-of-life care—a system that uses elements from the curative approach while ensuring that palliation of symptoms remains a major priority both for the patient and their carers. It is our belief that in this system general practice along with community services as well as hospital specialists should form the basis for quality end-of-life care [9,18].

References

1. UNAIDS Report: Towards Universal Access. Available at: http://www.unaids.org/en/aboutunaids/universalaccesstohivtreatmentpreventioncareandsupport/ (accessed July12, 2012).
2. *United Nations Report. 65th Session Agenda item No.10, 28 March 2011: Uniting for universal access towards zero new infections, zero discrimination and zero AIDS-related deaths: report of the Secretary-General.* Available at: http://www.who.int/hiv/pub/unsg_report_20110331.pdf (accessed on July 10, 2012).
3. World Health Organisation. *Key Facts on HIV/AIDS by the WHO.* Available at: http://www.who.int/features/factfiles/hiv/en/index.html (accessed on July 10, 2012).
4. UNAIDS. *Fact-Sheet: Eastern Europe and Central Asia. The Joint United Nations Program on HIV/AIDS.* Available at: http://www.unaids.org/en/regionscountries/regions/easterneuropeandcentralasia/ (accessed on July 12, 2012).
5. *New HIV and AIDS diagnoses and deaths in the United Kingdom in 2011.* Available at: http://www.hpa.org.uk/hpr/archives/2012/news1612.htm (accessed July 6, 2012).
6. *HIV in the United Kingdom: 2011 Report.* Available at: http://www.hpa.org.uk/webc/HPAwebFile/HPAweb_C/1317131685847 (accessed on July 6, 2012).
7. Health Protection Agency. *BHIVA/BASHH/BIS UK National Guidelines for HIV Testing 2008.* Available at: http://www.bhiva.org/HIVTesting2008.aspx (accessed June 29, 2012).
8. Health Protection Agency. *Largest Ever Annual Number of New HIV Diagnoses in MSM.* Available at: http://www.hpa.org.uk/webw/HPAweb&HPAwebStandard/HPAweb_C/1317131680627 (accessed July 12, 2012).
9. Madge S, Matthews P, Singh S, et al. *HIV/AIDS in Primary Care.* London: MedFASH Publications, 2011. Also available at: http://www.medfash.org (accessed July 6, 2012).
10. Public Health Agency of Canada. *HIV and AIDS in Canada. Surveillance Report to December 31, 2010.* Surveillance and Risk Assessment Division, Centre for Communicable Diseases and Infection Control, Public Health Agency of Canada, 2010. Available at: http://www.phac-aspc.gc.ca/aids-sida/publication/epi/2010/1-eng.php (accessed July 12, 2012).
11. Centers for Disease Control and Prevention (CDC). *HIV at a glance (2010 figures).* Available at: http://www.cdc.gov/hiv/resources/factsheets/PDF/HIV_at_a_glance.pdf (accessed July 12, 2012) Also available at: http://www.cdc.gov/hiv/topics/surveillance/resources/factsheets/pdf/HIV_overview_2012.pdf
12. World Health Organization. *AIDS Treatment and Care: Clinical protocols for the WHO European region,* 2007. Available at: http://www.who.int/_data/assets/pdf_file/0004/78106/E90840.pdf (accessed July 12, 2012).
13. Harding R, Simms V, Krakauer E, et al. Quality HIV care to the end of life. *Clin Infect Dis* 2011; 52(4): 553–554.
14. Thomas K. Improving end of life care: a matter of life and death. *Lond J Prim Care* 2009; 2: 89–92.
15. Gold Standards Framework. Available at: www.goldstandardsframework.org.uk/About_GSF(accessed July 12, 2012).
16. Gysels M and Higginson IJ. *Improving supportive and palliative care for adults with cancer: the manual.* London: National

Institute for Clinical Excellence, 2004. Also available at: http://www.nice.org.uk/nicemedia/live/10893/28816/28816 .pdf (accessed on July 4, 2012).

17. Harding R, Easterbrook P, Higginson IJ, et al. Access and equity in HIV/AIDS palliative care: a review of the evidence and responses. *Palliat Med* 2005; 19: 251–258. Also available at: http://pmj.sagepub.com/content/19/3/251 (accessed on July 7, 2012).

18. Singh S, Dunford A, and Carter Y. Routine care of people with HIV infection and AIDS: should interested general practitioners take the lead? *Br J Gen Pract* 2001; 51: 399–403.

19. General Medical Council. *Good Medical Practice*, 4th edition. London: General Medical Council, 2006. Also available at: http://www.gmc-uk.org/static/documents/content/GMP_ 0910.pdf (accessed December 11, 2012).

20. General Medical Council. Confidentiality guidance: disclosure after a patient's death. Available at: http://www.gmc-uk.org/static/documents/content/Confidentiality_0910.pdf (accessed July 12, 2012).

21. Health Protection Agency. *HPA Migrant health guide.* Available at: www.hpa.org.uk/MigrantHealthGuide July 12, 2012).

22. Larue F, Fontaine A, and Colleau SM. Underestimation and undertreatment of pain in HIV disease: multicentre study. *BMJ* 1997; 314: 23–28.

23. Breitbart W, Rosenfeld BD, Passik SD, et al. The undertreatment of pain in ambulatory AIDS patients. *Pain* 1996; 65: 243–249.

24. Twycross R and Wilcock A. *Palliative Care Formulary.* Nottingham: Palliativedrugs.com, 2007.

25. Terrence HigginsTrust. *Dealing with death and bereavement – Losing someone:* http://www.tht.org.uk/myhiv/HIV- and-you/Relationships/Losing-someone (accessed July 12, 2012).

26. National Association of Funeral Directors. Available at: http://www.nafd.org.uk/funeral-advice/funeral- advice-home.aspx (accessed on July 12, 2012).

27. Berlin A. Death certification: topical tips for GPs. *Lond J Prim Care* 2009; 2: 130–137.

28. Ellershaw J, Dewar S, and Murphy D. Achieving a good death for all. *BMJ* 2010; 341: c4862.

29. Palmer EM. Palliative care: importance of keeping both hands open. *BMJ* 2011; 342: d2887.

30. Reid C. Palliative care is not the same as end of life. *BMJ* 2011; 342: d2735.

Further reading

Gazzard B (ed.). *AIDS Care Handbook*, 2nd edition. London: Mediscript, 2002.

Harding R, Stewart K, Marconi K, et al. Current HIV/AIDS end-of-life care in sub-Saharan Africa: a survey of models, services, challenges and priorities. *BMC Public Health* 2003; 3: 33.

Miller R and Murray D. *Social Work and HIV/AIDS– Practitioner's Guide.* Birmingham: Venture Press, 1998.

Sherr L (ed.). *Grief and AIDS.* Chichester: John Wiley & Sons, 1995.

Singh S and Madge S. Caring for People with HIV: A Community Perspective. Aldershot: Ashgate Publications, 1999.

Wood CG, Whittet S, and Bradbeer CS. ABC of palliative care. HIV infection and AIDS. *BMJ* 1997; 315: 1433–1436.

Appendix A

Precautionary measures at home [12]

When palliative care is offered at home, the health-care provider (doctor or nurse) should counsel the home care provider (family member, friend, or other service provider) on the following points:

Family members and other caregivers can safely care for AIDS patients. There is an extremely low risk of HIV transmission to health-care providers and household contacts if the following hygienic practices are respected:

- Wear latex gloves when in contact with blood and bodily fluids.
- Keep wounds covered (on both caregivers and persons living with HIV (PLHIV)); if they become wet with blood or other body fluids, change dressings and dispose of properly.
- Clean up blood, faeces, and urine with ordinary household bleach while wearing gloves.
- Keep clothing and sheets that are stained with blood, faeces, or other body fluids separate from other household laundry. Use a piece of plastic or gloves to handle soiled items.
- Do not share toothbrushes, razors, needles, or other skin-piercing instruments.
- Wash hands with soap and water after changing soiled bedsheets and clothing and after any contact with bodily fluids.

There is no risk from casual household contact (no gloves needed).

Cutlery and other food items, unsoiled clothing and linens, toilets, baths, showers, and so on can be cleaned with ordinary cleaning products.

Handbook of Palliative Care, Third Edition. Edited by Christina Faull, Sharon de Caestecker, Alex Nicholson and Fraser Black.
© 2012 by John Wiley and Sons, Inc. Published 2012 by John Wiley & Sons, Inc.

15 Palliative Care for Children

Harold Siden[1], Camara van Breemen[2]

[1]Canuck Place Children's Hospice and University of British Columbia
[2]Canuck Place Children's Hospice, Vancouver, Canada

Introduction

The death of a child is recognised as one of the greatest tragedies that can happen to a family. The family's grief and distress are intense and long lasting and, now that death in childhood is so uncommon in the developed world, many families are never exposed to it. In these settings, parents can experience considerable isolation. Parents' expectations and plans barely even acknowledge the possibility of a child dying and society as a whole has become unfamiliar and uncomfortable with death in childhood and the ways to offer support. This includes medical and nursing staff too, who are affected not only emotionally but often also by their lack of experience and confidence.

This chapter can only offer an overview of pediatric palliative care (PPC). It will identify the children for whom palliative care is appropriate, discuss some of their needs, particularly where these differ from the needs of adults, and consider how services can be provided for them. The aim of this chapter is to provide an insight into the problems of the sick child and their family, and provide practical advice to primary care clinicians who are caring for these children and their families.

What kinds of children receive palliative care? Is it just children with cancer?

In developed nations, children enjoy unprecedented good health; over the past 100 years, infant and child mortality rates have plummeted. The common diseases, mostly infectious, that contributed to widespread child mortality have been eliminated through improved water and food safety, immunisation, and the availability of antibi-

> **Box 15.1 The range of life-limiting conditions affecting children**
>
> - Cancer.
> - Cardiopulmonary (cardiac and respiratory diseases).
> - Chromosomal abnormalities or gene abnormalities leading to multiorgan involvement.
> - Primary CNS condition, which includes primary dysgenesis of the brain, hypoxic-ischemic encephalopathy, and neurodegenerative diseases.
> - Infectious and immunological diseases.
> - Biochemical (metabolic) disorders of enzymatic pathways.
> - Neuromuscular diseases affecting peripheral neurons and muscles.

otics. Cancer is the number one disease-related cause of mortality in children in industrialised countries, but it actually is a rare disease with a high cure rate [1]. Other lethal diseases, while not cured, are amenable to aggressive and intensive long-term therapy; for example, the median survival age for cystic fibrosis (CF) is now 46.7 years [2]. The success in treating diseases such as cancer or prolonging life in CF represents a marvellous achievement. There still are rare diseases that lack curative therapies. In these conditions, treatment directed toward symptoms will prolong life. Our ability to maintain survival for many years in severe conditions which are ultimately terminal, for example, neurodegenerative diseases, or some forms of congenital heart disease means that palliative (comfort-focused) care must be provided for a long time.

The range of life limiting conditions (LLCs) that affect children is wide (Box 15.1). Palliative care needs to be considered for all these children, not just those with

Handbook of Palliative Care, Third Edition. Edited by Christina Faull, Sharon de Caestecker, Alex Nicholson and Fraser Black.
© 2012 by John Wiley and Sons, Inc. Published 2012 by John Wiley & Sons, Inc.

Quadrant 1

Conditions that can be cured but have the possibility of death (e.g., cancer)

Quadrant 2

Conditions requiring intensive therapy to prolong life that are ultimately terminal (e.g., cystic fibrosis, HIV-AIDS)

Quadrant 3

Conditions that have no cure but whose symptoms can be managed (e.g., metabolic disease)

Quadrant 4

Severe neurological impairments where complications lead to early death (e.g., severe cerebral palsy)

Figure 15.1 Canuck Place four quadrants model. Canuck Place Children's Hospice, Vancouver, Canada. (Adapted from [3].)

cancer. Most of the illnesses are specific to paediatrics and many are very rare; some are familial and many have a protracted course. Four broad groups can be identified (Figure 15.1). The original four categories of diseases to be considered for PPC services were described in a joint report of the British Association for Children's Palliative Care (ACT) and the Royal College of Paediatrics and Child Health (RCPCH) [3]. The four-category model is not intended to be exact, but instead a conceptual model that helps describe the span of diseases seen in PPC. It also suggests that as medicine advances diseases will shift from one category or "quadrant" to another. For example, enzyme replacement therapy has shifted some metabolic diseases from quadrant 3 (noncurable, nontreatable) to quadrant 2 (noncurable, treatable). The exception is quadrant 4, where in absence of being able to prevent the causes of static encephalopathy (such as trauma), there are not yet curative approaches.

In recent years, there has been increasing attention to a fifth group, not found in the original ACT/RCPCH report or the Canuck Place four quadrants model, namely, perinatal palliative care. In this group, attention is directed toward a foetus identified prenatally with life-threatening conditions [4–6]. Several outcomes are possible, including elective termination, stillbirth, death in the immediate delivery period, and a shortened life lasting hours, days, or weeks only. For these families, care begins at the time of *in utero* diagnosis. It requires careful planning and development of an integrated plan involving primary care/family physicians, obstetricians/midwives, geneticists, and/or other subspecialists (e.g., cardiol-

ogists), neonatologists/general paediatricians, delivery room nurses/midwives, and community nurses.

When is the right time for the clinician to consider palliative care for a child?

The four quadrants model, with the new addition of perinatal palliative care, is a starting point to understand when to introduce the elements of palliative care. Significant evolution of the field has reaffirmed that palliative care is an overarching umbrella, within which end-of-life or terminal care is only one specific phase. Palliative care, in our definition, applies to children with life-threatening illnesses, in other words those living with the following circumstances:
• The condition or disease is acquired in the span of childhood (defined as foetal life through adolescence).
• The condition is progressive, and is likely to result in the person's death before they reach full adulthood.
• There is no effective treatment directed toward the pathophysiology of the child's disease or if there is a treatment, it is failing in this patient.

One simple way to think about the condition is to ask the question, "Would the physician be surprised if this child died before they reached their mid-20s?" The answer to this question helps to conceptualise that the patient may benefit from the use of some of the elements of PPC as described in this chapter. The provision of PPC means balancing complex, chronic care with consideration of end-of-life care.

Does palliative care in children allow "curative" treatments to be continued?

It should be clear that PPC is provided in a complementary manner with curative care in children. In part, this is based on a strong philosophy of family-centred care now found throughout paediatrics. Families often choose aggressive curative or life-prolonging therapy when it is offered, even when it is apparent that the likelihood of cure, recovery, or prolongation is remote. Strong hope is fundamental for parents, leading to heroic efforts to save their children. Arguing that palliative care requires a cessation or discontinuation of these attempts is futile, and only establishes grounds for an unproductive relationship. Parents need active support in providing curative therapies even at the end of life. These treatments are only stopped when it is clear that they cause more harm than good. Second, aside from cancer and some conditions such as pretransplant conditions, most of the childhood life-threatening illnesses actually do not have curative treatments. Prolongation of life in noncurable conditions actually happens through simple interventions such as artificial enteral nutrition (gastrostomy tubes), antibiotics, seizure control, oxygen, and so on. It is these "simple" interventions that usually make the difference, not the implementation or discontinuation of a single disease targeted therapy. In this context, elements of PPC can be provided at any point along the trajectory, and not all elements need to be introduced at the same time.

Families whose children are experiencing diseases and conditions that hold a chance for a cure frequently seek it up until the very end of life. They often come to palliative care reluctantly; it almost always occurs late in an illness when the disease is obviously progressing and symptoms are becoming a major issue. It is important for these families to see how care providers can balance curative treatment with palliative treatment. For example, Canuck Place Children's Hospice in British Columbia, Canada does not require a Do Not Attempt Resuscitation/Permit Natural Death (DNAR/PND) order to be in place before a child and their family can be accepted on to the palliative care program. Many families never sign such an order, and yet at the end of life they are willing and able to acknowledge the onset of death, and do not request any resuscitation.

Thus, in the field of PPC a dichotomy exists. The dichotomy is between situations where families experience living with a child with likely death at an uncertain time, and families who experience treating a disease where cure and/or living into adulthood are possibilities. Regardless of which "quadrant" a child falls into, the decision to implement palliative care usually arises after a long process of discussion between families and physicians, social workers, nurses, and other care providers. It is important for families to know that when palliative care is instituted, especially when a DNAR/PND order is written, that viable options of ongoing comprehensive care directed toward comfort are available and will be provided right up to the time of the child's death. They should also be aware that involvement with a palliative care team continues afterward through bereavement.

What symptoms are children likely to have?

The symptoms encountered in children will not be substantially different than those encountered in adults with similar diseases and in moments of crisis. Children, like adults, can experience pain, dyspnoea, and any of the symptoms associated with significant and terminal illness. Cancer symptoms in one major study included fatigue, unrelieved pain, dyspnoea, poor appetite, or nausea, with 89% of children experiencing significant suffering from one or more symptoms [7]. It is important to remember that at least half of the children receiving palliative care (i.e., living with LLCs) will have conditions affecting the nervous system rather than cancer. Therefore, pain may not be the single most common symptom a clinician needs to deal with. Instead, a broad range of symptoms is often encountered, and problems may be respiratory (dyspnoea, secretions, and aspiration), GI (reflux, vomiting, feeding intolerance, and constipation), and neurological (insomnia, irritability, and seizures) [8].

How do I deal with developmental differences in assessing symptoms?

The greatest challenge for the clinician is not the symptoms, but the assessment of them. Symptom assessment must occur through a developmental lens; it is helpful to consider development as occurring along two tracks: typical and atypical (sometimes called delayed or impaired). In typical development, there is a progression from infancy through early and then mid-childhood, on to pubescence, adolescence, and young adulthood. At each of these phases, a child's communication ability will be different, and distinct approaches are needed for symptom assessment. For example, infants are essentially without language, but pain will be obvious with crying, tears, thrashing, and grimacing; however, the causes of pain will not be known, nor will the child localise it. Other symptoms, such as dyspnoea, which is a subjective sensation, will be even harder to assess. It is axiomatic in paediatrics to trust the parent's concerns and descriptions; even when it may be a challenge for a clinician to assess pain, parents are reliable reporters of their child's pain or other symptoms.

The task of symptom assessment becomes easier with mid-childhood (age 5+) and upward. It must be remembered that adolescence will pose its own challenges in terms of cooperation with assessment and the focus of adolescents on privacy. They may not describe their symptoms because of issues regarding trust, confidentiality, or a desire to avoid a sick role.

For a child with severe neurological impairment, regardless of underlying aetiology, the language-based developmental trajectory will be very different. Development is often uneven in these situations with language, cognition, and fine and gross motor skills moving at different speeds or arrested at different stages. It is clear that these children experience the same spectrum of symptoms described for any of the diseases, but the nature of the personal experience for any given child is virtually unknown. Their parents and caregivers, based on close observation, are the most helpful sources of information in identifying symptoms, assessing the intensity, and interpreting the experience.

Are there any tools to help with symptom assessment?

Across the developmental ranges described, tools exist for some, but not all symptoms. The greatest amount of work has been done in the field of pain. For typically developing children, there are a number of well-validated, easy-to-use assessment tools. It should be understood that these tools do not determine if pain is present; that is, they do not rule it in or out, but instead provide a scoring system against which one can measure the effect of interventions. To slavishly score a child's pain when there are no changes to analgesics or interventions is pointless. Box 15.2 lists available tools for assessing pain. In nonverbal patients, there are also valid and reliable tools. These were developed by undertaking collaborative research with parents who described their child's response to painful experiences.

For some of the common symptoms besides pain, such as dyspnoea, secretions, and insomnia, tools are under development, but none have reached widespread use. Constipation can be tracked with the Bristol Stool Chart, as checking consistency of faeces is important. However, assessment tools do not exist for some of the other problems such as reflux, vomiting, feeding intolerance, and seizures. In these situations, it helps to use a simple charting tool to capture frequency of episodes.

General principles for symptom management in children

It should be remembered that medication is only one aspect of symptom management. For each and every symptom, regardless of whether it is pain, respiratory symptoms, vomiting, or other symptoms, one must understand the context and the environment and make

---

Box 15.2 The assessment of pain in children and the tools that are available to support this

Specific assessment tools
3 years and up
- Faces Pain Scale—Revised (available at: http://www.usask.ca/childpain/fpsr).

School-age child
- Visual Analogue Scale (straight line, +/− numbers).
- Colour a body chart (different colours for different pains).

Adolescent
- Any of the above.
- Numerical rating scales.

Nonverbal children
- Direct questioning.
- Non-Communicating Children's Pain Checklist (NCCPC) [9] (available at: http://pediatric-pain.ca/files/02/78/NCCPCR_200901.pdf).
- Paediatric Pain Profile (PPP) [10] (available at: http://www.ppprofile.org.uk).
- FLACC Pain Scale (Face, Legs, Activity, Cry, Consolability Behavioral Scale) [11] (available at: http://www.med.umich.edu/1libr/pa/UMPedsPain.pdf).

Ask the parents
- They know their child the best.
- But they may lack confidence in their own assessment.

Consider contributory factors
- Meaning of the pain and underlying disease to the child and family.

---

modifications accordingly. This is simpler to do in a responsive adolescent who can provide a detailed description of the antecedents and relieving interventions for the symptom. Moreover, we expect that adolescents will be able to adjust their environment and schedules to their own liking. The same is not true for infants, young children, or nonverbal patients. This is one reason why PPC is a time-consuming activity. One must carefully develop with the family a detailed description of the setting, timing, and influences on a symptom's presentation.

Aside from medication, one always considers nonmedication interventions. Adopting a holistic approach that addresses the psychological, social, and spiritual concerns of the child and family is likely to achieve better symptom management than medication alone. Children have great powers of imagination and distraction that can be brought to bear in managing symptoms. This is especially well understood for treating pain, but has importance for other symptoms such as sleep disruption:

• *Care over positioning and the environment:* Sometimes the parents can address this, but at other times an occupational therapist or a physiotherapist can be helpful.

• *Distraction, imagery, and relaxation techniques:* These can be introduced to the child and the family with the assistance of a psychologist or other therapist. In Canada, every tertiary care children's hospital has a child life department available for consultation.

• *Play, art, and music therapy:* Counselling therapists with specific training in these techniques can provide these modalities.

Parents fear that they will not have the skills and confidence to relieve the pain and other symptoms that their child may experience. It is therefore important to provide them with detailed and honest information about the management of their child's current symptoms and any others that may be anticipated. Both they and the sick child need to take an active part in planning a practical and acceptable regimen of care, where possible retaining their confidence and control. It may help to draw out a flow-sheet algorithm for families showing when to give medications, when to phone for assistance, and so on.

Symptom patterns

Children dying from cancer are likely to have a final illness lasting only a few weeks or months, although brain tumours tend to have a more protracted course. These children often experience pain, depending on the site and spread of the tumour. Other problems include GI symptoms such as nausea, vomiting, and constipation. Bone marrow involvement is common in childhood cancer, so anaemia and bleeding are often concerns. Dyspnoea, anxiety, agitation, and seizures may also occur.

In contrast, children with slower degenerative diseases suffer a different spectrum of problems over a much longer period. Feeding difficulties, impaired intellect and communication, seizures, and poor mobility are common. These increase as the illness progresses and respiratory difficulties and excess secretions may develop. It can be difficult to distinguish intermittent bouts of severe symptoms from an end-of-life episode. The underlying nature of the neurological and metabolic conditions is quite different from cancer; rather than steady downward trajectory as may be seen with cancer, symptoms crises may be intermittent with returns to baseline in-between.

Notes about some specific symptoms

Pain

Pain can be due to nociceptive-inflammatory causes, such as direct tumour invasion, fractures, or pressure sores. Some cancers have a propensity to generate neuropathic pain via direct damage to neurons. In children with neurological, metabolic, and other gene-level conditions, a syndrome of pain behaviour and irritability is very common. There is no set nomenclature for this entity, with some authors referring to it as "neuropathic pain" while others call it "central pain." In any event, it is clearly a distressing symptom identified as a diagnosis of exclusion once all identifiable nociceptive-inflammatory causes have been ruled out. In the case of the noncancer patient, careful and thorough history-taking, physical examination, laboratory and imaging studies evaluate these nociceptive-inflammatory causes. Entities such as reflux disease, occult fracture, hip dysplasia, constipation, and hypertonicity need to be considered. In the end, one may be left with a patient with a syndrome of "pain/irritability of unknown origin." Management of this syndrome is not straightforward and may require the assistance of a paediatric subspecialist skilled in symptom management.

Feeding

For parents, an inability to feed and to nourish their child is very upsetting and often makes them feel they are failing in their role. Children with neurodegenerative diseases and brain tumours often have problems with eating because of neurological damage. Others, such as those with cancers, will lose their appetite. Nutritional goals aimed at some idealised weight gain and growth often remain primary in the family's mind, rather than becoming secondary to comfort and enjoyment as disease progresses. Clinicians should reframe the discussion to focus on comfort, even if that means minimal food intake. Assisted feeding, via a nasogastric (NG) tube or gastrostomy, may be the entirely correct choice for those with slowly progressive disease, but inappropriate for a child with a rapidly progressing tumour.

One of the most challenging subjects within PPC is withdrawal or not initiating assisted feeding. This can occur within many contexts, ranging from neonates who have never been fed, to dwindling appetite for the child with cancer, and to feed intolerance for the child reliant on tube feeds. One of the first questions is whether it is "ethical" to withhold or withdraw feeding for a child. This question has been recently addressed by both the

Canadian Pediatric Society and by the American Academy of Pediatrics, who have concluded that there are circumstances related to terminal illness where the cessation of feeding is ethical [12,13]. Their statements have outlined the elements of practice and process that need to be undertaken, including consensus among professionals, the family, and at times, the involvement of a bioethicist or clinical ethics committee.

The topic of feeding withdrawal is one that needs to be brought up sensitively, and involve a discussion with the parents and the entire care team. The most common indication is that the child, whether orally or tube fed, is no longer tolerating food. This can be seen with worsening symptoms such as nausea or vomiting. In the case of nonverbal, tube-fed children, reflux often becomes worse as well as pain behaviours, coughing, secretions, and hypertonic spasms. Parents and the team need to consider whether feeds make the symptoms worse. In our experience, most children do better with lower levels of feeding and hydration at end of life, and seem to live longer but with fewer symptoms than those cases where food is "pushed," More research needs to be done to address this issue [14].

Often, parents opt to reduce feeds to a minimum level, even with an electrolyte solution alone—this may ameliorate their concern that they are denying any food to the child. Extended family needs to be brought into the discussion as well, as they are often the major source of questions to the parents as to the wisdom of the decision. In withholding feeds, parents often change their minds, so that the discussion may have to occur more than once, with brief trials of reinitiating feeds to test against symptom severity.

Seizures

Watching a child have a seizure is frightening for parents and they should be advised about its management if there is any possibility it may happen. Children with neurodegenerative diseases often develop seizures as part of their ongoing disease and will already be taking routine anticonvulsants. These drugs can be adjusted when the pattern of seizures changes. Acute seizures can be treated with benzodiazepines. Country-specific guidance varies as to which drug should be given first, second, and third line: rectal diazepam, buccal or intranasal midazolam, or sublingual/buccal lorazepam. Regardless of drug choice, parents need teaching to administer these medications, which should be done at the time of prescribing them. We find the use of a box and arrow algorithm diagram

helpful for parents in advising them when and how to give medications for symptoms (Figure 15.2).

Respiratory symptoms

Dyspnoea, cough, and excess secretions can all cause distress to children and anxiety for their parents. If the underlying cause of the symptom can be relieved, even temporarily, this may be appropriate.

Excess secretions are often a problem for children with chronic neurodegenerative diseases as their illness progresses and they become less able to cough and swallow. This may also occur in other terminally ill children as they approach death. Oral glycopyrrolate, atropine, or hyoscine hydrobromide (also given by transdermal or subcutaneous (SC) routes) can all help to reduce the secretions but guidelines will vary as to which drug is the preferred local or country choice and of course best choice for the individual child. Routine and frequent chest physiotherapy and changing the child's position often provides temporary relief. It is tempting to use oral pharyngeal suctioning, but this can make the secretions more copious by stimulating the salivary glands.

What medications can I use in children and what doses?

When planning treatment, the preferences of the child and family need to be taken into account. It is important to find the most acceptable route for the child and to be flexible to changing situations. The key issues in deciding on routes of administration are as follows:

• The oral route is often preferable; however, one must plan alternate routes. At some point, a child may no longer be able to swallow. In that case, planning for medications that can be given by NG tube, intravenous (IV) infusion, or SC infusion needs to be done. Other important routes are rectal, sublingual/buccal, and intranasal. This planning should be done well in advance, rather than scrambling at the last minute. Working with a pharmacist who has a background in compounding is helpful in choosing medications and routes.

• Although rectal drugs are not commonly used, they can play a role; some children prefer them to using any needles. Rectal route should be a choice made by the child—there is usually an alternative, parenteral option (SC/IV) once a child's conscious level has decreased such that they cannot take medications by mouth. It may be helpful if other nonoral routes are not acceptable.

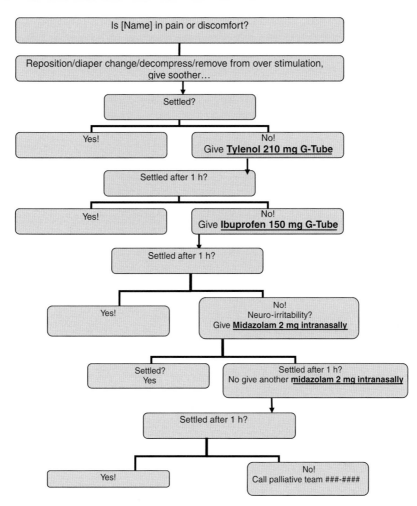

Figure 15.2 An example algorithm for parents to aid their management of seizures. From Canuck Place Children's Hospice, Vancouver, Canada.

- If parenteral drugs are needed, they can be usually given by continuous SC infusion, not as bolus doses; alternatively, an IV line can be used if it is already in place, especially when a vascular access device has been inserted.
- For children with neurological impairment using gastrostomy or jejunostomy routes, these devices make medication delivery easy. However, very close to end of life, digestion and motility may be compromised. In that situation, we have found SC routes to be useful.
- Intramuscular drugs are painful and not necessary.

Many of the drugs used in palliative care have not been recommended formally for use in children but a body of clinical experience has developed in the absence of many trials or extensive pharmacokinetic data. There are now several paediatric drug formularies available. In the United Kingdom, clinicians use the British National Formulary for Children [15] and the Association for Paediatric Palliative Medicine Master Formulary [16]. In Canada and the United States, practitioners often rely upon the *HSC Handbook of Paediatrics* [17] and the Harriet Lane Handbook [18]. Doses of drugs for children are calculated according to their weight on a mg/kg basis. Neonates need reduced doses relative to their size because of the immaturity of the metabolic enzymes in the liver for many drugs. Infants and young children may need comparatively higher doses and at shorter intervals than adults, especially for opioid analgesics. There is no scientifically agreed-upon approach for changing from the mg/kg basis used in childhood to the standardised doses used for adults. This becomes a problem with older children and young teens. One rule of thumb is to use 50 kg weight as a cut-off. Another rule of thumb is to calculate the mg/kg dose of the medication: if that dose exceeds the dose generally given to adults, then switch to the adult dose.

A note about opioids

Opioids are used extensively in managing pain in PPC. They form the mainstay of therapy for pain and respiratory symptoms. When prescribing strong opioids for children, the following points should be borne in mind:

• Long-acting (sustained release) oral preparations (morphine and sometimes hydromorphone) and transdermal fentanyl are effective and convenient.

• Short-acting (NR) preparations are required for breakthrough pain. This could be the same opioid as the child is having in a sustained release format or fentanyl can be given sublingually or buccally to provide fast and short-acting analgesia combined with an opioid every 4 h or with long-acting preparations given every 8 or 12 h. While fentanyl lozenges are available, the dosing adjustments needed for smaller children often mean that providing the IV form for buccal or intranasal administration is often easier; unpleasant tastes can be masked with flavouring. Children need to be reminded to keep the medicine under their tongue or in their cheek rather than swallowing it.

• Where oral administration is difficult or impossible, the use of transdermal patches (e.g., fentanyl or buprenorphine) has proved invaluable; other routes include NG tube, gastrostomy tube, SC, and IV.

• Studies of the pharmacokinetics of opioids and their metabolites suggest that in young children metabolism is more rapid than in adults and they may require both more frequent and relatively higher doses for analgesia.

• Neonates and infants under 3 months of age, however, require a lower starting dose of opioids because of their reduced metabolism and increased sensitivity.

• Recent evidence argues against the routine use of codeine, especially in children under 7 years of age who may be poor metabolisers of the drug. In the general population, up to 10% of people may not fully metabolise codeine; the figure is much higher in children [19]. Tramadol is a good substitute as a weak opioid, or one may use morphine or hydromorphone as a starting point.

Side effects of opioids and clinician concerns

Many doctors and nurses lack experience of using opioids in children, which often leads to unnecessary caution, underdosing, and inadequate pain control. Side effects from opioids tend to be less marked than in adults. Nausea and vomiting are rare and routine use of antiemetics is not needed. Constipation is the most common side effect and regular laxatives should always be prescribed. The majority will require a stimulant in addition to a softener (e.g., co-danthrusate or senna and magnesium sulphate), or polyethylene glycol (PEG).

A common concern is respiratory depression. The evidence base is clear that there is a low risk of adverse events, from both adult and paediatric literature and our 15-year experience in a paediatric palliative program supports these findings [20,21]. Respiratory depression with strong opioids is not a problem in children with severe pain, provided that certain practices are followed. Hypoventilation rarely occurs when opioids are prescribed in the context of pain that is increasing in intensity as happens with progressive cancers. The key to safe use is attentive observation of the patient after any increases; basing increases on prior utilisation, specifically the pattern of use of breakthrough doses; and knowledge of the basic pharmacokinetics of the different opioids such as their half-lives and bioavailability.

The risk of addiction is similarly overplayed in common perception. Physicians need to explain to families the distinctions between tolerance (the need for additional medication because of changes in pharmacokinetics/pharmacodynamics), dependency (a pattern where acute drug cessation leads to adverse effects), and addiction (a syndrome involving psychological alterations such as cravings, risky behaviour, and illegal or antisocial activities to acquire and use drugs). Addiction has genetic, environmental, and social substrates [22]. We have not seen an addiction syndrome in our work at Canuck Place despite extensive use of opioids. Physical dependency is a possible concern; the literature is not very helpful in this regard, but suggests that following 7–10 days of constant (round-the-clock) exposure to opioids, dependency will ensue. In this situation, acute cessation of the drug will lead to a withdrawal syndrome with escalation of the underlying pain, in addition to arthralgia/myalgia, diarrhoea, nausea, chills, rigors, and photophobia. Again, we have seen this very infrequently, primarily because if we

Box 15.3 Resources and directories of PPC providers and information

- Canada: Canadian Network of Palliative Care for Children (http://www.cnpcc.ca)
- The United Kingdom: ACT (http://www.act.org.uk) and Together for Short Lives (http://www.togetherforshortlives.org.uk/)
- The United States: National Hospice Palliative Care Organization, Children's Project on Palliative/Hospice Services (ChiPPS) (http://www.nhpco.org)
- International: International Children's Palliative Care Network (http://www.icpcn.org.uk)
- PPC Group ListServe:
  - ← (http://health.groups.yahoo.com/group/ palliativecare_ pediatric)
  - ← (http://lists.act.org.uk/mailman/listinfo/ paedpalcare)

stop opioids we wean them down over a course of several days to weeks.

Opioids need to be started at a dose based on formulary standards, but should be rapidly escalated upward to control the pain. It is useful to remember that experienced PPC doctors and nurses are available through local and regional programs in the United Kingdom, Canada, and the United States. There are also clinicians available worldwide who welcome contact by e-mail, Web-based bulletin board, or telephone for consultation on such matters. A list of resources is shown in Box 15.3.

Parental concerns over opioids

Parents may be reluctant for their child to have strong opioids. It is important to establish exactly what their concerns are. Parents may be anxious about the side effects in which case it will be helpful to reassure them that these too can be treated. They may also be worried that if opioids are started "too early" there will be nothing left for later. In such a situation, it would be necessary to explain that there is no upper dose limit to strong opioids, and that other medications are also available to treat different types of pain. A third concern is addiction, but this behavioural pattern is very rare in children; regardless of whether the question regarding addiction is raised, we review the issue with every family as part of starting opioids.

However, another common difficulty for parents is the feeling that by agreeing to start opioids they are acknowledging that their child is really going to die. They may even be concerned that this step represents them as giving up hope—something they would find unacceptable. This clearly requires sensitive discussion and support. It may be helpful to encourage them to focus again on the immediate needs of the child. With anticipatory discussion of these issues between clinicians and families, their perception will change such that their child can again receive the analgesia that he or she requires.

How do I make a reliable prognostication for a child?

Prognostication is very difficult in children, even close to end of life, and should be avoided. Even skilled PPC providers who attempt to give likely ranges of time are wrong more often than they are right. Prognosticating is complicated by the number of rare conditions encountered, and by the fact that the disease process occurs within the context of an overall healthy and growing individual. In other words, while one organ system may be functioning very poorly due to the disease, all other organs are working well—unlike the situation in many adults. This means that there is an underlying resilience in children. In a recent study, more than 66% of children referred to PPC were still alive after 1 year [23].

As death approaches, parents will need and value further information, including the possible modes of death. Professionals can sometimes be reluctant to undertake such frank discussion, but knowing what to expect and having a clear plan of what to do as the situation changes can enable families to cope better. Indeed, it is essential if the child is being cared for at home.

The possibility of distressing symptoms (such as seizures, dyspnoea, tachycardia, or agitation) should be discussed. The team should ensure that emergency drugs (i.e., anticonvulsants, strong analgesics, and sedatives) are available in the house, or are easily accessible if the child is in hospital. Suitable doses via appropriate routes must be calculated ahead of time, so that medication can be given as soon as it is needed. If the child is at home, the medication doses and the route of administration should be such that the parents will be able to give the drugs themselves; it should be clearly noted that the parents have been taught to prepare and administer these drugs. As shown in Figure 15.2, the use of a box and arrow algorithm diagram is helpful. We make these specifically for each individual child and they sometimes run to several pages; they are updated constantly and shared with all of the teams involved. Finally, there should always be a professional available 24 h a day who parents and the nonspecialist professionals who support them can contact for additional support.

Does the primary care provider have a role in caring for children with complex conditions?

It remains vitally important that the needs of each child and family are considered individually, both in the context of the illness and of what is available locally. Families may build up very close relationships with various members of the hospital staff and can become heavily reliant on them.

As a consequence of this, the primary health-care team can easily feel superfluous and marginalised. This is exacerbated by the fact that most family doctors will see relatively few children with life-limiting illnesses, each of whom is likely to have a different, rare, and complex illness. It is therefore difficult for the family doctor to gain experience and confidence in PPC, and to define his or her role in the care of such a child. This can be misinterpreted by the family as a lack of interest, thereby perpetuating the lack of contact with the primary care team.

The active involvement of the primary health-care team is vital. It is essential that the primary care team receive support from professionals with experience in PPC as well as professionals with knowledge and experience of the child's underlying disorder.

What is the best way to work with families of children in palliative care?

Support for the child and family begins at the time of diagnosis and continues as the illness progresses, through the child's death and into bereavement. All the family—the sick child, the parents, siblings, and the wider family—will be affected by the illness and may need help, both as a family unit and as individuals.

Care for children with life-limiting/threatening conditions and their family can span weeks to years and requires care providers who understand development, family systems, effective communication, and have the ability to be present in the face of grief and sadness. Families and the children themselves have incredible resources and innate abilities to love and live with a multitude of challenges. However, with each change and in the experience of deteriorating health, families describe their ongoing journey as one with "uncharted territory" [24]. Finding a new normal and adjusting to the vast changes in function, care, and symptoms are made easier with caring and knowledgeable care providers who listen, value their expertise, and explore hopes and fears.

How do I advise parents to talk to their children about the illness?

Some parents may be reluctant to discuss the diagnosis with their children and may need encouragement and help to do so. Goals of care should be discussed regularly and be based on a relationship that includes understanding the child's condition and current wellness and challenges, the family's and the child's hopes and own understanding of the condition, and the aspects that enhance or impact quality of life. A health-care provider who can balance hoping for the best (taking a trip, having another birthday, participating in the school play, graduating) while planning for the "what ifs?" (what if: "there is another aspiration pneumonia?"/"the feeds are no longer tolerated?"/ "the palliative chemo does not help?") empowers the family to have a plan of care that enables them to live each day more meaningfully. Even if a particular "decision" has not been made regarding the many aspects of care (advance decisions, treatment options, location of care), these ongoing discussions and relationship provide a foundation on which to evolve with the child and family as the child becomes more ill and symptomatic.

Most families employ some avoidance and denial as part of their coping strategy, including avoiding discussion and reminders of the illness. This is normal behaviour that helps protect them from extremes of emotion. It allows them to live with the illness and function day to day, while coming to understand and recognise the situation gradually. This needs to be recognised and respected; frequent discussions about the disease at this time may prove burdensome rather than supportive. Although families may be reluctant to be open with children about their progressive illness, encouraging children to talk, express feelings, and ask questions through ongoing conversations, engaging in drawing, sand tray, and play enhances the children's sense of security and ability to cope [25].

In addition to this, parents often want health professionals to maintain some hope (with them) as long as their child is alive. This has to be expressed in the context of honest information about the progression of the disease, but this is also what parents would expect [26]. Truth-telling and respect are essential as treatment and care decisions shift from active treatment to more intense symptom management and end-of-life care. However, it can prove very challenging to get the balance right for each individual family.

On the other hand, children know when adults are withholding information; and often they know that their illness is progressing. Furthermore, lying to children through omission or commission can severely alter the parent–child bond and the child's sense of security [27].

However, it is clear that children understand and learn about their illness and its implications whether the parents and the professionals encourage it or not. This can go unnoticed, as it is common for the children to "protect" their parents by keeping their worries to themselves. It is therefore important to provide opportunities for the sick child to discuss what is actually on his or her mind. Parents (and health professionals) can be surprised by the nature of the child's fears: rather than being scared of death *per se*, it is more common that they are scared of situations that they can be genuinely reassured about. That is not to deny that open discussion with children, particularly when death is a real possibility, can be a daunting prospect and very difficult to establish in practice.

Children may not be able to guide all decisions; however, by sharing information with them in a manner that is developmentally appropriate and by listening to their views, their inherent worth is preserved and valued [28]. Care providers can model this respect for children and increase communication and understanding by including them in care meetings (or parts of) with their family and other care providers. Opportunities for conversation and exploring thoughts and feelings arise naturally when there is a change in care routine, when making decisions about investigations, when children have a change in ability or function, or when pain or other symptoms arise. Care providers who help to acknowledge the changes and create space for expressing intense feelings assist children and their family's access their voice and strengths.

Should families try to continue their routines, or is it better to focus on the ill child?

As the illness progresses, the family has to live with the underlying conflict of maintaining some hope and semblance of day-to-day life in spite of persistent uncertainty. The parents may develop depression, anxiety, and sleep disturbance, although they are often reluctant to speak of these problems unless asked specifically. Marital discord

and loss of libido are also common. Parents often find difficulty in handling the children, particularly in maintaining discipline and boundaries for the sick child, and in balancing their time and emotions between the sick child and well siblings. If frequent hospital admissions are involved, there are practical problems of travel, separation, and finance. If the child has heavy nursing needs, with physical disability and/or developmental delay, the burdens of care can be considerable. Parents may have very little time to themselves or to devote to well brothers and sisters, and the opportunity for some respite care for the sick child, either at home or away from home, becomes essential.

The sick child may continue to experience regular hospital visits and treatment, while developing increasing symptoms and disability. Trying to encourage as normal a life as possible—maintaining friendships, education, and outside activities—within the confines of the illness—is a continual but important struggle. Children themselves are usually surprisingly keen to attend school as much as they can. However, as the illness progresses, extra support, special facilities, and home education may need to be introduced.

Is it helpful to tell siblings everything that is happening?

An important issue at this time for parents is what to discuss with the child who is sick and with their other children. Parents, understandably, are usually reluctant to discuss with the sick child that they are not getting better from their disease. Their aim in this is to protect their children.

Having a sick brother or sister has a great impact on siblings and they should be included in care planning and support [29]. Providing opportunities to hear their perspective, express the range of feelings experienced, and address questions, hopes, and fears are essential for family-centred care. Parents may need guidance and support in integrating and providing opportunities for the well sibling to connect with and love his or her brother or sister while still having time to enjoy life, experience things that the sick sibling may not be able to (and not carry guilt), and work toward individual goals.

Communicating with children must take into consideration their level of understanding about illness and the concept of death [30]. It also will be influenced by the child's previous experiences, the family's style of communication, and their own personal defences. Some approaches to helping families toward a more open and honest pattern of communication include:

- shifting the emphasis from "telling" to "listening";
- helping them identify the child's indirect cues as well as obvious questions;
- discovering the child's fears and fantasies;
- maintaining the child's trust through honesty;
- building up the whole picture gradually; and
- explaining that communication need not rely on talking—drawings, stories, and play are often more effective and easier for children.

Siblings may feel isolated and left out by their parents and, noticing the differential treatment they are receiving, can come to resent their sick brother or sister. They may also feel less worthy and develop low self-esteem as a result. This is less likely if they have opportunities to talk about their feelings and are given honest answers to their questions about what is happening. They also benefit from being involved in the day-to-day care of their brother or sister, and later by having a role in planning and attending the funeral and by being allowed to keep some of their sibling's possessions [31,32].

The final stages

Eventually, it becomes clearer that not only is death inevitable but that the time of death is becoming closer. This may be apparent from gradual deterioration in a long progressive illness or more abruptly, such as after a relapse in cancer. The emotional impact at this time may be dramatic for parents, particularly for those who have held a very positive and "fighting" approach throughout the treatment. For others, it is just a confirmation of what they have dreaded and known was inevitable all along. Sometimes there is a sense of relief that the uncertainty and suffering will soon be over, alongside the distress and sadness.

As well as information and discussion about the child's care, parents need an opportunity to explore their own feelings and express their emotions. They may be able to talk to each other openly and offer each other support, but more often they will cope in different ways and find that the whole experience is so physically and emotionally exhausting that they have little strength left to offer support either to each other or to their other children. Both the parents and well siblings often value the opportunity to talk to someone outside of the immediate family during this time [33].

Many parents have never seen anyone die and will value the opportunity of talking about what may happen at the moment of death. They also appreciate information about the practical details of what to do after a person has died. Most will have been anticipating the funeral in their mind and are relieved to be able to acknowledge this and make some plans before the child has died.

The bereaved family

After children die, families value ongoing connection with those who provided care. Telling their story and reflecting on their children's life is helpful and a normal process of grieving. Ongoing contact also allows the health-care provider opportunities to assess the family's coping, referring to more intense support if symptoms are beyond the range of normal grief. Siblings who are not experiencing joy, having extended periods of poor sleep or appetite, self-isolating, or not engaging in any conversation related to their sibling should be assessed by a professional who has expertise in grief. Parents who have intrusive memories of their child's suffering that do not decrease over time and fail to have periods of less intensity in their grief should also be referred. Again, assessing for ability to carry out day-to-day activities, connections with others, and feeling hope are vital for ongoing health. A depression tool such as the Patient Health Questionnaire (PHQ) can be a good screen and barometer of how the parent is coping (Figure 15.3) [34,35].

Though families do not get over the death of a child, learning to live differently is a process that takes many years. The ability to hold hope and look forward, as well as reflect on the past joys and difficult times of their deceased child, demonstrates healing. With new life experiences, grief may resurface and caring professionals will again listen and reflect the experience. The intensity and the duration of that intensity should, over time, be less.

With time, there is usually less involvement of health-care professionals providing bereavement support, while other informal supports through extended family and friends become more important for families. For primary care providers, the families may continue to be in contact at various times for their primary care needs but their needs for support for the grief will lessen. Paediatric hospices often offer ongoing support that decreases over time but will still be available when families experience resurgence of grief or questions about themselves or other family members. Having both informal and formal ways to remember their child often becomes part of the

PATIENT HEALTH QUESTIONNAIRE (PHQ)

This questionnaire is an important part of providing you with the best health care possible. Your answers will help in understanding problems that you may have. Please answer every question to the best of your ability unless you are requested to skip over a question.

Name_____ Age_____ Sex: ☐ Female ☐ Male Today's Date_____

1. During the <u>last 4 weeks</u>, how much have you been bothered by any of the following problems?	Not bothered	Bothered a little	Bothered a lot
a. Stomach pain	☐	☐	☐
b. Back pain	☐	☐	☐
c. Pain in your arms, legs, or joints (knees, hips, etc.)	☐	☐	☐
d. Menstrual cramps or other problems with your periods	☐	☐	☐
e. Pain or problems during sexual intercourse	☐	☐	☐
f. Headaches	☐	☐	☐
g. Chest pain	☐	☐	☐
h. Dizziness	☐	☐	☐
i. Fainting spells	☐	☐	☐
j. Feeling your heart pound or race	☐	☐	☐
k. Shortness of breath	☐	☐	☐
l. Constipation, loose bowels, or diarrhea	☐	☐	☐
m. Nausea, gas, or indigestion	☐	☐	☐

2. Over the <u>last 2 weeks</u>, how often have you been bothered by any of the following problems?	not at all	Serveral days	More than half the days	Nearly every day
a. Little interest or pleasure in doing things	☐	☐	☐	☐
b. Feeling down, depressed, or hopeless	☐	☐	☐	☐
c. Trouble falling or staying asleep, or sleeping too much	☐	☐	☐	☐
d. Feeling tired or having little energy	☐	☐	☐	☐
e. Poor appetite or overeating	☐	☐	☐	☐
f. Feeling bad about yourself — or that you are a failure or have let yourself of your family down	☐	☐	☐	☐
g. Trouble concentrating on things, such as reading the newspaper or watching television	☐	☐	☐	☐
h. Moving or speaking so slowly that other people could have noticed? Or the opposite — being so fidgety or restless that you have been moving around a lot more than usual	☐	☐	☐	☐
I. Thoughts that you would be better off dead or of hurting yourself in some way	☐	☐	☐	☐

FOR OFFICE CODING Som Ds if at least 3 of #1a-m are *a lot* and lack an adequate biol explanation.
Maj Dep Syn if answers to #2a or b and five or more of #2a-i are at least "More than half the days" (count #2i if present at all).
Other Dep Syn if #2a or b and two three, or four of #2a-i are at least "More than half the days" (count #2i if present at all).

PHQ 1/3

Figure 15.3 Patient Health Questionnaire (PHQ). (Developed by Drs. Robert L. Spitzer, Janet B.W. Williams, Kurt Kroenke and colleagues, with an educational grant from Pfizer, Inc. No permission required to reproduce, translate, display, or distribute.)

family culture and enables the child to be remembered while continuing to live and love.

Ideally, the professionals who know the family well and have been involved throughout the sick child's life should continue to be available through their bereavement. Grief is likely to continue over many years, and its depth and persistence is often underestimated. Parents value continuing contact with professionals who have known their child and the opportunity to talk about the child and their grief when others in the community expect them to "have come to terms with it" [31]. This support, initially more frequent and gradually decreasing, helps facilitate the normal tasks of mourning. Help can be offered for brothers and sisters and information provided about appropriate literature, telephone helplines, and support organisations.

What kinds of professionals provide PPC?

This is an evolving question. Twenty years ago, there was no defined field of PPC. There are now some formal programs for doctors and training for nurses and psychosocial care providers (psychologists, social workers, and counsellors). At present, the care and support for children with life-limiting illnesses is provided by a variety of professionals who have acquired their skills and knowledge in several different ways. There is still no uniformity of service provision; hence, the service available to a child and family remains dependent on geographical location. There is a risk that families may be either neglected or receive inappropriate or uncoordinated help. Responsibility for care may fall to community providers, including paediatricians, adult palliative care doctors, family physicians, home care nurses, child therapists, and community pharmacists. One of the most important lessons that these professionals need to learn is how to function as a team and develop a shared communication strategy. An *ad hoc* community team, developed around the care of a specific child, can provide excellent care so long as there is a focus on team process. These *ad hoc* teams can rely on regional PPC teams, often based at a tertiary children's hospital or hospice. The key element is that PPC is inherently multidisciplinary; different relationships can exist within teams, but without physician, nursing, pharmacy, and psychosocial elements, PPC cannot be said to be available. This concept is inherent in the standards, norms, and guidelines that have been promulgated worldwide.

Where is PPC provided (and what difference does it make)?

Locations include hospital, home, and hospice, depending on services in the area. The full spectrum of care includes in-hospital, free-standing children's hospices, community hospice, and home. Ideally, there is a seamless experience of coordinated and integrated care provided to the family regardless of their physical location at any given time.

Families should be given a realistic idea of what to expect with regard to the needs of their child as they deteriorate and the support that is available. Those who are at home need access to advice and support 24 h a day, and this should be planned so that professionals caring for the child have backup from others with experience in PPC. Families should also be given some flexibility, so they can move between home, hospital, and hospice as they choose, without their care being compromised.

In 1982, the first freestanding hospice for children opened (Helen House, Oxford, UK). By 1995, there were six in the United Kingdom, and the first one opened in North America (Canuck Place Children's Hospice, Vancouver, Canada). Today, there are dozens of freestanding children's hospices across the United Kingdom, Europe, Russia, Canada, the United States, South Africa, and Australia.

In addition to the freestanding children's hospices, in some countries many tertiary care Children's Hospitals to have an in-house palliative care service providing a spectrum of care across in-hospital consultation to community in-home support. In the United States, some community hospice programs have expanded their care mandates and capabilities to care for children and their families, primarily with home-based support.

These choices and options are very dependent on national and regional policies, for example, insurance systems, and what has developed in a specific community and where public–private funding has been directed. Nevertheless, it is increasingly clear that the best option of families is the availability of all of the settings. Especially at end of life, families develop comfort with moving between settings. Many hospices staffed by expert nurses and specialist PPC physicians provide respite to stable but chronically ill children, but shift into the mode of palliative care units when there are symptom crises or an end-of-life situation. The conventional wisdom in the literature is that "families prefer to be at home" at end of life, often based on surveys and qualitative interviews [36].

However, when examined through epidemiological lenses, it appears that families assort themselves evenly across the settings of hospital, hospice, and home, when all three are available [37].

For most primary care clinicians practicing in North America and western Europe, it is likely that a PPC team is not far away. The majority of children with complex, chronic diseases are cared for by subspecialists at a Children's Hospital, at least some of the time. It is increasingly likely that such an institution will have a palliative consult team. Even if one's own region does not have a children's hospice or tertiary consultation team, many are just a phone call or e-mail away, and are likely willing to assist it. In Canada, a list of children's palliative programs can be found through the Canadian Network of Palliative Care for Children (www.cnpcc.ca) [38]. A similar list for the United Kingdom can be found through ACT (http://www.act.org.uk).

Conclusions

Helping to care for a child with a life-threatening illness, and for the family of such a child, is rarely easy. It presents many challenges both in terms of the professional tasks that may be required and to our own emotional resources. Though the task may seem daunting, families greatly value professionals who stay alongside them throughout their difficult journey, offering practical help and support in an almost intolerable situation. Parents will have a lasting memory of their child's death and as professionals we have the privileged opportunity to make this as good as it can be.

References

1. Canadian Cancer Society's Steering Committee on Cancer Statistics. *Canadian Cancer Statistics*. Toronto, ON: Canadian Cancer Society, 2011.
2. Stephenson A, Chilvers M, Durie P, et al. Canadian Cystic Fibrosis Patient Data Registry (CPDR) 2009 Report. Cystic Fibrosis Canada. Retrieved July 10, 2011, from http://www.cysticfibrosis.ca/assets/files/pdf/CPDR_ReportE.pdf
3. ACT/RCPCH. *A Guide to the Development of Children's Palliative Care Services: Report of the Joint Working Party*. Bristol: ACT/RCPCH, 1997.
4. Breeze AC, Lees CC, Kumar A, et al. Palliative care for prenatally diagnosed lethal fetal abnormality. *Arch Dis Child Fetal Neonatal Ed* 2007; 92(1): F56–F58.
5. Collier R. Providing hospice in the womb. *CMAJ* 2011; Mar 22; 183(5): E267–E268.
6. ACT. *A Neonatal Pathway for Babies with Palliative Care Needs*. Bristol: ACT, 2009
7. Wolfe J., Grier HE, Klar N, et al. Symptoms and suffering at the end of life in children with cancer. *N Eng J Med* 2000; 342(5): 326–333.
8. Hunt A, Mastroyannopoulou, Goldman A, et al. Not knowing—the problem of pain in children with severe neurological impairment. *Int J Nurs Stud* 2003; 40: 171–183.
9. Breau LM, McGrath PJ, Camfield CS, et al. Psychometric properties of the non-communicating children's pain checklist-revised. *Pain* 2002; 99(1–2): 349–357.
10. Hunt A, Goldman A, Seers K, et al. Clinical validation of the paediatric pain profile. *Dev Med Child Neurol* 2004; 46(1): 9–18.
11. Merkel SI, Voepel-Lewis T, Shayevitz JR, et al. The FLACC: a behavioral scale for scoring postoperative pain in young children. *Pediatr Nurs* 1997; 23(3): 293–297.
12. Tsai E. Withholding and withdrawing artificial nutrition and hydration. *Paediatr Child Health* 2011; 16(4): 241–242.
13. Diekema DS, Botkin JR, and Committee on Bioethics. Clinical report—forgoing medically provided nutrition and hydration in children. *Pediatrics* 2009; 124: 813–822.
14. Siden H, Tucker T, Derman S, et al. Pediatric enteral feeding intolerance: a new prognosticator for children with life-limiting illness?. *J Palliat Care* 2009; 25(3): 213–217.
15. *British National Formulary for Children*. BMJ group, Pharmaceutical Press, and RCPCH Publications Ltd, 2011.
16. Jassal S (ed.). *The Association of Paediatric Palliative Medicine Master Formulary*, 2011. Available at: http://www.act.org.uk/landing.asp?section=385&sectionTitle=The+Association+for+Paediatric+Palliative+Medicine+%28APPM%29 (accessed on: November 14, 2011).
17. Dipchand AI and Friedman J. *HSC Handbook of Pediatrics*, 11th edition. Canada: Saunders-Mosby, 2009.
18. Custer JW and Rachel ER (eds). *The Harriet Lane Handbook: A Manual for Pediatric House Officers*, 18th edition. St. Louis: Mosby-Year Book, 2011.
19. Williams DG, Hatch DJ, and Howard RF. Codeine phosphate in paediatric medicine. *Br J Anaesth* 2001; 86(3): 413–421.
20. Siden H and Nalewajek G. High dose opioids in pediatric palliative care. *J Pain Symptom Manage* 2003; 25(5): 397–400.
21. Walsh TD, Rivera NI, and Kaiko R. Oral morphine and respiratory function amongst hospice inpatients with advanced cancer. *Support Care Cancer* 2003; 11(12): 780–784.
22. Ballantyne JC and LaForge KS. Opioid dependence and addiction during opioid treatment of chronic pain. *Pain* 2007; 129(3): 235–255.
23. Feudtner C, Kang TI, Hexem KR, et al. Pediatric palliative care patients: a prospective multicenter cohort study. *Pediatrics* 2011; 127(6): 1094–1101.

24. Steele R. Experience of families in which a child has a prolonged terminal illness: modifying factors. *Int J Palliat Nurs* 2002; 8(9): 418–433.

25. Van Breemen C. Using play therapy in paediatric palliative care: listening to the story and caring for the body. *Int J Palliat Nurs* 2009; 15(10): 510–514.

26. Laakso H and Paunonen-Ilmonen M. Mothers' experience of social support following the death of a child. *J Clin Nurs* 2002; 11(2): 176–185.

27. Stillion JM and Papadatou D. Suffer the children: an examination of psychosocial issues in children and adolescents with terminal illness. *Am Behav Sci* 2002; 46(2): 299–315.

28. Carnevale FA. Listening authentically to youthful voices: a conception of the moral agency of children. In: Storch J, Rodney P, and Starzomski R (eds), *Toward a Moral Horizon: Nursing Ethics for Leadership and Practice*. Don Mills, ON: Pearson Education Canada, pp. 3960413.

29. Bluebond-Langner M. *The Private Worlds of Dying Children*. Princeton, NJ: Princeton University Press, 1978.

30. Stevens M. *Psychological Adaptation of the Dying Child*, 3rd edition. Oxford: Oxford University Press, 2004, pp. 799–806.

31. Foster C, Eiser C, Oades P, et al. Treatment demands and differential treatment of patients with cystic fibrosis and their siblings: patient, parent and sibling accounts. *Child Care Health Dev* 2001; 27(4): 349–364.

32. Pettle Michael SA and Lansdown RG. Adjustment to death of a sibling. *Arch Dis Child* 1986; 61: 278–283.

33. Laakso H and Paunonen-Ilmonen M. Mothers' experience of social support following the death of a child. *J Clin Nurs* 2002; 11(2): 176–185.

34. Spitzer RL, Kroenke K, and Williams JB. Validation and utility of a self-report version of PRIME-MD: the PHQ primary care study. Primary Care Evaluation of Mental Disorders. Patient Health Questionnaire. *JAMA* 1999; 282(18): 1737–1744.

35. Patient Health Questionnaire (PHQ) Screeners. Available at: http://www.phqscreeners.com (accessed on: September 12, 2011).

36. Hannan J and Gibson F. Advanced cancer in children: how parents decide on final place of care for their dying child. *Int J Palliat Nurs* 2005; 11: 284–291.

37. Siden H, Miller M, Straatman L, et al. A report on location of death in paediatric palliative care between home, hospice and hospital. *Palliat Med* 2008; 22(7): 831–834.

38. The Canadian Network of Palliative Care for Children. Retrieved July 10, 2011, from http://www.cnpcc.ca

Acknowledgements. We would like to acknowledge the work of Keith Sibson, Finella Craig, and Ann Goldman for the previous edition of this chapter, and Charlotte Mellor for her contribution to ensure that the chapter is consistent with UK practice.

16 Palliative Care for Adolescents and Young Adults

Daniel Kelly[1], Victoria Lidstone[2], Jacqueline Edwards[3], Jo Griffiths[4]

[1]Cardiff University, Wales, UK
[2]University Hospital of Wales, Cardiff, UK
[3]Heart of England NHS Foundation Trust Bordesley Green East Birmingham, UK
[4]Abertawe Bro Morgannwg Health Board, Swansea, Wales, UK

Introduction

> Laura was 15 when she was diagnosed and 19 when she died and during that time she struggled hard with her emotions and matured at an alarming rate leaving her friends behind, as they too struggled to come to terms with her illness—how she desperately fought the treatment and would not allow them to see her ill—she was such a clever actress never allowing many people to see the real Laura—in pain, vomiting, weak, high temperature, mouth full of ulcers—I could go on and on . . . [1].

The aim of this chapter is to highlight the particular needs of adolescents and young adults who are faced with a life-threatening illness. In health care, attention has only slowly shifted toward the care of those who can no longer be considered children, but who are neither fully independent adults. There is a current drive to improve services for this group whose needs have been recognised for some years as being "specific and different from both children and adults" [1]. Research is active in this area and many of the studies going forward are asking the young people themselves about their experiences, and what they want and need [2,3].

This chapter will examine the nature of some of these specifics to help professionals, families, or friends to understand the needs of young people whose lives are shortened by serious illness. It is not the intention to review the medical management of common symptoms that are covered elsewhere. Instead, the emphasis is placed on the "appropriate application" of such interventions—ensuring that the necessary medication is employed in line with the expectations of young people themselves. For the purpose of this chapter, a range of 13–24 years has been adopted as this has also been applied elsewhere [4]. More generally, challenges arise in this age group about the meaning of suffering, the emotional toll of symptoms, and the disclosure of prognosis, as well as the support needs of those closest to the patient. While these issues apply to all age groups, the nature of adolescence and young adulthood make them ever more acute in the face of impending death [5].

The disease trajectories of young people with life limiting conditions (LLCs) are diverse and numerous. While cancer diagnoses form a substantial subset, nononcological conditions account for the greater majority bringing new challenges to professionals working alongside young people and their families. As greater numbers of children with neurodisabling, metabolic, congenital, chronic respiratory, and neuromuscular conditions survive into young adulthood, palliative care teams must arm themselves with understanding a range of conditions, many of which are unique and not likely to be encountered regularly in a professional's working career. Such young people may have a long palliative phase with symptoms differing from those with cancer, including a higher prevalence of neurological and behavioural problems that place unique stresses on families and carers. In England, between 2001 and 2005, over 6,000 young people between the ages of 15 and 24 died from causes likely to have required palliative care: over 500 with congenital malformations, 1,000 with

Handbook of Palliative Care, Third Edition. Edited by Christina Faull, Sharon de Caestecker, Alex Nicholson and Fraser Black.
© 2012 by John Wiley and Sons, Inc. Published 2012 by John Wiley & Sons, Inc.

diseases of the nervous system, and 1,300 with diseases of the circulatory system [6].

The experience of young people and their families living with LLCs varies hugely and is dependent on a large number of factors, including social situation, family values and beliefs, previous experience (some LLCs are familial), and individual coping strategies. The life experience of those living with a diagnosis from birth (e.g., metabolic disorders, severe cerebral palsy, congenital anomalies) or a very young age Duchenne muscular dystrophy (DMD), is likely to be different from those for whom the diagnosis affects a previously healthy individual out of the blue (e.g., cancer). The latter group, for example, is often previously independent and may have had the opportunity to develop peer groups and support networks through employment; the point of diagnosis may be the first contact they have had with health-care services. For those young people with a later LLC diagnosis such as cancer, there has often been a period of intense treatment, sometimes with curative intent. There may have been a period of remission, sometimes years long, before relapse and further treatment. This roller coaster is harsh and may bring a different emotional experience compared with the other group of young people. Those young people who have more indolent disease progression and disability from a young age face different but equally complex social and emotional needs. Adolescence is a challenging time for all, and the issues of independence, emerging sexuality, and need for a purpose are no less important in those who are disabled. The challenge for professionals is how to work primarily with these young people, rather than their parents, even if this means finding alternative ways to communicate.

By the time they reach late adolescence, those with lifelong diagnoses are likely to have already experienced stepwise deteriorations and sequential losses, and the families will often have supported a significant burden of care for many years. They may have had complex interactions with many different care professionals (CPs) over a long period and are often significantly fatigued through "fighting their corner" by the time the young people reach adulthood. Some of these families will have lived with a knowledge of prognosis for a long time, and some will only have reached the point of a clearer, short, prognosis as adulthood approaches.

Prognostication in young people is notoriously difficult. This is particularly true for those with nonmalignant conditions: Acute and clinically significant deteriorations may occur on repeated occasions creating uncertainty and extreme distress, and survival may be felt unlikely, but does occur. For those with cancer, in whom there may be more tangible signs and symptoms aiding prognostication, the terminal phase can still be unexpectedly long. In either case, the uncertain situation, and "the wait" is extraordinarily hard to bear for young people, families, carers, and professionals.

Prognostication is not always welcome, and as with the giving of any bad news, it should be given carefully and with a great deal of forethought. For this group, there will be young people who will wish to have information, and those that do not, and those that need some of it but not all. Exploring how much and what a person wants to know at any one point is essential, and should always also involve a discussion with family where appropriate. Professionals (and families) should never assume they know what a young person wants to know. In the United Kingdom, once a young person reaches 18 years of age the basis of consent for information sharing changes, and professionals must remember that they need to seek the permission of the young person before holding discussions with the family. It is important to point out to young people that they have rights of confidentiality, as they may not be aware of this.

The dawning realisation that a young person is unlikely to reach adulthood is likely to provoke a crisis. Strong emotions, including anger and disbelief, may be expressed by the young person, as well as by family and friends [7]. The roots of such responses can be traced to social and cultural expectations about death and illness over the life course. Socially, we are poorly prepared to comprehend the death of those who are on the threshold of adulthood, and for whom the future usually holds promise. The focus of the resulting anger and confusion may often be the professionals involved in the young person's care—especially when delays or similarly frustrating events that characterise hospital life combine to provoke the expression of pent-up feelings.

From professionals, it requires pragmatism, sensitivity, and effective communication skills. A holistic approach is essential and psychological and spiritual support should be explored and sought, despite the fact that they are not always easy to identify or access. Regular, thorough, and creative review of practical support is essential and may involve reoffering services previously declined, that may now be useful and perhaps accepted. Caring for young people who are very ill may invoke strong emotional reactions among professionals, especially if they have had limited exposure to death in this age group during their career. It is important for all professionals involved to recognise this. For some, there may be a risk of overidentifying with the young patient's or the parent's situation [8]. Good team working is helpful but in such a situation it is easy for personal/professional boundaries to become blurred and some form of debriefing, supervision, or staff support should be available [9,10].

The challenge of providing palliative care for young people

Providing appropriate palliative care for young people presents professionals with a series of complex challenges. Young people have different needs from children, and older adults, and their care needs an approach that reflects this [11]. Paediatric services usually continue caring for children until they are at least 16 years old. After this point, there is enormous variability between specialties and some will refer to adult services at 16 years (e.g., cardiology and diabetes), while others will keep young people until 19 years (e.g., neurology and community paediatrics). Young people with nonmalignant LLC may be under the care of several specialties and may transfer care from each one at a different times. This is not necessarily a bad thing—transfer of all specialties at 16 years may be a bit of a shock—but it can make the process seem long and drawn out. Inpatient care is particularly affected in this respect—at 16 years, a young person may well no longer be admitted to the paediatric wards which can be difficult on several counts: First, the young person and their family may have a well-established relationship with the staff of the paediatric ward. Second, adult wards are not always well equipped, in terms of skills or facilities, for young people. This is particularly true in relation to young people with severe communication or behavioural difficulties, and those with complex needs. It is entirely predictable that care will transfer at a given point. But unfortunately, this is generally not done well [12,13]. Much can be done, however, to optimise care in the adult services by careful transition planning. There is helpful information and guidance available for transition planning in complex needs and disability [13], as well as transition in specific conditions [14]. The UK charity ACT (now "Together for short lives") published a *Transition Care pathway* [15] that summarises the needs, concerns, and necessary steps of the process and is a recommended starting point for any service looking to improve transition [16]. Recommendations in relation to good practice in transition are shown in Box 16.1.

Planning ahead can greatly improve the first and future experiences of a young person and their family and help start to build the trust that they will need to establish as the years go by. For example, in the United

Box 16.1 Recommendations for good practice in transition [16–18]

- The appointment of a key worker.
- Development of local policies and arrangements around transition.
- Training of paediatric and adult health professional in the issues, needs, and risks.
- Engagement and empowerment of young people in their own health care.
- Services to be designed around the needs of the young people not the needs of the service, that is, flexibility.
- Timely services.
- Multiagency collaboration.
- Person-centred services.

Kingdom, health-care professionals are starting to recognise the need for transition planning, and in some specialties (notably cardiology, renal, endocrine) there are named professionals who take responsibility for smoothing a young person's transition between services. All children with complex health needs or learning difficulties in the United Kingdom should have a transition plan from the age of 14, led by education and with input from social services. Health services should play a full and active role in this transition planning to help allay the fears of young people and their families.

One of the benefits of developing specialist centres for young people (such as young adult hospices and teenage cancer units) is that expertise will be developed to deal with the complex issues of death and dying. On the other hand, such centres may be so few in number that the young person has to travel so far that they become further isolated from their friends and family and transference of skills into the community is more limited [19].

One study suggests that the place of death should be used as a measure of the quality of supportive and palliative care [20]. Home deaths are less likely to be achieved for those lower in the social scale, or for those with leukaemia or lymphoma rather than solid cancers. This raises important questions about the quality of palliative services for these patient groups, and suggests the need to devote further attention to their needs. Similarly, areas in inner London (with higher rates of child poverty) were less likely to achieve home deaths than more "affluent" areas of England. Young people with brain tumours were also more likely to die in a hospice setting.

At present, the majority of young people likely to require palliative care die in hospital. Also those between 20 and 24 years of age are less likely to die at home, and more likely to die in hospice than those between the ages 15 and 19 years [6]. Although the literature is sparse, in the United Kingdom, it is likely that more young people with nonmalignant LLC die at home than those with malignancies. Many young people with nonmalignant diagnoses will have been cared for at home with the support of a care package for some time, and this may facilitate their dying at home if this is a choice they make. Two studies looking at place of death in oncology patients have reported that preferred place of death was achieved for the majority [21,22].

Decision making should involve the patient, family, and friends in ways that are meaningful to them. Toward the end of life, it is especially important that effective communication is promoted between all members of the care team to minimise misunderstandings and the frustrations within what is likely to be an already highly emotional situation. This relies on hospital staff passing on the history and care goals to primary care colleagues who will become more closely involved in provision of palliative care. At this stage, it is crucial that the multidisciplinary team (MDT) work together to achieve the best possible care at the end of life. Importantly, this will require professionals to confront the poignancy of an adolescent or young adult facing the end of their life. An understanding of the underlying psychology of this patient group, together with recognition of the personal impact on CPs is therefore essential.

In health, the transition from adolescence to young adulthood is characterised by growth, development, and the challenging of social norms [23]. The rate of such development varies widely between individuals, however, and is often unpredictable [24]. Particular cognitive functions, such as abstract thinking, develop at different rates as do the physical changes associated with puberty itself. Chronological age, therefore, may not always be the most appropriate indicator of whether a "young adolescent" with cancer would best be admitted to an adult or paediatric ward for a highly specialised surgical procedure. Similarly, age does not always correspond to physical or cognitive maturity. As the opening quotation suggests, young people facing a life-threatening illness often develop wisdom beyond their years, and they can usually detect when professionals are trying to avoid certain topics, or trying to protect them from bad news. Many of the young people with LLC will have complex neurodevelopmental difficulties with a cognitive age greatly below their chronological age. Despite being physically larger, their needs may best be served within a paediatric setting or in a setting with a similar philosophy. Regardless of where such care is pro-

vided, the main concern is the provision of appropriate psychosocial care. Flexibility is often needed in practice and open dialogue may offer the best approach when decisions are made with young people about their individual care needs.

The psychology of adolescence and young adulthood

The range of developmental changes that occur between adolescence and young adulthood means that this patient population will present with diverse support needs. An LLC brings about a change in the perceived natural order of events, and the challenge for palliative care services is to respond appropriately while remaining aware of the young person's stage of development. By the time adult palliative care services are involved, the young person may already have faced the disappointment of failed treatments and, possibly, a realisation that they are likely to die from their disease. This process takes time and will have occurred alongside the normal developmental tasks of adolescence and young adulthood (Tables 16.1 and 16.2).

Young people facing a serious illness may, for instance, want to maintain some degree of control over their lives—as they become more ill, their focus is likely to shrink to involve events and people in their immediate environment. At the same time, they will also need help to cope with a number of debilitating symptoms such as pain, breathlessness, nausea, and fatigue. A fine balance

Table 16.1 Developmental tasks of adolescence.

- Forming a clear identity
- Accepting a new body image
- Gaining freedom from parents
- Developing a personal value system
- Achieving financial and social independence
- Developing relationships with members of both sexes
- Developing cognitive skills and the ability to think abstractly
- Developing the ability to control one's behaviour according to social norms
- Taking responsibility for one's own behaviour

Source: Adapted from work of Joint Working Party on Palliative Care for Adolescents and Young Adults, 2001 [4].

Table 16.2 Stages of adolescent and young adult development and the impact of a life-threatening/life-limiting illness.

Age	Early adolescence 12–14 years (female) 13–15 years (male)	Middle adolescence 14–16 years	Young adult 17–24 years
Key issues and characteristics	Focus on development of body; most pubertal changes occur; rapid physical growth; acceptance by peers; idealism mood swings, contrariness, temper tantrums; daydreaming	Sexual awakening; emancipation from parents and figures of authority; discovery of limitations by testing limitation/boundaries; role of peer group increases	Defining and understanding functional roles in life in terms of career, relationships, and lifestyle
Social relationships, behaviours	Improved skills in abstract thought, foreseeing consequences, planning for future; physical mobility prominent; energy levels high; appetite increases; social interaction in groups; membership of peer group important	Relationships very narcissistic; risk-taking behaviour increases; intense peer interaction; most vulnerable to psychological problems	Increasing financial independence; planning for the future; establishment of permanent relationships; increasing time away from family
Impact of life-threatening illness	Concerns about physical appearance and mobility; privacy all-important; possible interference with normal cognitive development and learning (school absence, medication, pain, depression, fatigue); comparison with peers hindered, making self-assessment of normality difficult; possible lack of acceptance by peers; reliance on parents and other authorities in decision-making; hospitals perceived as very disturbing	Illness particularly threatening and least well tolerated at this stage; compromised sense of autonomy; emancipation from parents and authority figures impeded; interference with attraction of partner, fear of rejection by peers; limited interaction with peers may lead to social withdrawal; dependence on family for companionship and social support; hospitalisation, school absences interfere with social relationships and acquisition of social skills noncompliance with treatment	Absences from work, study; interference with plans for vocation and relationships difficulties in securing employment and promotion at work; unemployment hinders achieving separation from family and financial independence; discrimination in employment, health cover, and life insurance; loss of financial independence and self-esteem; concerns about fertility and health of offspring

Source: Adapted from work of Joint Working Party on Palliative Care for Adolescents and Young Adults, 2001 [4].

will need to be struck between becoming dependent on professionals for some things and retaining a degree of independence. An example of this concerns compliance with medication, which often needs careful negotiation, particularly if side effects are an issue. Achieving a balance can challenge even the most experienced parent or health professional, as frustration and exhaustion take their toll. In addition, related concerns such as being able to access appropriate expertise when at home (especially if symptoms suddenly worsen) or having skilled psychological support available, when needed, are practical concerns to be addressed. The challenges of providing effective palliative care for young adults are magnified as their condition deteriorates and they are faced with a range of interrelated physical, emotional, and existential needs.

An important aspect of adolescence and young adulthood that is often stressed is the forming of independent relationships apart from the family unit. While this is a potential challenge for all young people, it is more marked in those with pre-existing physical or learning difficulties. Life-limiting illness may mean this is more difficult to achieve due to deteriorating health and the need for constant additional support, resulting in frustration and conflict. Support from family members, however, is also crucial at other times. Researchers have found that informal support from family members is directly linked to the illness experience of young adults aged between the ages of 19 and 30 years with cancer and leads to a greater ability to cope with the demands of illness [25]. Therefore, there is a need to balance the challenge of living with cancer and its treatment with relationships, careers, and other life events. Those supported by family members felt more able to cope with such demands. It is likely that family members will also be experiencing significant life events and transitions. One theoretical approach for assessing family functioning in such situations is presented next [26,27].

Vulnerable families tend to show the following characteristics:

• Serious illness occurring alongside other major life transition can result in a loss of individual and family coherence/adaptability.
• The greater the match between the social character of the family and the developmental needs of its members, the better likelihood there is of adapting to serious illness.
• Middle-aged families with adolescents living with a chronic illness may show less family unity or achievement of developmental tasks.
• The older the family, the less the likelihood of disruption when a member becomes ill.

Despite the fact that variation should be anticipated, guidelines such as these may help to focus attention on the nature of family relationships in end-of-life care situations. Individual or family counselling may also be helpful for the young person and their family when necessary [28].

It is little wonder that those who find themselves in such a situation will express a wide range of emotions. At the same time, as their body and mind are developing, they are become increasingly dependent on others and face the possibility of death itself.

From health to illness

The experience of cancer for a young person has been described as a process of transition [1,29]. Edwards suggests that there are two dimensions of this transition. These are the following:

1. The transition from a state of perceived health to living with a life-threatening illness.
2. The transition from active treatment to palliative care—essentially moving from a "life-threatening" illness to a "life-limiting" one.

Major life events such as these will impact on all aspects of a young person's experience. For example, symptoms arising as a result of disease or treatment will mean time being lost from education or work. This, in turn, will mean less contact with peers while being more dependent on professionals or family. Once again it is clear that serious illness impacts as much socially as it does physically for a young person [30]. Advancing symptoms will also result in changes such as skin breakdown, the insertion of central venous catheters and weight loss or gain, which further threatens self-esteem and sense of personal control [31].

Adolescence and young adulthood can be a time of contradictions—seeking ways to be understood may be opposed by a reluctance to express feelings [32]. The desire to maintain control and independence while experiencing physical deterioration can be demoralising, frustrating, and confusing. A deteriorating physical condition can also result in being treated in a childlike way.

An example from practice helps to illustrate these points:

> Mary was 19 years old when she was diagnosed with acute myeloid laeukemia. Prior to this, she had taken a year out from her studies and had travelled the world. She enjoyed partying with friends and was due to return to university when she suddenly became unwell. The laeukemia chemotherapy treatment schedule was intense, which meant that very little time was spent out of the hospital environment. Side effects from the treatment left her feeling exhausted; she experienced weight loss and had to have a central venous catheter inserted. Gradually, she refused to see her friends because she felt more and more like a "freak." At the same time, she became so dependent on her mother that she asked her to stay with her in hospital every night.

The development of appropriate helping strategies in such a situation requires an awareness of the environmental, cultural, and historical factors as well as the biological, psychological, and social phenomena that are now impacting on the young person's life. Some may find having to be examined by a member of staff of a different gender particularly distressing. Having a parent present may be upsetting for some, while helpful for others. It is easy for carers to assume that a child with a disability is used to the assistance of others—nevertheless, with increasing age and body awareness, the same consideration to their dignity should be afforded, no matter how severe the disability.

Sexuality and fertility are also notoriously difficult issues for any young person to discuss with their parents [24]. While sexuality may be considered a taboo subject by some, early adolescence and young adulthood are times of intense sexual activity and development [33]. A life-threatening disease or pre-existing disability, no matter how severe, does not necessarily halt this process. Instead, sexual function can become a focus of concern for young people as a result of the disease, its treatment, or its side effects. For instance, failing to menstruate may be seen as a highly significant loss for some young women. Such concerns may be coupled with a lack of sexual experience before diagnosis and may result in resentment toward healthy peers who are developing in this way. Discussing such topics can be very difficult for parents, especially as friends and peers are the usual first choice [1]. It is important that this topic is not ignored because it is difficult to approach—for some young people, it is very much at the forefront of their minds and the loss of personal capacity to explore and fulfil their wishes, and the loss of peer groups with which to discuss them, can be very difficult. For professionals, training and support are available including a DVD produced by young people themselves and the UK charity ACT [34].

Different concerns may arise for young adults, particularly those involved in established relationships who, as a result of their illness or treatment, may face never having the opportunity to produce, or raise, their own children.

Promotion of intimacy and supportive personal relationships during the later stages of serious illness are important considerations. Privacy and space may be difficult to provide in hospital settings, or may be easily overlooked [35] though may be more achievable in hospice settings, where there may be more flexibility around residential visitors and where visiting hours are usually open. Those with young children, as the illness progresses, some may wish to leave something tangible behind for their children, such as a book of memories or a recording. Psychological support for the patient, their partner, children,

and other significant family members may be of benefit when considering creation of lasting memory legacies.

Young people and their families often report that it is hard for others to understand what they are going through, and, that talking to others with personal experience is very helpful. Douglas House, a young people's hospice in Oxford, UK runs a peer-support program for siblings, pre- and postbereavement, and reports that the mixing of the two groups has many advantages, including the possibility of hope as siblings meet those who have already been bereaved and are able to see that, for all the difficulties, they have moved through it. This approach also shows benefits for bereaved parents.

Quality of life

Living with an LLC can be frustrating and gruelling for everyone involved, but for the young people at the centre, there is an innate drive to cling to normality and above all else "join in" with life to their maximum potential:

> I am not interested in dying, I am interested in living. (Young person age 19 years).

In common with their healthy peers, the drive to push to extremes and risk take is present but perhaps more meaningful to young people aware of their own mortality. This can create some challenges for parents and professionals but often this drive is a part of coping and allows the family to focus on more positive goals through a period of extreme distress. Continuing education is an important part of life in this age group, and supporting a young person who wants to do this can be very rewarding. Allowing plenty of time for planning is key here, as is finding the right people to support education. A detailed understanding of the situation and capabilities and goals should lead to the creation of a plan that is likely to succeed. Flexibility is fundamental and advocating for the young person can require patience and persistence.

Young adults may also seek "normality" in other ways, such as seeking to return to employment, to a role in which they felt productive and useful. A mother, in Grinyer [1], recounts the following account of her son Steve's experience:

> Work was always so important to you Steve, especially when your life was threatened. Work was a place where customers asked you for help and didn't ask you about the cancer.... Now I am reliving the last three months, exactly twelve weeks to the day when we knew it had really got you and was in your bones, back to normality while you could. How sensible, how

mature. . . . Your pain is unbearable, you can only work for short bursts, but as you say at least on the shop floor people treat me normally, they ask me for help. You go on, what strength you have.

Being treated as an individual is important to each of us. However, it can be seen as even more significant to the young person still be seeking to find their identity as they come to transition.

In terms of care, this requires a different approach to that of younger children and older adults:

We may have had two or three hundred young people with Duchennes come through our doors over the last 13 years, but each one, and the one that will come next week, is an individual (Sister Frances Dominica, Helen & Douglas House Hospice, Oxford, UK).

Those working with young people should have training to enable them to support individuality, and not rely on intuition [17,18]. Listening well is at the heart of care for these young people. Ascertaining their priorities and the priorities of their families (which are usually different, but nonetheless important to address) is a helpful way to work. These priorities will change, sometimes frequently, but often allow explorations of further concerns that might otherwise remain hidden. Insights from the 2010 UK National Cancer Patient Experience Survey suggest that cancer patients aged 16–25 years had less positive views about their treatment than middle-aged groups. Specifically, the need for information given in a way that is helpful and mindful of their lack of contact with services before illness is highlighted. This may be an important consideration if their condition does progresses as any perceived dissatisfactions early in their illness experience may be magnified over time [36].

Toward the end of life

As death approaches, a variety of reactions and needs should be anticipated. No two people will react in the same way, regardless of their age, background, or situation. There may be a point at which there is a realisation that cure is no longer possible, or it may be that current interventions are no longer giving benefit. In either scenario, feelings of abandonment and failure are common—patients may feel they have somehow "failed" those working to cure them and professionals may find it difficult to acknowledge that their interventions have been unsuccessful. There may also be a sense of guilt on the part of parents that more could have been done to recognise

the disease earlier (such as in the case of cancer), or a sense of failure that they have been unable to protect their child from the illness itself. Conversely, parents of young people with complex disability may have faced potential "end-of-life" crises many times. Such experiences can lead to them doubting whether they have done the right thing in helping their child to live through exacerbations and feelings of guilt about the same. Exploring these emotions can be helpful at the time and into bereavement. Indeed, support prebereavement can impact positively on the experience of families postbereavement. Young people and families may feel abandoned if their care is passed on to other teams at this point, and so this transition needs careful handling. Robust joint working between acute services and palliative care services can improve this. Rather than transferring end-of-life care from one team to another, members of the MDTs from the specialty, working in partnership with palliative care services and community staff, can deliver a coordinated package of supportive care [30].

Not all individuals will have the emotional capacity to comprehend the enormity of the situation [31], and this can impact on the way that symptoms such as pain, anxiety, and restlessness are experienced, often escalating them, and thus the management of these symptoms should always include explorations of their meaning to the young person [37]. An individual's willingness to engage in decisions about symptom control is likely to mirror their own, and their family's, coping strategies. Some may ask for every detail to be explained, while others prefer deferring to professional opinions. The significance of symptoms should not be underestimated as this has been found to be linked with how life-limiting illness is perceived by young people and their families [28,38,39]. Carers who witness a young person's suffering yet feel unable to provide adequate relief may also experience frustration [40].

Planning ahead around management of acute or slow deteriorations, and end-of-life care can be beneficial for young people, families, and services [41]. It can provide an opportunity to air concerns that may otherwise remain hidden, and to explore personal values and wishes. It can provide a professional with a structured way of approaching difficult issues and recording them in a manner in which they will be retained and respected when needed. Many young people will have grown up with plans detailing specific intervention for particular medical emergencies. This may have included plans for management of respiratory arrest and/or CPR. In essence, paediatric plans often provide an option for limited resuscitation measures (such as bag and mask only) and do not represent a clear

Yes/No "DNR" decision commonly found in adult health-care settings. Young people with plans in place like this are now living to adulthood and these plans are moving from the paediatric to the adult sector. It is essential that careful discussion occurs at this point. The plans will need review and in some cases, as authority passes from parent to young people, they may change. The importance here is that the young person is approached and offered discussion, that information is given in a sensitive and appropriate (to understanding rather than age) way, and that changes, once negotiated, are respected. All efforts must be made to establish a young person's wishes, even those young people with the most challenging communication issues, providing that they have capacity to make decisions in this area. For young people without capacity, in the United Kingdom, best interest decisions can be made. These are usually made through a multidisciplinary route with involvement of the families/principal carers; the involvement of advocates in this process should be explored when a young person does not have capacity. Chapter 8, *Advance care planning*, provides more detail on this aspect.

Young people's preferences for specific treatment interventions will be influenced by social and emotional maturity, as well as past experiences and cultural and spiritual beliefs. While some wish to be involved in decision-making throughout their illness, others may prefer to rely upon carers to decide on their behalf. Some may also wish to be involved in some areas of care but not others. This situation can result in family discord as protective instincts may challenge the young person's need to remain independent. Professionals need to be sensitive to the dynamics and tensions in such situations, and adopt practical strategies such as encouraging both parties to spend time away from each other. End-of-life care for adolescents and young adults (whether provided in the home or hospital/hospice setting) requires openness, honesty, flexibility, and responsiveness to meet the many individual needs that will arise in each situation.

Research findings suggest that there are two key issues that benefit those assisting young people and their families in making end-of-life decisions. The first is clarity and honesty when information is being imparted. The second involves trust in, and having the support of, the health-care team [10]. From interviews with bereaved parents of young people with cancer, adolescents, and staff, key concerns included knowing that all that could be done had been done to achieve a cure, no acceptable treatment options remained untried, and, as a result, long-term survival was unlikely. Decisions made by parents and families were judged according to the balance struck between quality of life, treatment toxicity, and other adverse outcomes, as well as estimations of suffering and the patient's individual preferences. Such findings may be helpful in practice—especially when the boundaries between cure and care, or between experimental therapy and palliation, become blurred [10].

Conclusions

This chapter has explored the particular challenges that professionals face in providing effective palliative care to young people. Awareness of developmental needs, as well as the disruption that serious illness causes at this stage of life, may help to ensure that we respond appropriately to this unique patient group. An issue of crucial importance is the need for effective channels of communication between the young person, family, hospital, and primary care professionals to ensure that all parties are working together to achieve the same goals [42]. Growing awareness of these issues demands a greater evidence base on which to base care, and a creative approach to service provision.

Practical expertise needs to be combined with appropriate education and research to ensure that adolescents and young adults who are facing death are provided with appropriate care and support.

References

1. Grinyer A. *Cancer in Young Adults: Through Parents' Eyes.* Buckingham: Open University Press, 2002.
2. Marie Curie Cancer Care. Young people: life-limiting conditions but life-enhancing choices. *PublicServiceWorks*, April 2011.
3. York University Social Policy Research Unit. *Supporting health transitions for young people with life limiting conditions: researching evidence of positive practice.* York University Social Policy Research Unit.
4. Joint Working Party on Palliative Care for Adolescents and Young Adults. *Palliative Care for Young people Aged 13–24.* Bristol: Association for Children with Life-Threatening Conditions and Their Families, 2001. ISBN 1 898447 06 3.
5. Bisset M, Hutton S and Kelly D. Palliation and end of life care issues. In: Kelly D and Gibson F (eds), *Cancer Care for Adolescents and Young Adults.* Oxford: Blackwell Publishing Ltd, Chap 9, 2008.
6. Department of Health. *Palliative care statistics for children and young adults.* Department of Health, 2007

7. Grinyer A and Thomas C. Young adults with cancer: the effects on parents and families. *Int J Palliat Nurs* 2001; 7: 162–170.

8. Evans M. Interacting with teenagers with cancer. In: Selby P and Bailey C (eds), *Cancer and the Adolescent*. London: BMJ Publishing Group, 1996, pp. 251–263.

9. Pearce S. The impact of adolescent cancer on health care professionals. In: Kelly D and Gibson F (eds), *Cancer Care for Adolescents and Young Adults*. Oxford: Blackwell Publishing Ltd, Chap 4, 2008.

10. Emold C, Schneider M, Meller I, et al. Communication skills, working environment and burnout among oncology nurses. *European Journal of Oncology Nursing* (2011); 15: 358–363.

11. Craig F and Lidstone V. The special needs of adolescents and young adults. In: Goldman A, Hain R, and Liben S (eds), *Oxford Textbook for Palliative Care for Children*, 2nd edition. Oxford University Press, in press.

12. Gleeson H and Turner G. Transition to adult services. *Arch Dis Child Educ Pract Ed* 2011.

13. Department of Health. *Transition: moving on well: a good practice guide for health professionals and their partners on transition planning for young people with complex needs or a disability*. Department of Health, 2008.

14. Muscular Dystrophy Campaign. *Becoming an adult: transition for young men with Duchenne muscular dystrophy*. Muscular Dystrophy Campaign, 2010.

15. The ACT Transition Care Pathway. *A framework for the development if integrated multi-agency care pathways for young people with life-threatening and life-limiting conditions*. Bristol: ACT, 2007.

16. *Palliative Care Services for children and young people in England. An independent review for the secretary of State for health by Professor Sir Alan Craft and Sue Killen*. Department of Health, 2007.

17. Royal College of Nursing. *Lost in transition: moving people between child and adult healthcare services*. Royal College of Nursing, 2007.

18. Department of Health. *Transition: moving on well*. Department of Health UK, 2008.

19. Kelly D, Mullhall A, and Pearce S. Adolescent cancer: the need to evaluate current service provision in the UK. *Eur J Oncol Nurs* 2003; 7: 53–58.

20. Higginson I and Thompson M. Children and young people who die from cancer: epidemiology and place of death in England (1995–9). *BMJ* 2003; 327: 478–479.

21. Vickers J, Thompson A, Collins GS, et al. Place and provision of palliative care for children with progressive cancer: a study by the Paediatric Oncology Nurses' Forum/United Kingdom Children's Cancer Study Group Palliative Care Working Group. *J Clin Oncol* 2007; 25(28): 4472–4476.

22. Dussel V, Kreicbergs U, Hilden JM, et al. Looking beyond where children die: determinants and effects of planning a child's location of death. *J Pain Symptom Manage* 2009; 37(1): 33–43.

23. Brannen J, Dodd K, Oakley K, et al. *Young People, Health and Family Life*. Buckingham: Open University Press, 1994.

24. Silverman RP. *Never Too Young to Know. Death in Children's Lives*. Oxford: Oxford University Press, 2000.

25. Lynam MJ. Supporting one another: the nature of family work when a young adult has cancer. *J Adv Nurs* 1995; 22: 116–125.

26. Rankin SH and Weekes DP. Life-span development: a review of theory and practice for families with chronically ill members. *Sch Inq Nurs Pract* 2000; 14: 355–373.

27. Weekes DP and Rankin SH. Life-span developmental methods: application to nursing research. *Nurs Res* 1988; 37: 380–383.

28. Rose K, Webb C, and Wayers K. Coping strategies employed by informal carers of terminally ill cancer patients. *J Cancer Nurs* 1997; 1: 126–133.

29. Edwards J. A model of palliative care for the adolescent with cancer. *Int J Palliat Nurs* 2001; 7: 485–488.

30. Woodgate RL. A different way of being: adolescents' experiences with cancer. *Cancer Nursing* 2005;15: 8–18.

31. Ritchie MA. Psychosocial functioning of adolescents with cancer: a developmental perspective. *Oncol Nurs Forum* 1992; 19: 1497–1501.

32. DeMinco S. Young adult reactions to death in literature and life. *Adolescence* 1995; 30: 179–185.

33. Muuss RE. *Theories of Adolescence*, 6th edition. London: The McGraw-Hill Companies, Inc, 1996.

34. *Let's Talk About Sex* (DVD). Bristol: ACT, 2009.

35. Searle E. Sexuality and people who are dying. In: Heath H and White I (eds), *The Challenge of Sexuality in Health Care*. London: Blackwell Science, 2002.

36. Department of Health. *National Cancer Patient Experience Survey Programme—2010 National Survey Report*. London: Department of Health, 2010.

37. Woodgate R and McClement S. Symptom distress in children with cancer: the need to adopt a meaning-centred approach. *J Pediatr Oncol Nurs* 1998; 15: 3–12.

38. Hockenberry M, Hooke M. Symptom clusters in children with cancer. *Seminars in Oncology Nursing* 2007; 23:152–157.

39. Woodgate RL and Degner F. A substantive theory of keeping the spirit alive: the spirit within children with cancer and their families. *J Pediatr Oncol Nurs* 2003; 20: 103–119.

40. Hinds PS, Oakes L, Furman W, et al. End-of-life decision making by adolescents, parents, and health care providers in pediatric oncology. *Cancer Nurs* 2001; 24: 122–135.

41. Rabow MW, Hauser JM, and Adams J. Supporting family caregivers at the end of life: "they don't know what they don't know". *JAMA* 2004; 291(4): 483–491.

42. George R and Hutton S. Palliative care in adolescents. *Eur J Cancer* 2003; 39: 2662–2668.

17 Palliative Care for People with Advanced Dementia

Rachael E. Dixon

Dove House Hospice, Hull, UK

Introduction

Dementia is an umbrella term describing the symptoms of memory loss, cognitive decline, and others that occur when the brain is affected by certain diseases or conditions. People with dementia may wait years for a diagnosis and some never receive one. Doctors often defer the diagnosis because they think it is futile, that the condition is not treatable, that it carries stigma, and that it will leave people feeling hopeless. There is however much that can be done in providing optimal quality of care for both people with advanced dementia and their families, some of whom live together and many of whom are forced into separation by the behavioural and other impacts of dementia.

About two-thirds of patients with dementia die in nursing or residential care and up to 70% of care home residents have a varying degree of dementia. The general practitioner (GP) is often best placed to ensure an integrated and coordinated approach to meet the wishes of the patient and family. The reality is however that often the GP will not have known them before their arrival in the care home. Even if the GP has known them, communication can be particularly difficult in advanced dementia. Knowing the wishes of the person with dementia and incorporating the knowledge of families are vital in directing care.

This chapter will consider ethical and symptomatic issues and advance care planning (ACP) that is crucial in a condition where patients will lose capacity. It will also consider what is different about palliative care in advanced dementia in comparison to patients with other illnesses and suggest how we may also need to respond differently to our patients and their carers.

Types of dementia

Alzheimer's disease

This is the most common cause of dementia. Plaques and tangles develop in the brain leading to cell death. There is also a disturbance of several neurotransmitter systems, including the cholinergic, somatostatinergic, serotonergic, noradrenergic, and possibly dopaminergic. People become confused and frequently forget names and appointments, have mood swings, and have difficulty carrying out everyday activities. Over time, more parts of the brain are affected and the symptoms become more severe. In the vast majority of cases, there does not appear to be a pattern of inheritance; however, carriers of the ApoE4 gene variant have a much higher chance of developing Alzheimer's disease as do people with Down's syndrome.

Vascular dementia

Brain cell death from loss of blood supply is related to high blood pressure, high cholesterol, diabetes, and smoking. There are two main types of vascular dementia, one affecting larger blood vessels caused by strokes and one caused by smaller vessel disease. People have difficulty concentrating and may have periods of acute confusion. They may also experience a more stepped progression with symptoms remaining stable then suddenly deteriorating.

Dementia with Lewy bodies

Lewy bodies are tiny spherical protein deposits found in nerve cells. Their presence disrupts the normal message

Handbook of Palliative Care, Third Edition. Edited by Christina Faull, Sharon de Caestecker, Alex Nicholson and Fraser Black.
© 2012 by John Wiley and Sons, Inc. Published 2012 by John Wiley & Sons, Inc.

processes of the brain involving dopamine and acetyl-choline. Lewy bodies are also found in the brains of patients with PD. Patients with Lewy body dementia tend to have some symptoms similar to Alzheimer's disease—problems with attention, spatial awareness, and executive function. They may also develop symptoms of PD, including loss of facial expression, muscle stiffness, and a tendency to shuffle when walking. They may also experience detailed and convincing visual hallucinations, which are typical to Lewy Body dementia.

Frontotemporal dementia

This covers a range of conditions including Pick's disease, frontal lobe degeneration, and dementia associated with Motor Neuron Disease. This is a rarer type of dementia but is more common in younger people, being the second most common cause of dementia in people under the age of 65. There is a family history in one-third to a half of all cases of frontotemporal dementia. During the initial stages, memory remains intact but their personality and behaviour changes. In the later stages, the damage to the brain becomes more progressive and symptoms are similar to Alzheimer's disease.

There are other rarer causes of dementia, including progressive supranuclear palsy (PSP), HIV/AIDS, Korsakoff's syndrome, Huntington's disease (HD), and Binswanger's disease.

Epidemiology

Currently, it is estimated that there are around 750,000 people in the United Kingdom suffering from dementia, out of which 15,000 are under the age of 65 [1]. Over the next 30 years, the numbers are expected to double. A mapping exercise into dementia diagnosis levels across the United Kingdom has shown that by 2021 half a million people with the condition will not have received a diagnosis. The estimated median survival time from the onset of dementia is 4.1 years for men and 4.6 years for women. Patients without comorbidities may however live considerably longer.

Worldwide up to 30 million people are thought to be affected by dementia, with this expected to rise to over 100 million by 2050. Due to few studies in the developing world, there is more uncertainty about the frequency of dementia. In North America, the prevalence figures are similar to western Europe with a slightly larger percentage of the population over 85 being affected [2].

Estimates for the prevalence of dementia (%) per WHO region and age range are as follows [9]:

WHO region description	60–64	65–69	70–74	75–79	80–84	85+
Western Europe	0.9	1.5	3.6	6.0	12.2	24.8
North America	0.8	1.7	3.3	6.5	12.8	30.1

How is palliative care in advanced dementia different?

Palliative care in advanced dementia aims to maximise the quality of life rather than to extend its length. The differences are that the patient is likely to have lost the ability to communicate verbally, and discussing treatment options with the patient is unlikely to be possible. Patients may have severe expressive and receptive problems but emotional receptivity does not necessarily disappear. Tactile communication or simply being there with the patient can be helpful.

Communication with the family and/or care team is vital. Even when patients can no longer communicate verbally and are completely reliant on others for all care, the people who work with them closest are often able to tell whether they are content or distressed. They may also have developed ways of encouraging patients to take medications and so on. At present, few people, in the United Kingdom at least, have advance care plans; therefore, discussions around treatment often take place with the family and it is important they are aware what may happen as the disease progresses.

The disease trajectory tends to be much longer and more unpredictable than that of cancer. For families, it can be difficult to live with this uncertainty and some older relatives may fear that they will die before the patient, leading to concerns about their future.

Health professionals may also struggle with the longer disease trajectory and deciding when it is no longer appropriate to actively treat and develop a purely palliative approach. Because of this, decisions such as resuscitation status may not be taken as readily as they are with a patient with advanced cancer.

Prognostic indicator guide

One of the major barriers to good end-of-life care is that people approaching the end of their life are not recognised at an early enough stage. This is a particular problem for dementia as it often does not follow as predictable disease trajectory as cancer. The Prognostic Indicator Guidance developed by the GSF team aims to assist in helping identify patients approaching the end of their illness, anticipate needs, and plan ahead.

Prognostic Indicator Guide in Dementia (taken from GSF 2008):

- Unable to walk without assistance.
- Urinary and faecal incontinence.
- No consistently meaningful verbal communication.
- Unable to dress without assistance.
- Barthel score <3 (the Barthel scoring system comprises 10 basic daily living activities with the scores for each item ranging from 0 (completely dependent) to 3 (independent) [3]).

Plus any one of the following:

- Ten percent weight loss in previous 6 months without other causes.
- pyelonephritis or urinary tract infection.
- serum albumin 25 g/L or less.
- severe pressure ulcers.
- recurrent fevers.
- reduced oral intake/weight loss.
- aspiration pneumonia.

Communication issues

Nonverbal communication becomes particularly important in a patient with dementia who is losing their language skills. When a person with dementia behaves in a way that makes things difficult for those caring for them, it may be because they are trying to communicate something. It is important to correct any factors that may be affecting their communication such as making sure hearing aids are turned on and that they are wearing glasses if needed. Trying to eliminate excess background noise could help establish what they are trying to say. Remain calm, respectful, and unhurried in your approach. It can be frustrating when you seem to be getting nowhere but do not be tempted to speak over them to other family members/carers as this can cause more distress.

Becoming more emotional

As we become more emotional and less cognitive, it's the way you talk to us, not what you say, that we will remember. We know the feelings, but don't know the plot. Your smile, your laugh and your touch are what we connect with. Empathy heals. Just love us as we are. We are still here, in emotion and spirit, if only you could find us!
[Christine Bryden. *Dancing with Dementia*. Jessica Kingsley Publishers 2005].

Advance care planning

This can be very helpful for people with dementia and can take place even when people have fairly advanced disease as long as they have capacity for the specific decisions being explored—the ability to understand and speculate about the treatment decision to be made (see mental capacity discussion in Chapter 8, *Advance Care Planning*). People with early dementia are often keen to participate in ACP discussions and this can help to improve satisfaction with care, both for the patients and their families.

Discussions usually need to take place on more than one occasion and be unhurried. Information should be clearly given using words that are easy to understand. Individuals need to be given sufficient information about their possible options and under what circumstances their plan would be activated. They need to be able to understand what the consequences of their decision will be. Summarising and checking understanding helps clarify what people want. ACP is discussed in detail in Chapter 8, *Advance Care Planning*.

Caring for the carers

The majority of care for people with dementia is delivered by unpaid carers. Many of them are elderly and frail themselves. There is evidence that carers of people with dementia experience greater strain, distress, and higher levels of psychological morbidity than carers of other older people. Caring for someone 24 h a day, 7 days a week, particularly if they have a disrupted sleep pattern is mentally and physically exhausting. Their own health needs can be neglected as they are unable to leave their loved one alone to attend GP/hospital appointments. Carers may be reluctant to ask for help, seeing it as their duty with many not aware what help is available. Finding out about local volunteer services such as sitting services can give the carer a few hours break to either sleep or leave the house. Investigating whether the patient is entitled to continuing health care could enable a care package to be put in place or respite to allow the carer a chance to have a complete break. Their hard work needs to be acknowledged and should the patient need to be cared for in a residential/nursing home, the carers must not be made to feel like this is a failure on their part. They need to be aware that if, for example, the patient has very disruptive behaviour, nobody would be able to continue to manage this 24 h a day by themselves without help, as even larger teams can struggle with this scenario.

If the person with dementia is in a home and the relative spends many hours a day visiting, they can also become socially isolated as other areas of their life are neglected; conversely, when the person dies, they lose the social contact and support from visiting the home.

It is important that the carers have all the information they require to make choices about the future. This may involve the GP discussing at an early stage what is likely to happen during the illness. It is also vital to acknowledge that the carers have a vast knowledge of the person and dementia and can impart this to health professionals.

Carers report facing difficult moral decisions throughout the dementia journey. This ranges from deciding when to get involved and take over day-to-day tasks, to decisions such as placing a relative in residential care or choosing palliative care over more aggressive management. Despite being well informed about dementia and its progression, very few are well prepared for having to make end-of-life decisions [4]. GPs, residential and nursing home staff often have regular contact with the person with dementia and their family over a significant period of time and are often in a good position to advise and support them. In the absence of advance care plans and discussions about end of life, families are often left making decisions under the pressure of time and distress.

Spirituality in dementia

The spiritual needs of people with end-stage dementia are often ignored, but addressing them can give great comfort. Suffering caused by dementia can often last a long time and cause relatives and carers to ask deep and searching questions about the meaning of life. Music is something that can reach people at an emotional level even in very advanced disease when they can appear otherwise unable to interact with the world. Pets and babies can also bring out an unexpected and "happy" emotional experience for people (Box 17.1).

> **Box 17.1 Lost Chord, a charity reaching people with dementia through music**
>
> Last year the doctors gave up on my father, who was suffering from a deadly and painful combination of ailments. He was cut-off from fluids and nutrition and we all had to wait in our own agony as we watched him fade away. He was in terrible pain and shuddered and gasped, unable to communicate. Over my tears, I took his hand and started singing. His breathing calmed, his eyes focused and his hand held mine. He looked like my father again. My experience with Lost Chord had enabled me to give the only gift my father could receive. [Patricia Hammond. www.lost-chord.org.uk]

Common physical symptoms in people with advanced dementia

The majority of patients with dementia are likely to be elderly and may have multiple comorbidities. Establishing what is causing the problem is complicated as a clear history will be difficult to obtain from the patients and reliant upon input from the family and carers to help piece together what is going on.

The general rules of pharmacological symptom management, irrespective of the specific symptoms, are the following:
- Give as few medications as possible.
- Start medications at low doses and gradually increase.
- Consider route on an individual basis; for example, tablets, liquids, dispersible, patches, depending on extent of disease and what the patient can tolerate.
- Regularly review medications and stop unnecessary tablets.

Pain

In a small series of people with dementia, 59% had pain. A larger series of 170 people with dementia showed that they had needs comparable to cancer patients; however, pain is often underestimated [5].

It is not acceptable to start an analgesic without making some assessment of the likely cause and even in severe dementia this can be possible. There are a number of tools that have been used for assessing pain and distress, such as Abbey, DOLOPLUS, Pain Assessment in Advanced Dementia (PAINAD), and Disability Distress Assessment Tool (DisDAT). The PAINAD scoring system (which is derived from DisDAT) is quick and simple to use and is able to reliably indicate improvements in pain with

Table 17.1 Pain Assessment in Advanced Dementia (PAINAD) scale.

Items	Characteristics			Score
	0	1	2	
Breathing independent of vocalisation	Normal	Occasional laboured breathing, short period of hyperventilation	Noisy, laboured breathing; long period of hyperventilation; Cheyne-Stokes respirations	
Negative vocalisation	None	Occasional moan or groan, low level speech with a negative or disapproving quality	Repeated troubled calling out, loud moaning or groaning, crying	
Facial expression	Smiling or inexpressive	Sad, frightened, frown	Facial grimacing	
Body language	Relaxed	Tense, distressed, pacing, fidgeting	Rigid, fists clenched, knees pulled up, pushing or pulling away, striking out	
Consolability	No need to console	Distracted or reassured by voice or touch	Unable to console, distract or reassure	
			Total	

Total scores range from 0 to 10 with a higher score indicating more pain; for example, 0 = no pain; 10 = severe pain.

treatment (Table 17.1). The DisDAT helps identify distress cues in people with severely limited communication. It looks at a broader array of signs and the clinical decision checklist can be used to decide upon the cause of the distress. Both tools are useful; however, the PAINAD also picks up distress not caused by pain and could potentially lead to false ascriptions of pain [6].

After establishing that pain is present, the character should be assessed. It may be a constant pain, or a pain related to movement secondary, for example, to osteoporosis or fracture, or only on sitting perhaps due to pressure sores. If there are wounds, then dressing changes may cause a period of distress. Colicky pain may be due to constipation, and opioids may worsen the situation. The WHO analgesic ladder approach should be used including adjuvants if necessary (see Chapter 9, *Pain and Its Management*). Nonsteroidal anti-inflammatory drugs can be used but due to the increased risk of dehydration in this group of people and the high prevalence of comorbidities, paracetamol should be tried first to avoid the risk of adverse renal effects.

Nonpharmacological measures should also be considered. Massage can be a very effective alternative as the act of touch may calm the patient and help ease aches and pains. Positioning may allow relief from a painful sore and advice from an occupational therapist with regard to pressure relieving and mobility aids can be helpful.

Compliance with medication may be an issue with patients sporadically taking painkillers, leading to poor symptom control. Low-dose buprenorphine transdermal patches, which start at 5 mg/h and are changed weekly, are an alternative to codeine (approximately equivalent to 60 mg codeine per 24 h) or very low dose morphine (5 mg per 24 h). They ensure the patient is getting a constant level of analgesia. Fentanyl patches are more appropriate where higher doses of opioids are required as the lowest dose (12 mg/h) is broadly equipotent with 40 mg morphine over 24 h. If pain is related to a specific activity such as dressing changes, a low dose of NR opioid, 15–20 min before the procedure, can be beneficial. Carers will need educating about providing the correct medications at the correct time.

Constipation

In advanced disease, it becomes common to eat less. Passing hard stool is a better indicator of constipation than the frequency of bowel openings. Constipation can be caused by reduced fibre intake, decreased mobility, decreased fluid intake, and medications such as morphine and antidepressants. Altering diet or increasing fluid intake is unlikely to be an option. If mild, lactulose may help in low doses such as 5 ml bd, but greater than this can lead to abdominal bloating. More severe constipation is likely to require a combination of softener (e.g., docusate) and stimulant (e.g., dulcolax or senna), all of which are available as liquids. Patients are unlikely to be able to tolerate the volume of liquid required with macrogols. Suppositories may be the most effective route to clear hard stool.

Behavioural symptoms of dementia

Up to 90% of people with dementia will develop some behavioural/psychiatric symptoms during their illness [7]. These include agitation, mood disorders (depression, anxiety, apathy), and psychotic symptoms (delusions and hallucinations). Agitation is the most frequently occurring symptom. Guidelines recommend a careful physical and psychological assessment and that nonpharmacological management should be tried first. Pharmacological treatments are only indicated when other strategies have failed.

Symptoms of depression are common occurring in approximately 20% of people with Alzheimer's disease and a higher proportion of people with vascular dementia or dementia with Lewy bodies. TCAs are not appropriate as the cholinergic side effects are likely to worsen the severity of the cognitive and functional impairments. One of the SSRIs is probably the drug of choice in Alzheimer's disease, but it is slightly less clear for people with vascular dementia. An expert opinion should be sought.

Nonpharmacological management of behavioural and psychological symptoms

Apart from cognitive decline, the most common symptom associated with dementia, agitation, aggression, and abnormal vocalisation can also cause problems as the disease progresses. Rather than using medications, other alternatives can be considered.

Music therapy

This may involve engagement by playing an instrument or singing a song or merely listening to songs and music. Several studies have reported benefits including increases

in the level of well-being, better social interaction, and improvements in autobiographical memory [8]. There was also found to be a significant reduction in agitation in people played an individualised music programs compared to standard relaxation music.

Art therapy

Art therapy can provide meaningful stimulation and improve social interaction. It allows people to exercise some choice with regard to colour and theme compared to other aspects of their life.

Aromatherapy

Aromatherapy can help agitation and can be used for bathing and inhalation as well as massage. Inhalation may be more helpful for a patient who is particularly restless.

Feeding difficulties

People with dementia often lose weight because they are not eating enough. It is important that families realise that loss of interest in food and weight loss in advanced dementia is part of the natural history and not a sign of neglect if a person is in a care home.

Forgetfulness, poor concentration, and distractibility may make people leave much of their meal uneaten. Feeding dyspraxia may mean they hold food in their mouth and forget to chew and swallow it. A change in their diurnal rhythm can leave them unable to identify meal times. Where possible small amounts of food left out in bowls allows patients to graze at any time of the day and this is often more effective than set meals. There is little point in asking ahead what meal they would prefer. It can be more beneficial to offer a choice of two dishes at meal times.

Highly flavoured foods and drinks and drinks which are hot or cold (not tepid) provide more stimulation within the mouth and are more likely to trigger a stronger swallow. Unskilled or hurried feeding can be counterproductive and increase weight loss. Poor dentition, dry mouth, and candidiasis can also interfere with feeding and should be treated. The key principle is never to force food onto someone who does not want it.

In very advanced dementia, people often develop swallowing difficulties and may start to aspirate. This may be due to behavioural problems such as vocalising while swallowing, a reduced awareness of food in their mouth, and an inability to both chew and swallow effectively. At this point, nasogastric (NG) or percutaneous endoscopic gastrostomy (PEG) feeding may be considered. There is however very little evidence showing that this improves nutritional status, prolongs life, improves quality of life, or indeed reduces the risk of aspiration pneumonia. What needs to be considered are the very large risks of gastrostomy insertion. If patients have infection or pressure sore at the time of insertion, the median survival is 32 days [7]. It should be remembered that people with end-stage dementia have a terminal condition with a limited life expectancy that cannot be reversed by tube feeding. It is important to emphasise to families that the patient is dying of dementia, not starvation.

Using a PEG in dementia might be expected to show an improvement in certain outcomes, including aspiration pneumonia, prevention of malnutrition, prevention/improvement in pressure ulcers, and decreased infections, but there is no clear evidence of reduced risk for any of these. PEG feeding cannot reduce the risk of aspiration from oral secretions and there are no data to show it reduces the risk from regurgitated gastric contents. They have not been shown to make patients with dementia more comfortable and may cause more problems than they relieve [9]. Guidance from the Royal College of Physicians is helpful in supporting these discussions [10].

The most appropriate management is to discuss what is happening with the family, making them fully informed about the situation. Options include allowing the patient to continue to take small amounts of pureed food and thickened fluids using maximum precautions. Placing the patient nil by mouth is occasionally the apparent best option.

Terminal care

Terminal care for patients with dementia follows the same principles as for other conditions. One of the most common causes of death is aspiration pneumonia and treating this with antibiotics has only been shown to extend survival by 7 days.

Medications used in the terminal phase are the following:

Anxiolytics	Haloperidol 1.5 mg sc prn
	Diazepam suppositories 5–10 mg
	Midazolam 2.5–5 mg sc prn
Analgesics	Paracetamol suppositories 1 g every 4 h
	Morphine 2.5 mg sc prn
	Leave analgesic patches in place and continue appropriate prn dose

As people deteriorate and enter the dying phase, care home staff require support to ensure the patient is not admitted to hospital at this point. Staff may have known the patient for months or even years and can often accurately predict that the resident is approaching the end of life but lack confidence that they can continue caring for them in their home. Explaining what is likely to happen to the patient and prescribing anticipatory medications for common symptoms will help provide reassurance to both the staff and family. District nurses may be required if a syringe driver is started and community Macmillan nurses can provide advice if problematic symptoms occur. Daily visits from the GP could prevent crisis admissions, and where appropriate thanking staff for the care they have given or how well they may have dealt with a particularly difficult situation.

Admiral nurses

These are primarily registered mental health nurses specialising in dementia care. They are named after Joseph Levy who had vascular dementia and was known as Admiral Joe because of his love of sailing. His family inspired the creation of Dementia UK.

They offer skilled assessments and provide information and practical advice to family/carers. They work from diagnosis, throughout the journey providing psychological and emotional support, as well as collaborating with other professionals and organisations to coordinate care. Dementia UK provides information about accessing Admiral nurses. Unfortunately, at present they are not available in all regions.

Conclusions

This chapter outlines the difficulties that people with dementia may encounter. The key points are as follows:
- Get involved early while patient's still have the ability to communicate their wishes.
- Consider the use of assessment tools to aid with identifying pain.
- Be aware of the impact on families, the length of time they have spent caring for a loved one, and the difficult decisions they may have to make on their behalf.
- Be aware of experts/agencies that can help.

References

1. Xie J, Brayne C, Matthews FE, et al. Survival times in people with dementia: analysis from population based cohort study with 14 year follow-up. *BMJ* 2008; 336: 258–262.
2. Alzheimer's Disease International. *The prevalence of dementia worldwide.* Available at: www.alz.co.uk/adi/pdf/prevalence.pdf (accessed in July 2011).
3. Mahoney FI and Barthel DW. Functional evaluation: the Barthel Index. *Md State Med J* 1965; 14: 61–65.
4. Livingston G, Leavey G, Manela M, et al. Making decisions for people with dementia who lack capacity: qualitative study of family carers in UK. *BMJ* 2010; 341: c4184. doi:10.1136/bmj.c4184.
5. Lloyd-Williams M. An audit of palliative care in dementia. *Eur J Cancer Care (Engl)* 1996; 5 (1): 53–55.
6. Jordan A, Regnard C, O'Brien J, et al. Pain and distress in advanced dementia: choosing the right tools for the job. *Palliat Med* 2011 (Epub ahead of print).
7. McCarthy M, Addington-Hall J, and Altmann D. The experience of dying with dementia: a retrospective study. *Int J Geriatr Psychiatry* 1997; 12: 404–409.
8. Killick J and Allan K. The arts in dementia care: tapping a rich resource. *J Dementia Care* 1999; 7: 35–38.
9. Light VL, Slezak FA, Porter JA, et al. Predictive factors for early mortality after percutaneous gastrostomy. *Gastrointest Endosc* 1995; 42: 330–335.
10. Royal College of Physicians. *Oral Feeding Difficulties and Dilemmas: A Guide to Practical Care, Particularly Towards the End of Life. Report of a Working Party.* London: Royal College of Physicians, 2010.

Further reading

Hughes J (ed). *Palliative Care in Severe Dementia.* London: Quay Books, 2005.
National Council for Palliative Care. *Out of the Shadows: End of Life Care for People with Dementia.* London: National Council for Palliative Care, 2009.

Useful resources

www.disdat.co.uk DisDAT Tool.
www.dementiauk.org Links to local Admiral Nurses.
www.alzheimers.org.uk Alzheimer's Society in the United Kingdom.
www.alz.org Alzheimer's Society in the United States.
www.alzheimer.ca Alzheimer's Society in Canada.
www.alzheimers.org.au Alzheimer's Society in Australia.

18 Palliative Care in Advanced Heart Disease

Ryan Liebscher, Fraser Black

Victoria Hospice, Victoria, Canada

Introduction

Although death rates due to cardiovascular disease (CVD) have declined in the past decade [1], 1 out of every 2.9 deaths in the United States or 34.3% of all deaths in 2006 were attributed to CVD, which is more than that from cancer, chronic lower respiratory tract disease, and accidents combined [1]. In the United Kingdom in 2009, over 180,000 people died from CVD—one in three of all deaths [2]. There has however also been increased survival, which has resulted in a greater prevalence of chronic heart failure (HF), often resulting in high symptom burden, poor quality of life, and many other challenges related to end-of-life care [3].

This chapter will not only address the common physical symptoms and psychosocial distress that patients with advanced cardiac disease face but also examine the barriers that often limit access to quality symptom management and palliative care for these patients living with advanced cardiac disease.

HF, often referred to as congestive heart failure (CHF), is the only cardiac condition with increasing prevalence. This is as a result of an aging population, improvements in prolonging survival in patients suffering coronary events, and improvements in preventing secondary cardiac events [4]. All of these events result in more people suffering with HF and dying from it rather than for some what was a sudden death due to an acute cardiac event. The estimated direct and indirect cost of HF in the United States for 2010 is $39.2 billion [1].

Patients with HF have a similar symptom burden to those with malignant disease yet relatively few HF patients receive palliative care [3,5]. Interestingly, as has been seen with patients with some cancer diagnoses, a retrospective cohort study showed that end-stage HF patients had improved survival when using hospice services compared with not having received those services [6], but a minority of people with HF receive such services [7,8].

Heart failure

HF is a chronic progressive syndrome usually associated with a structural abnormality of the heart with compensatory haemodynamic, inflammatory, and neurohormonal changes. These result in typical symptoms and signs of fatigue, breathlessness, exercise intolerance, and fluid retention [9]. There is no cure. HF is most commonly a consequence of hypertension, coronary artery disease (CAD), valve abnormality, diabetes, or cardiomyopathy. The severity of HF is useful to classify, such as described by the New York Heart Association (NYHA) (Table 18.1) [10].

Almost 6 million Americans are currently diagnosed with HF and, in 2006, 1 out of every 8.6 death certificates mentioned HF [1]. The prevalence of HF rises steeply with age. At 40 years of age, the lifetime risk of developing HF is 1 in 5 [1]. The prevalence of HF in 70- to 80-year olds is 10–20%, with the mean age of persons with HF in the developed world being 75 years [4].

Acute HF is the most common cause of hospitalisation in those over 65 years of age in the United States, Europe, New Zealand, and Australia [11], and it accounts for 10% of patients in hospital beds [4]. In developed countries, the mean age of patients admitted to hospital

---

Table 18.1 New York Heart Association (NYHA) classification of heart failure severity.

NYHA class	Description
1	No limitation in physical activity. Ordinary physical activity does not cause undue fatigue, palpitation, or dyspnoea
2	Slight limitation of physical activity. Comfortable at rest, but ordinary physical activity results in fatigue, palpitation, or dyspnoea
3	Marked limitation of physical activity. Comfortable at rest, but less than ordinary activity causes fatigue, palpitation, or dyspnoea
4	Unable to carry out any physical activity without discomfort. Symptoms of cardiac insufficiency at rest. If any physical activity is undertaken, discomfort is increased

Source: Reproduced from Reference 10.

with HF is 76 years and elderly patients with HF often have multiple comorbid conditions, including diabetes, renal failure, chronic obstructive pulmonary disease (COPD), depression, anaemia, and cognitive impairment [3,12]. The advanced age and complex medical problems faced by this population with HF contribute to their unpredictable disease trajectory and prognosis.

Prognosis and prognostic models

The trajectory of HF (Figure 18.1) can be quite variable but typically includes a slow progressive overall decline accompanied by a gradual worsening of dyspnoea, fatigue, and function with a decreased quality of life. With time, patients will experience exacerbations of acute HF and the frequency of cardiac decompensation increases with a need for more hospitalisations and further decline in quality of life. Families and patients grow accustomed to this course of illness and often do not foresee dying, thus, patients frequently die in an acute facility [13].

HF is associated with a poor but generally uncertain prognosis. Fifty percent of patients diagnosed with HF die within 4 years and 40% of those admitted with HF die or are readmitted within 1 year [4]. Further, sudden cardiac death occurs in approximately half of all deaths in patients with HF [4]. The variable trajectory coupled with high rates of sudden unpredictable cardiac death makes prognostication very difficult [1].

Accurate prognostication can aid clinical decision-making and help patients and families with expectations and advance care planning (ACP) [14]. Multiple studies have shown many factors to have some predictive value. The practical use of these models for individuals, however, is limited and they are infrequently used in clinical practice [15].

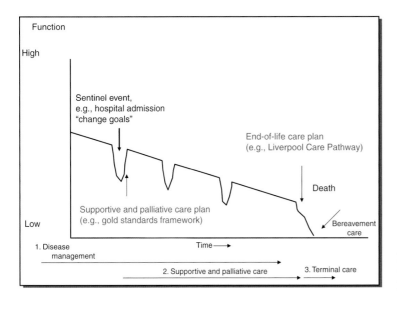

Figure 18.1 Model of heart failure trajectory. (Reproduced from Reference 14.)

Clinical factors shown to predict increased mortality are as follows [16]:

- Frequent emergency visits or hospitalisations
- Symptoms at rest (NYHA class 4)
- Dependency with activities of daily living
- >10% nonfluid weight loss
- Symptomatic arrhythmias
- Low systolic blood pressure
- Ejection fraction <20%
- Peripheral arterial disease
- Prior cardiopulmonary resuscitation (CPR)
- Syncope
- Embolic stroke

Laboratory measures shown to be prognostic include albumin <2.5 g/dL, elevated growth differentiation factor-15 [17], low sodium, anaemia [18], increased blood urea nitrogen (BUN) [16], circulating cardiac troponin levels [19], and persistent elevation in BNP [20].

These factors individually have limited utility, however, and this information has led to the creation of many prognostic models for HF. Some examples include the Heart Failure Survival Score used for those being selected for cardiac transplantation [21] and the Seattle Heart Failure Score that can be accessed on the Internet (http://depts.washington.edu/shfm/) as an online calculator to predict mortality at 1, 2, and 5 years [22].

Box 18.1 lists the elements of a validated risk score for determining in-hospital mortality, independent of left ventricular systolic function [15].

These easy to obtain parameters on hospital admission may be useful to risk stratify patients and may encourage necessary discussions around advanced directives (advanced decisions) and end-of-life care if the patient is at increased risk of dying.

An alternative approach in the elderly is advocated by Jaarsma et al.: irreversible decline indicated by progressive renal dysfunction, cardiac cachexia, and intractable NYHA class 4 symptoms with escalating diuretic doses [3]. At the very least, these features should prompt a discussion and a transition to a more palliative approach.

Interventional aspects of care

Specialist cardiac care may coordinate additional interventions that can be considered.

Automatic implantable cardioverter defibrillators (AICDs) are increasingly being used and have been shown to decrease sudden cardiac death and improve symptoms and quality of life [23]. In the United States, over 10,000 devices are implanted per month [24]. All of these patients will at some point become critically ill and the burdens of these therapies will outweigh the benefits. Patients may not understand that their AICD can be deactivated and may have concerns and misunderstandings regarding deactivation and its consequences and benefits. If in advanced disease, quality of life is no longer acceptable to the patient and goals of care no longer include life prolongation, AICDs must be reprogrammed and inactivated to prevent painful, repeated firing of unwanted shocks near death. This is usually done by a cardiologist or one of their team members and ideally this is preplanned between the patient and their health-care provider during a discussion regarding goals of care. Often a cardiac resynchronisation device or pacemaker that may accompany the AICD will be continued for palliation to avoid symptomatic deterioration. It is very important to tell patients with AICDs that deactivation itself is not painful nor will it result in immediate death. AICD reprogramming should be considered in those who request it, those who are near to death, those who have a do not resuscitate (DNR) order in place, and in whom sudden death would be welcome [3]. If the AICD is not able to be reprogrammed and death is imminent, a large magnet may be held over the device to prevent painful shocks; surgical removal is not recommended [24]. Fortunately, it is now recommended that device deactivation be discussed with patients before its implantation [24].

Inotropes may be used as a bridge to heart transplant or for intermittent or chronic use. There is no survival benefit with inotropes and, in fact, they are quite costly and are associated with high mortality, but, may improve symptoms [25]. They have a class 2B indication by the American College of Cardiology/American Heart Association given that there is no survival benefit [25].

Heart transplant and left ventricular assist devices are interventions infrequently available at present but provide

---

Box 18.1 Elements of a validated risk score for determining in-hospital mortality

Presence of advanced age
Elevated BUN
Low systolic blood pressure
Elevated heart rate
Low serum sodium
Presence of COPD
Being of a non-black race

Source: Reproduced from Reference 15.

both palliation of symptoms and extension of life for some. Heart transplants are limited to otherwise healthy individuals and only 5,000 or so occur each year [3]. A left ventricular assist device is a battery-operated blood pump that is implanted into either ventricle to decrease the workload of the struggling ventricle. They provide mechanical circulatory support and can serve as a bridge to transplant or used on a long-term basis but are costly and available to very few at present. Ethical dilemmas exist and invariably there will be a tension between measures seen by some to be more aggressive than palliative. Further discussion on these topics is beyond the discussion of this chapter.

Barriers/challenges in extending palliative care to patients with HF

People living with HF have multiple palliative care needs with a high symptom burden, spiritual, social, and psychological distress resulting in a poor quality of life for many [5,26,27]. However, because prognostication in these patients is very difficult, clinicians may be hesitant to discuss palliative care services with patients, refer to palliative care services or apply for benefits such as the Medicare Hospice Benefit (a 6-month prognosis criterion), or complete a "DS1500" form in the United Kingdom (which triggers prompt assessment of benefit entitlement). This is especially so in countries where an "either-or" approach is mandated and palliative care services are not to be accessed in parallel with more curative approaches. To restrict palliative care services based on prognosis alone can result in important needs not being met for a significant period of time. Palliative care as a philosophy should be integrated into the various stages of HF management based on individual need and not reserved for those actively dying.

A recent retrospective case comparison study of hospice use in HF and cancer patients in the United States showed that those persons with HF were found to receive longer periods of hospice care than may be allowed for in funding systems or service criterion. Over 7% of persons with HF utilised hospice services greater than 6 months and 19% of those receiving services were discharged from hospice care with some clinical stability. HF patients were much older than those persons with cancer (more than 75% of patients were over the age of 80) and those with HF were more likely to reside in long-term care facilities [8].

The prognostic uncertainty in HF can prevent effective ACP [14]. Patients and families often have unrealistic expectations as to survival, prognosis, and benefits of CPR and have little insight into the severity of their disease [3,28]. Clinicians have difficulty anticipating the terminal phase of HF [3] and may, therefore, not appreciate the futility or appropriateness of interventions and continue the use of aggressive acute therapies when a palliative approach may be more prudent. The curative focus typically taken with HF can delay or prevent end-of-life conversations as well as a transition to a palliative approach [5].

Further, there may be a lack of physician communication skills and confidence to discuss prognosis, dying, and end-of-life care [3,29]. Clinicians often fear taking away hope [14,29], and there is a lack of knowledge of when to refer to palliative care [29] and as to the meaning of palliative care [30]. Perhaps, compounding this is that research outcomes have focused on mortality benefits to medications and interventions and less so on quality of life measures.

Another barrier to the delivery of good palliative care to patients with HF is that there is little evidence as to the best model of care [26]. This elderly population often has multiple medical comorbidities and accesses multiple providers of care, and the ability of primary care alone to manage and coordinate all their complex issues may be compromised due to a lack of professional time and resources [13,14].

Case Study

BB is a 94-year-old female who lives alone with minimal home supports in a two-storey house with three supportive adult children in town. She has NYHA class 4 HF, hypertension, CAD with previous coronary artery bypass graft (CABG), pulmonary hypertension, atrial fibrillation and sick sinus syndrome with pacemaker placement earlier in the year, severe aortic stenosis, osteoporosis with recent T12 compression fracture, chronic kidney disease (CKD) with baseline glomerular filtration rate (GFR) of 40 ml/min, and recurrent urinary tract infections. She has been followed closely by her primary care family physician who has been coordinating her cardiac care. He has been working closely with a home care nurse in the community to optimise BB's condition and quality of life. With the recognition of recurrent hospital admissions, increased dyspnoea at rest and decreased quality of life and function with a palliative performance scale (PPS) of 40%, BB's physician discussed with BB and her family the benefits of registering her with the hospice/palliative care team.

Palliative care delivery in HF

Proposed models of care for HF often involve the integration of active treatment and life-prolonging therapies along with palliative therapies because of the unpredictable end-of-life phase and significant palliative care needs of patients with HD [14,31,32]. Indeed, many active treatments are good palliative treatments but the benefits and burdens will vary with the individual and their stage of HF. The degree of palliative intervention and decisions about who would provide that care would depend on the severity of disease, frequency of exacerbations, symptom burden, and patient goals of care. Boyd et al. developed a HF care framework based on perspectives from patients, caregivers, and clinicians with key stages and services to help in providing the best coordinated care that recognises and manages stage-specific needs [14]. They emphasise that services be coordinated by a key health-care professional in the community using an integrated approach to care planning that considers the unique challenges of HF and not base services on what they call "restrictive prognostic judgements" (Table 18.2) [14]. Primary care clinicians can provide the majority of palliative care in HF with the support of palliative and cardiology services to provide best comprehensive care as necessary [32]. To assist the primary care physician, "trigger points" have been identified to prompt a transition to a more palliative approach (Table 18.3) [3].

Major national heart associations are providing recommendations to address some of the palliative care needs of these patients. The HF Association of the European Society of Cardiology issued a position statement and recommendations (Table 18.4) in 2009 to increase the awareness of the need of palliative care for patients with HF [3]. The goal was to improve accessibility and quality of palliative care services to this population while promoting the development of HF-orientated palliative care services across Europe [3]. The 2010 HF Society of America guidelines emphasise early communication with patients and families regarding prognosis and ACP at end of life and readdressing changing preferences. They recommend that:

> Patients with HF receiving end-of-life care should be considered for enrollment in hospice (ie. referral to palliative care) that can be delivered in the home, a nursing home, or a special hospice unit [28].

Canadian Cardiovascular Society 2006 Heart Failure Guidelines recommend early discussions with prognosis, substitute decision making, advanced directives and goals of care to be reviewed regularly. They suggest a need to balance quality and quantity of life, that palliative care consultation be considered, and emphasise the need to address psychosocial and family/caregiver issues [33].

Case continued

BB was admitted to the hospice/palliative care unit from home 1 month later with severe dyspnoea, poor appetite, mild confusion, and probable support for death. She presented with a respiratory rate of 36, gross peripheral oedema, ascites, and pulmonary oedema, recent weight gain of 9 kilos, and a PPS of 30%. BB had already established with her family physician a preference not to be resuscitated with CPR. BB's goals expressed on admission included management of dyspnoea and pain and if possible to treat any reversible contributors to her decline if minimally invasive, in hopes she would survive the exacerbation and possibly return home. The palliative care team discussed the guarded prognosis with BB and her three daughters.

Symptom management

Patients with HF have a symptom burden similar to those with malignant disease. To ensure good palliation of symptoms and best patient care, a systematic symptom assessment should be performed. Special attention should be given to patient preferences and goals of care.

Optimal HF management combines both symptom- and disease-modifying therapies and as patient goals of care change, the benefits of some medications will need to be revisited. Many patients with HF have refractory symptoms such as pain, dyspnoea, fatigue, cough, nausea, limited mobility, falls, depression, anxiety, insomnia, constipation, and loss of appetite [3,7,26]. In the community, these persons experience a loss of independence with increased dependence on others [26]. The management of symptoms should consider patient goals and preferences, subjective experience, and disease-specific factors such as available and appropriate therapies, performance status, and prognosis.

Dyspnoea

Dyspnoea is the most common reason for patients with HF to seek medical attention and hospital admission

Table 18.2 A framework for coordinated care of people with heart failure.

Stage 1: Chronic disease management phase: (NYHA Classes I–III)
- *Performance status*: good; no advanced comorbidities.[a]
- *Goals of care*: active monitoring, evidence-based treatment to prolong survival, symptom control, patient and carer education, supported self-management.
- *Information*: name of condition and what that means, course of the illness/treatment.
- *Primary care team*: coordinates regular monitoring and review using local protocols derived from national guidelines; practice register/database for chronic illness triggers and monitors service provision.
- *Hospital specialists (cardiologists and/or geriatricians)*: diagnostic review, assessment and specialist treatment/advice for complex cases; specialist support to primary care team.
- *Heart failure nurse specialists*: short-term interventions to aid patient self-management; support, advice and education for the primary care team.

Stage 2: Supportive and palliative care phase: (NYHA Classes III–IV)
- *Performance status*: deteriorating due to heart failure and/or advanced comorbidities; disease specific prognostic indicators used as an aid to professional judgement.[b]
- *Goals of care*: tertiary prevention; maintaining optimal symptom control and quality of life.
- Information: discuss changing condition, goals and preferences for future care; anticipatory care planning with patient and family.
- *Primary care team*: move patient to Supportive Palliative Care register; identify a key professional; ensure regular holistic, multidisciplinary assessment of patient and carer health and social care needs; treatment and medication review in consultation with hospital specialists; plan for acute crises including liaison with out-of-hours services.
- *Hospital specialists*: assessment and specialist treatment review for complex cases; specialist support to primary care team; planned admission and rapid triage if hospital inpatient or outpatient care needed; coordinated discharge planning.
- *Heart failure nurse specialists*: specialist advice to primary care team on heart failure medicines management and monitoring; hospital/community liaison for patients needing secondary care.
- *Palliative care specialists*: support for primary care team and hospital specialists; specialist advice or short term interventions for symptom control, complex communication and advance care planning.

Stage 3: Terminal care phase: (NYHA Class IV)[c]
- *Performance status*: frail and largely bedbound despite maximal therapy; no reversible problems, or life threatening co-morbidity. Dying period may range from days to weeks; clinical indicators: renal impairment, hypotension/tachycardia, persistent oedema, anaemia, hyponatremia.
- *Primary care team*: coordinate comprehensive health and social care package for patients who remain at home; plan for management of acute deteriorations; clarify resuscitation status; withdraw medication not for symptom control; carer support including bereavement care.
- *Hospital specialists/specialist nurses*: advice/management of treatment withdrawal (e.g., defibrillators); optimise end-of-life care of patients dying in hospital (integrated care pathway).
- *Palliative care specialists*: advice and support for end-of-life care in hospital and community; advice on complex symptom control in end-stage organ failure.

Source: Reproduced from Reference 14.
[a]WHO performance status 0/1 or modified Karnofsky performance status 80–100.
[b]WHO performance status 2/3 or modified Karnofsky performance status 50–70.
[c]WHO performance status 4 or modified Karnofsky performance status 40 or less.

Table 18.3 Trigger points for palliative transition.

- Recurrent episodes of decompensation within 6 months despite optimal therapy
- Occurrence of malignant arrhythmias
- Need for frequent or continual intravenous therapies
- Chronic poor quality of life
- Intractable NYHA class 4 symptoms
- Signs of cardiac cachexia (e.g., body wasting)

Source: Reproduced from Reference 14.

[34]. Compared with primary or metastatic lung cancer, persons with HF and other noncancer causes of dyspnoea have significantly higher levels of dyspnoea in the last 3 months of life, which remains relatively constant until death [35].

Management includes searching for and treating reversible causes (if this aligns with the patient's goals of care) including anaemia, infection, dysrhythmias, pulmonary embolism, comorbid pulmonary disease, and decompensated HF while ensuring good symptom control as will be discussed next.

In the management of pulmonary oedema, good evidence exists for the use of diuretics, long-acting nitroglycerin formulations, and hydralazine to give some relief, but sometimes, in end-stage disease, the use of these medications is limited by symptomatic hypotension [25]. There is some evidence for the use of hawthorn berry extract for symptomatic relief in HF [36]. Optimal management must include excellent palliation of dyspnoea regardless of cause.

Nonpharmacological palliating strategies for dyspnoea may include salt and water restriction in HF (depending on patient preferences), raising the head of bed, providing a fan to the facial area, breathing training and exercise programmes, and anxiety management [37]. Oxygen may be useful if hypoxemic. A recent randomised controlled trial of palliative oxygen versus room air via nasal cannula for breathlessness in patients with refractory dyspnoea without hypoxia, however, showed no additional benefit with oxygen [38]. However, only a small proportion of these patients had cardiac disease and a trial

Table 18.4 Recommendations from the palliative care workshop of the Heart Failure Association of the European Society of Cardiology.

- The expected or anticipated course of the illness, final treatment options, treatment preferences, living wills, and advanced directives should be discussed with patients and their families at an early stage of disease.
- Goals of care should be evaluated repeatedly during disease progression, anticipating that patients may frequently want to modify their decisions.
- Close to the end of life, any life-prolonging treatment not contributing to symptom control should be carefully evaluated and possibly withdrawn and additional palliative care measures introduced as appropriate.
- Patients should understand that withdrawal of previously applicable conventional treatment does not mean withdrawal of care.
- Discussion with patients and families should focus on what will be provided rather than what will be discontinued.
- Optimal coordination and continuity of care for those patients who are often readmitted under a variety of medical specialties or who are unable to visit the outpatient department. Collaboration with primary care services is vital.
- Patient education should be regularly reinforced.
- Communication skills should be included in staff training.
- Joint educational opportunities should be available for heart failure (HF) and palliative care professionals (CPs) working with advanced HF patients.
- Cardiac palliative care should be incorporated in the postgraduate palliative care training of general practitioners (GPs).
- Treatment coordination for advanced HF patients is essential to help reduce the risk of care fragmentation and potential conflicts commonly encountered when many health professionals and multiple agencies are involved.
- Further research is required to assess how patients needing a palliative care approach can best be identified and how that care can best be planned and coordinated throughout their illness.
- Further research is needed to determine optimal treatment strategies and care models for end-stage HF patients across the whole spectrum of those affected from young individuals to the elderly with comorbidity.
- Research gaps in pharmacological and nonpharmacological treatment of symptoms have been identified and should be addressed.

Source: Reproduced from Reference 3.

of oxygen therapy may be considered on an individual basis.

Pharmacological management includes optimising cardiac medications, especially diuretics and transdermal or sublingual nitrates [25]. Furosemide may be administered subcutaneously [39] in the home or hospice to control congestive symptoms. The use of opioids, however, is the cornerstone of prompt palliation of dyspnoea; there is convincing evidence that morphine is safe and has been used with benefit for dyspnoea in HF and other causes [25,40,41]. Although evidence is lacking, anxiolytics such as short- or medium-acting benzodiazepines may be tried if panic or anxiety is associated with dyspnoea. Drainage of pleural effusion is rarely necessary in the setting of HF.

Case continued

On admission, BB's heart rate was 78/min, blood pressure 112/72 mmHg, oxygen saturation was 94% on 4 L of oxygen with a respiratory rate of 36/min, and she had a temperature of 36.5°C. Auscultation of her lungs revealed bilateral crepitations and she had ascites and significant peripheral oedema. Her cardiac medications included clopidogrel 75 mg, bisoprolol 2.5 mg od, furosemide 80 mg bid, spironolactone 50 mg od, and nifedipine XL 30 mg od. She stated she was "allergic" to morphine and was on no regular opioids or nitrates. Her electrolytes were in the normal range, GFR was 41 ml/min, cardiac troponins were negative, and she was diagnosed with an exacerbation of her HF, cause not determined.

Acutely, BB received high-dose parenteral furosemide and sublingual nitroglycerin. She was also administered hydromorphone 0.25 mg subcutaneously every 4 h and as needed for dyspnoea and a dose of lorazepam 0.5 mg sublingually for panic associated with her dyspnoea. She continued with oxygen at 4 L via nasal prongs for the first 24 h. A Foley catheter was placed *in situ* as accepted by BB for expected diuresis.

The following day her spironolactone was increased to 100 mg od, metolazone 5 mg od was added, and nifedipine was discontinued. Her furosemide was continued at 80 mg po bid. After 24 h, BB no longer required the hydromorphone regularly but used it for dyspnoea only on a PRN basis.

BB continued to improve and after 8 days she had lost 10 kg and her peripheral oedema and ascites had significantly decreased. Her electrolytes and GFR remained within normal range. Metolazone was discontinued to prevent overdiuresis. Physical and occupational therapists worked with BB to optimise her mobility and her PPS improved to

40% but she remained deconditioned. The geriatric team also assessed BB.

She developed a symptomatic urinary tract infection and opted for antibiotic treatment.

Pain

Pain has a significant impact on quality of life and occurs in about 60% of those with end-stage heart disease [34]. It may be caused by angina, peripheral vascular disease, gout, diabetic peripheral neuropathy, or musculoskeletal and other comorbidities [34]. One should attempt to treat the underlying cause and nonpharmacological, physical, or psychological strategies may be attempted. Often in the management of advanced stage disease, however, pain is best palliated with analgesics.

Colchicine and low-dose steroids (use cautiously watching for fluid retention) are beneficial for the treatment of gout. For angina, ensure that cardiac medications such as nitrates, beta-blockers, and calcium channel blockers are optimised; coronary revascularisation may be considered in those with refractory symptoms in well-selected patients. Tricyclic antidepressants (TCAs) and gabapentinoids may be useful for peripheral neuropathy although TCAs should be used with caution as they may prolong the QT interval leading to tachyarrhythmias. Calcitonin or bisphosphonates [42,43] may be considered for acute compression fractures.

In general, it is best to start with the WHO analgesic ladder (see Chapter 9, *Pain and Its Management*) with paracetamol (acetaminophen) first line for mild pain; one should generally avoid nonsteroidal anti-inflammatory drugs (NSAIDs) in this population because of fluid retention and renal toxicity. Opioids are tolerated well and do not cause end organ damage and for moderate or severe pain, these are considered first line [25]. Doses should consider comorbid renal or hepatic impairment. Opioids should be used for refractory angina pectoris and peripheral vascular disease. In advanced renal failure, opioids with active metabolites such as morphine and codeine should be avoided [44]. Methadone is safe in renal failure, may have further benefit in neuropathic pain, and is well tolerated. However, it can have unpredictable pharmacokinetics, may prolong the QT interval at high doses, and specific drug–drug interactions should be considered [45]. If a patient is overburdened by a significant number of pills, the use of a transdermal opioid such as a fentanyl patch can be useful for dyspnoea or pain once opioid needs have been established and titrated to effect. All regular opioids should be accompanied by an "as needed" breakthrough dose for uncontrolled pain and a laxative to prevent constipation.

Case continued

During her admission, BB also complained of back pain at the location of her recent T12 compression fracture. She was initially treated with 1,000 mg of paracetamol (acetaminophen) regularly but with minimal benefit. Intranasal calcitonin and oral methadone 0.5 mg tid were then started for this pain and the methadone was increased to 1 mg tid with good analgesic effect and tolerated well. Senokot was started regularly to prevent constipation. After 1 month and shortly before her discharge, the calcitonin and methadone were titrated down and discontinued without loss of analgesia.

Fatigue

The management of fatigue should include an attempt to identify reversible causes such as anaemia, infection, obstructive sleep apnoea, electrolyte abnormalities, and renal failure. One should exclude depression, thyroid abnormalities, and psychosocial contributors and ensure the optimal treatment of HF. Exercise training programmes may have a role for persistent fatigue [13,25] depending on patient performance status and safety. A recent randomised controlled trial showed that a nurse-coordinated multidisciplinary HF cardiac rehabilitation programme significantly improved exercise tolerance and functional status in addition to improved quality of life measures and decreased hospital readmission rates [46]. Educating patients on how to time their activities to periods of peak energy may be useful. There is evidence for the use of stimulants such as methylphenidate for cancer-related fatigue [47] but no such evidence in HF patients exists. It may be reasonable to consider these therapies but important to be mindful of potential adverse effects such as an increased heart rate and blood pressure.

Anaemia

The prevalence of anaemia in HF patients depends on the severity but can affect up to 50% [48]. It is associated with poor outcomes and most commonly is attributed to renal dysfunction, nutritional deficiencies, anaemia of chronic disease, haemodilution, decreased erythropoietin (EPO) levels, or resistance to EPO in the bone marrow and medications [48]. Anaemia not only causes the symptom

burden of breathlessness and fatigue, but can also worsen HF itself, the cardiorenal anaemia syndrome [48]. One should treat iron and B_{12} deficiencies if found. There is now some evidence that intravenous (IV) iron and EPO therapy can improve NYHA functional class [49]. Three small studies have shown IV iron to improve cardiac function, exercise capacity, and quality of life with an acceptable side effect profile [48,50]. A Cochrane review on erythropoiesis-stimulating agents for anaemia in HF showed improvement in anaemia, NYHA class and exercise tolerance, decreased hospitalisations and symptoms, and has benefits on quality of life [51]. Additional, larger studies are needed but so far no increase in adverse events or mortality has been found. This is in contrast to prior studies in those with CKD which showed these therapies were associated with an increase in mortality, arteriovenous thrombosis, and hypertension [48]. Large studies to assess the benefits and safety of EPO therapy are ongoing [49]. Blood transfusions may provide temporary relief in specific cases but are associated with risks, especially fluid overload in this population [49]. These interventions are included here more for completeness than as a recommendation, because they are not yet the standard of care and one must seriously weigh the risks and benefits to ensure quality of life is not compromised by being overly aggressive. As with all palliative therapeutic strategies, one must consider patient goals and potential benefits and risks of therapy.

Oedema/ascites

The management of oedema requires excellent skin care to prevent pressure and other skin ulcers and cellulitis. Compression stockings may be useful and raising legs when not mobilising will give symptomatic relief. Optimal management of HF is necessary and discontinuing medications associated with fluid retention such as dihydropyridine calcium channel blockers, thiozolidinediones, NSAIDs, steroids, and others may help. Optimal dosing of diuretics considering electrolyte balance depending on goals and prognosis is the mainstay of medication management. Similarly, ascites secondary to right-sided HF is best managed with diuretics; paracentesis could be considered rarely if refractory [25].

Psychological/psychosocial

Depression is very common among HF patients, especially those with many comorbid conditions [3]. Depression occurs in 21–36% of patients with HF [25], the frequency of which correlates with HF severity. It is associated with decreased quality of life, hospital admission, higher mortality, and increased economic cost [3,25,52–54]. Self-rated depression using the Beck Depression Inventory is independently associated with higher long-term mortality in HF patients [53]. Given the high prevalence and burden, it is recommended that HF patients should be screened for depression [55].

Treatment of depression must be holistic, addressing physical, psychological, spiritual, and social needs. People with HF at the end of life face social isolation, hopelessness, significant frustration, challenges of working with the formal health-care system, life disruption, high symptom burden, and uncertainty about prognosis and symptoms [26,56]. Social and psychological decline has been shown to follow physical decline and those persons with worse physical symptoms also have more spiritual distress [19]. Spiritual contentment affects depression in HF patients [3,57], with greater spiritual well-being associated with less depression [57].

In patients with CAD, interventions such as cardiac rehabilitation, stress management, education, music therapy, psychosocial counselling, and exercise have had positive effects on depression [55]. At present, there are no randomised controlled trials on psychological interventions for depression and HF [58].

Selective serotonin reuptake inhibitors (SSRIs) are recommended first line as pharmacological agents for depression [55]. Although only a few studies have been done, the use of SSRIs has been shown to improve quality of life but effects on mortality and hospitalisations are not known [55]. However, the recently published and long awaited double-blind randomised controlled trial of sertraline versus placebo in depressed HF patients showed safety of treatment but did not show any difference in the reduction in depression or improvement in cardiovascular status [59]. Interestingly, both groups had very high response rates, perhaps attesting to the benefits from the extensive nursing involvement; this population has increased support needs that can respond to supportive care. Antidepressant use in HF patients is associated with an increased mortality, lower doses of beta-blockers, and increased class of HF [60]. It is recommended not to avoid beta-blockers in this population as there is no evidence these agents worsen depressive symptoms [55].

Further, it is important not to forget the challenges that caregivers experience. Many caregivers of elderly patients with HF are themselves elderly and often experience poor health. These caregivers have high rates of depression, relationship strain, social isolation, and need for increased supports [61].

Case continued

BB declined transfer to a rehabilitation unit for a preference to return home as soon as possible in spite of risks that she would not regain her mobility and be mostly limited to her bed. She accepted the risks and wanted to spend the last chapter of her life in the comfort of her own home. BB and her daughters met with spiritual care and a counsellor for life review and discussions about goals and care preferences.

She was discharged home with excellent symptom control at rest. She remained fatigued but focused what energy she had on her most important tasks. She was screened for depression but her mood remained stable in spite of recognising her uncertain prognosis. She continued with a PPS of 40% and was unable to descend her stairs with the urinary catheter left *in situ*, which was acceptable to her. After being discharged, she was followed closely by her home care nurse and family physician, and in the event of exacerbation, instructed to follow-up with the palliative care community response team if after hours. As part of her advanced care planning, she stated a preference for death at home.

Discontinuing medical therapies

Beta-blockers, ACEI, and aldosterone antagonists have all been shown to improve symptoms, decrease hospitalisations, and decrease mortality in advanced HF [37]. Digoxin decreases hospitalisations and may improve symptoms but has not been shown to affect survival [37].

As the patient transitions to a more palliative stage and approach, however, the merits of some medications, side effects, and the burdens of polypharmacy should be considered. Symptomatic hypotension may warrant discontinuing beta-blockers and angiotensin-converting enzyme (ACE) inhibiting or angiotensin receptor blocking (ARB) medications. Refractory fluid overload or symptomatic bradycardia may benefit from discontinuing or decreasing beta-blockers. Kidney failure may limit the use of angiotensin-converting enzyme inhibitor (ACEI) or ARBs, aldosterone antagonists, and affect digoxin and diuretic doses. As a transition to a more palliative approach is taken, one must weigh the risks and benefits of what medications are continued and for what benefit. Indeed, some patients are all too happy at this point to minimise medications and anecdotally often feel better on minimal therapies.

End-of-life care

It is of the utmost importance that physicians discuss advanced directives (advance decisions) and care planning with their patients, including DNR orders and deactivation of AICDs when the time is appropriate. This discussion is best carried out in an outpatient setting rather than during an acute exacerbation in the emergency department. Studies show that HF patients often prefer resuscitation and are ten times less likely to have a DNR order compared to those with cancer [37].

In the SUPPORT, only 23% of advanced HF patients admitted for an exacerbation of HF stated they did not want to be resuscitated and only 25% reported having discussed resuscitation/preferences with their physicians. Interestingly, the physician perception of preference disagreed with actual patient preference in 24% of cases. Significant correlates of not wanting to be resuscitated included older age, perception of a worse prognosis, poorer functional status, and higher income [62]. Physicians are not obliged to provide a futile intervention but clear discussions should occur around advanced directives (advance decisions) and resuscitation status with realistic expectations. The health-care team can assist or obstruct the transition between an aggressive and palliative approach. HF patients may wish to die at home or hospice although this is not often the case [7] and this requires recognition of the terminal phase.

When death is imminent and comfort is the primary goal, a reassessment of symptom burden, psychosocial, informational, and other needs must be done. Opioids with or without benzodiazepines via subcutaneous (SC) route of administration for dyspnoea are used. Medications must be re-evaluated and patients may benefit from admission to hospice or palliative care unit if home is unmanageable for symptomatic or psychosocial reasons. Grief and bereavement support for families is a necessity.

Case conclusion

The palliative care team did not hear from BB for 2 months time and called to find she was as stable as in her discharge, with good symptom control and acceptable quality of life and was planning for Christmas. Her family physician and home care nurse had been seeing to her needs. She managed living for a number of additional months with daily visits from her daughters and received twice daily home support help. She slowly deteriorated with a PPS of 30% and then found her quality of life to become strained beyond her

wishes and expressed a desire to discontinue all life-prolonging therapies. She was well supported by her family, primary care physician, and home care nurse. She continued on her diuretics and was placed on regular hydromorphone at low doses with titration to effect for relief of dyspnoea and started on a bowel protocol. Lorazepam 0.5 mg was used for panic and anxiety and haloperidol 1 mg used twice daily for hypoactive delirium. She declined over the following weeks and utilised the support of the palliative response team who assisted with a change of medication administration to SC route, titration of doses to comfort, and provided glycopyrrolate subcutaneously at a PPS of 10% for the treatment and relief of upper respiratory secretions. The three daughters had gathered around their mother for her last weeks and received grief and bereavement counselling.

Conclusion

The prevalence of HF patients is increasing and so are their symptom, caregiver, informational, social, psychological, and spiritual needs. Earlier identification of these palliative care needs will help bring improved quality of life to this growing population. Primary care physicians will provide or coordinate the majority of palliative care services for these patients with consultation as necessary. Recommendations for hospital-based clinical practice to meet the needs of chronic HF patients include improving methods of providing information to patients, introducing protocols for cardiology and palliative care staff, and providing training and education to enhance cardiologists' palliative care skills and palliative care physicians' abilities to manage advanced HF [29]. There is a need for the development of specific HF care pathways with mutually determined referral criteria [29]. Discussions with patients and families about the anticipated course of the disease, prognostic uncertainty, goals of care, and advanced directives (advance decisions) including preference for resuscitation orders and place of death need to be revisited along the trajectory. Recognition of end-stage disease is crucial to meet patient goals and optimise care, but palliative care is not simply "terminal care" in this population and should be introduced earlier along with active care depending on identified needs. A patient and family-centred multidisciplinary approach with improved integration and communication between primary, palliative, and cardiology care will likely serve patients best.

Aside from the clinical management of these patients, further research must be done to better define when to transition to a more palliative approach and how to implement effective models of care delivery. There must be education and training of health-care professionals in end-of-life planning and care and the development of evidence-based guidelines and standards of care. It has been suggested to identify and measure key, well-defined performance indicators to guide evidence-based care and assess quality of care [7]. There is a need to increase resources, accessibility, and better support community-based palliative care delivery and end-of-life care for HF patients and their families [7]. HF patients are no less deserving of good palliative care and with the initiatives, increased research, and direction of care noted above these patients will surely see more benefit in the near future.

References

1. Lloyd-Jones D, Adams RJ, Brown TM, et al. Heart disease and stroke statistics—2010 update. A report from the American Heart Association. *Circulation* 2010; 121(7): 948–954.

2. British Heart Foundation Statistics Database. Available at: www.heartstats.org (accessed on: October, 2010).

3. Jaarsma T, Beattie JM, Ryder M, et al. Palliative care in heart failure: a position statement from the palliative care workshop of the Heart Failure Association of the European Society of Cardiology. *Eur J Heart Fail* 2009; 11: 433–443.

4. Dickstein K, Cohen-Solal A, Fillippatos G, et al. ESC Guidelines for the diagnosis and treatment of acute and chronic heart failure 2008. *Eur J Heart Fail* 2008; 10: 933–989.

5. O'Leary N, Murphy NF, O'Loughlin C, et al. A comparative study of the palliative care needs of heart failure and cancer patients. *Eur J Heart Fail* 2009; 11: 406–412.

6. Connor SR, Pyenson B, Fitch K, et al. Comparing hospice and non hospice patient survival among patients who die within a three year window. *J Pain Symptom Manage* 2007; 33: 238–246.

7. Howlett J, Morin L, Fortin M, et al. End of life planning in heart failure: it should be the end of the beginning. *Can J Cardiol* 2010; 26(3): 135–141.

8. Bain KT, Maxwell TL, Strassels SA, et al. Hospice use among patients with heart failure. *Am Heart J* 2009; 158: 118–125.

9. Krum H and Abraham WT. Heart failure. *Lancet* 2009; 373: 941–955.

10. The Criteria Committee of the New York Heart Association. *Nomenclature and Criteria for Diagnosis of Diseases of the Heart and Great Vessels*, 9th edition. Boston, MA: Little, Brown & Co, 1994, pp. 253–256.

11. Fonarow GC. Epidemiology and risk stratification in acute heart failure. *Am Heart J* 2008; 155(2): 200–207.

12. Dahlström U. Frequent non-cardiac comorbidities in patients with chronic heart failure. *Eur J Heart Fail* 2005; 7(3): 309–316.

13. Johnson MJ. Extending palliative care to patients with heart failure. *Br J Hosp Med (Lond)* 2010; 71: 12–15.

14. Boyd KJ, Worth A, Kendall M, et al. Making sure services deliver for people with advanced heat failure: a longitudinal qualitative study of patients, family carers, and health professionals. *Palliat Med* 2009; 23(8): 767–776.

15. Peterson PN, Rumsfeld JS, Liang L, et al. A validated risk score for in-hospital mortality in patients with heart failure from the American Heart Association get with the guidelines program. *Circ Cardiovasc Qual Outcomes* 2010; 3: 25–32.

16. Huynh BC, Rovner A, and Rick MW. Identification of older patients with heart failure who may be candidates for hospice care: development of a simple four-item risk score. *J Am Geriatr Soc* 2008; 56: 1111–1115.

17. Anand IS, Kempf T, Rector TS, et al. Serial measurement of growth differentiation factor-15 in heart failure. *Circulation* 2010; 122: 1387–1395.

18. Groenveld HF, Januzzi JL, Damman K, et al. Anemia and mortality in heart failure patients. A systematic review and meta-analysis. *J Am Coll Cardiol* 2008; 52: 818–827.

19. Kociol RD, Pang PS, Gheorghiade M, et al. Troponin elevation in heart failure prevalence, mechanisms, and clinical implications. *J Am Coll Cardiol* 2010; 56: 1071–1078.

20. deFilippi CR, Christenson RH, Gottdiener JS, et al. Dynamic cardiovascular risk assessment in elderly people: the role of repeated N-terminal pro-B-type natriuretic peptide testing. *J Am Coll Cardiol* 2010; 55: 441–450.

21. Zugck C, Kruger C, Kell R, et al. Risk stratification in middle-aged patients with congestive heart failure: prospective comparison of the Heart Failure Survival Score (HFSS) and a simplified two-variable model. *Eur J Heart Fail* 2001; 3: 577–585.

22. Levy WC, Mozaffarian D, Linker DT, et al. The seattle heart failure model: prediction of survival in heart failure. *Circulation* 2006: 113: 1424–1433.

23. Mark DB, Anstrom KJ, Sun JL, et al. Quality of life with defibrillator therapy or amiodarone in heart failure. *N Engl J Med* 2008; 359(10): 999–1008.

24. Padeletti L, Arnar DO, Boncinelli L, et al . EHRA Expert Consensus Statement on the management of cardiovascular implantable electronic devices in patients nearing end of life or requesting withdrawal of therapy. *Europace* 2010; 12: 1480–1489.

25. Adler ED, Goldfinger JZ, Kalman J, et al. Palliative care in the treatment of advanced heart failure. *Circulation* 2009; 120: 2597–2606.

26. O'Leary N. The comparative palliative care needs of those with heart failure and cancer patients. *Curr Opin Support Palliat Care* 2009; 3: 241–246.

27. Iqbal J, Francis L, Reid J, et al. Quality of life in patients with chronic heart failure and their carers: a 3 year follow-up study assessing hospitalization and mortality. *Eur J Heart Fail* 2010; 12: 1002–1008.

28. Heart Failure Society of America, Lindenfeld J, Albert NM, et al. HFSA 2010 Comprehensive Heart Failure Practice Guideline. *J Card Fail* 2010; 16(6): e1–e194.

29. Harding R, Selman L, Beynon T, et al. Meeting the communication and information needs of chronic heart failure patients. *J Pain Symptom Manage* 2008; 36: 149–156.

30. Hupcey JE, Penrod J, and Fogg J. Heart failure and palliative care: implications in practice. *J Palliat Med* 2009; 12(6): 531–536.

31. Hupcey JE, Penrod J, and Fenstermacher K. A model of palliative care for heart failure. *Am J Hosp Palliat Care* 2009; 26(5): 399–404.

32. Goodlin SJ. Palliative care in congestive heart failure. *J Am Coll Cardiol* 2009; 54: 386–396.

33. Arnold JM, Liu P, Demers C, et al. Canadian Cardiovascular Society consensus conference recommendations on heart failure 2006: diagnosis and management. *Can J Cardiol* 2006; 22: 23–45.

34. Opasich C and Gualco A. The complex symptom burden of the aged heart failure population. *Curr Opin Support Palliat Care* 2007; 1: 255–259.

35. Currow DC, Smith J, Davidson PM, et al. Do the trajectories of dyspnea differ in prevalence and intensity by diagnosis at the end of life? A consecutive cohort study. *J Pain Symptom Manage* 2010; 39: 680–690.

36. Pittler MH, Guo R, and Ernst E. Hawthorn extract for treating chronic heart failure. *Cochrane Database Syst Rev* 2008; (1): CD005312.

37. Goldfinger J and Adler ED. End-of-life options for patients with advanced heart failure. *Curr Heart Fail Rep* 2010; 7: 140–147.

38. Abernethy AP, McDonald CF, Frith PA, et al. Effect of palliative oxygen versus room air in relief of breathlessness in patients with refractory dyspnea: a double blind, randomized controlled trial. *Lancet* 2010; 376: 784–793.

39. Verma AK, da Silva JH, and Kuhl DR. Diuretic effects of subcutaneous furosemide in human volunteers: a randomized pilot study. *Ann Pharmacother* 2004; 38: 544–549.

40. Johnson MJ, McDonagh TA, Harkness A, et al. Morphine for the relief of breathlessness in patients with chronic heart failure—a pilot study. *Eur J Heart Fail* 2002; 4(6): 753–756.

41. Hochgerner M, Fruhwald FM, and Strohscheer I. Opioids for symptomatic therapy of dyspnea in patients with advanced chronic heart failure—is there evidence? *Wien Med Wochenschr* 2009; 159(23–24): 577–582.

42. Armingeat T, Brondino R, Pham T, et al. Intravenous pamidronate for pain relief in recent osteoporotic vertebral compression fracture: a randomized double-blind controlled study. *Osteoporos Int* 2006; 17(11): 1659–1665.

43. Knopp JA, Diner BM, Blitz M, et al. Calcitonin for treating acute pain of osteoporotic vertebral compression fractures: a systematic review of randomized, controlled trials. *Osteoporos Int* 2005; 16(10): 1281–1290.

44. Dean M. Opioids in renal failure and dialysis patients. *J Pain Symptom Manage* 2004; 28: 497–504.

45. Fredheim OMS, Moksnes K, Borchgrevink PC, et al. Clinical pharmacology of methadone for pain. *Act Anaesthesiol Scand* 2008; 52: 879–889.

46. Davidson PM, Cockburn J, Newton PJ, et al. Can a heart failure-specific cardiac rehabilitation program decrease hospitalizations and improve outcomes in high risk patients? *Eur J Cardiovasc Prev Rehabil* 2010; 17: 393–402.

47. Peuckmann V, Elsner F, Krumm N, et al. Pharmacological treatments for fatigue associated with palliative care. *Cochrane Database Syst Rev* 2010; (11): CD006788.

48. Van der Meer P and van Veldhuisen DJ. Anaemia and renal dysfunction in chronic heart failure. *Heart* 2009; 95: 1808–1812.

49. Anand IS. Anemia and chronic heart failure implications and treatment options. *J Am Coll Cardiol* 2008; 52: 501–511.

50. Anker SD, Comin Colet J, Filippatos G, et al. Ferric carboxymaltose in patients with heart failure and iron deficiency. *N Engl J Med* 2009; 361: 2436–2448.

51. Ngo K, Kotecha D, Walters JA, et al. Erythropoiesis-stimulating agents for anaemia in chronic heart failure patients. *Cochrane Database Syst Rev* 2010; (1): CD007613.

52. Rutledge T, Reis VA, Linke SE, et al. Depression in heart failure a meta-analytic review of prevalence, intervention effects, and associations with clinical outcomes. *J Am Coll Cardiol* 2006; 48(8): 1527–1537.

53. Jiang W, Kuchibhatla M, Clary GL, et al. Relationship between depressive symptoms and long term mortality in patients with heart failure. *Am Heart J* 2007; 154: 102–108.

54. Sullivan M, Simon G, Spertus J, et al. Depression-related costs in heart failure care. *Arch Intern Med* 2002: 162(16): 1860–1866.

55. Watson K and Summers KM. Depression in patients with heart failure: clinical implications and management. *Pharmacotherapy* 2009; 29(1): 49–63.

56. Hopp FP, Thornton N, and Martin L. The lived experience of heart failure at the end of life: a systematic literature review. *Heath Soc Work* 2010; 35(2): 109–117.

57. Bekelman DB, Dy SM, Becker DM, et al. Spiritual well-being and depression in patients with heart failure. *J Gen Intern Med* 2007; 22: 470–477.

58. Lane DA, Chong AY, and Lip GY. Psychological interventions for depression in heart failure. *Cochrane Database Syst Rev* 2005; (1): CD003329.

59. O'Connor CM, Jiang W, Kuchibhatla M, et al. Safety and efficacy of sertraline for depression in patients with heart failure: results of the SADHART-CHF (Sertraline Against

Depression and Heart Disease in Chronic Heart Failure) trial. *J Am Coll Cardiol* 2010; 56(9): 692–699.

60. Veien KT, Videbæk L, Schou M, et al. High mortality among heart failure patients treated with antidepressants. *Int J Cardiol* 2011; 146(1): 64–67.

61. Selman L, Beynon T, Higginson IJ, et al. Psychological, social and spiritual distress at the end of life in heart fail-ure patients. *Curr Opin Support Palliat Care* 2007; 1: 260–266.

62. Krumholz HM, Phillips RS, Hamel MB, et al. Resuscitation preferences among patients with severe congestive heart fail-ure: results from the SUPPORT project. Study to Understand Prognoses and Preferences for Outcomes and Risks of Treat-ments. *Circulation* 1998; 98(7): 648–655.

19 Palliative Care in Advanced Renal Disease

Deb Braithwaite

Community Lead Victoria Hospice, Victoria, Canada

Introduction

End-stage renal disease (ESRD) is the last stage of chronic kidney disease (CKD) and occurs when estimated glomerular filtration rate (GFR) drops below 15 ml/min and becomes inadequate to support daily living. Although renal patients represent a small portion of the current palliative population, their numbers and impact are growing. Palliative care is increasingly involved with renal patients across a variety of settings, including conservative management, dialysis therapy, end-stage decline, and dialysis withdrawal.

Over the past two decades, the incidence of ESRD has risen with the aging population, and increased occurrence of predisposing disease such as diabetes and atherosclerosis. As survival times have improved, so has the prevalence of patients with complex medical problems and high symptom burdens. As we plan to meet the needs of ESRD patients and families in the future, the question arises: how might palliative care best support renal patients at end of life?

Patient needs in ESRD are common to other palliative populations and include control of physical symptoms, emotional support for patients and families, triage of goals and priorities, and practical support across diverse care settings. Renal patients require all the above and more, given the many complex medical and psychological challenges they encounter in advanced illness and decline. Optimal care of this population requires the combined efforts of family physicians, nephrologists, palliative physicians, and associated renal and palliative teams.

ESRD management

Until the mid-1960s, all ESRD management was medical and conservative, but with the advent of haemodialysis, patients could be supported over the long term. Dialysis was initially available only for those awaiting kidney transplantation, but as technology improved and dialysis became more available, it was increasingly employed as permanent renal replacement.

However, dialysis is not appropriate for everyone, and a portion of ESRD patients receive conservative management today, either by choice or because they are poorly suited to replacement therapy.

Given the dramatic differences between treatment options, patients and families require clear information and understanding of choices to make informed decisions. Full consideration of prognosis, lifestyle, and symptom management allows planning that best reflects individual priorities and goals.

Conservative management

Conservative management in ESRD is medically active and aimed at delay and control of disease and associated symptoms, without use of renal replacement therapy. It is holistic in nature and includes coordinated medical and emotional support for patients and families across disease trajectory. It is most appropriate for patients in whom dialysis proves the greatest burden with the least benefit to quality of life, comfort, and survival.

Handbook of Palliative Care, Third Edition. Edited by Christina Faull, Sharon de Caestecker, Alex Nicholson and Fraser Black.
© 2012 by John Wiley and Sons, Inc. Published 2012 by John Wiley & Sons, Inc.

Table 19.1 Conservative management of ESRD.

Uraemic syndrome	Symptoms and sequela	Management
Chronic anaemia	Dyspnoea, fatigue, worsening CHF	Iron, EPO, RBC transfusion
Fluid overload	Peripheral and pulmonary oedema, encephalopathy	Diuretics, fluid, and sodium restriction
Acidosis	Fatigue and malaise	Sodium bicarbonate, diuretics
Electrolyte disorders	Pruritus, cardiac arrhythmia, elevated potassium and phosphate	Protein restriction, sodium polystyrene sulphonate (e.g., Kayexalate)

This population is generally over 80 years of age, with limited prognosis due to age and high comorbidity scores. Incidence and severity of end-stage symptoms are comparable to other advanced conditions such as cancer, CHF, and COPD [1–3] and managed in a similar manner. Conservative management in the setting of ESRD is presented in Table 19.1.

While conservatively managed patients may survive months and even years, death inevitably occurs once GFR falls below 5 ml/min. However, those who opt for less aggressive management may enjoy improved quality of life as they avoid the arduous burdens of routine dialysis, repeat hospitalisations, and the sense of "suspended living" in drawn out decline [4].

Patient case study

Mrs. S is a 79-year-old female with long-standing insulin-dependent diabetes mellitus, peripheral vascular disease, and progressive renal failure. She and her husband live independently at home with extended family close by. She was referred to nephrology several years ago for management of CKD, but falling GFR has now raised the question of renal replacement therapy. As she is not a candidate for renal transplantation, Mrs. S and her family recently met with the nephrologist to discuss treatment options and next steps.

At the meeting, the risks and benefits of conservative management versus haemodialysis were discussed, along with the patient's current goals and priorities. She and her family had many questions about how haemodialysis would impact things, such as prognosis, disease management, and quality of life. The patient's husband seemed to support haemodialysis, but Mrs. S requested additional time to consider her options.

The trend toward conservative management appears to be increasing, as the limitations of kidney replacement therapy become better understood. Today, many renal clinics provide specific programs for patients forgoing dialysis that focus on education, family support, disease management, and symptom control until death.

Patient case study

On further discussion with her family physician and family, Mrs. S decided to opt for conservative management. She clearly understood the potential consequences to her prognosis, but felt her quality of life would be improved on balance. Mrs. S indicated she might reconsider haemodialysis in the future, but preferred to manage CKD progression in a conservative manner for the time being.

The patient was therefore referred to the renal outpatient clinic for advice regarding management of fluids and diet, initiation of iron and erythropoietin (EPO) to treat chronic anaemia, and referral to counselling for family support.

Effective communication regarding clinical and lifestyle implications of conservative management requires input from skilled nephrologists and renal teams. Conservative care should also include access to palliative supports at end of life.

Renal replacement therapy

Renal replacement takes several forms, including kidney transplantation, peritoneal dialysis, and haemodialysis. Though transplantation is usually favoured for long-term management of ESRD, the relative scarcity of donor

Table 19.2 Expected remaining lifetime (years) of general population and those on haemodialysis by age, US Renal Data System 2008 [5] (Abridged).

Age	General population	Dialysis
60–64	21.0	4.6
65–69	17.2	3.9
70–74	13.8	3.3
75–79	10.8	2.8
80–84	8.2	2.3
85+	4.4	1.9

kidneys for initial or repeat transplantation requires many patients to rely on dialysis for ongoing survival. While renal replacement offers indefinite maintenance in theory, in reality, survival is profoundly decreased in both dialysis and transplant populations (Table 19.2).

Actively treated ESRD patients die under a number of circumstances, including graft failure, progressive cardiovascular morbidity, sudden cardiac death during dialysis, or unrelated secondary diagnosis. Consideration of treatment withdrawal may be prompted by any significant decline in comfort, function, or quality of life, and remains a common trigger for palliative consultation.

Kidney dialysis is accordingly most appropriate in patients with reversible disease, those awaiting transplantation and ESRD patients with few comorbidities and the greatest chance of life prolongation. Renal consultation should be considered early in CKD as research shows nephrology referral, rather than early dialysis, is most associated with improved patient outcomes and survival [6].

Patient case study

Mrs. S has done well with conservative management over the past year but recently developed a chronic left foot ulcer secondary to vascular insufficiency. She presented as an emergency 6 weeks ago with bacteraemia and delirium secondary to peripheral cellulitis and was successfully treated with IV fluids and antibiotics. She subsequently developed acute on chronic renal failure, and her caregivers choose temporary haemodialysis, in hope of renal recovery. Unfortunately, she has remained dialysis dependent, and is now complaining of multiple discomforts during dialysis including bilateral lower limb pain and uncontrolled nausea.

Renal dialysis controls most symptoms associated with uraemia. Regular treatments maintain electrolyte and fluid balances, controlling problems such as oedema, fluid overload, acidosis, and pruritus. However, dialysis brings its own burdens including time and schedule restrictions, vascular access maintenance, anticoagulation risks, and associated dialysis effects such as fatigue, pruritus, headache, and abdominal cramps. Long-term effects include progressive vascular insufficiency contributing to peripheral ischaemia, CHF, vascular dementia, calcific uraemic arteriolopathy, and neuropathic pain. Timely adjustments to dialysis compounds and prescriptions along with effective symptom management offer patients the best in ongoing maintenance and comfort.

For all the above reasons, dialysis decisions also require careful vetting and review over time. In-depth discussions regarding dialysis initiation or withdrawal are generally welcomed by patients with CKD and provide additional guidance for substitute decision-makers at times of medical crisis and stress [7,8].

Symptom management in ESRD

The scope and severity of symptoms in ESRD have been significantly underestimated in the past by both patients and medical care providers, but this is rapidly changing. Research aimed at caregiver attitudes and identification of patient priorities regarding symptom management and quality of life has led to new initiatives in care. Over the past decade, renal end-of-life guidelines have been developed to include standards for shared decision making, identification of goals, and symptom control in end-stage disease [8–10].

We now understand that renal patients experience symptom burdens that are severe and entirely comparable to other end-stage conditions such as CHF, COPD, and cancer as outlined in Table 19.3. ESRD patients experience major symptoms of pain, nausea, dyspnoea, and delirium common to other palliative populations, as well as renal-related problems such as pruritus, vasculopathy, and heightened drug effects [3].

The combination of major symptoms and increased drug sensitivity creates complex management problems in CKD. Optimal control requires a good understanding of common symptoms, focused physical assessment, and an informed approach to medications.

Table 19.3 Comparison of symptoms in ESRD and other chronic disease [1,2].

Symptom	Overall prevalence (%)	ESRD with dialysis (%)	COPD/CHF (%)	Cancer (%)
Pain	53	47	49	63
Nausea	26	33	28	45
Dyspnoea	61	37	86	23
Constipation	35	53	30	34
Pruritus	74	55	26	27
Fatigue	76	71	84	73

Pain

Until recently, pain was not considered a major problem in ESRD, but recent research finds it common and frequently severe. Davison and others have shown that between 50% and 76% of renal patients experience pain in advanced disease and that intensity is severe in over half of those surveyed. Of the patients studied, 30% received no analgesic therapy and the remainder described poor pain control 75% of the time. The association between uncontrolled pain, insomnia, and chronic depression was also noted, prompting some patients to consider dialysis withdrawal as a result [11,12].

Pain in ESRD is often multifactorial and can be somatic, neuropathic, or a combination of both. Aetiology ranges from musculoskeletal (arthritis, osteoporosis, fracture, and renal osteodystrophy) to vascular (peripheral oedema, ischaemia, and necrosis) to neuropathic (polyneuropathy) to dermal (xerosis and calciphylaxis) to dialysis related. Mixed aetiologies are most common and require careful analgesic and adjuvant selection for optimal control.

Non-opioid analgesics

Non-opioid analgesics are appropriate for mild to moderate pain, especially in patients experiencing musculoskeletal discomfort.

Paracetamol (acetaminophen) is a good first choice and requires no dose adjustment in renal disease. Like most analgesics, it should be taken routinely in divided doses of 1,000 mg three or four times a day.

Nonsteroidal anti-inflammatory preparations are also useful, either alone or in combination with paracetamol (acetaminophen). Dosing should also be routine, but conservative, due to increased risks of progressive renal insufficiency, hypertension, electrolyte imbalance, and bleeding. It may be given orally or rectally and is most appropriate for short-term use, unless the patient is close to death.

Opioid analgesics

Opioid use for the control of moderate to severe pain is necessary in a significant portion of ESRD patients over time. Opioids are safe and appropriate when carefully chosen, titrated, and monitored, and are useful in the settings of boney fracture, peripheral neuropathy, vascular ischaemia, or painful skin conditions such as calciphylaxis. However, use is constrained in terms of dosing and interval in renal disease, due to prolonged metabolism and length of analgesic action, prolonged elimination, and retention of physiologically active metabolites. These factors combine to make renal patients "chemically sensitive" (see Figure 19.1) to the effects of opioids and limit the choices that are considered "most appropriate" in this setting.

In this section (as in Chapter 9, *Pain and Its Management*), formulations of opioids that have a prolonged

Dosing opioids in "chemically sensitive" patients

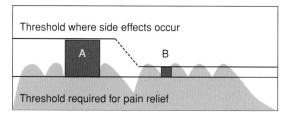

A. Normal "window of comfort"

B. Small "window of comfort" in sensitive pts

Figure 19.1 "Chemically sensitive" patient. (Reproduced with permission from Dr. Michael Downing, Victoria Hospice, Victoria, Canada.)

duration of effect are referred to as "MR" and this should be taken to mean the same as "extended release" or "sustained release." Opioid formulations that have not been adapted to deliver over a prolonged period of time are referred to as "NR," which means the same as "immediate release."

First-line opioids

While there is no single opioid that is the "best first choice" in the setting of renal failure, there are "better" or "worst" choices. Options for first-line opioids would include hydromorphone, tramadol, transdermal fentanyl, and buprenorphine. These opioids are described in detail in Chapter 9, *Pain and Its Management*, but also discussed briefly below.

Hydromorphone may be considered in ESRD as it is partially cleared during dialysis and has an improved side effect profile (decreased incidence of nausea, pruritus, and sedation) in renal disease. It should be initiated in small doses of 0.5–1 mg every 6 h and gently increased over time as tolerated. It is available in a variety of formulations for different routes of administration as well as in normal and MR preparations and is suitable for control of moderate to severe pain. It should always be initiated in NR form, as the strength and duration of MR versions are difficult to predict in CKD.

Tramadol has both opioid and non-opioid properties with a side effect profile akin to other opioids. It has some advantages in CKD as although it is metabolised in the liver to O-desmethyltramadol (M1) that is itself an active substance, it then undergoes further biotransformation into an inactive form that is then excreted by the kidneys. It should however be prescribed conservatively in renal patients to a maximum of 50 mg twice a day [13].

Fentanyl is a good choice in ESRD and is widely prescribed by family physicians, nephrologists, and palliative care physicians alike. It is partially cleared by dialysis and has a low side effect profile in terms of nausea, sedation, and pruritus (non-histamine releasing). The patch is popular with patients due to its transdermal route and long 72-h duration of action, but fentanyl is also available in short-acting parental form. The transdermal patch is best suited to control stable chronic pain and is considered appropriate in both somatic and neuropathic management. Disadvantages include cost and fixed dose limitations. Conversion to fentanyl patch usually occurs following titration with an alternative, short-acting opioids or other agents such as the buprenorphine transdermal patch. Patients who require reversal on fentanyl patch have opioid in their systems for 18–24 h following

patch removal and often require prolonged monitoring and repeated naloxone during that time. Chapter 9, *Pain and Its Management*, gives further detail on initiating, titrating, and discontinuation of fentanyl.

Fentanyl injectable formulation may also be administered by continuous SC infusion and in some settings alfentanil (a potent injectable opioid) is also used in patients with renal failure. The UK PCF 4e [14] and the Web-based resource palliativedrugs.com provide more information on these agents and if their use is considered, advice should be sought from the specialist palliative care team.

Buprenorphine transdermal patch is another option, but it should be noted that differing strengths and formulations exist in different countries. In the United Kingdom, there are multiple strengths available and the option for either 4- or 7-day patch formulations (see Chapter 9, *Pain and Its Management*). Currently, in Canada, the buprenorphine transdermal patch is available in 5, 10, and 20 μg/h strengths and comes in a 7-day patch formulation. Buprenorphine transdermal 5 μg/h patches can be initiated in an opioid naïve patient.

Second-line opioids

Oxycodone is similar to hydromorphone in terms of side effects, but opinions vary as to its suitability in ESRD. It has been used in the past for ESRD patients with excessive CNS sedation associated with other opioids. As with all strong analgesics, it requires gentle titration and careful monitoring, starting at 2 mg every 6–8 h.

Third-line opioid—option for use but may require specialist supervision

Methadone is considered an excellent choice in renal disease as it is primarily metabolised in the liver and excreted via the gut. It can be prescribed by itself or in combination with other medications, for the control of severe somatic or neuropathic pain. It has an interesting duration of action as it becomes therapeutic in approximately 30 min, but provides analgesia for 8–12 h on average. In ESRD, methadone is usually started at 2 mg three times a day, alone or in combination with other opioids and adjuvants.

Unfortunately, methadone has some distinct drawbacks. Titration is complicated by a double peak of absorption that occurs in the first week and has led to overdose deaths in the past. It should be prescribed carefully in patients with cardiac problems as Q-T prolongation may occur. Electrocardiography is suggested before methadone initiation followed by weekly testing until a stable dosing is achieved [15,16]. Due to the above risks, methadone prescribing in Canada is limited by special license and its use in most countries is generally confined to palliative and other pain care specialists with specific expertise.

Opioids that should be avoided

Morphine, codeine, and meperidine are effective analgesics, but considered poor choices in renal disease, due to prolonged elimination and accumulation of physiologically active metabolites [9]. Some in this group are inadequately cleared during dialysis, leading to retention of metabolites, increased risk of opioid neurotoxicity, and associated CNS effects of somnolence, confusion, myoclonic jerking, and uncontrolled pain.

Topical opioids

Open skin lesions are common in ESRD and topically applied opioids allow local analgesia with little systemic absorption. Pain may be caused by renal manifestations such as metastatic calcification, or in association with comorbid conditions such as diabetes, CHF, and peripheral vascular disease. Vascular insufficiency produces ischaemic lesions of the toes, feet, and legs and decreased mobility increases the incidence of painful decubiti. Opioid formulations designed for parental administration, such as morphine 10 mg/ml injectable, can be dripped or atomised across painful lesion edges, or combined with carrier creams during dressing changes, to provide 12–16 h of local analgesia, following application [17].

Adjuvants

Adjuvant medications are typically combined with analgesics for improved control of complex pain and may be derived from a range of separate drug categories. Adjuvants used for neuropathic pain management typically affect the CNS and may require dose reduction.

Carbamazepine has been used successfully in CKD and requires little dose adjustment. The usual starting dose of 200 mg twice daily is generally well tolerated in renal populations and can be further titrated as required. Tricyclic medications are also useful but require careful monitoring, especially in cardiac patients. Nortriptyline and desipramine are both good choices. Desipramine should be started at 10 mg at bedtime and titrated to a maximum of 150 mg until control or intolerable side effects occur [9].

Gabapentin is often prescribed for neuropathic pain and restless legs, but accumulates easily in CKD, resulting in profound sedation and myoclonic jerking. It should be initiated at 50 mg twice a day and slowly increased to a

daily maximum of 300 mg. Pregabalin may be started at 25 mg a day and titrated up to 100 mg a day [9].

Gastrointestinal

ESRD patients experience a variety of GI complaints in end-stage disease. Chronic anorexia, nausea and vomiting, diarrhoea, or constipation often go under-recognised and undertreated in renal patients, but are a frequent source of distress in advancing disease.

Bowels

Many renal patients experience diarrhoea on dialysis. This may be due to multiple causes and is sometimes improved by adjusting dialysis parameters and medications. Persistent diarrhoea should initially be investigated for a coincidental cause unrelated to the chronic renal disease and if no other correctable cause is found it should be treated symptomatically with loperamide (Imodium) or the lowest tolerated dose of an appropriate opioid. Bear in mind that fentanyl, which is favoured in renal patients, actually causes less constipation than other opioids and so may not prove so useful in reducing the tendency to diarrhoea.

Conversely, constipation is also common in ESRD. Aetiology includes fluid restriction, altered diet, decreased mobility, and constipating medications. Patients should maximise fibre in their diet as far as this can be tolerated and also require laxatives to be prescribed and titrated to effect alongside opioid medication. Macrogols (such as polyethylene glycol (PEG)) are well tolerated and effective but may prove difficult for patients with fluid restrictions or swallowing difficulties. Softening agents, such as docusate sodium or lactulose, and stimulant laxatives such as senna, are safe and effective in renal patients and should be taken on a daily basis.

Nausea and vomiting

Nausea and vomiting are common symptoms in uraemia, but also occur in 5–15% of patients during haemodialysis [18]. In advanced disease, approximately 30% of patients experience nausea and vomiting associated with renal toxicity, haemodialysis, and the effects of emetogenic medications (opioids, antibiotics, oral iron, and so on) [1]. Accordingly, portions of patients require routine antiemetic as part of end-stage management.

Antiemetics to consider include neuroleptics such as levomepromazine (methotrimeprazine) and haloperidol. This group is effective for the control of nausea and vomiting associated with metabolic imbalance or opioid effects and is usually tolerated at conservative standard doses. Haloperidol may be started at 1 mg bd and titrated as required, but as with other neuroleptics, requires dose reduction if GFR is less than 10–15 ml/min. Levomepromazine should be used in low doses (starting at 6.25–12.5 mg once daily) because side effects include sedation and hypotension.

Metoclopramide is most appropriate for nausea associated with gastric stasis, but the standard dose of 10 mg four times daily should be reduced if GFR drops below 15–20 ml/min. If extrapyramidal symptoms develop with metoclopramide, consider domperidone as an alternative. Dexamethasone may also be considered if the above antiemetics are not wholly effective. It should be initiated at 2–3 mg bd with the awareness that steroid increases hypertension and bleeding in renal patients.

Patient case study

Mrs. S has been attending haemodialysis three times a week for 6 months. She initially experienced generalised peripheral pain and nausea during haemodialysis, but has been well controlled with hydromorphone 2 mg and haloperidol 1 mg before and during dialysis as required. More recently, she has developed neuropathic pain in both feet secondary to diabetic neuropathy and now requires hydromorphone 4 mg every 6 h and gabapentin 75 mg three times a day. Mrs. S notes progressive difficulty attending her dialysis sessions due to rising fatigue, dyspnoea on exertion, and increased foot and leg pain with weight bearing. Her family describes her as increasingly forgetful and occasionally confused at night.

Dyspnoea

The incidence of dyspnoea is generally low in dialysed patients but more frequent in those receiving conservative care alone. However, it is very common when ESRD combines with comorbid disease such as CHF and COPD, and surveys show that 30% of renal patients have significant dyspnoea at end of life [1].

Depending on aetiology, dyspnoea may be improved through a number of measures including careful management of comorbid disease, red blood cell transfusion, continuous oxygen, diuretics, and ultrafiltration (haemodialysis for fluid removal only). Equally important are general comfort measures such as lowered room temperature, brisk airflow via a fan or opened window, loose clothing, and elevated head of bed.

In addition, patients find significant improvement with low dose opioids and benzodiazepines. As stated earlier, opioids and adjuvants must be carefully selected and adjusted in ESRD. In the imminently dying patient, the benefit/risk profile should be reviewed with the patient to ensure adequate symptom relief with doses titrated and given regularly even if symptom relief is associated with an element of sedation. Transdermal fentanyl using a patch is appropriate for stable dyspnoea, but short-acting opioids are more useful in patients with evolving symptoms. Lorazepam, 0.5–1 mg administered sublingually or subcutaneously, provides rapid short-term relief of dyspnoea that occurs suddenly or in association with activity. When dyspnoea is severe, midazolam 2.5 mg SC hourly can provide relief and comfort in final hours [9]. Midazolam may also be administered by a continuous SC infusion. For an overview of symptom management in the terminal phase (last days of life), see Chapter 21, *Terminal Care and Dying*.

Delirium

The incidence of delirium is high in all palliative populations, but renal patients face additional risk as GFR falls. Patients with pre-existing cerebral vascular disease or dementia are especially vulnerable to the CNS consequences of metabolic aberration, altered drug metabolism, or haemodialysis. In early ESRD, delirium should be reviewed for reversible aetiology, including sepsis, hypoxia, and medication effects. Pharmaceuticals with CNS effects such as opioids, benzodiazepines, steroids, or gabapentin should be reduced, rotated, or discontinued whenever possible. However, neuroleptics should be considered in any patient with severe agitation or terminal delirium. Haloperidol 1–2 mg every 8 h may settle early delirium but more agitated states require stronger sedation such as midazolam 2.5–5 mg/h. If physical restlessness persists despite routine neuroleptic, consider additional measures such as lorazepam 1–2 mg every 2–4 h, for improved safety and control.

Seizures and myoclonic jerking

Although seizure activity in terminal uraemia does occur, it is less frequent than commonly assumed. Grand mal seizures occur in approximately 10% of ESRD patients [19] and some require antiseizure prophylaxis following. Phenytoin is commonly prescribed but dose reduction and careful blood level monitoring is required.

Myoclonic jerking is very common in uraemic decline, and is thought to be caused by retention of metabolic and pharmaceutical by-products. Twitching tends to become more pronounced in the imminently dying patient, and can cause distress to the patient, family, and medical team. This symptom is fortunately well controlled with benzodiazepine, such as lorazepam 0.5–2 mg every 2–4 h as required or midazolam given by continuous SC infusion.

Skin

Skin problems are common in CKD with most patients experiencing one or more dermatological disorders. Manifestations range from mild to severe and include changes such as easy bruising, Raynaud's phenomenon, peripheral vascular breakdown, and metastatic calcification. However, the most common complaints are pruritus and xerosis.

Pruritus

Pruritus occurs in up to 50% of renal patients during the course of their illness. Elevated calcium phosphate is thought to contribute to pruritus, but excitation of cutaneous sensory nerve endings due to retained urochrome may also play a role [20]. Pruritus related to CKD increases with the severity and duration of renal failure, but tends to resolve with renal replacement treatment. However, it may additionally occur during dialysis if the patient develops allergies to one or more dialysis compounds.

Pruritus can be local but is more often generalised. Mild to moderate itching is usually managed through a combination of topical emollients, moisturisers, and UVB light treatment. If localised, topical agents such as capsaicin may also help. Progressive pruritus requires the addition of antihistamine or gabapentin 50–100 mg three times daily or on days following dialysis. In severe cases, consider cholestyramine 5 g twice daily [20].

Xerosis

Xerosis, or dry roughened skin, also contributes to pruritus in renal disease. Of dialysis patients, 50–75% complain of xerosis, which typically occurs along the extensor surfaces of arms and legs [20]. It is thought to relate to dysfunction of the dermal barrier, which predisposes patients to painful fissures, ulcers, and infections. Most dialysis patients improve with routine moisturisers and keratolytics.

Calciphylaxis

Metastatic dermal calcification is a rare but serious complication in ESRD, related to altered calcium and phosphate metabolism. It occurs in 1–4% of renal patients but is associated with 60–80% mortality [21]. Calciphylaxis develops when calcium salts precipitate in normal tissues. When this occurs in dermal vasculature, it results in ischaemic pain and widespread tissue necrosis. Lesions initially present as painful purpuric areas that progress to ecchymosis, then cordlike nodules. In advanced disease, ischaemic bullae form on top of these areas spreading superficially and then resulting in deep ulcers progressing to necrosis and gangrene. Lesions can occur anywhere but proximal lesions carry the poorest prognosis.

Calciphylaxis usually presents in late renal disease and tends to progress despite intervention. Early treatment includes normalisation of calcium and phosphate levels through diet, phosphate binding, and parathyroidectomy, if indicated. In advanced calciphylaxis, good wound care and antibiotics help control sepsis, but patients also require excellent management of pain. The discomfort of calciphylaxis is typically severe, so palliative consultation should be considered.

End of life

Despite advances in care, ESRD has a mortality rate of around 23% per year [22]. Patients reach end of life under various circumstances, including treatment failure, associated comorbidity, separate terminal diagnosis, and treatment withdrawal. Yet many enter advanced disease without previous consideration of end-stage goals or priorities. This may occur due to physician avoidance or the perception that patients resist end-of-life discussions. However, new research has challenged this assumption. In 2008, ESRD patients were studied to discover patient preferences in advance care planning (ACP). Researchers found that less than 10% of patients had discussed end-of-life concerns with their nephrologist in the previous year, despite having advanced disease and receiving regular renal care. It also found that patients generally welcomed these discussions and wanted medical caregivers to initiate them without direct prompting. Patient concerns included a better understanding of prognosis, natural history of disease, and when appropriate, access to palliative services and support at end of life [22].

Given the high incidence of cognitive deficits, progressive comorbidities, and sudden decline in ESRD, ACP should begin ideally at diagnosis and repeat as disease progresses. Because disease outcomes vary widely, end-of-life discussions should be incorporated into care routines at regular time or treatment intervals to ensure that patient priorities are identified and met.

Patient case study

Renal clinic staff report that Mrs. S is increasingly exhausted and disorientated during haemodialysis and appears to be declining quickly. Formerly pleasant and cooperative, she is now withdrawn and often asks to be "left alone to die." Her family physician recently met with the patient, family, and medical care team to discuss the changes. All agreed that the patient's quality of life was declining and future improvements were unlikely. Mrs. S repeated her desire to discontinue haemodialysis and return home for death. Her family supported this decision but had many questions about expected end-stage symptoms, length of prognosis, and palliative resources in the home. Over the next few days, they met with the renal and palliative teams for additional information and planning and following a final dialysis treatment, Mrs. S was discharged home for end-of-life care.

Withdrawal from dialysis

Studies show that up to 60% of patients regret the decision to initiate dialysis and that 30% of this group eventually withdraw from treatment [22]. In recent years, increased attention has been focused on the complex issues surrounding initiation and withdrawal of treatment and organisations such as the Renal Physicians of America have developed guidelines to encourage better informed, shared decision making between patients, families, and medical caregiver [8].

Withdrawal decisions usually centre on issues of symptom management, decreased quality of life, and the impact of chronic progressive disease. Many patients are relieved following the decision, as it allows freedom from dialysis routines and the opportunity to focus on end-stage concerns. Dialysis withdrawal also provides some prognostic predictability. Length of survival varies with residual kidney function, age, and comorbidity but averages 8–12 days once treatment is discontinued. Whether supportive care is planned for home, hospital, or hospice, palliative planning is best completed before final withdrawal. This area is discussed in more detail in Chapter 8, *Advance Care Planning*.

Continued renal replacement

Patients with previous transplantation or ongoing dialysis may die of unrelated causes, but most succumb to associated morbidity. This population maintains treatment close to death, either by choice or because ACP has not addressed palliative care alternatives. Whether terminal decline is due to CVD, COPD, cancer, or uraemia, control of associated end-stage symptoms remains paramount. This is especially true for patients with severe problems related to sepsis, vascular necrosis, and complex neuropathy. Such patients are end stage and require ongoing palliative support and symptom management, regardless of continuing dialysis.

Conclusions

ESRD is rising in our population and presents many complex issues involving treatment paths, resource allocation, and ethical decision-making. Palliative care is ideally suited to address the myriad physical and emotional needs of renal patients at end of life, including effective symptom management, social and spiritual support, and clarification of priorities. Palliative consultation is increasingly common in advanced renal disease as patients, families, and care teams seek improved outcomes in the provision of compassionate care and comfort, at end of life.

References

1. Saini T, Murtagh FEM, Dupont PJ, et al. Comparative pilot study of symptoms and quality of life in cancer patients and patients with end stage renal disease. *Palliat Med* 2006; 20(6): 631–636.
2. Tranmer JE, Heyland D, Dudgeon D, et al. Measuring the symptom experience of seriously ill cancer and non cancer patients near end of life with the memorial symptom assessment scale. *J Pain Symptom Manage* 2003, 25(5): 420–429.
3. Murtagh FE, Addington-Hall JM, Edmonds PM, et al. Symptoms in advanced renal disease; a cross sectional survey of symptom prevalence in stage 5 chronic kidney disease managed without dialysis. *J Palliat Med* 2007; 10: 1266–1275.
4. Calvin AO. Haemodialysis patients and end of life decisions; a theory of personal preservation. *J Adv Nurs* 2004; 46(5): 558–566.
5. US Renal Data System, USRDS. *Annual Data Report, Atlas of Chronic Kidney Disease and End-Stage Renal Disease in the United States.* National Institutes of Health, National Institute of Diabetes and Digestive and Kidney Diseases, Bethesda, MD, 2008. Available at: www.usrds.org/2008/view/esrd'06.asp.
6. Clark WF, Na Y, Rosansky SJ, et al. Association between estimated glomerular filtration rate at initiation of dialysis and mortality. *CMAJ* 2011; 183(1): 47–53.
7. Davison S and Simpson C. Hope and advance care planning in patients with end stage renal disease: qualitative interview study. *BMJ* 2006; 333(7574): 886.

8. Renal Physicians of America. *Shared Decision-Making in the Appropriate Initiation Of and Withdrawal From Dialysis.* Rockville, MD: Renal Physicians of America, 2010. Available at: www.renalmd.org. Search-Shared Decision Making Recommendation Summary (accessed on July 13, 2012).

9. Kidney End-Of-Life Coalition. *Clinical Algorithms and Preferred Medications to Treat Pain in Dialysis Patients.* Available at: www.kidneyeol.org./Files/PainBrochure9-09.aspx (accessed on July 13, 2012).

10. *Robert Wood Johnson Foundation ESRD Peer Workgroup Report.* Available at: www.promotingexcellence.org/esrd/ (accessed on July 13, 2012).

11. Davison SN. Pain in haemodialysis patients: prevalence, etiology, severity and management. *Am J Kidney Dis* 2003; 42(6): 1239–1247.

12. Davison SN and Jhangri GS. The impact of chronic pain on depression, sleep, and the desire to withdraw from dialysis in haemodialysis patients. *J Pain Symptom Manage* 2005; 30(5): 465–473.

13. Twycross R and Wilcock A (eds). *Palliative Care Formulary,* 4th edition. Nottingham: Palliativedrugs.com.

14. College of Physicians & Surgeons of British Columbia. *Recommendations for the use of methadone in pain.* Vancouver: College of Physicians & Surgeons of British Columbia, 2005.

15. Krantz MJ, Martin J, Stimmel B, et al. QTc interval screening in methadone treatment. *Annals of Internal Medicine* 2009; 150(6): 387–395.

16. Black F and Downing MG. *Medical Care of the Dying,* 4th edition. 2006, Chap 7, p. 234.

17. Holley JL, Berns JS, and Sheridan AM. Acute complications during haemodialysis. *UpToDate 19.1.* Available at: www.uptodate.com/contents/acute-complications-during-hemodialysis (accessed on July 13, 2012).

18. Neely KJ and Roxe DM. Palliative care/hospice and the withdrawal of dialysis. *J Palliat Med* 2000; 3: 57–67.

19. Lynde C and Kraft J. End stage renal disease and the skin. *Parkhurst Exchange* Sept 2009; 48–50.

20. Lynde C and Kraft J. Skin manifestations of kidney disease. *Parkhurst Exchange* Feb 2007; 95–100.

21. Poppel DM, Cohen LM, and Germain MJ. The renal palliative care initiative. *J Palliat Med* April 2003; 6(2): 321–326.

22. Davison SN. End of life care preferences and needs: perceptions of patients with chronic kidney disease. *Clin J Am Soc Nephrol* 2010; 5: 195–204.

20 Pressure Ulcer Care and the Management of Malignant Wounds

Mary Walding

Katharine House Hospice, Banbury, UK

Introduction

This book focuses on the holistic nature of palliative care, exploring the impact that a limited prognosis may have on an individual and their family. Physical symptoms cause great distress, which can increase the psychological impact. This is particularly true of pressure ulcers and malignant wounds. Not only can they cause pain and discomfort but they are also a visible reminder of the impact of the disease on the individual. It is difficult to ignore such an obvious reminder of one's illness, and developing a wound may precipitate grieving for all that an individual is losing.

Denial is often associated with coping with this loss, and individuals may resist pressure-relieving strategies, or present with advanced fungating tumours that have previously been ignored. Treatment should respect the physical and psychological consequences and should always be what is acceptable to the individual. Box 20.1 identifies some of the factors to consider when assessing a patient's needs. The aim is to provide appropriate care that respects the patient's wishes and causes minimal disruption to their lifestyle.

Pressure ulcers

Pressure ulcers are also sometimes known as decubitus ulcers, pressure sores, or bed sores. The internationally recognised term is pressure ulcer [1] and will therefore be used in this text. A pressure ulcer is an area of localised damage to the skin and underlying tissue caused by pressure, sheer, friction, and/or a combination of these. It is difficult to assess the extent of the problem in the community, but the prevalence of pressure ulcers in the general hospital population is 4–32% [2], with a higher rate being generally reported in palliative care populations (26–38% [3]). This is due to the multiple factors involved in the maintenance and healing of normal skin that are compromised in the individual who is seriously ill.

Pressure ulcers rarely occur in those who are healthy because an individual will react to discomfort and alter position. Propensity to develop pressure ulcers is related to the following:

- Reduced mobility or immobility
- Sensory impairment
- Acute illness
- Level of consciousness
- Extremes of age
- Vascular disease
- Severe chronic or terminal illness
- History of pressure damage
- Malnutrition and dehydration

Development of pressure ulcers is exacerbated by some medications and moisture to the skin. Areas of the skin most likely to develop a pressure ulcer are those that tend to be in contact with support surfaces:

- Heels
- Sacrum
- Ischial tuberosities
- Femoral trochanters
- Elbows
- Temporal region of the skull (including ears)

Handbook of Palliative Care, Third Edition. Edited by Christina Faull, Sharon de Caestecker, Alex Nicholson and Fraser Black.
© 2012 by John Wiley and Sons, Inc. Published 2012 by John Wiley & Sons, Inc.

Box 20.1 Possible impact of skin damage on patients who are dying

Physical	Psychological
Pain	Anxiety
Fatigue	Depression
Odour	Grief
Immobility	Feeling that the wound dominates their life
Lifestyle restrictions	Fear

Box 20.2 Pressure ulcer reduction measures

- Nutritional support (consider involving the dietician).
- A mobility assessment by a physiotherapist.
- A review of manual handling procedures (how do the family manage?). Work with the physiotherapist to recommend moving and handling techniques.
- Pain control (as this may improve mobility).
- Skin hygiene.
- Assessment and treatment of any incontinence problems (this may require a specialist referral).
- Assessment of need for pressure-relieving support surfaces.
- Regular observation of vulnerable pressure points, as possible.
- Review of medication.

- Shoulders
- Back of head
- Toes

Signs of incipient pressure ulcer development include persistent erythema; non-blanching hyperemia; blisters; discolouration; and localised heat, oedema, or induration. It is recommended that all health-care professionals are aware of these signs and document and act upon them, including that health-care organisations recognise that any pressure ulcer of stage two or above should be treated as a clinical incident [1,4].

Risk assessment and risk reduction

Using knowledge of aetiology of pressure ulcers, assessment tools have been developed to assist health-care professionals in identifying those most at risk. The usefulness of these has been much debated within the nursing press. A major flaw with risk assessment tools is that they appear to be performing most poorly in settings where preventative care is most effective [5]. The value of assessment tools are primarily as aides-mémoire and as a guide to getting resources.

Using pressure ulcer risk assessment tools, most palliative care patients will be indicated as at "high risk" of developing a pressure ulcer. It is important that these scores are related to the clinical picture and incorporated into care plans that are realistic and acceptable to the patient. It may not be possible or appropriate to persuade a patient with a short prognosis to comply with all care, particularly when they only see a health-care professional for a brief time at home. However, they have a right to be given the information required for them to make an informed choice.

Measures that can be used to reduce the risk of pressure ulcers will depend on the needs and circumstances of the individual patient. Appropriate considerations are shown in Box 20.2.

Areas vulnerable to pressure ulcer development are those that are in contact with a support surface. One of the ways of reducing the risk of developing pressure ulcers is to encourage the patient to move regularly, certainly as soon as they begin to feel uncomfortable. However, many patients receiving palliative care require assistance to move and this will be restricted by carer availability, particularly in the community. A change in position, however minimal, should be suggested each time a carer has contact with a patient.

Pressure relief

A standard hospital mattress offers no pressure-relieving properties, neither is there evidence to suggest that soft mattress overlays are useful in preventing pressure sores. Guidelines state that all individuals assessed as being vulnerable to pressure ulcers should, as a minimum provision, be placed on a high-specification foam mattress with pressure-relieving properties [1,4]. It is important that patients at risk of pressure ulcer development also have a seating assessment undertaken by a physiotherapist or occupational therapist [6].

Pressure-relieving devices either use a conforming support surface to distribute body weight over a large area or are powered to create areas of low or zero pressure on body surfaces. These can be categorised as following:

- *High-specification foam mattresses*: There is consistent evidence of effectiveness with these, but they are not the ideal support surfaces for immobile patients [7].

• *Static air-filled*: These work by distributing the body weight evenly over a large area. Fluid-filled mattresses also work on the same principle, but have the disadvantage of weight.

• *Alternating pressure*: These consist of a system of cushions that are inflated and deflated in a preset alternating pattern, the cycle lasting several minutes. This relieves pressure and creates a pressure gradient that enhances blood flow. A wavelike motion may occasionally be felt, which can distress nauseated patients.

• *Air-fluidised systems*: These suspend the individual on a cushion of air, creating low interface pressure. They tend to be large, expensive, and cumbersome, but are effective if an individual is bedbound and immobile. The systems tend to be either cushion-based or bead-based. While the individual will require assistance to move on bead-based beds, the advantage is great if a patient has a wound that produces a lot of exudate, or if incontinence is a problem, as fluids will sink to the bottom of the bed and be removed later without infection risks. Maintenance costs and storage problems mean that most units will hire these when needed. It is unlikely that these will be used in the community setting.

The price and sophistication of these mattresses varies widely and the most expensive or technological is not necessarily the best. Each choice should be individual for the patient, taking into account their needs, abilities, and expectations.

Treatment of pressure ulcers

The aim of wound care is to minimise patient distress and discomfort, and where possible to promote healing. This can only be achieved through the holistic approach discussed earlier that considers the psychological and social issues alongside the physical problems.

Pain is often associated with pressure ulcers, and it should be addressed regardless of other proposed treatment options. Patients will often require extra analgesia about half an hour in advance of a dressing procedure.

It should not be assumed that pressure ulcers in a palliative care population will not improve; they have been seen to heal even in individuals who were within weeks of death [8]. However, many of the systemic factors that lead to pressure ulcer development will also inhibit wound healing [9]. The patient's care record should contain a detailed assessment of the status of all wounds, which is updated regularly [1]. Issues to be considered as part of an assessment are shown in Box 20.3.

National Pressure Ulcer Advisory Panel and European Pressure Ulcer Advisory Panel emphasise the need to use standardised staging criteria for effective communication between health-care professionals about pressure ulcers.

Box 20.4 suggests dressings that are suitable for certain wound criteria.

Box 20.3 Areas to consider within an assessment

- Location
- Size (width, length, depth)
- Presence of any sinuses
- Colour and type of wound tissue
- Exudate (amount and colour)
- Odour
- Condition of wound margins
- Condition of surrounding skin
- Pain
- Dressing management
- Patient perceptions of wound and wound management

Box 20.4 Suggested dressings for pressure ulcers

Appearance	Treatment
Intact skin, discoloured, erythema	Consider using a hydrocolloid dressing for protection. If it is possible to avoid pressure/friction and contact with urine or faeces, a transparent film may suffice
Damaged epidermis, slight damage to dermis	Hydrocolloid dressing. Leave *in situ* for 5–7 days if possible. If bleeding occurs, use an alginate dressing and a film dressing. Change daily
Full thickness, skin loss	Fill cavity with a hydrocolloid paste and cover with a hydrocolloid dressing
Slough or necrotic tissue	Autolysis may be facilitated by maintaining a moist wound environment. Use a collagen or hydrogel
Highly exuding wounds	Use hydrophilic foam sheets or cavity dressings. Use extra padding and film dressings to contain exudate. Wound drainage bags are also available

Wounds should not be routinely cleaned during dressing changes as this can cause physical damage, which disrupts the healing process. If debris or old dressing material needs to be removed this should be through irrigation with warmed isotonic (0.9%) sodium chloride [9].

Wounds are often colonised by a variety of bacteria, but this only constitutes an infection if there is evidence to suggest that the body's own defence systems cannot cope with the bacterial load—for example, there is increased erythema, increased exudate, malodorous exudate, pain, or pyrexia [4,10]. The decision to swab a wound to identify appropriate antibiotic therapy should only be taken if the patient's prognosis indicates this or if the effects of the infection are difficult for the patient.

Malignant wounds

A fungating malignant wound arises when malignant tumour cells infiltrate and erode through the skin. They develop most commonly from the following cancers: breast, head and neck, skin, and genital cancers. The incidence of these wounds in patients with cancer is poorly recorded, but it has been estimated that about 5% of patients with metastatic cancer will develop a malignant wound [11].

The spread tends to be through tissues that offer the least resistance—between tissue planes, along blood and lymph vessels, and in perineural spaces [12]. Abnormalities in tissue growth in malignant tumours lead to areas of tissue hypoxia and consequent infection of the nonviable tissue. It is this that results in the characteristic malodor and exudate of malignant wounds.

It may be possible to control tumour growth to prevent further problems associated with an invasive tumour. The options include the following:
- Radiotherapy.
- Chemotherapy (including topical miltefosine, for which there is weak evidence [13]).
- Hormone manipulation.
- Surgery.

However, tumours do not always respond to palliative treatment, and in these situations, it is necessary to manage the wound to minimise its impact on the patient. A malignant wound will affect social, emotional, mental, spiritual, and sexual well-being and the psychological impact for the patient and family may be great. Healthcare professionals must work with the patient and family as a team, to comprehensively assess needs and provide a plan of care. There are likely to be many professionals involved, and it is often helpful to identify a key worker to link with the patient so that information is shared appropriately and efficiently.

Physical manifestations need to be controlled as well as possible. Malignant wounds are very unlikely to heal [12], so conventional treatments to aid wound healing are less important than the priority of controlling odour and exudate. However, this is difficult to achieve, with many wounds requiring frequent dressing changes. These wounds are also complicated by their rapidly changing nature; therefore, dressing plans will need to be flexible.

A summary of symptom control considerations for malignant wounds is provided in Box 20.5.

As with all wounds, it is important to document an assessment of a malignant wound, so that all health professionals who are involved are aware of the state and requirements of the wound [11]. This also allows changes in the wound status to be noted and the effectiveness of dressing regimes to be evaluated.

Box 20.5 Summary of symptom control approaches for malignant wounds

Aim	Action
Control tumour growth	Consider radiotherapy, surgery, chemotherapy, low-powered laser therapy, hormonal treatment
Control malodor	Use occlusive dressings and charcoal pads. Consider the use of antibiotic therapy. Consider de-sloughing the wound. Use an air freshening unit and pleasant aromas. Consider the use of aromatherapy
Control pain	Review analgesia, consider the need for coanalgesics. Consider use of TENS. Involve complementary therapists
Control exudate	Use highly absorbent dressings and padding. Occlude wound if possible. Consider the use of wound drainage (or ileostomy) bags. Consider the use of radiotherapy
Control bleeding	Consider radiotherapy. Consider using adrenaline 1:1,000 soaks. Use padding and haemostatic dressings. Consider the use of silver sulphadiazine or sucralfate paste. Is there a risk of tumour infiltrating a vessel? If so, consider potential patient and family needs.

TENS, transcutaneous electronic nerve stimulation.

Dressings used for malignant wounds should be occlusive as this will help to control odour and exudate. This can be difficult to achieve as the wounds are not of a uniform size and shape, often being difficult to dress. It is important that the dressings do not adhere to the wound. If a malignant wound produces little exudate, a hydrocolloid dressing may be useful. Control of exudate is best achieved with hydrophilic foam, alginates, hydrofiber dressings, and semipermeable film dressing.

Large amounts of padding with absorbent materials are sometimes helpful, as is the use of wound drainage or colostomy bags if the wound can be contained and the bags will adhere. It can be helpful to use medical adhesive (and remove with a suitable solvent).

It is important that the skin surrounding the malignant wound is well protected. It is vulnerable to breakdown through infiltration, maceration due to the wound exudate, and damage caused during removal of dressings. "Second skin" dressings may be helpful and consideration may be given to some of the barrier preparations used around stomas. Stoma therapists are skilled in protecting skin around stoma sites and are a useful resource if difficulties are encountered. It may also be appropriate to use a thin hydrocolloid sheet cut to fit around the wound to provide protection.

The malodor associated with malignant wounds can cause great distress as the individual feels permanently unclean and may isolate themselves for fear of offending others. It may also cause nausea and associated problems with appetite. Where possible, the wound should be kept occluded, so odour escape is limited as much as possible. It is also possible to use charcoal dressing pads as an outer barrier as these will help neutralise odour. However, they become ineffective when wet.

The odour is caused by the anaerobic bacteria, which inhabits hypoxic and necrotic tissue. Metronidazole 200 mg orally t.d.s is sometimes an option. However, the incidence of nausea associated with this drug often reduces compliance and there is a possibility that effective dosage may be compromised by inconsistent vascular perfusion of the wound. It may be more effective to apply the antibiotic topically in the form of a gel. The disadvantage of this is cost, lack of available evidence about quantities to apply [14], and the fact that this mode of application may be of little use when there are large quantities of exudate.

De-sloughing the wound, that is, removing the devitalised tissue, is also worth considering [15], although this should be done with extreme caution as de-sloughing may uncover further problems, such as bleeding, in a malignant wound.

It is often helpful to provide an air-conditioning unit for individuals with fungating wounds, or consider the use of air fresheners or aromatherapy oils.

Fungating (proliferating) wounds are usually vascular and are thus prone to bleeding. The padding that is often necessary to contain exudate also has a useful protective function. If there is localised capillary bleeding, then one of the following may be used:

- Alginate dressings (these have some haemostatic properties).
- Topical adrenaline 1:1,000, applied to a dressing pad.
- Silver sulphadiazine (should be avoided during radiotherapy as it can disperse the rays).
- Sucralfate paste (crush a 1 g tablet and mix with 5 ml hydrogel).
- Prophylactic use of tranexamic acid 1 g tds orally or sometimes topically.

Malignant wounds can cause the rupture of a major blood vessel. The team caring for the individual should be aware of this and the consideration given to the need to inform the patient and their family, particularly if cared for in the community. It is sensible to follow precautions similar to any situation where a haemorrhage may be considered likely: to have a dark or red blanket to hand; to have gloves and pads; and to ensure there is adequate sedation and analgesia prescribed as required. It is also important to ensure that carers know who to call for support.

Malignant wounds are often associated with pain that is difficult to control. The pain may be potentiated by the impact of the tumour and the experience for an individual. It is important to involve the wider multidisciplinary team, including the complementary therapists.

The patient may require large doses of opiates, as well as the use of adjuvant drugs; nonsteroidal anti-inflammatory drugs are also important. If pain is uncontrolled, it is possible to apply opiates directly to the wound, using a 0.1% solution dissolved in a carrier hydrogel (10 mg morphine in 8 ml hydrogel, giving a 0.125% morphine solution [16,17]). However, this has limitations in highly exuding wounds and is not always effective. The pain may also have a neuropathic component, due to the effect of the tumour distorting nerve tissue. TCAs and TENS can be helpful. The latter is also of use in relieving the pruritus related to some malignant wounds.

Conclusion

Wounds may be seen as the most obvious indicator of an individual's disease. However, there are strategies available to reduce the impact on the patient and family. The use of creative, patient-centred, multidisciplinary management can maximise effectiveness of health-care professionals in this area.

References

1. European Pressure Ulcer Advisory Panel and the National Pressure Ulcer Advisory Panel. *Prevention and Treatment of Pressure Ulcers: Quick Reference Guide* Washington, DC: National Pressure Ulcer Advisory Panel, 2009.

2. Kaltenthaler E, Whitfield MD, Walters SJ, et al. UK, USA, and Canada: how do their pressure ulcer prevalence and incidence data compare? *J Wound Care* 2001; 10: 530–535.

3. Galvin J. An audit of pressure ulcer incidence in a palliative care setting. *Int J Palliat Nurs* 2002; 8(5): 214–221.

4. National Institute for Health and Clinical Excellence. *Pressure Ulcers: The Management of Pressure Ulcers in Primary and Secondary Care (CG29)*. London: NICE, 2005.

5. Moore ZEH and Cowman S. Risk assessment tools for the prevention of pressure ulcers. *Cochrane Database Syst Rev* 2008; (3): CD006471.

6. National Collaborating Centre for Nursing and Supportive Care. *The Use of Pressure Relieving Devices (Beds, Mattresses and Overlays) for the Prevention of Pressure Ulcers in Primary and Secondary Care*. London: National Institute for Clinical Excellence, 2003.

7. McInnes E, Bell-Syer SEM, Dumville JC, et al. Support surfaces for pressure ulcer prevention. *Cochrane Database Syst Rev* 2008; (4): CD001735.

8. Walding M and Andrews C. Preventing and managing pressure sores in palliative care. *Prof Nurse* 1995; 11(1): 33–38.

9. Hess CT and Kirsner RS. Uncover the latest techniques in wound bed preparation. *Nurs Manage* 2003; 34(12): 54–56.

10. Thomas S. *Wound Management and Dressings*. London: The Pharmaceutical Press, 1990.

11. Alexander S. Malignant fungating wounds: epidemiology, aetiology, presentation and assessment. *J Wound Care* 2009; 18(7): 273–280.

12. Grocott P. The palliative management of fungating malignant wounds. *J Wound Care* 1995; 4(5): 240–242.

13. Adderley UJ and Smith R. Topical agents and dressings for fungating wounds. *Cochrane Database Syst Rev* 2007; (2): CD003948.

14. Enck R. The management of large fungating tumours. *Am J Hosp Palliat Care* 1990; 7(3): 11–12.

15. Benbow M. Fungating malignant wounds and their management. *J Community Nurs* 2009; 23(11): 12–18.

16. Chief Medical Officer. *Topical Morphine Guidelines*. Auckland: Auckland District Health Board, 2006.

17. East Lancashire Drugs and Therapeutics Committee. *Topical Morphine for Painful skin Ulcers in Palliative Care*, 2009. Available at: www.elmmb.nhs.uk.

Further reading

Grocott P and Robinson V. Skin problems in palliative care: nursing aspects. In: Hanks G, Cherny N, Christakis N, Fallon M, Kaasa S, Portenoy R (eds), *Oxford Textbook of Palliative Medicine*, 4th edition. Oxford: Oxford University Press, 2010.

Twycross R, Wilcock A, and Stark Toller C. Skin care. In: *Symptom Management in Advanced Cancer*, 4th edition. Nottingham: Palliativedrugs.com Ltd, 2009.

21 Terminal Care and Dying

Christina Faull[1], Alex Nicholson[2]

[1] University Hospitals of Leicester and LOROS, The Leicestershire and Rutland Hospice, Leicester, UK
[2] South Tees Hospitals NHS Foundation Trust, Middlesbrough, UK

Introduction

Patients who are entering the last phase of their illness and for whom life expectancy is very short (days) require particular focus and expertise. A combination of a rapidly changing clinical situation and considerable psychological demands poses challenges to professionals that can only be met through competence, commitment, and human compassion. The patient's family requires a great deal of support, not only because they are losing someone that they love but also because providing care for someone who is very ill is incredibly challenging and tiring. One of the main reasons that people who wish to die at home are unable to do so is because family carers cannot continue to support this, either emotionally or because they are simply exhausted. It is also important to remember that the experience and memory of what actually happens during the last days of life has particular consequences for the bereaved [1].

Enabling patients to die with dignity, in comfort, and in the place of their choice is a very valuable skill bringing benefit to patients and also immense professional satisfaction:

> We celebrated his life by singing "All You Need is Love" by the Beatles. Palliative care helped him to die entirely on his own terms. I felt honoured to be involved in his care [2].

Furthermore, recent guidance from the General Medical Council (GMC) in the United Kingdom clarifies the expectation that doctors document that they have considered end-of-life care, discussed it with the patient or their representative, liaised and communicated within any multidisciplinary team (MDT), and recorded the results in an unambiguous and accessible way [3].

This chapter is concerned with how to care for patients whose health has deteriorated to the point when death is imminent. It includes how to recognise the terminal phase and how to manage the physical, psychological, and social needs of patients and their families or close carers including reference to the use of an integrated care pathway. A summary of physical symptom management is given in Figure 21.1.

Helping people to achieve the preferred place for their death

Most people say that they would ideally like to die at home [4]. However this is not true of everyone (about 25% of people say they want to die in a hospice) and the preference often depends on the patient's symptom burden, characteristics of their disease [5], previous experience of care, and social factors. For example, many people with COPD may prefer to be in hospital where they know the staff well and especially if there is even a small chance that they may recover from yet another acute exacerbation of their condition. Perhaps social circumstances are the most important because unless the close family is supportive of the patient being at home this may be difficult to achieve [6]. Psychological factors are also a key determinant and a high level of anxiety or fear may make people feel unsafe at home. In addition, many people do not want to feel a burden to their family or leave "bad memories."

Asking people where they want to die is not straightforward [7]. Many practitioners find discussing preferred place of death a difficult area of practice, unless the patient broaches the subject. Also perhaps as many as 30% of patients change their mind about their preference as they progress through their illness [8]. Preferences for place of death are typically dynamic, evolving as the circumstances and their impacts unfold with progression toward

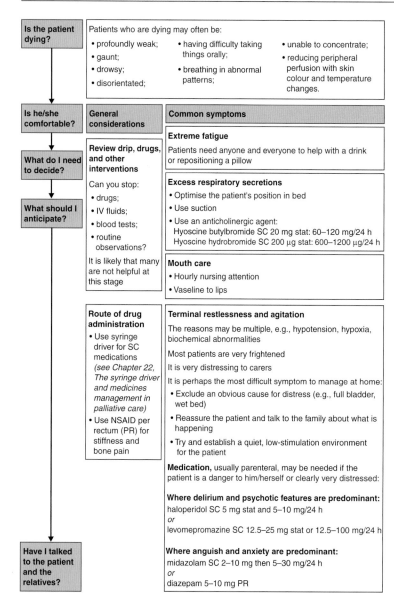

Is the patient dying?	Patients who are dying may often be:

- profoundly weak;
- gaunt;
- drowsy;
- disorientated;
- having difficulty taking things orally;
- breathing in abnormal patterns;
- unable to concentrate;
- reducing peripheral perfusion with skin colour and temperature changes.

Is he/she comfortable?

General considerations

Common symptoms

Extreme fatigue

Patients need anyone and everyone to help with a drink or repositioning a pillow

What do I need to decide?

Review drip, drugs, and other interventions

Can you stop:
- drugs;
- IV fluids;
- blood tests;
- routine observations?

What should I anticipate?

It is likely that many are not helpful at this stage

Excess respiratory secretions
- Optimise the patient's position in bed
- Use suction
- Use an anticholinergic agent:
  Hyoscine butylbromide SC 20 mg stat: 60–120 mg/24 h
  Hyoscine hydrobromide SC 200 μg stat: 600–1200 μg/24 h

Mouth care
- Hourly nursing attention
- Vaseline to lips

Route of drug administration
- Use syringe driver for SC medications (see Chapter 22, The syringe driver and medicines management in palliative care)
- Use NSAID per rectum (PR) for stiffness and bone pain

Terminal restlessness and agitation

The reasons may be multiple, e.g., hypotension, hypoxia, biochemical abnormalities

Most patients are very frightened

It is very distressing to carers

It is perhaps the most difficult symptom to manage at home:
- Exclude an obvious cause for distress (e.g., full bladder, wet bed)
- Reassure the patient and talk to the family about what is happening
- Try and establish a quiet, low-stimulation environment for the patient

Medication, usually parenteral, may be needed if the patient is a danger to him/herself or clearly very distressed:

Where delirium and psychotic features are predominant:
haloperidol SC 5 mg stat and 5–10 mg/24 h
or
levomepromazine SC 12.5–25 mg stat or 12.5–100 mg/24 h

Where anguish and anxiety are predominant:
midazolam SC 2–10 mg then 5–30 mg/24 h
or
diazepam 5–10 mg PR

Have I talked to the patient and the relatives?

Figure 21.1 A summary of the management of physical symptoms in the dying patient. (Adapted from Faull C and Woof R. *Palliative Care: An Oxford Core Text*, 2002, with permission from the Oxford University Press.)

the final days of life and unexpected problems arise (e.g., coping with severe agitation). Preferences can also often be vague or only partially formed. Only some patients voice very clear preferences that are unwavering (e.g., "definitely want to die at home") [9].

A large number of patients who die do not appear to have had a discussion or have not been able to express a preference. In a snapshot of primary care in England in 2009, only 27% of people that died had been identified in advance and put on the practice register. Of these, only 58% were offered a discussion about preferences for end-

of-life care and 42% actually had a preference recorded (i.e., 11% of all deaths) [10].

However, even allowing for change of heart and the difficulties of accurate prognostication there is a big gap between what patients seem to want and what is achieved. Social support and health-care inputs have been found to be the most important factors enabling people to stay at home [11]. Patients need:
- family or other lay carers;
- adequate nursing care;
- night sitting service;

- good symptom control;
- confident committed GPs;
- access to specialist palliative care;
- a clear plan of wishes and preferences, including resuscitation status;
- effective coordination of care;
- sufficient information for family and carers; and
- effective out-of-hours medical and nursing services.

Is home "best"?

For many patients home is indeed "best." They want to be at home, their family wishes to assist them in this, and support from health and social care can make this experience the best possible.

Many people, however, change their minds when the reality of the situation for both themselves and their carers is apparent [8]. Dying can, even with great symptom management and lots of support, turn out to be much more difficult than people anticipate. Our understanding of this time and its struggles for patients and carers is becoming more sophisticated. The palliative care provided for patients with cancer or cardiopulmonary disease was studied in two practices in Leicestershire, UK [12]. Roughly one out of five people died at home and one out of two people in hospital. Fifteen percent of patients with cancer died in the hospice but none of the patients with cardiopulmonary disease. In this retrospective study, 41% of relatives indicated that the patients had expressed a preference in where they wanted to die, 95% indicating home. Although less than half of those that expressed a preference were able to achieve this, 77% of carers felt that, on balance, the place that the patient had died had been the best place for them to die, irrespective of whether it was their preferred place of death or not.

The potential advantages and disadvantages of the various settings of care for the dying patient are shown in Table 21.1.

When is a patient terminally ill?

To achieve all the quality outcomes of terminal care (preferred place of death, successful symptom management, spiritual care, and a good experience for the carers), the first step is actually to recognise that someone is dying. While this seems an obvious statement, failure to recognise the onset of the last days of life features prominently in many reports looking at improving end-of-life care:

Sixty three per cent of patients who died in hospital had the fact that death was expected recorded in their notes. In most

of these cases, however, this assessment was made less than one week before death. The timing of this assessment may have left insufficient time for an appropriate care package to be arranged [19].

This is not just a failure in the hospital setting. In this report by the National Audit Office, nearly three-quarters of those people who died in hospital were admitted from their own home. Just under a quarter were admitted from a care home, the majority of whom were already receiving nursing care. Most admissions involved self-referral in some form or another (e.g., a 999 call was the source of referral in 36% of cases) and GP involvement in the admission of patients who subsequently died in hospital was limited (19% of cases).

Professionals require sophisticated clinical acumen to make the distinction between inevitable decline and potentially reversible deterioration. This dilemma is most pronounced in patients with nonmalignant illness where episodic, life-threatening deterioration is part of the "normal" progressive disease trajectory (e.g., heart failure (HF) and chronic obstructive airways disease). These are difficult distinctions to make in practice, requiring clinical wisdom, experience and expertise, and should be made as a team. Indeed, the most important element in diagnosing dying is that the members of the multiprofessional team caring for the patient agree that the patient is likely to die. Where there is disagreement between team members, opposing goals of care are sought and then mixed messages are presented to patient, carer, and wider team members, resulting in poor patient management and confused communication. Barriers to making these decisions are shown in Box 21.1.

> ## Key point
>
> Recognising that a patient is probably dying is perhaps "the" most important factor in enabling achievement of all the factors we associate with a "good death."

HF is the most common cause of death in many hospital wards. Experienced clinicians can recognise a subgroup of patients, admitted to hospital because of worsening HF, whose prognosis seems to be particularly poor. These patients are often characterised by

- previous admissions with worsening HF; the absence of any identifiable reversible precipitant for the current exacerbation; already being treated with optimised conventional drugs titrated to maximum tolerable levels;

Table 21.1 Advantages and disadvantages of different care settings.

Setting	Advantages	Disadvantages
Home	• Often preferred by patients [13] • Familiar surroundings and a nonmedical environment • Family life maintained • Patient in control (e.g., decisions, visitors, cultural/spiritual needs) • Home is generally a more peaceful environment • Familiar with medical staff (GP and district nurse)	• Pain control may be inadequate [14] • Specialist palliative care services not always available for nonmalignant disease • Professional help not as accessible • Patients may not be protected from unwelcome visitors • Burden of caregiving falls on the relatives and friends who may be unable or unwilling to cope • Disruption of family life • Financial consequences to care at home • Critically ill patients may need intensive support (e.g., daily or twice daily visit by GP)
Nursing/residential home	• Immediate access to nursing care (except in residential care) • The family is relieved of the burden of care • Familiar GP will have ongoing responsibility for medical care	• Financial implications for patients and families • Standards of care may be variable, being limited by resources • Surroundings are unfamiliar • Families may experience guilt; "don't put me in a home" • Staff knowledge on symptom control may be limited [15] • Families may feel there is a lack of specialist medical and nursing attention [16,17]
Hospital	• Medical and nursing expertise is readily available • Burden of care is removed from the family • Patients and families may feel safe knowing that doctors and nurses are available	• Patients and families may feel isolated on a busy unit [18] • Nursing care may be limited by resources • Symptoms may be poorly controlled [18] • Care is more orientated to cure • Unfamiliarity with staff • Family may not be encouraged to participate in the care of the patient • Visiting hours may be restricted
Hospice	• Immediate access to specialised staff, within a multidisciplinary team • Palliative care philosophy is widely applied • Most have a higher staff ratio of qualified nurses • Generally less noisy, more peaceful environment than hospitals • Bereavement support is generally more available	• Hospices may be perceived as "a place to die" • Unfamiliar surroundings • Some hospices may be perceived as being too "religious" • Many hospices may not meet the needs of patients from ethnic minority groups (although this could be true of other settings)

deteriorating renal function; and failure to respond within 2 or 3 days to appropriate changes in diuretic or vasodilator drugs.

While others steadily improve, such patients often continue to worsen, although they may survive for a week or more [20]. For these patients and for others with chronic conditions who have deteriorated to the point where recovery from an acute or subacute illness seems very uncertain, the likelihood of recovery and the justification for continuing invasive treatments or monitoring should be reviewed and discussed with patients and carers and between primary and secondary care doctors.

Some hospitals have adopted tools to help clinicians work with the parallel curative and palliative approaches to a very sick patient. The AMBER care bundle© [21] (Figure 21.2) has been developed and piloted in a number of acute hospital settings. The AMBER care bundle provides a systematic approach to manage the care of hospital patients who are facing an uncertain recovery and who are at risk of dying in the next

1–2 months. Evidence suggests the AMBER care bundle results in:

- improved decision making (including care escalation and resuscitation);
- a positive impact on multiprofessional team communication and working;
- increased nurses' confidence about when to approach medical colleagues to discuss treatment plans;
- greater clarity with patients around uncertainty, preferences, and plans with daily review of these; and
- significantly lower emergency readmission rates.

Recognising the onset of dying

It is useful to look for the following signs as indicators of irreversible decline. This process is often gradual, but progressive:

- Profound weakness
- Gaunt appearance
- Drowsiness
- Disorientation
- Diminished oral intake
- Difficulty taking oral medication
- Poor concentration
- Skin colour changes
- Temperature change at extremities

How to assess the needs of a terminally ill patient

Ideally, needs should be defined by the patient and be managed in terms of quality of life. However, in terminal care, it is not usually appropriate to make exhaustive assessments. In addition, communication with the patient may be difficult and accounts from carers can be inaccurate. Skills in nonverbal assessment of pain and distress are important [22] but a high degree of uncertainty may exist. Professionals therefore have to shoulder and share

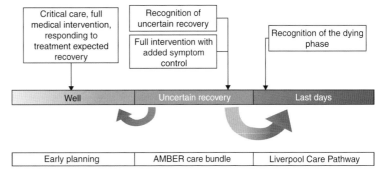

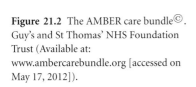

Figure 21.2 The AMBER care bundle©. Guy's and St Thomas' NHS Foundation Trust (Available at: www.ambercarebundle.org [accessed on May 17, 2012]).

greater responsibility when making difficult decisions in these situations. This can make practitioners feel outside their "comfort zone" and be a key factor leading to inappropriate and unwanted hospital admissions. The wise practitioner is able to use professional experience combined with knowledge of the patient (previous symptoms, concerns, wishes), and information from team colleagues, to perform a sensitive, problem-focused assessment.

Psychosocial needs of patients

When assessing patients' needs, it is important to remember that some psychosocial problems may present as poorly controlled physical symptoms (e.g., total pain, terminal agitation, and sick with fear). Some of the common problems experienced are outlined in Box 21.2.

Also, factors such as personality, relationships, and coping mechanisms are important to consider. Giving patients time and encouraging them to express their feelings is particularly important. Some, however, will not appreciate unrequested "counselling" and should be allowed the option of denial as a legitimate coping mechanism.

In responding to patient concerns and providing emotional support, it is helpful to use the following guidelines:

- Consider where the patient wants to die and whether this is this likely to be possible.
- Involve the patient in decision-making for as long as possible.
- Answer the patient's questions honestly, giving him/her time. Explanations may need to be repeated on several occasions.
- Patient confidentiality should be assured. There may be things that they do not want to share with their family, or certain family members.
- Allay any fears about dying (such as uncontrolled symptoms, prolonged process, being alone, and lack of warning).

Box 21.2 Psychosocial needs: what to look for

- Fear, for example, mode of death and drug side effects
- Guilt, for example, becoming a burden and past life experiences
- Anger, for example, loss of dignity, missed opportunities, and loss of independence
- Uncertainty, for example, spiritual questions, prognosis, and the future of the family

---

- Space and privacy should be provided if the patient wishes.
- Consider the patient's spiritual needs. Respect culture and religious views.
- Reassure patients that their family will be offered bereavement support.
- Do not let the medical process obstruct the expression of affection between loved ones.
- Make careful enquiries about the patient's will and other important tasks.

Importance of religion and ritual in dying

For those patients who possess a strong religious conviction as part of their spirituality, rituals around death are very important. Professionals should be respectful of this and act with sensitivity to these requirements. Table 21.2 gives a brief outline of some of the traditional practices of the main religious and cultural groups in the United Kingdom. It is beyond this book to give a detailed account of all beliefs and rituals. It is hoped that this introduces professionals to what they may encounter in their care of dying patients. We all have values, beliefs, and rituals that influence the way we experience and cope with life and death. Enquiring about the religious needs of patients can be especially appreciated by both patients and their families (see Chapter 24, *Spirituality in palliative care*). What is of vital importance in culturally safe care is that we ask and explore as we would in any other aspect of care. For example:

> Can I ask you please what your faith means to you at this time? Is there anything that you need or that you particularly don't want?
>
> People like to be cared for in different ways in their last days and after that. We want to get this right for you all. Could you possibly talk me through what you as a Jewish person want to do and who you might want to be involved?

It is also important to remember that in a pluralistic society such as the United Kingdom, religious law can be interpreted in various ways. Consequently, religious practices may be applied differently by each and every individual and should never be assumed.

Clinical care at the end of life

Principles of management

The care of people who are dying often requires a change of emphasis [23]. To provide quality terminal care as defined

Table 21.2 Overview of rituals around death for main UK religious/cultural groups.

Religion/culture	Death rituals	Disposal of the body
Christianity	• Traditionally a priest performs the last rites before death (prayers of forgiveness and sacrament if possible) • Individuals may wish to pray with the dying patient	• Body can be touched by non-Christians • Body is cleaned and covered with a white sheet • Body can be buried or cremated • Funeral directors assist in much of this preparation • The religious component of bereavement occurs at the funeral service
Islam	• Patient should face Mecca if possible • May keep beard once they have been on pilgrimage to Mecca & wear a topi (head gear). Not to be removed • May prefer to die at home as hospital is seen as for cure only • Mullah (religious leader) may whisper prayers in patient's ear	• Traditionally the body should not be touched by non-Muslims • Washing and preparing the body follows precise rules • Burial should occur within 24 h or as soon as possible • Postmortems and organ donation are resisted • Burial is the traditional means of disposal of the body
Hinduism	• Brahmin priests may perform rituals that allow forgiveness of sins • A thread may be left around the wrist to show that the patient has received a priest's blessing • Devout Hindus may wish to die on the floor, being close to mother earth	• Correct funeral rites are believed to be important for the salvation of the deceased's soul • Body is washed and put in normal clothes • Only men can perform funeral rites, preferably the eldest son • Cremation is used to dispose of the body • Bereavement involves 10 days of mourning, each day has a particular ceremony
Sikhism	• A reader from the temple will recite hymns, if the patient is too weak to do this personally • At death attendants may utter words of praise (Wonderful lord, Wonderful lord)	• The body is washed and placed in a shroud • Religious artefacts worn by patient will be left on the body—"the 5 K's": Kangha, wooden comb; Kara, iron wrist band; Kirpan, short sword; Kachha, undershorts; and Kesh, uncut hair • Traditionally Sikhs are cremated • Friends and family consider visiting the bereaved as a duty and may provide food
Judaism	• Psalms are recited and the patient should not be left alone • Pillows should not be removed from beneath the head (is believed to hasten death)	• The body should be left for 10 min after death • The body may be laid on the floor, with feet pointing to the door • Preparation of the body can be precise and is performed by Jews who specifically deal with the dead • Burial should occur within 24 h of death • Bereavement is structured with religious ceremony

(continued)

Table 21.2 (*Continued*)

Religion/culture	Death rituals	Disposal of the body
Buddhism	• The patient will wish to die with a "clear mind" and may use chanting to achieve this. This influences the nature of the next incarnation • There may be a wish to avoid distractions, for example, sedating drugs, overcrowding of room, intrusions • Most Buddhists believe that consciousness remains in or near the body for 8–12 h after death. This may mean that some Buddhists would prefer the body not to be touched during this period	• Ideally the body should not be moved or washed before the arrival of a Buddhist monk • Disposal of the body may be by burial, cremation, or embalming, depending on the nationality of the deceased
Rastafarianism	• Rastafarians are reluctant to undergo treatments it may contaminate God's temple (their body) • Western style medicine may come second to CTs such as herbalism • Blood transfusion and organ transplant are not acceptable	• Orthodox members show their symbol of faith through a dreadlocks hairstyle, which is not cut at all • After death, Rastafarians have 10 days of scripture reading and praying • Prayers are said in the name of Ras Tafari, the new Messiah

by the National Institute for Clinical Excellence [24], the principles outlined in Chapter 1, *The context and principles of palliative care*, need to be applied in a focused and rigorous way. Dying people require a truly holistic approach to their care. Consider the patient and their family and friends as the unit of care, and encourage participation from all of these people. It is vital to offer frequent information and support to patients and families. Every effort should be made to reduce the morbidity due to bereavement among family and friends. If the patient is in hospital, explore whether they would rather be cared for at home and what will be needed to achieve this.

A clinical pathway approach has been shown to be particularly effective in enabling high-quality care. For example the *Liver Care Pathway (LCP) for the Dying Patient* is a systematic approach to defining and monitoring the needs of patients, together with guidance for interventions that are commonly required [20,25,26]. However, it is important to ensure that the use of such a tool does not reduce dying to a "tick-box" exercise. The concerns of the family that might arise from misinterpretation of a "dying pathway" need to be specifically addressed. Maintaining comfort and dignity with the use of medication including judicious use of analgesics and sedatives is good clinical

practice and most emphatically not euthanasia. This needs to be clear.

It is important to perform a systematic physical assessment (see Box 21.3) and relieve the patient's physical symptoms promptly bearing in mind these may be multifactorial and remembering the psychosocial component (e.g., fear) of certain symptoms. Avoiding unnecessary medical intrusion ("First do no harm") is paramount.

Box 21.3 Physical assessment checklist: what to look for

• Pain
• Shortness of breath
• Nausea/vomiting
• Agitation/restlessness/confusion
• Myoclonus and epilepsy
• Noisy breathing
• Urinary incontinence or retention
• Constipation
• Pressure areas/skin care
• Dry/sore mouth
• Difficulty in swallowing
• Reversible complications/comorbidity

Medication should be reviewed and all unnecessary drugs discontinued.

Resuscitation status and decisions

In most care settings, documentation of the resuscitation status of the patient will be required. As the patient is dying of their disease, resuscitation is clinically futile and any decision that resuscitation will not be attempted (do not attempt cardiopulmonary resuscitation [DNACPR]) is clinically led [27]. A DNACPR form or order will need to be kept with the patient. Sensitive discussion of the rationale behind this decision, as of all components of the management plan, should be undertaken with the patient, provided this is not deemed unduly burdensome in the context of the patient's condition. Consideration should be given to sharing this information also with the family. This is of particular importance for patients at home where the form will be in the house and available for all to see. Remember this is a sharing of information and an opportunity to identify and explore concerns. The clinician is sharing information about resuscitation status *with* a patient or carers, not asking for a decision to be made on the status *by* the patient or carers (see Chapter 5, *Ethical issues in palliative care*, and Chapter 8, *Advance care planning*). Box 21.4 highlights key steps in any resuscitation discussion.

Box 21.4 Suggested steps in a discussion about resuscitation

- Clarify the patient/carer understanding of the current medical condition.
- Clarify that the future expected course of the illness is further deterioration in strength and ability with increasing fatigue giving way to exhaustion and increasing periods of time spent sleeping.
- Emphasise aspects of the care being given, including regular review of symptoms, administration of symptom relief medication, and support to the patient and carers.
- Explain that as the illness progresses further the body systems will gradually slow down so that there comes a point when the heart will no longer beat, breathing will stop, and life will end.
- Explain that emergency treatments that might apply in other medical emergencies, such as "electric shock treatments to restart the heart," will not be given in this situation because they will not work.
- Explain that to avoid intrusive and inappropriate treatments, appropriate paperwork needs to be put in place to make sure all professionals involved understand what to do and what not to do.

Anticipating future needs

Anticipatory planning, follow-up, continuity, and 24-h emergency cover are key. The team should plan thoroughly to pre-empt future problems, in what is likely to be a rapidly changing clinical picture. There are five common symptoms in the terminal phase that are encountered regardless of diagnosis. These symptoms and their management are discussed more later in this chapter. It is good practice to make sure the drugs that may be needed to manage these symptoms are in the home (or care home or ward) and appropriate prescribing authorisation is in place for whichever clinician is called. Involve all necessary resources for extra support at an early stage and ensure good communication, especially with out-of-hours services.

Communication with emergency and out-of-hours services

Many health communities have developed systems to communicate across services about potential problems for dying patients. In the United Kingdom, these include referral forms to emergency or "out-of-hours" duty doctor and community nursing organisations and notification documents to providers of ambulance or emergency response services. The intention is that if these services are called by the family in a crisis, there is useful background information provided by the patient's own regular medical and/or nursing team, which will help guide the clinician called to attend to the patient outside routine working hours.

General care at the end of life

Depending on where the dying patient is being cared for, nursing care will be delivered by a combination of professional and lay carers. Supporting and involving family members in this care, provided they are physically and emotionally able to participate in a "hands-on" way, can be very empowering. This is important at a time when the relatives/carers may otherwise feel excluded or not in control.

Positioning and pressure care

Careful positioning of the patient to ease discomfort and contribute to good pressure area care, with appropriate pressure relieving mattresses, is crucial at a time when the vast majority of patients will spend all their time in bed. Continence problems compound risks to skin integrity exacerbated by poor nutrition and deteriorating circulation.

Mouth and eye care

Several factors result in potentially poor oral hygiene, dryness, and odour in the last days of life. Many drugs, especially opioids and those with anticholinergic effects, reduce salivary secretion. Mouth breathing and oxygen flow further increase water loss from the mucosal surface. Dry crusted uncomfortable secretions may accumulate and the perception of thirst worsen. Regular mouth care with sips of water if feasible, or sponges soaked with water applied carefully onto the tongue and inside the cheeks, may relieve crusting and thirst, and support maintenance of a fresh pink mucosal surface and reduced halitosis. Vaseline or other moisturiser applied to the lips provides relief. These measures can be offered by the family/carers, helping them to feel involved in nurturing the patient.

Careful eye care to remove dried tears and mucus may comfort the patient and maintain their dignity and appearance.

Bladder and bowel care

It is important to remember these fundamental elements of care because without attention to them, other needs are harder to fulfil.

Urinary problems are common in the terminal phase and must be excluded in any patient who demonstrates agitation in the last phase of life.

Incontinence arises due to immobility and generalised weakness. A patient who is left to lie in wet clothing or bedding will become agitated and distressed, skin integrity will be compromised, and dignity lost. Simple practical measures including attentive nursing, use of pads, provision of a commode for the patient who can still be transferred from bed to chair, and penile sheaths may help. In many cases, catheterisation will be appropriate to the situation and should be offered and the potential benefits explained carefully to the patient/carer.

Retention of urine is also common. Causes include prostatic outflow obstruction, constipation, and the anticholinergic effects of medication. Where possible, predisposing factors should be excluded but in the last days of life some of the culprit drugs may be specifically indicated for control of respiratory secretions or intestinal colic. Again, the option of catheterisation may be most practicable.

Constipation is a problem for many frail patients and this is just as true in the last days of life. A combination of drugs, inability to take oral laxatives, reduced food and fluid intake, electrolyte changes, and poor mobility combine to increase the risk of constipation substantially. In severe cases, there may be faecal impaction resulting in anorectal pain and agitation. As for urinary problems, constipation should always be excluded as a cause of agitation before sedatives are administered. Even in a frail patient, significant relief may be obtained from rectal intervention.

Decision making about nutrition and hydration

Ethical principles and guidance

In considering the ethical and legal aspects of nutritional support, an expert report commissioned by the UK NICE [28] states:

> a distinction has to be drawn between those cases where a patient's life can be prolonged indefinitely by treatment or provision of nutrition, but only at a cost of great suffering, and those cases where the 'incompetent' patient is in the final stages of life and although treatment would prolong the dying process this would be at the cost of comfort and dignity.

Detailed and explicit guidance is available from the GMC (London) End-of-Life guidance [3] (see www.gmc.org.uk). The recommendations are not reproduced here but emphasise the need for careful decision-making, including acknowledging the patient's wishes, and a need to weigh the benefits and burdens of intervention. The need for careful explanation of decisions made, regular review, and the requirement that a second opinion be offered if there is disagreement are key principles.

Fluids

The evidence base for and against artificial hydration (fluid supplementation given by the subcutaneous (SC) or intravenous (IV) route) is equivocal. There is a range of professional's views and a variety of evidence or lack of it to support these. There are arguments for and against thirst being associated with dehydration in the terminally ill. There are also suggested benefits (reduced oedema, urine output and therefore incontinence, and reduced respiratory secretions) that need to be set against disadvantages (risk of delirium and impaired clearance of opioid metabolites) in relation to symptom control for dying patients who are dehydrated (Box 21.5). Harlos [29] advises:

> helping navigate the 'path of least regret' is an important task in the terminal phase.

It is important to bear in mind that treatment decisions may have a bearing on the place in which it is possible to care for a patient, and this may be an overriding consideration, and there are times when a trial of intervention for a defined period of time before reviewing evidence of efficacy may be considered appropriate.

Box 21.5 Considerations on artificial hydration at the end of life

For	Against
May reduce thirst	May prevent care being delivered at home—even if SC fluids are proposed
May support renal clearance of drugs/metabolites lessening risk of adverse effects of accumulation	Infusion sites may be painful
Reduces risk of agitation due to dehydration	Additional infusion sites and giving sets to manage (alongside SC infusions of symptom medication)
Reduces anxieties about "giving up" or "letting die"	Possible exacerbation of peripheral and pulmonary oedema
Reduces lay and professional carer concerns about accusation of neglect in patients whose terminal phase is prolonged (e.g., noncancer)	Risk of "medicalising" last days of life
Limited evidence to support intervention	Limited evidence to support withholding
	Risk of giving a mixed message or false hope to patient and family

If a decision is made in favour of supplemental fluids, SC administration (known as hypodermoclysis) is recommended over IV infusion. The advantages of hypodermoclysis include [29] the following:
- No requirement to secure a cannula in a peripheral vein when veins are fragile and skin thin and easily bruised.
- Convenient access points provided edematous and lymphoedematous areas are avoided.
- Avoids the risk of thrombophlebitis.
- SC access may be secured and used intermittently to suit patient's day/night routine.

Artificial nutrition (nasogastric, percutaneous endoscopic gastrostomy, and percutaneous endoscopic jejunostomy feeding)

As indicated in the National Collaborating Centre report [28], neither total parenteral nutrition (TPN) nor enteral feeding is recommended to be commenced in the last days of life. TPN should be withdrawn as the risks far outweigh the benefits. Central lines can be kept in place. There needs to be a clear rationale for continuing enteral feeding because this is of some harm to the patient and unlikely to be of any benefit. Families may find this hard as it may feel as though it is hastening death or increasing suffering. An explanation that the body cannot use the nutrition and that it may worsen nausea and abdominal pain and potentially increase the risk of aspiration pneumonia is helpful reassurance. Sometimes it is appropriate to replace enteral feeding with enteral clear fluids only. The GMC guidance on this area of practice is helpful [3].

Therapeutics at the end of life

Review and rationalisation of medication

In the weeks preceding the last days of life, regular review by the clinical team should include rationalisation of medication. Treatments which are preventative in intent for chronic conditions including those listed below, should have been discontinued with a supportive explanation to the patient:
- hypercholesterolaemia/hyperlipidaemia;
- osteoporosis;
- vitamin and iron deficiencies;
- disease-modifying treatments, for example, for motor neuron disease (MND) and dementia; and
- hormonal antagonists treating some cancers (e.g., breast and prostate cancer).

The patient's clinical deterioration, weight loss, reduced activity, and general frailty means that further drug groups should be reviewed. The extent to which the drug controls possible day-to-day symptoms (such as breathlessness due to pulmonary oedema) rather than disordered physiology (such as antihypertensives) will influence which medication is reduced, by how much, and when. Examples include:
- antihypertensives;
- antianginals;
- oral antidiabetic agents; and
- diuretics, angiotensin-converting enzyme inhibitors (ACEIs), and other cardiac drugs.

Table 21.3 Medicines management approaching end of life.

Treatment	Recommendation
Antiepileptic medication	Replace with midazolam SC infusion starting dose 30 mg/24 h
	Prescribe rectal diazepam 10 mg as needed for frank convulsion
	Any recurrence of seizures indicates need to increase midazolam dose to 30–40 mg/24 h
	Further problems—seek specialist advice
Corticosteroids	In the last few days of life, these serve no purpose for most patients. Some, who have a very slow decline, may benefit from avoiding the symptoms of hypoadrenal crisis (exacerbation of weakness/malaise) by dexamethasone 2 mg given subcutaneously once daily. A few patients need them to continue to prevent fits or headaches recurring. An oral to SC conversion ratio of 1 mg:1 mg is appropriate
Oxygen	If the patient is unresponsive in terminal phase care, slowly reduce and withdraw oxygen over 1–2 h. If withdrawal appears to prompt symptoms (agitation or breathlessness), small doses of rescue opioid or benzodiazepine (see below) may be given
Diabetes management	See algorithm—Appendix 7

With further deterioration as prognosis shifts from weeks to days and the patient struggles to take oral medication, wisdom and pragmatism require that remaining drugs are either discontinued or changed to an alternative route (Table 21.3). Management of current symptoms now becomes paramount. The team must feel confident to stop drugs such as thyroxine, aspirin, and antidepressants. Some drugs/treatments require special consideration.

Symptom management in the last days of life

Symptom management in the last days of life involves two key elements: (1) maintenance of existing symptom control and (2) anticipation of new symptoms.

Ongoing symptom management

In the last months and weeks of life, multiple symptoms are common. In a detailed review [30] of studies of symptom prevalence in patients with advanced disease, pain, depression, anxiety, breathlessness, insomnia, nausea, constipation, and diarrhoea were among the most common symptoms whatever the diagnosis, be it cancer or noncancer. At this stage, patients are often taking several different drugs in a combination that has been adjusted to control their symptom burden. As the deteriorating patient weakens and struggles to take oral medication, review of the treatment plan requires use of alternative routes, wherever possible, to ensure that symptoms continue to be controlled.

The SC route is favoured in palliative care practice (see Chapter 22, *The syringe driver and medicines management in palliative care*).

Ongoing symptom control of pain, nausea, vomiting, breathlessness, anxiety, and insomnia is possible with a switch from oral to SC medication.

Some drugs (e.g., opioids) require a dose adjustment when the route of administration changes. Some will require a change of agent. Others can be switched with a direct substitution from oral to parenteral formulation (see Table 21.4). It is not inevitable that pain will worsen as the patient enters the last days of life but rescue analgesia should be prescribed by the nonoral route and requirements continue to be reviewed to guide titration of analgesia against pain. For guidance on how to manage patients with fentanyl patches for pain see Appendix 1.

Anticipatory prescribing for common symptoms in the last days of life (see Appendixes 2–6)

Five symptoms are common at the end of life:
1. Pain
2. Breathlessness
3. Nausea and vomiting
4. Respiratory secretions
5. Restlessness and agitation/delirium.

These may already be present, and worsen, or appear as new problems. While quoted prevalence rates vary depending on study methodology, patient population,

Table 21.4 Guidance on switching agent and route of typical drugs for symptom management of pain, nausea and vomiting, breathlessness, and anxiety in the last days of life.[a]

Oral treatment (dose/24 h)	Nonoral (CSCI) option (dose/24 h)	Notes
Analgesics [31]		
Morphine 30 mg	Morphine 15 mg	Based on approximate opioid dose equivalences
Morphine 30 mg	Diamorphine 10 mg	
Oxycodone 20 mg	Oxycodone 10–15 mg	
Hydromorphone 16 mg	Hydromorphone 8 mg	
NSAIDs	Ketorolac 30–90 mg	Consider suppositories such as diclofenac
Regular paracetamol or low-dose codeine/paracetamol combinations	Morphine 5 mg Diamorphine 2.5–5 mg	Pragmatic recommendation; use clinical judgement
Codeine or dihydrocodeine 240 mg	Morphine 10 mg Diamorphine 7.5 mg	Based on approximate opioid dose equivalences; use clinical judgement
Tramadol 400 mg	Morphine 20 mg Diamorphine 15 mg	
Coanalgesics for neuropathic pain	Midazolam 10–20 mg	If previous coanalgesic regime involves more than one agent, and/or moderate to high doses—seek specialist advice
Antiemetics		
Cyclizine, metoclopramide, haloperidol, levomepromazine	Use same total dose of injectable formulation	
Prochlorperazine	Cyclizine 150 mg	
Domperidone 60 mg	Metoclopramide 30–60 mg	Ensure no history of metoclopramide-induced dyskinesia
Anxiolytics—for anxiety or breathlessness		
Diazepam 10 mg/lorazepam 1 mg	Midazolam 10 mg	
Antipsychotics	Haloperidol or levomepromazine	Either may be combined with midazolam. Specialist advice recommended

Use conversion factors to guide prescription switches—if in doubt, seek specialist advice.
CSCI, continuous subcutaneous infusion; NSAID, nonsteroidal anti-inflammatory drug.
[a]For compatibility of drug combinations in syringe driver and guidance on diluent choice and volume, see Chapter 22, *The syringe driver and medicines management in palliative care*, and consult online resources such as palliativedrugs.com

and setting, the key message is that these symptoms are "common" regardless of underlying diagnosis (see Table 21.5).

The clinical relevance is that anticipatory prescribing of treatment for "all" these symptoms is essential whatever the underlying diagnosis or care setting. Care pathways for the last days of life, such as the LCP [32], include specific recommendations for management of these symptoms and regular monitoring in the care pathway documentation. Availability of drugs in the home is important. The use of the so-called emergency boxes is one way this has been addressed [33].

Table 21.5 End-of-life symptoms and what to exclude depending on prognosis.

Symptom and prevalence	Causes to exclude/reverse/treat according to clinical situation	
Symptom and prevalence in last days of life	*Prognosis h/days*	*Prognosis several days or more*
Pain 40% [34]–99% [35]	Poor absorption of analgesics Inadequate dose titration or dose conversion on changing route	Full pain assessment
Breathlessness 50%[34] – 80%[29]	Physical position Anxiety Hypoxia Pulmonary oedema	Venous thromboembolism Infection Pleural effusion Lymphangitis
Nausea/vomiting Up to 70% [35]	Omission of previous antiemetic Bowel obstruction (physical examination only) Anxiety	Full assessment especially metabolic abnormalities (hypercalcaemia, uraemia) Infection Drug adverse effects Oropharyngeal candidiasis
Respiratory "secretions" Up to 80% [36]	Fluid overload Physical position Oropharyngeal pooling	Infection/aspiration
Restlessness and agitation/delirium 28–83% [37]	Uncontrolled fear/anxiety/pain Faecal impaction Urinary retention/incontinence	Metabolic abnormality (hypercalcaemia, uraemia, hepatic encephalopathy, hyponatraemia) Accumulation of opioid metabolites Other drug causes Cerebral metastases Spiritual distress

When prognosis appears to be in the range of hours to small numbers of days, the opportunity for, and appropriateness of, investigation for underlying causes is limited, potentially counterproductive and often futile. Drawbacks include:

• difficulty gaining access to venous blood sampling to exclude biochemical abnormalities or markers of infection;

• focus on investigations that create a false hope that the patient may improve;

• attention diverted to investigation may distract from attentive symptom management;

• some investigations may require transfer away from home with risk of exhaustion, further deterioration, and death away from the preferred place of care; and

• investigation results leading to clinical dilemmas about managing an abnormal result, possibly necessitating hospitalisation.

Nevertheless, the importance of excluding simple, reversible causes must be emphasised.

Four questions should go through the clinician's mind:
1. Would I transfer this patient for investigation?
2. Will I be able to offer successful treatment for an abnormality that I discover?
3. What are the burdens and losses of transfer, investigation, and treatments?
4. What difference will it make?

Sound clinical judgement exercised on a case-by-case basis is crucial in this phase of patient care but Table 21.5 is intended to give some broad guidance depending on estimated prognosis.

All decisions that are made for and against investigation must be sympathetically explained to the patient (if possible) and to the family/carers.

Management of diabetes

The management of patients with diabetes, whether with insulin or oral antidiabetic agents, causes concern at the end of life and there is often uncertainty about what the correct management plan should be. Appendix 7 offers pragmatic guidance on the management of diabetic patients who are thought to be in the last days of life.

Emergencies in the last days of life—crisis management

General points about symptom crisis management

Throughout all stages of the management of patients reaching the end of life, exploration of concerns and fears has been emphasised. Specific enquiry about fears of the dying stage should be explored gently and sensitively. This will guide whether it is likely to be helpful for the individual patient to ask directly about fears of an exacerbation of pain or breathlessness, or of bleeding or choking, or loss of dignity and confusion. In the authors' experience, such enquiry is far more often helpful than a cause of anguish, and patients are almost invariably relieved to gain reassurance for themselves and their families that such problems will be anticipated and that treatment will be available.

A particular anxiety often prevails, however, over how much detail to go into regarding the risk of major haemorrhage. On the one hand, the clinician will not wish to frighten a lay carer about the possibility of haemorrhage with the results that they spend the last days (or longer) of the patient's life in a state of nervous exhaustion anticipating a grotesque and gory final hour, but on the other hand, there is nothing more dreadful than having to cope with a major bleed at home, perhaps alone with the patient, and having no idea what to expect. As always, sensitive communication and careful exploration are critical. Specialists will be more than ready to provide support to the host clinical team in this particular challenge:

For a patient being cared for at home, the following must be assured:

• Medication is available and prescribed on appropriate documents to allow community health-care professionals to administer it.
• Use and doses of drugs that can be given by the family have been explained with a written plan.

• Telephone numbers for on call professionals are correct and available.
• Daytime and on call services have been primed about possible emergencies that may occur and the treatment that has been left in the home.
• Resuscitation status and future care plans are documented and understood by family and community professionals alike.

Possible emergencies at the end of life

Depending on the underlying illness, potential emergencies are listed below and guidance on management indicated:

• Bleeding (see Appendix 8).
• Severe pain (see Chapter 9, *Pain and its management*, p. 135–136). Pain management at the end of life is also covered in Appendix 2.
• Severe agitation (see Appendix 6).
• Extreme breathlessness (see Appendix 3).
• Seizures (see Section "Management of seizures").

Management of seizures

In the last days of life, the goal of all management is to prevent patient distress and this applies in the management of seizures. Earlier in the course of illness, the management will be different reflecting the anticipated prognosis.

A patient on regular antiepileptic medication reaching the terminal phase and no longer able to swallow will have been converted onto an SC infusion of midazolam as described earlier. If a seizure occurs despite this, crisis medication should be administered and the dose of maintenance treatment reviewed. Specialist advice may be appropriate in this situation.

Crisis medication options:
• SC midazolam 5–10 mg, repeated if necessary after 10 min.
• Buccal midazolam 10 mg, either using a specific buccal formulation or the standard injectable preparation administered from a syringe (without a needle) into the sulcus between the cheek and lower gums. This allows treatment to be given by the family (with appropriate prior guidance and if they feel able), and other carers, enhancing a sense of being in control.
• Diazepam rectal solution 10 mg PR, repeated after 10–15 min.

If a seizure occurs, the clinical team must review the maintenance/prophylactic treatment with attention to the following:
• Check that the maintenance treatment has actually been prescribed and at the appropriate dose and infusion rate.

• Check that the SC infusion is running correctly and that there is no problem with the syringe driver/infusion pump, power supply, the administration line, the site of infusion, or the connections.

If problems persist, specialist advice on use of additional or alternative anticonvulsant medication, for example phenobarbital, should be sought. See PCF 4e (2011) (palliativedrugs.com) for further guidance.

Special needs of family and lay carers during the last days of life

General needs of family/friends

The team members may be so focused on the patient that family and friends have little opportunity to express concerns. Often, all that is required is a recognition of the family's position and an expression of understanding. However, in certain circumstances, it is important to explore difficulties at a greater depth. This assessment should cover physical (e.g., fatigue), psychological (e.g., depression; alcohol use), and social (e.g., finances) needs.

The family and/or friends should have access to professionals, both for information and to meet their own health needs. Information should be given, whenever patient confidentiality allows, even if this feels somewhat repetitious to the professional. The information needs of family/carers will vary and must be explored sensitively with explanations tailored to their needs and ability to understand. Many will imagine situations that may be far more graphic or horrific than reality. They need to be reassured that the questions they ask and, even more importantly, those questions that they are afraid to ask, are valid and common concerns of all people involved in such a difficult time of life. Gentle prompts to explore these issues may begin with expressions such as:

Many people wonder how things will change at this time. Do you have any questions you would like to ask?

or

People I meet often begin to imagine what will happen next.

I wonder what is going through your mind.

Family and carers must understand what to do in an emergency, and be advised of the different professional support services available over each 24-h period. The strain on the family and carers should be acknowledged and support offered as appropriate. It may be helpful for team members to determine the family's previous experience of death.

If the patient is not at home, families and carers often need to feel helpful and to know that their contribution is valued. This may include physical care (e.g., bathing, mouth care). Families and friends should not be made to feel like intruders in the care of their loved one. They must be given every opportunity to stay with the patient, and visiting arrangements should be flexible. Reassure family members who find it too difficult to be at the bedside that the patient will not be left alone. Explain that even if comatose, the patient may be aware of the family's presence and may even hear and recognise the voices of those around them.

Explanation of focus of care

It is important to emphasise that the goals of care are to maintain/achieve dignity, comfort, and symptom relief. Clarify that assessment of patient's needs is now based on careful observations—including the validity of those of the family/lay carers—and responding to these, and not on taking blood tests, ordering scans or measuring the temperature, pulse, and blood pressure. For carers who have perhaps spent months or years waiting for the results of tests or observing clinical staff measuring vital signs, this will feel like a big change and give rise to the concern that "nothing is being done."

Explanation about nutrition, hydration, and medication decisions

We can't just let him starve to death.

In the last days of life, the patient's inclination and ability to take food and fluids by mouth declines. At the same time the disease processes bring about increasing weakness and fatigue, and in some conditions the physical manifestations associated with the anorexia-cachexia syndrome become increasingly apparent. Artificial hydration or nutrition that depends on maintenance of venous access and careful monitoring of blood parameters will be discontinued. As the patient deteriorates, families may question whether the withdrawal is responsible for the decline and may seek to have these treatments resumed. Patients with NG, gastrostomy, or jejunostomy feeding regimes are easier to manage at home—and this may be familiar to the care team—but conversations about rationalising volume or feed frequency as the illness progresses will be needed. In patients who have been eating and drinking normally until the onset of the terminal phase, questions may be asked about how nutrition and hydration may be provided as they take less for themselves. Exploring and instituting artificial feeding is not recommended in the final days of life.

In all cases, careful and sensitive discussion is required. Carers may feel frustrated or helpless observing deterioration and minimal intake running in parallel and these feelings may give rise to anger or suspicion. The feelings must be acknowledged and discussed, not avoided.

Explanation about medication

Careful explanations should be offered about the medication changes that are made in the last days of life. Regular prescriptions that formed part of the mainstay of management of chronic conditions such as hypertension, hypercholesterolaemia, ischaemic heart disease, diabetes, and others are often held to be of great importance. Concordance with these treatments will have been emphasised to patient and carer over many years. The fact that they are no longer of value needs to be explained clearly and compassionately.

Newly commenced regular or "as required" prescriptions also require explanation. It is very important to establish from the start that treatment for pain and agitation with parenterally administered opioids and benzodiazepines will be given in sufficient dose to relieve symptoms but not in excess to cause, or risk causing, harm. Dose adjustment by judicious, proportionate titration must be emphasised. With ongoing media discussions about assisted suicide or "mercy killing," and because of outrages such as those perpetrated by the UK GP Dr Harold Shipman [38], some people believe that the symptom control measures used in end-of-life care are actually a form of euthanasia.

Ongoing reassurance that physical changes are due to the deteriorating condition, and that the medication is adjusted and reviewed to achieve symptom control for the comfort and dignity of the dying patient, is essential.

Explanation about physical changes at time of death

It can be helpful to prepare the family/carers for the changes that occur as the patient dies. In the hours before death, the patient will show reduced levels of consciousness and less interaction. Oral intake will reduce to nothing. Skin may change in colour and temperature beginning at the extremities, the pulse becomes weaker and more difficult to locate.

Respiratory changes include alteration in depth and frequency of respiration with shallower breaths, more frequently, and use of the accessory muscles.

Later still the breathing pattern may demonstrate Cheyne–Stokes respiration with gasping breaths separated by periods of apnoea. The breathing will stop before the heart stops beating.

Care after death

Diagnosing death

It was traditionally the responsibility of a doctor to diagnose death, but in some health-care organisations senior nursing staff are now able to verify an expected death. Confirmation of somatic death is made by observing the following:
- fixed dilated pupils;
- absence of heart sounds;
- absence of respiratory effort; and
- absent pulse.

Care of the body after death

Relatives should be allowed the choice to see and spend time with the deceased person, not only during dying but also afterward. They may need a lot of support in this and preparation of the body may play a part in this support. Some relatives may wish to be involved in the "laying out" of the body. Institutional policies with regard to laying out should be followed with sensitivity to the wishes of family and friends. In particular, different cultural or religious practices should be respected (see Table 21.2).

Wounds should be covered with waterproof dressings and pads used to absorb body fluid and leakage. Catheters and infusion lines should be removed (unless the case is being referred to the coroner). Those handling the body should be warned of any risk of infection and some bodies may need to be placed in body bags.

In some cases, preparation for end of life will have included consideration of care after death and a funeral director may already have been chosen and other arrangements agreed. Community health-care professionals who attend the patient and family at the time of death may support with the immediate practical arrangements. Undertakers are available 24 h a day, can prepare the body, and arrange transfer to the funeral parlour.

Organ donation

Patients carrying a donor card, or whose family consent, may be able to donate various organs and tissues. If the last days of life have been managed by an end-of-life care pathway, clarification of wishes over donation should already have been achieved. Commonly tissue and organ donation is rarely considered and often overlooked. Although many terminally ill patients may not satisfy the criteria, this does not apply universally and families should be given an opportunity to provide consent, if they wish. For instance, corneal donation is most likely to be possible, with certain restrictions. Some patients may have made plans in advance to donate organs for research (e.g., donation of the CNS for research into MND).

It is important for professionals to be fully conversant with local policy and approach relatives with appropriate sensitivity. Additional advice is provided by local tissue transplant coordinators. They are able to speak to relatives and arrange tissue retrieval.

Postmortem

A postmortem may be a mandatory requirement (e.g., cases referred to the coroner). This is a legal requirement and cannot be refused. Postmortems can also be requested to clarify medical details of the death. Relatives can refuse these even if the patient had wished it.

Conclusions

Care for patients who have reached the terminal phase of their illness poses many challenges to professionals. Good quality care at this point often requires increased professional support of patients and their loved ones. The development of care pathways has provided a method to improve the quality of such care in the last days and hours of life. Following a death, there are certain practical requirements that need to be dealt with professionally and with sensitivity to the feelings of the bereaved.

References

1. Wright AA, Keating NL, Balboni TA, et al. Place of death: correlations with quality of life of patients with cancer and predictors of bereaved caregivers' mental health. *J Clin Oncol* 2010; 28(29): 4457–4464.

2. O'Connor S, Schatzberger P, and Payne S. A death photographed: one patient's story. *BMJ* 2003; 327: 233. doi: 10.1136/bmj.327.7408-233.

3. General Medical Council. *Treatment and Care Towards the End of Life: Good Practice in Decision-Making.* London: GMC, 2010.

4. Bell CL, Somogyi-Zalud E, and Masaki KH. Methodological review: measured and reported congruence between preferred and actual place of death. *Palliat Med* 2009; 23(6): 482–490.

5. Gomes B and Higginson IJ. Factors influencing death at home in terminally ill patients with cancer: systematic review. *BMJ* 2006; 332(7540): 515–521.

6. Fukui S, Kawagoe H, Masako S, et al. Determinants of the place of death among terminally ill cancer patients under home hospice care in Japan. *Palliat Med* 2003; 17(5): 445–453.

7. Barclay S and Maher J. Having the difficult conversations about the end of life. *BMJ* 2010; 341: c4862.

8. Agar M, Currow DC, Shelby-James TM, et al. Preference for place of care and place of death in palliative care: are these different questions? *Palliat Med* 2008; 22(7): 787–795.

9. Munday D, Petrova M, and Dale J. Exploring preferences for place of death with terminally ill patients: qualitative study of experiences of general practitioners and community nurses in England. *BMJ* 2009; 339: b2391.

10. OMEGA End of life care in primary care: National snapshot. 2009. Available at: http://www.omega.uk.net/end-of-life-care-p-21.htm (accessed on February 23, 2011).

11. Murray MA, Fiset V, Young S, et al. Where the dying live: a systematic review of determinants of place of end-of-life cancer care. *Oncol Nurs Forum* 2009; 36(1): 69–77.

12. Exley C, Field D, McKinley RK, et al. *An Evaluation of Primary Care Based Palliative Care for Cancer and Non-Malignant Disease in Two Cancer Accredited Primary Care Practices in Leicestershire.* Leicester: Department of Epidemiology and Public Health, University of Leicester, 2003.

13. Townsend J, Frank AO, Fermont D, et al. Terminal cancer care and patients' preference for place of death: a prospective study. *BMJ* 1990; 301: 415–417.

14. Cartwright A. Changes in life and care in the year before death 1967–1987. *J Public Health Med* 1991; 13(2): 81–87.

15. Duncan JG, Forbes-Thompson S, and Bott MJ. Unmet symptom management needs of nursing home residents with cancer. *Cancer Nurs* 2008; 31(4): 265–273.

16. Maccabee J. The effect of transfer from a palliative care unit to nursing homes. Are patients' and relatives' needs met? *Palliat Med* 1994; 8(3): 211–214.

17. Thompson GN, Menec VH, Chochinov HM, et al. Family satisfaction with care of a dying loved one in nursing homes: what makes the difference? *J Gerontol Nurs* 2008; 34(12): 37–44.

18. Addington-Hall JM and O'Callaghan AC. A comparison of the quality of care provided to cancer patients in the UK in the last three months of life in in-patient hospices compared with hospitals, from the perspective of bereaved relatives: results from a survey using the VOICES questionnaire. *Palliat Med* 2009; 23(3): 190–197.

19. National Audit Office. *End of Life Care. Report by the Comptroller and Auditor General.* London: National Audit Office, 2008.

20. Ellershaw JE and Ward C. Evidence based guidelines on symptom control, psychological support and bereavement are available to facilitate a 'good death'. *BMJ* 2003; 326(7379): 30–34.

21. AMBER (Assessment, Management, Best practice, Engagement for patients when Recovery is uncertain). Southwark and Lambeth Modernisation Initiative End of Life

Care Programme, 2009. Available at: www.gsttcharity.org
.uk/projects/eolc.html (accessed on May 17, 2012).

22. Commission for Health Improvement. *Investigation into the
Portsmouth Healthcare NHS Trust Gosport War Memorial
Hospital.* London: Commission for Health Improvement,
2002.

23. Clinical Guidelines Working Party. *Changing Gear: Guidelines for Managing the Last Days of Life,* 2nd edition. London:
National Council for Palliative Care, 2006.

24. National Institute for Clinical Excellence. *Improving Supportive and Palliative Care for Adult Patients with Cancer.* London: National Institute for Clinical Excellence,
2004.

25. Ellershaw J and Wilkinson S. *Care of the Dying. A Pathway
to Excellence.* Oxford: Oxford University Press, 2003.

26. Veerbeek L, van Zuylen I, Swart SJ, et al. The effect of the
Liverpool Car Pathway for the dying: a multi-centre study.
Palliat Med 2008; 22(2): 145–151.

27. Resuscitation Council UK. *Resuscitation Guidelines.* London:
Resuscitation Council UK, 2010.

28. National Collaborating Centre for Acute Care. *Nutrition
Support in Adults. Oral Nutritional Support, Enteral Tube
Feeding and Parenteral Nutrition.* London: National Collab-
orating Centre for Acute Care, 2006.

29. Harlos M. The terminal phase. In: Hanks G, Cherny NI,
Christakis NA, Fallon M, Kaasa S, and Portenoy RK (eds),
The Oxford Textbook of Palliative Medicine. Oxford: Oxford
University Press, 2009. Section 19.

30. Solano JP, Gomes B, and Higginson IJ. A comparison of
symptom prevalence in far advanced cancer, AIDS, heart
disease, chronic obstructive pulmonary disease and renal
disease. *J Pain Symptom Manage* 2006; 31(1): 58–69.

31. *Palliative Care Formulary,* 3rd edition. palliativedrugs.com
Ltd. 2000–2011.

32. Ellershaw J, Foster A, Murphy D, et al. Developing an integrated care pathway for the dying patient. *Eur J Palliat Care*
1997; 4(6): 203–207.

33. Thomas K. *Out of Hours Palliative Care in the Community.*
London: Macmillan Cancer Relief, 2001.

34. Lynn J, Teno JM, Phillips RS, et al. Perceptions by family
members of the dying experience of older and seriously ill
patients. SUPPORT investigators. Study to understand prognoses and preferences for outcomes and risks of treatment.
Ann Intern Med 1997; 126(2): 97–106.

35. Fainsinger R, Miller MJ, Bruera E, et al. Symptom control
during the last week of life on a palliative care unit. *J Palliat
Care* 1991; 7(1): 5–11.

36. Wee B and Hillier R. Interventions for noisy breathing in
patients near to death. *Cochrane Database Syst Rev* 2008;
(1): CD005177. doi: 10.1002/14651858.CD005177.pub2.

37. Casarett DJ, Inouye SK, and American College of Physicians-
American Society of Internal Medicine End-of-Life Care
Consensus Panel. Diagnosis and management of delirium
near the end of life. *Ann Intern Med* 2001; 135(1): 32–40.

38. The Shipman Inquiry. *First report. Crown copyright.* The
Shipman Inquiry, Norwich: The Stationery Office, 2002.

Acknowledgement. We would like to acknowledge the work of Brian Nyatanga for the previous edition of this chapter.

Appendices[1]

[1] Appendices 1–7 are adapted from the North of England Cancer Network Palliative Care Guidelines (2009) with permission.

Appendix 1: Management of Pain with Fentanyl Transdermal Patches at End of Life

Fentanyl patches in the dying/moribund patient

It is recommended to continue fentanyl patches in these patients. Remember to carry on changing the patch(es) every 72 h—this is sometimes forgotten.
If pain occurs, give rescue doses of morphine or an alternative opioid as recommended by the specialist palliative care team.
Correct rescue doses should be calculated from locally agreed opioid dose equivalence charts/guidelines.
If the preferred/recommended injectable opioid is not available seek specialist advice about an alternative.

Adding a subcutaneous infusion alongside a patch
If two or more rescue doses of opioid are needed in 24 h, start a subcutaneous infusion with the chosen opioid and continue the patch(es).
The dose of opioid in the subcutaneous infusion should equal the total of the opioid rescue doses given in the previous 24 h. Many specialists suggest that this infused dose initially be a maximum of 50% of the opioids equivalence of the existing fentanyl patch dose. This is to provide a safety margin in titration.
The 50% limit, subject to specialist advice, should be applied in ongoing titration.
Remember to use the dose of the patch and the dose in the syringe driver to work out the new rescue dose each time a change is made.

Handbook of Palliative Care, Third Edition. Edited by Christina Faull, Sharon de Caestecker, Alex Nicholson and Fraser Black.
© 2012 by John Wiley and Sons, Inc. Published 2012 by John Wiley & Sons, Inc.

Appendix 2: Management of Pain at the End of Life

This algorithm assumes use of morphine. For the appropriate doses of other opioids, see the opioid dose conversion tables in Chapter 9, *Pain and its Management*

	Yes	Is patient already on opioid drugs?	**No**	

Patient on morphine sulphate
- Divide 24 h total dose of current oral morphine *(regular + prn)* by 2 and prescribe this as morphine (mgs) by subcutaneous (SC) infusion over 24 h
- Prescribe 1/6th morphine infusion dose for breakthrough/rescue medication to be given SC up to hourly if needed
- Start SC infusion driver 4 h before next oral opioid dose would have been due (or immediately if a dose has been missed)
- Discontinue oral opioid

Review within 24 h
If extra medication has been needed for pain:
- Increase SC infusion dose by total amount of rescue morphine given or by 50%, whichever is less
- Adjust rescue/breakthrough dose to 1/6th of SC infusion morphine dose to be given SC up to hourly if needed

If pain is controlled, make no changes

Continue to review regularly

Patient on weak opioid
(codeine, tramadol, dihydrocodeine)
- Stop oral weak opioid
- Start morphine 10 mg/24 h by SC infusion soon after last oral dose
- Prescribe morphine 2.5 mg SC hourly if needed for rescue/breakthrough pain

Review regularly and adjust as above

Scenario 1: "Planning ahead"
Patient not in pain
- Prescribe morphine 2.5 mg SC hourly if needed
- If patient later develops pain, proceed to next box.

Scenario 2: "Act now"
Patient in pain
- Give morphine 2.5 mg SC stat
- If effective prescribe and start morphine 10 mg/24 h by SC infusion
- Prescribe morphine 2.5 mg SC for rescue/breakthrough pain to be given up to hourly if needed

Review within 24 h
If extra medication has been needed for pain:
- Increase SC infusion dose by total amount of rescue medication given or to 20 mg/24 h, whichever is less
- Increase rescue/breakthrough dose of morphine to 5 mg SC to be given

Review within 24 h
If extra medication has been needed for pain:
- Increase SC infusion dose by total amount of rescue morphine given or by 50%, whichever is less
- Adjust rescue/breakthrough dose to 1/6th of SC infusion morphine dose to be given SC up to hourly if needed

If pain is controlled, make no changes

Continue to review regularly

Handbook of Palliative Care, Third Edition. Edited by Christina Faull, Sharon de Caestecker, Alex Nicholson and Fraser Black.
© 2012 by John Wiley and Sons, Inc. Published 2012 by John Wiley & Sons, Inc.

Appendix 3: Management of Breathlessness at the End of Life

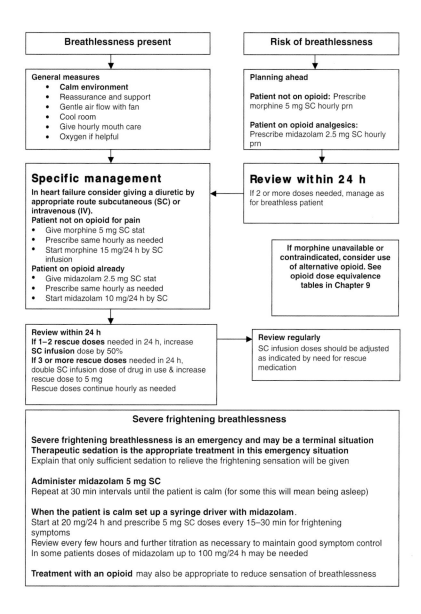

Breathlessness present	Risk of breathlessness
General measures • **Calm environment** • Reassurance and support • Gentle air flow with fan • Cool room • Give hourly mouth care • Oxygen if helpful	**Planning ahead** **Patient not on opioid:** Prescribe morphine 5 mg SC hourly prn **Patient on opioid analgesics:** Prescribe midazolam 2.5 mg SC hourly prn

Specific management

In heart failure consider giving a diuretic by appropriate route subcutaneous (SC) or intravenous (IV).

Patient not on opioid for pain
• Give morphine 5 mg SC stat
• Prescribe same hourly as needed
• Start morphine 15 mg/24 h by SC infusion

Patient on opioid already
• Give midazolam 2.5 mg SC stat
• Prescribe same hourly as needed
• Start midazolam 10 mg/24 h by SC

Review within 24 h
If 2 or more doses needed, manage as for breathless patient

If morphine unavailable or contraindicated, consider use of alternative opioid. See opioid dose equivalence tables in Chapter 9

Review within 24 h
If 1–2 rescue doses needed in 24 h, increase **SC infusion** dose by 50%
If 3 or more rescue doses needed in 24 h, double SC infusion dose of drug in use & increase rescue dose to 5 mg
Rescue doses continue hourly as needed

Review regularly
SC infusion doses should be adjusted as indicated by need for rescue medication

Severe frightening breathlessness

Severe frightening breathlessness is an emergency and may be a terminal situation
Therapeutic sedation is the appropriate treatment in this emergency situation
Explain that only sufficient sedation to relieve the frightening sensation will be given

Administer midazolam 5 mg SC
Repeat at 30 min intervals until the patient is calm (for some this will mean being asleep)

When the patient is calm set up a syringe driver with midazolam.
Start at 20 mg/24 h and prescribe 5 mg SC doses every 15–30 min for frightening symptoms
Review every few hours and further titration as necessary to maintain good symptom control
In some patients doses of midazolam up to 100 mg/24 h may be needed

Treatment with an opioid may also be appropriate to reduce sensation of breathlessness

Handbook of Palliative Care, Third Edition. Edited by Christina Faull, Sharon de Caestecker, Alex Nicholson and Fraser Black.
© 2012 by John Wiley and Sons, Inc. Published 2012 by John Wiley & Sons, Inc.

Appendix 4: Management of Nausea and Vomiting at the End of Life

---

New nausea/vomiting in a patient not currently using an antiemetic

ASK: Is a chemical cause possible?

    If YES prescribe haloperidol 1.5–3 mg daily by SC injection (SC infusion if preferred)
    Also prescribe cyclizine 50 mg prn SC maximum 150 mg/24 h

    If NO prescribe cyclizine 150 mg/24 h via SC infusion
    Also prescribe haloperidol 1.5 mg SC prn, maximum three doses in 24 h

REVIEW AFTER 24 h:

    If symptoms are controlled, continue as before

    If either nausea or vomiting persists, please contact the Specialist Palliative Care Team

---

Uncontrolled nausea/vomiting in a patient already on an antiemetic

Review the possible causes but do not delay changing the antiemetic regime or arrange burdensome investigations in an end-of-life care situation.

If a combination of cyclizine and haloperidol fails to control nausea/vomiting replace them with levomepromazine 12.5 mg/24 h SC via SC infusion

Also prescribe levomepromazine 6.25 mg SC prn up to 4 doses per 24 h

---

Nausea/vomiting already controlled

Continue existing antiemetic but switch to the SC route
    (this may require a change of agent if prochlorperazine or domperidone is in use)
Also prescribe levomepromazine 6.25 mg SC prn up to 4 doses per 24 h

REVIEW THE SYMPTOM CONTROL ACHIEVED ON A REGULAR BASIS

Notes on levomepromazine

The effects of this drug may last up to 24 h—once daily SC dosing may be an alternative to SC infusion

The maximum antiemetic effect may be achieved at doses of 25–50 mg per 24 h.

Doses above 25 mg per 24 h (or lower in patients who are sensitive) have a sedative effect.

The sedative effect may be clinically useful—this drug is also used the management of terminal agitation and restlessness

---

Handbook of Palliative Care, Third Edition. Edited by Christina Faull, Sharon de Caestecker, Alex Nicholson and Fraser Black.
© 2012 by John Wiley and Sons, Inc. Published 2012 by John Wiley & Sons, Inc.

Appendix 5: Management of Respiratory Secretions at the End of Life

Secretions "death rattle" are easier to control early than late. Treat promptly.

Hyoscine salts are most commonly prescribed to try to control secretions at the end of life. There are two forms of hyoscine.
Hyoscine **butylbromide is nonsedating** and should therefore be considered in a conscious patient. (NB *hyoscine butylbromide is incompatible with cyclizine when given by SC infusion*).
Hyoscine **hydrobromide has sedative effects** that *may* be useful.
Some palliative care services use **glycopyrrolate** as the preferred antisecretory agent to avoid sedation.

Consider these details and local experience when deciding what to prescribe.

Secretions present	**Secretions absent**

General management
- **Give explanation and reassurance to relatives**
- Alter position to shift secretions
- Consider stopping parenteral fluids
- Give hourly mouth care

Anticipatory prescribing is crucial to allow early and better control of this symptom

When a patient starts on the end-of-life pathway always prescribe hyoscine up to hourly SC as needed.

Use either hyoscine butylbromide 20 mg or hyoscine hydrobromide 400 mcg

Specific management – three actions

Give stat dose SC
Either hyoscine butylbromide 20 mg
Or hyoscine hydrobromide 400 mcg

Start SC infusion
Either hyoscine butylbromide 60 mg/24 h
Or hyoscine hydrobromide 1.2 mg/24 h

Ensure rescue doses up to hourly SC as needed
Either hyoscine butylbromide 20 mg
Or hyoscine hydrobromide 400 mcg

Review after no longer than 24 h
If two or more doses needed, manage as for "secretions present"

Review after 24 h or sooner
If rescue doses needed, increase 24 h dose
Either hyoscine butylbromide 120 mg/24 h
Or Hyoscine hydrobromide 2.4 mg/24 h

Continue rescue medication up to hourly as needed

Difficult cases
In heart failure, pulmonary odema may cause a rattle. Consider giving diuretic by an appropriate route

Do not hesitate to seek specialist advice if needed

Handbook of Palliative Care, Third Edition. Edited by Christina Faull, Sharon de Caestecker, Alex Nicholson and Fraser Black.
© 2012 by John Wiley and Sons, Inc. Published 2012 by John Wiley & Sons, Inc.

Appendix 6: Management of Restlessness and Agitation/Delirium at the End of Life

Consider common causes of restlessness, for example, urinary retention, faecal impaction, and pain. Manage these appropriately. Also consider whether sedation is acceptable or not.
Patients on regular or long-term benzodiazepines who enter the terminal phase should continue to receive a benzodiazepine as midazolam by subcutaneous (SC) infusion to prevent rebound agitation/withdrawal.
The doses given here are a guide. If symptoms are problematic, seek specialist advice.

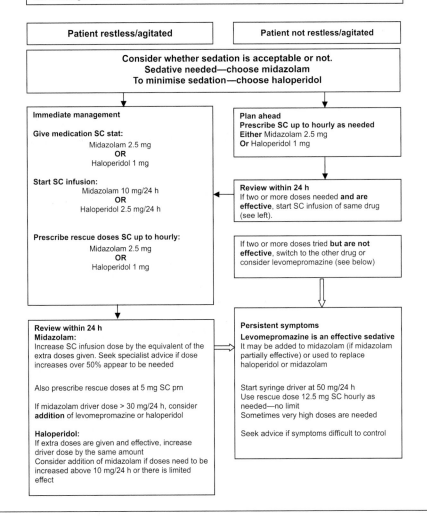

| **Patient restless/agitated** | **Patient not restless/agitated** |

Consider whether sedation is acceptable or not.
Sedative needed—choose midazolam
To minimise sedation—choose haloperidol

Immediate management

Give medication SC stat:
Midazolam 2.5 mg
OR
Haloperidol 1 mg

Start SC infusion:
Midazolam 10 mg/24 h
OR
Haloperidol 2.5 mg/24 h

Prescribe rescue doses SC up to hourly:
Midazolam 2.5 mg
OR
Haloperidol 1 mg

Plan ahead
Prescribe SC up to hourly as needed
Either Midazolam 2.5 mg
Or Haloperidol 1 mg

Review within 24 h
If two or more doses needed **and are effective**, start SC infusion of same drug (see left).

If two or more doses tried **but are not effective**, switch to the other drug or consider levomepromazine (see below)

Review within 24 h
Midazolam:
Increase SC infusion dose by the equivalent of the extra doses given. Seek specialist advice if dose increases over 50% appear to be needed

Also prescribe rescue doses at 5 mg SC prn

If midazolam driver dose > 30 mg/24 h, consider **addition** of levomepromazine or haloperidol

Haloperidol:
If extra doses are given and effective, increase driver dose by the same amount
Consider addition of midazolam if doses need to be increased above 10 mg/24 h or there is limited effect

Persistent symptoms
Levomepromazine is an effective sedative
It may be added to midazolam (if midazolam partially effective) or used to replace haloperidol or midazolam

Start syringe driver at 50 mg/24 h
Use rescue dose 12.5 mg SC hourly as needed—no limit
Sometimes very high doses are needed

Seek advice if symptoms difficult to control

Handbook of Palliative Care, Third Edition. Edited by Christina Faull, Sharon de Caestecker, Alex Nicholson and Fraser Black.
© 2012 by John Wiley and Sons, Inc. Published 2012 by John Wiley & Sons, Inc.

Appendix 7: Management Diabetes in the Last Days of Life: A Pragmatic Approach[2]

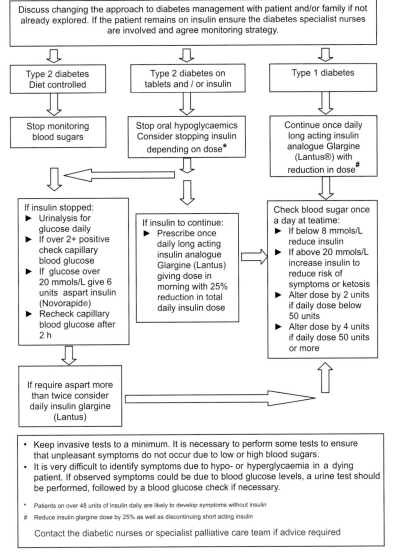

Discuss changing the approach to diabetes management with patient and/or family if not already explored. If the patient remains on insulin ensure the diabetes specialist nurses are involved and agree monitoring strategy.

Type 2 diabetes Diet controlled

Type 2 diabetes on tablets and / or insulin

Type 1 diabetes

Stop monitoring blood sugars

Stop oral hypoglycaemics Consider stopping insulin depending on dose*

Continue once daily long acting insulin analogue Glargine (Lantus®) with reduction in dose#

If insulin stopped:
- ▶ Urinalysis for glucose daily
- ▶ If over 2+ positive check capillary blood glucose
- ▶ If glucose over 20 mmols/L give 6 units aspart insulin (Novorapid®)
- ▶ Recheck capillary blood glucose after 2 h

If insulin to continue:
- ▶ Prescribe once daily long acting insulin analogue Glargine (Lantus) giving dose in morning with 25% reduction in total daily insulin dose

Check blood sugar once a day at teatime:
- ▶ If below 8 mmols/L reduce insulin
- ▶ If above 20 mmols/L increase insulin to reduce risk of symptoms or ketosis
- ▶ Alter dose by 2 units if daily dose below 50 units
- ▶ Alter dose by 4 units if daily dose 50 units or more

If require aspart more than twice consider daily insulin glargine (Lantus)

- • Keep invasive tests to a minimum. It is necessary to perform some tests to ensure that unpleasant symptoms do not occur due to low or high blood sugars.
- • It is very difficult to identify symptoms due to hypo- or hyperglycaemia in a dying patient. If observed symptoms could be due to blood glucose levels, a urine test should be performed, followed by a blood glucose check if necessary.

* Patients on over 48 units of insulin daily are likely to develop symptoms without insulin

\# Reduce insulin glargine dose by 25% as well as discontinuing short acting insulin

Contact the diabetic nurses or specialist palliative care team if advice required

[2] Diabetes in Palliative Care Guidelines, November 2010. MacLeod, J. et al. North Tees and Hartlepool NHS Foundation Trust, Hartlepool Primary Care Trust, Stockton-on-Tees Teaching Primary Care Trust. (Reproduced with permission from Dr Jean MacLeod.)

Appendix 8: Management of Bleeding at the End of Life

1. Recognition
- Bleeding of all types occurs in 14% of patients with advanced disease.
- Haemorrhage causes death in approximately 6% patients.
- Catastrophic external haemorrhage is less common than internal unseen bleeding

Clinical presentation
- Cardiovascular compromise—hypotension, tachycardia (>100 beats/min = significant recent bleed).
- Identifiable bleeding source, for example, haematemesis, meloena, hoemoptysis, PV or PR bleeding, haematuria
- Erosion of an artery by a malignant ulcer or superficial/fungating tumor

2. Anticipatory management
- Massive haemorrhage is often preceded by smaller bleeds. Oral/topical treatment may help (see below).
- Review resuscitation status and document decision.
- Consider stopping warfarin or switching to low molecular weight heparin.
- Always monitor INR closely if warfarin continues. Correct any coagulation disorder.
- Consider referral for radiotherapy or embolisation if patient has an erosive tumour.
- Try to discuss possibility of haemorrhage with the patient/family. This may enable discussion of options for preferred place of care if haemorrhage occurs or risk of haemorrhage increases.
- Dark towels should be available nearby to reduce the visual impact of blood if haemorrhage occurs.
- Midazolam/diazepam (see below) should be prescribed and made available.
- Prescription charts for community staff to administer these emergency drugs should be signed.

3. Immediate action
If a patient is close to death from underlying cancer, it is usually appropriate to regard major haemorrhage as a terminal event and not to intervene with resuscitation measures.
   Advance decisions or statements regarding preferred place of care should be observed.

If resuscitation is inappropriate

- Administer midazolam 10 mg IM (*IV if in hospital and access available*). Buccal midazolam could be used depending on source of bleeding. Rectal diazepam 10 mg is an option but not very practical.
- Stay with the patient, giving as much reassurance/explanation as possible.
- Try to remain calm. This will help a dying patient to achieve a peaceful death.

If resuscitation is appropriate

- Admit as emergency. Secure IV access.
- Start rapid infusion of 0.9% saline.
- Cross match and follow local hemorrhage protocols.
- Apply local pressure to any obvious bleeding.
- Seek specialist help on further management.

4. Follow up
- Ensure support available for family and staff following experience of haemorrhage.
- If the patient survives the hemorrhage and remains stable for 24--48 h, consider transfusion.
- To prevent rebleeding: **ORAL**: Tranexamic acid 1g every 8 h (avoid in haematuria) or etamsylate 500 mg every 6 h. **TOPICAL**: Sucralfate paste applied direct to ulcer under nonadherent dressing; adrenaline 0.1% (1 mg/ml) soaks (10 ml on gauze); tranexamic acid (500 mg/5 ml of injectable formulation).
- Consider diathermy, radiotherapy, or embolisation.

Handbook of Palliative Care, Third Edition. Edited by Christina Faull, Sharon de Caestecker, Alex Nicholson and Fraser Black.
© 2012 by John Wiley and Sons, Inc. Published 2012 by John Wiley & Sons, Inc.

22 The Syringe Driver and Medicines Management in Palliative Care

Christine Hirsch[1], Maria McKenna[2]

[1]University of Birmingham, Birmingham, UK
[2]Newcastle upon Tyne Hospitals NHS Foundation Trust, UK

Introduction

Palliative care encompasses a diverse range of patients, diagnoses, and symptoms. Medications, often in complex combinations, are a significant component of the holistic approach to symptom management. Within this chapter, we will explore the role of the pharmacist within palliative care and some of the prescribing issues unique to the palliative care setting, namely, utilisation of drugs beyond licence and the syringe driver.

Pharmacist in palliative care: a key team member

Palliative care, by definition, requires a multidisciplinary approach [1]. In the United Kingdom, National Institute for Clinical Excellence guidelines [2] specifically recommend that an effective specialist palliative care team incorporates the range of expertise provided by a pharmacist. The role of a palliative care pharmacist comprises "clinical, educational, administrative, and supportive" responsibilities [3,4].

Clinically, pharmacists advise on drug therapy and supply both standard and nonstandard formulations. Palliative care practitioners are skilled in "precision pharmaco-palliation" [5], appropriately rationalising medications to maximise positive and minimise adverse effects. The pharmacist provides support with this, as well as proficiency in the process of drug discontinuation.

Pharmacists participate in education of other healthcare professionals, patients, relatives, and carers, around prescription and administration of medication. The role in counselling patients about their drugs is particularly important, as on average, palliative care patients regularly take 5–6 different medications and it has been reported that 60% are noncompliant with their medication regimen at home [6]. In addition, particularly in palliative care, pharmacists need to understand any psychosocial issues that may influence the drug management for a patient. For example, a patient with underlying anxiety may overuse opioid analgesics with the consequent risk of opioid toxicity. The pharmacist can recommend alternative strategies or drug classes to optimise pain control in conjunction with an multidisciplinary team (MDT) approach to the patient's care [7].

Through provision of and advice on cost-effective drug formulations and doses, as well as support in rationalisation of medications, pharmacists may play a role in reducing financial expenditure within an organisation [8]. Furthermore, palliative care pharmacists often contribute to patient safety and clinical governance: through medicines reconciliation, investigation of errors, development of evidence-based guidelines, and local formularies and participation in audit.

Use of drugs beyond licence

In palliative care, medications are routinely prescribed outside the terms of their product licence or "off-label." Examples of this include prescribing antidepressant agents for pain control, the administration of some drugs by continuous subcutaneous (SC) infusion, and administration of medication via feeding tubes. In the United Kingdom,

Handbook of Palliative Care, Third Edition. Edited by Christina Faull, Sharon de Caestecker, Alex Nicholson and Fraser Black.
© 2012 by John Wiley and Sons, Inc. Published 2012 by John Wiley & Sons, Inc.

25% of prescribing in palliative care was found to be off-label [9,10] and in an Australian study, 22% in an acute oncology setting [11].

Any new medicines intended for use in Europe are first evaluated by the Committee for Medicinal Products for Human Use of the European Medicines Agency (EMEA). In the United Kingdom, the Medicines and Health-care products Regulatory Agency (MHRA) regulates the licencing of drugs by the pharmaceutical companies. It does not restrict prescribing or administration by qualified medical practitioners, or nurse- or pharmacist-independent prescribers, as long as they are prescribing within their area of competence. In many cases, pharmaceutical companies may not have applied for extensions to the terms of the product licence for the product for economic reasons.

A position statement was prepared on behalf of the Association for Palliative Medicine of Great Britain and Ireland and the Pain Society, which addressed the use of drugs beyond licence in palliative care and pain management. This recommends that:

> The use of drugs beyond licence should be seen as a legitimate aspect of clinical practice. . . . is currently both necessary and common. . . . Health professionals should inform, change and monitor their practice. . . . in the light of evidence from audit and published research [12].

It is important that the prescriber appreciates and is aware when a medicine is being prescribed "off-label" and understands the medical, legal, and ethical implications. It is recommended that the prescriber should ensure that the patient is fully informed, the reason for the decision to prescribe should be documented in the patient's medical records, and where possible, the patient and or family should be given sufficient information to allow them to give informed consent. It is recognised that in palliative care to adhere to all of these recommendations, when "off-label" use is often current best practice, would not always be achievable. However, patients usually receive "patient information leaflets" with their dispensed medicines that may be a cause of anxiety and confusion for the patient or carer if the written information regarding the indications and dosage is inconsistent with verbal information from their prescriber. It may also be important to inform other health-care professionals involved in the patient's care when prescribing "off-label."

Administration of drugs via feeding tubes is an unlicenced activity (for most drugs), but necessary for those palliative care patients unable to swallow. There is little published data about the administration of drugs via feeding tubes and in many areas local policies have been developed. Guidance should be sought from the pharmacist on the suitability of formulations, possibility of interaction with other medication and feed, and maintaining tube patency [13,14].

Occasionally, patients require drugs that are available only as unlicenced "specials," or on a named patient basis from the pharmaceutical industry. Community pharmacists may have to call on the local hospital pharmacy department, or pharmaceutical manufacturing specialist, to obtain these medicines. Time and advanced warning are particularly important in these situations.

Prescribing and administration of medicines "off-label" also extends to mixing medicines, for example, in syringe drivers. Recent discussion with regard to this has resulted in temporary legislation enabling the mixing of medicines in palliative care in the United Kingdom, and this will be discussed further under Sections "Drugs used in syringe drivers" and "Combining drugs in syringes."

Medication compliance aids

Patients taking a large number of different medicines may have difficulty, for a variety of reasons, in adhering to the correct regimen. This is a complex issue that can be approached in a variety of ways tailored to each individual [15,16]. Some patients may find compliance aids helpful such as blister packs or plastic boxes that contain tablets for the day, indicating the time to be taken. An example is the "Redidose" box (see Figure 22.1). Some of these

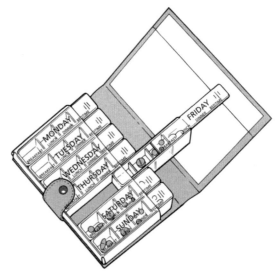

Figure 22.1 The Redidose 7-day pill dispenser.

devices include alarms and electronic dispensers. Patients interviewed about their use of multicompartment medication compliance aids reported that most had purchased the systems because taking multiple medicines did not fit well in their lives and some found them helpful in giving them more control over their medicines. Rather than reminding them "to take" medication, the devices allowed patients to check whether "they had taken" medication and thus relieved the anxiety. Often, other measures were employed in addition to the compliance aid itself [17]. The stability of tablets outside of the manufacturers' original packaging should be checked with pharmacy and consideration should be given to issues such as availability of "as required" medication, for example, breakthrough analgesia that may not be appropriate to include in restricted access packaging and the safety of some medications due to licenced scheduling. No system is optimal for all patients and their ability to cope at home with a particular device should always be assessed before recommending [18]. The pharmacist may be able to offer alternative solutions to individual problems such as the use of large print labels, diaries, and charts.

Use of the "syringe driver" for continuous infusion in palliative care

When patients become unable to take medications via the oral route, drug administration by continuous infusion can be an alternative way to achieve symptom control. In the United Kingdom, the SC route is typically used for continuous infusion as this is well tolerated by patients and easily achievable in the community setting particularly if the rectal or transdermal route is not appropriate. SC administration is also preferable to the intravenous (IV) or intramuscular routes. It is less painful than intramuscular administration and more convenient than IV access that may be difficult to achieve in patients at the end of life because of difficulty securing a suitable vein, limitations imposed on place of care if venous access needs to be maintained, and potential additional risk of infection. The method of delivery is by using a portable lightweight device called a syringe driver, which is discussed, with detail on specific indications, in more detail later. Clinicians outside the United Kingdom may be more familiar with different infusional devices.

In UK palliative care, the role of the syringe driver has been firmly established to administer SC infusions of drugs for symptom control. This may include analgesics, antiemetics, sedatives, or anticholinergic drugs [19–25]

administered either as single agents or in combinations according to recognised compatibilities of different drugs. The syringe driver provides "steady-state" plasma concentrations of drugs, avoiding the necessity for repeated injections or for admission to an inpatient unit for IV treatment. Prescribing for continuous SC infusion via the syringe driver involves anticipation of the patient's drug requirements over the next 24 h. Any alteration in symptoms may necessitate additional injections to supplement the infusion regimen; therefore, medication should also be prescribed, and be available, for immediate administration in case of breakthrough symptoms. This is sometimes referred to as "rescue" medication.

Overenthusiastic and indiscriminate use of the syringe driver should be avoided. For those who can take and absorb oral medication, an SC infusion delivered by a syringe driver is unlikely to improve symptom control. Some drugs with long half-lives, for example, levomepromazine or dexamethasone, may be given by bolus SC injections. Other characteristics make certain drugs less suitable for continuous infusion. For example, dexamethasone has the potential to cause psychological stimulation so that infusion overnight may disturb sleep, and the injectable version that is formulated as a suspension commonly poses problems in terms of its compatibility with other drugs in the syringe driver. Alternative nonoral routes such as sublingual, buccal, rectal, or transdermal should also be considered. Long-term use is rarely indicated, but if required, may be maintained as long as necessary. Once symptoms are controlled, it is often possible to reconvert medications to the oral formulations.

Syringe drivers commonly used in palliative care in the United Kingdom are lightweight, portable infusion pumps, usually electrically or mechanically operated, capable of delivering precise doses of medication over a set period of time, most commonly 24 h. An example is the McKinley T34 syringe driver (see Figure 22.2).

However, the use of these devices is not without risk. Between January 1, 2005 and June 30, 2010, the NPSA in the United Kingdom received reports of 8 deaths and 167 reports of nonfatal incidents involving ambulatory syringe drivers [26].

Following concern expressed over the risk for errors with certain models of syringe driver involving incidents due to rate calculation error, together with issues around lockable covers, a harmonised European Standard (BS EN 60601-2-24 1998) was drawn up identifying features of ambulatory syringe drivers that would reduce the risk of incidents in practice. New Zealand and Australia no longer use millimetre calibrated syringe drivers, and the United

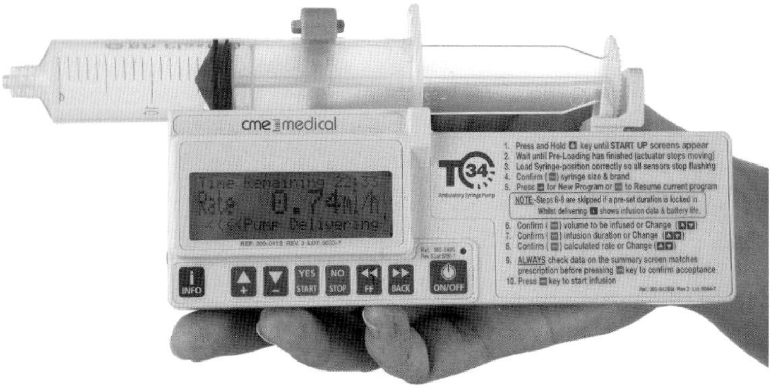

Figure 22.2 McKinley syringe driver.

Kingdom has set a target date of 2015 for all ambulatory syringe drivers to be calibrated in millilitres per hour.

In addition to rate setting in millilitres per hour and comprehensive training other desirable safety features include:

- mechanism to stop the infusion if connections and fittings are incorrect;
- alarms to indicate if the syringe becomes disconnected from the pump;
- locks to prevent tampering; and
- internal log memory to record pump events.

Indications for using the syringe driver

The syringe driver may be indicated in the following situations:

- Persistent nausea or vomiting
- Oral/pharyngeal lesions
- Difficulty in swallowing
- Poor alimentary absorption
- Intestinal obstruction
- Profound weakness/cachexia
- Comatose or moribund patient.

Explanation to the patient and carers

Before commencing an infusion, time should be spent with the patient and their carers explaining the nature and intention of the procedure. Some patients find the syringe driver obtrusive and disconcerting; many have reservations and some fear that the institution of a syringe driver equates with impending death. Questions should be invited, anxieties acknowledged, and appropriate reassurance given.

Drugs used in syringe drivers

This section discusses the drugs more commonly used in symptom management and highlights some of the impor-

tant issues to be considered when prescribing drugs for SC infusion. See Table 22.1 for more specific detail on these drugs, doses, and indications. The choice of drug may be directed by local or national guidelines. Other chapters in this book should be consulted for more detail about the use of drugs in symptom management. Advice should be sought from local palliative care specialists on unusual drugs or combinations, and there are several sources of readily available information on drugs, and combinations, which may be successfully used in syringe drivers including local guidelines [27–30]. If drug dosages need to be altered, a new syringe should be set up rather than the infusion rate altered. Alteration of the rate will deliver all of the drugs at an increased or decreased rate. It will also alter the time of next refilling of the syringe, risking a period with no infused medication if the supply runs out before the next district or community nursing visit.

Changing the infusion rate can potentially lead to an overdosage (or underdosage) if the rate is not checked and reset at each syringe recharge. It also complicates the calculation of the actual dose of each drug the patient is receiving daily.

Combining drugs in syringes

Diamorphine was traditionally the opioid of choice for use in syringe drivers in the United Kingdom because it has high water solubility. The maximum recommended concentration for single-agent diamorphine is 250 mg/ml. However following supply problems over recent years, many centres in the United Kingdom turned to morphine as the most cost-effective alternative, reserving diamorphine for those patients who require higher doses.

Many different drug and dosage combinations have been used in syringe drivers. A survey of UK hospices in 2001 [31] found that 19 drugs were being used in combination in a syringe driver compared to 29 reported

Table 22.1 Drugs used in syringe drivers.

Medication	Trade name and ampoule size	Indication	Dose range per 24 h	Comments
Analgesics				
Morphine [27]	10, 15, 20, 30 mg/ml (1 and 2 ml amps)	Pain, dyspnoea	Start: One-half total daily dose of oral morphine; 10–20 mg in opioid naive patients; increase as necessary by 30–50% increments; no maximum dose	• In some areas may be first-line opioid of choice for SC infusion
Diamorphine hydrochloride [56]	Crystalline powder 5, 10, 30, 100, 500 mg; reconstitute with water	Pain, dyspnoea	Start: One-third total daily dose of oral morphine; 10–20 mg in opioid naive patients; increase as necessary by 30–50% increments; no maximum dose	• Alternative opioid to morphine if high doses required, which restricts volume in syringe driver • Highly soluble • Do not exceed 250 mg/ml • Loading dose (equivalent to 4 h) may be required initially SC
Hydromorphone‡	10, 20, 50 mg/ml	Diamorphine intolerance, on the recommendation of palliative care specialist	Start 1/2 dose of oral hydromorphone	Unlicensed, available as a special order from Cardinal Health–Martindale Products; chemically incompatible with hyaluronidase [57]
Oxycodone [47]	10 mg/ml, 1 and 2 ml, 50 mg/ml, 1 ml	Diamorphine intolerance	7.5 mg in 24 h in opioid naive patients; one-half of oral oxycodone dose	If mixing with cyclizine, do not exceed 3 mg/ml cyclizine
Alfentanil† [28]	1 mg/2 ml, 5 mg/10 ml, 5 mg/ml	Alternative to diamorphine on advice of palliative care specialist, particularly in renal failure	Opioid-naive patients start 0.5–1 mg over 24 h	Incompatibility may occur with cyclizine
Methadone [58,59]‡	10 mg/ml 1, 2, 3.5, and 5 ml	Only on recommendation of palliative care specialist	Seek advice from palliative care specialist	• Can have unacceptable adverse reactions at injection site • Wide variation in individual plasma concentration • Long half-life tendency to accumulate • Rectal route an alternative

(continued)

Table 22.1 (*Continued*)

Medication	Trade name and ampoule size	Indication	Dose range per 24 h	Comments
Ketamine [60–62][†]	Ketalar 10 mg/ml/20 ml vial, 50 mg/ml/10 ml vial, 100 mg/ml/10 ml vial	Difficult cancer pain, especially of neuropathic origin on recommendation of palliative care specialist	Seek advice from palliative care specialist	• Inhibits NMDA receptor • Psychotomimetic side effects (may need midazolam/haloperidol cover) • Contraindicated in raised intracranial pressure and fits • Caution in hypertension/cardiac problems • Available in the community on named patient basis only; irritant therefore dilute with sodium chloride 0.9% to largest possible volume
NSAIDs				
Ketorolac[†] [27]	Toradol 10, 30 mg/ml	Bone pain on recommendation of palliative care specialist	30–60 mg	• Well tolerated • Caution in renal failure • Can be nephrotoxic • Short-term use only (few days because of nephrotoxicity) • High incidence of upper GI bleeding, coprescribe gastroprotective drug • Irritant therefore dilute with largest possible volume 0.9% sodium chloride • Very alkaline, high risk of precipitation in combination
Antiemetics				
Metoclopramide*	Maxolon and nonproprietary 5 mg/ml, 2 and 20 ml	Impaired gastric emptying	30–100 mg	• Dopamine receptor antagonist • Nonsedating • Large volume • Possibility of extrapyramidal/dystonic side effects or tardive dyskinesia with prolonged use in younger women
Haloperidol*	Haldol and nonproprietary 5 mg/ml, 1 ml	Drug-induced nausea; metabolic causes; antipsychotic	2.5–10 mg	• Central dopamine receptor antagonist • Mildly sedating • Settles agitation and psychosis

Cyclizine*	Valoid 50 mg/ml, 1 ml	Intestinal obstruction; movement-induced nausea	50–150 mg	• Antihistamine (H_1) and anticholinergic • Drowsiness can be a problem • Compatibility problems; do not dilute with sodium chloride
Ondansetron[‡]	Zofran and nonproprietary 2 mg/ml, 2 and 4 ml	Chemotherapy or radiotherapy-induced vomiting (not usually SC route)	8–24 mg	• $5HT_3$ antagonist If not effective in 3 days discontinue • Expensive
Sedative and antiemetic Levomepromazine* [27]	Nozinan 25 mg/ml, 1 ml	Nausea; restlessness/agitation; psychosis	6–12.5 mg increasing to 25 mg for nausea (doses above 25 mg cause significant sedation and are rarely necessary for nausea); starting dose 25 mg SC single dose or 50–75 mg/24 h CSCI for restlessness/agitation; titration according to response. Very rarely doses as high as 200 mg/24 h are needed for severe terminal agitation but seek specialist advice	• Effective antiemetic • Extremely useful for terminal agitation • Occasional skin reactions • If used as a single agent may be diluted with 0.9% sodium chloride
Sedative Midazolam [63]	Hypnovel and nonproprietary 1 mg/ml 2, 5, and 50 ml; 2 mg/ml 5 ml; 5 mg/ml 2 and 10 ml	Anxiety; terminal restlessness; dyspnoea; anticonvulsant myoclonus	10–90 mg (common range 10–30 mg)	• Water-soluble benzodiazepine • Large interindividual variability in steady-state plasma level
Clonazepam[†]	Rivotril 1 mg/1 ml	Anxiety; terminal restlessness; anticonvulsant neuropathic pain	0.5–8 mg	• Less water soluble than midazolam • Irritant • May cause confusion

(continued)

Table 22.1 (Continued)

Medication	Trade name and ampoule size	Indication	Dose range per 24 h	Comments
Anticholinergic				
Hyoscine hydrobromide‡	0.4 mg/ml 1 ml; 0.6 mg/ml 1 ml	Terminal bronchial secretions and additional sedation	0.6–2.4 mg	• Dry mouth—extra attention to oral hygiene
Hyoscine butylbromide† [27]	Buscopan 20 mg/ml 1 ml	Severe colic Intestinal obstruction	20–120 mg	• Less likely to cause sedation than hydrobromide
Glycopyrronium bromide [42]	Robinul 0.2 mg/ml, 1 and 3 ml amps	Terminal secretions	0.6–1.2 mg	• Less likely to cause confusion than hyoscine hydrobromide. Slower onset than hyoscine hydrobromide
Steroids				
Dexamethasone†	Dexamethasone as sodium phosphate 4 mg/ml 1 ml amp;	Spinal cord compression, cauda equina compression	12–16 mg	• Compatibility difficulties (see Table 22.2) • Administer by SC bolus or via a separate syringe driver if possible
	Dexamethasone sodium phosphate 3.3 mg/ml 1 and 2 ml vial	Raised intracranial pressure	8–16 mg	
		Reduction in peritumour oedema	4–16 mg	
Anticonvulsants				
Clonazepam†	See above			
Midazolam*	See above			
Miscellaneous				
Octreotide [41]†	Sandostatin 50 µg; 100 µg/ml 1 ml 200 µg/ml 5 ml 500 µg/ml 1 ml	Reduces GI secretions; volume of vomit in intestinal obstruction; volume of enterocolic fistula	500 µg initially, if ineffective stop after 48 h, if effective titrate to lowest effective dose (range 50–600 µg)	Expensive

This list is not exhaustive; it covers many of the drugs used in palliative care. See other chapters for specific indications and usage. CSCI, continuous subcutaneous infusion; GI, gastrointestinal; SC, subcutaneous.

*Frequently used; †Sometimes used; ‡Rarely used; §Solubility of morphine salts: diamorphine HCl = 625 mg/ml, morphine acetate = 400 mg/ml, morphine tartrate = 100 mg/ml, morphine sulfate = 45 mg/ml. Contraindicated: the following are all too irritant to be used subcutaneously; diazepam, prochlorperazine, and chlorpromazine.

combinations in 1992 [32]. Although there was no explanation given for the reduction in the different number of drug combinations used, some of the drug mixtures reported were only prescribed in a small number of units. With the advent of an increase in the compatibility data available and the advent of care pathways, the results may indicate a tendency toward a more standardised approach to end-of-life drug treatment. At the time of the surveys, diamorphine was the most commonly administered analgesic in the syringe driver usually in combination with an antiemetic and/or sedative. In the United Kingdom, in 2006 a smaller Web-based survey of syringe driver drug combinations was conducted via users of a palliative care information website who were invited to respond [33]. Results indicated that a majority of syringe drivers from the sample of 328 contributed by respondents contained a combination of two or three drugs with only one-fifth containing a single drug. There is however still limited evidence regarding compatibility or stability of drug combinations. An additional complication under the current UK Medicines Act 1968 is that mixing drugs together, where one drug is not a vehicle of administration of the other as detailed in the summary of product characteristics, creates an unlicenced medicine. This was addressed by an amendment following a public consultation (MLX356) when the MHRA together with the Commission on Human Medicines recommended that changes should be made to medicines legislation, which apply to palliative care and other clinical areas where mixing of medicines is accepted practice. The law will be amended to allow doctors and dentists to mix medicines and to allow nonmedical prescribers to prescribe unlicenced medicines in the same way as doctors and supplementary prescribers [34].

In the United Kingdom, drugs are usually diluted with water for injection unless there is a specific requirement to use sodium chloride. In particular, 0.9% saline should not be used to dilute cyclizine or higher concentrations of diamorphine ($\geq$40 mg/ml) as there is a high risk of precipitation. The number of drugs combined in a single syringe should be kept to a minimum, checking compatibility data and seeking advice from specialist palliative health-care professionals, and specialist medicines information pharmacists. Examples of other useful resources are shown in Box 22.1.

Recognising and responding to possible compatibility problems

If the contents of the syringe become cloudy or discoloured before or during infusion, the syringe should be discarded immediately. Should incompatibility problems

Box 22.1 Information resources: drug compatibility in palliative care

Dickman A, Schneider J, and Varga J. *The Syringe Driver: Continuous Subcutaneous Infusions in Palliative Care.* Oxford: Oxford University Press, 2005.
www.palliativedrugs.com
www.pallmed.net
www.sign.ac.uk

persist and alternative drugs or routes are not available, then a second syringe driver may be required to infuse drugs separately. Alternatively, the use of bolus SC injections may be considered if the drug has a longer duration of action, provided that the patient's skin condition will make bolus injections tolerable.

Correct storage temperatures should be observed for all drugs. Where high concentrations of drugs are being infused, change in temperature (particularly cold) can reduce solubility. The syringe driver contents should also be protected from light by placing in an opaque pouch, holster, or pocket to prevent photodegradation.

Compatibility and stability

Consideration of the compatibility of drugs is vital to ensure efficacy of therapy. Interactions between drugs can be difficult to predict and may produce a number of effects, including a reduction in stability or changes in solubility resulting in precipitation or crystallisation. This may cause the infusion cannula to become blocked, the injection site to become inflamed, and the treatment to be ineffective. Physical examination of the contents (looking for cloudiness or discolouration), although a guide to compatibility, does not guarantee absence of chemical reaction. Ideally, all combinations would be chemically analysed for active ingredients and any toxic breakdown products across the range of physical environments in which drugs may be administered or stored. This is costly in terms of time and resources and has not been done for the many different combinations of drugs and doses tailored to individual symptoms.

Most drugs used in syringe drivers are water soluble and can be mixed. However, some drugs, for example, phenobarbital (made up in propylene glycol), are immiscible with aqueous solutions and should not be used in the same syringe as other drugs.

The major factor leading to incompatibility is the relative concentration of each drug. Other factors include pH, storage conditions, temperature, and ionic strength.

Many salts in aqueous solution undergo degradation: for example, diamorphine is hydrolysed to 6-monoacetylmorphine and morphine. The stability of diamorphine, morphine, and oxycodone in syringe drivers under a variety of conditions has been examined [35–47]. Table 22.2 indicates the compatibility and stability of two-drug mixtures for at least 24 h. Higher concentrations may lead to lower efficacy due to instability or precipitation of drugs.

Site of the infusion

An appropriate choice of infusion site as indicated later will help to minimise site problems. Change the infusion site only when necessary, that is, if it is painful, or appears to be inflamed or swollen. The frequency of this will vary between patients and depend on the combination of drugs used. Single-agent diamorphine or morphine infusions can last for several days, whereas if cyclizine or levomepromazine is used, daily changes may be necessary. The extension set and needle should generally be changed at each resiting [48].

Should there be persistent problems with irritation at the injection site, consider the following options:
• Reducing the concentration of drugs (i.e., larger volume).
• Changing the drug or considering an alternative route.
• Mixing drugs with 0.9% saline (if compatible).
• Using a plastic (Teflon or Vialon) cannula.
• Applying hydrocortisone 1% cream to the skin around the needle entry site, and covering it with an occlusive dressing [27].
• Adding dexamethasone 0.5–1 mg to the infusion (if compatible). Dexamethasone should not be routinely added to infusion solutions unless there is a specific problem with infusion sites [49].

Choice of site for the infusion cannula

Suitable sites for placement of the butterfly needle include the upper chest, outer upper arm, anterior abdomen, and thighs. The exact placement may be influenced by the patient's preference, by the disease process, and by common sense. The area over the scapula may be used in confused or disorientated patients.

Care should be taken to avoid the deltoid area in bedbound patients who require regular turning and sites over bony prominences in cachectic patients. Also avoid broken skin, areas of inflammation, recently irradiated areas, sites of tumour, and oedematous/lymphaedematous areas.

Management of the subcutaneous infusion: regular checks

It is essential that the following checks are made regularly throughout the period of use, preferably using a dedicated syringe driver monitoring chart:
• Drug and doses.
• For signs of irritation or inflammation at the injection site.
• For evidence of leakage at the various connections.
• That the driver is working (light flashing/intermittent motor noise).
• That the set rate is correct and the corresponding amount of fluid infused.
• For signs of crystallisation or precipitation (cloudiness).
• That the tubing is not kinked.

Obtaining the drugs for the palliative care patient—seamless care at the hospital/hospice/community interface

Although palliative care patients may spend some periods in a hospital or hospice, the majority of patients receive palliative care in the community. It is vital that drugs required for symptom control are easily accessible within the community and that the necessary communication channels exist for responding to changing requirements.

Domiciliary or home care services

Many community pharmacists offer a home delivery service for patients without carers or those who are too frail or unwell to collect medicines from the pharmacy. Some operate prescription collection services or repeat medication services where a pharmacy receives prescriptions directly from a general practitioner (GP) surgery. This service must be requested by the patient or carer.

Drugs used frequently in palliative care

The range of drugs often required to treat palliative symptoms is not routinely stocked by all community pharmacies. In the United Kingdom, in an attempt to resolve this issue, various service development initiatives have been adopted in different geographical areas to enable access to necessary medicines required for symptom control when these are required, including provision of a service by specified pharmacies that hold a locally agreed list of palliative care drugs. The patient and their carers may need assistance in organisation of supplies so that essential equipment and medications are always available.

Table 22.2 The compatibility of drugs combined in a syringe for SC infusion.

	Morphine	Diamorphine	Metoclopramide	Haloperidol	Cyclizine	Levomepromazine	Midazolam	Hyoscine hydrobromide	Hyoscine butylbromide	Dexamethasone**	Octreotide	Glycopyrronium	Oxycodone
Morphine		N	c√√	√√	c√√	√√	√√	√√	√√	c	√√	√	N
Diamorphine	N		c‡√√	√√	*√√	√√	√√	√√	√√	c	√√	√√	N
Metoclopramide	c√√	c‡√√		N	N	N	√	N	N	√√	√	N	√√
Haloperidol	√√	√√	N		√	N	√√	√	√	p	√	No data	√√
Cyclizine	c√√	*√√	N	√		√	c	c	p	p	NO	No data	p§
Levomepromazine	√√	√√	N	N	√		√	√	√	p	NO	No data	√√
Midazolam	√√	√√	√	√√	c	√		√	√	p	No data	√	√√
Hyoscine hydrobromide	√√	√√	N	√	c	√	√			N	No data	No data	√√
Hyoscine butylbromide	√√	√√	N	√	p	√	√	N		No data	No data	N	√√
Dexamethasone**	C	c	√√	p	p	p	p	No data	No data		p	NO	√√
Octreotide	√√	√√	√	√	NO	NO	No data	No data	√	p		No data	No data
Glycopyrronium	√	√√	N	No data	No data	No data	√	N	N	NO	No data		No data
Oxycodone	N	N	√√	√√	p§	√√	√√	√√	√√	√√	No data	No data	

√√, no problems at usual therapeutic concentrations—published evidence.

√, compatible at usual therapeutic concentrations—common usage but no published evidence. Seek specialist advice before use.

c, caution at higher concentrations.

p, occasionally precipitates. Seek specialist advice before use.

NO, definite compatibility problems. These drugs must "never" be combined.

N, generally not a clinically useful combination (same group of drug or counteracting effects).

*Stable with diamorphine up to 20 mg/ml + cyclizine up to 20 mg/ml. Higher concentrations of diamorphine are probably only stable with lower concentrations of cyclizine. Diamorphine any concentration + cyclizine up to 6.7 mg/ml (i.e., maximum 50 mg of cyclizine in 8 ml infusion with diamorphine >160 mg: maximum 100 mg of cyclizine in a 16 ml infusion with diamorphine >320 mg in 16 ml).

‡Stable with diamorphine up to 25 mg/ml + metoclopramide up to 5 mg/ml (i.e., diamorphine 200 mg is stable with up to 40 mg of metoclopramide in an 8 ml infusion).

§Cyclizine concentrations should not exceed 3 mg/ml when mixed with oxycodone injection, either diluted or undiluted.

**Dexamethasone has a long half-life. To avoid potential compatibility problems, it should be administered where possible by SC bolus. 1 mg dexamethasone = 1.3 mg dexamethasone sodium phosphate.

Box 22.2 Examples of prescription medicines that are sometimes only stocked by community pharmacists participating in a palliative care scheme

- Large quantities or high dosages of morphine-containing analgesics.
- Alternative strong opioids (diamorphine injection, transdermal fentanyl, oxycodone, hydromorphone).
- Midazolam injection.
- Levomepromazine injection.
- Haloperidol injection.
- Metoclopramide injection.
- Dexamethasone tablets in high doses and injection.
- Hyoscine hydrobromide, butylbromide, or glycopyrronium injection.
- Diazepam suppositories or rectal liquid.

Examples of prescription medicines commonly used in palliative care but which are sometimes not routinely stocked by community pharmacists are shown in Box 22.2.

The complexity of medicines used in the care of terminally ill patients in the community serves to highlight the importance of careful planning of the discharge of a patient from secondary to primary care, or from hospice to home. Good communication between health-care professionals is the key to the smooth operating of such systems. This applies equally when patients are discharged from hospital or specialist palliative care units. Faxing medication details (where a patient has identified a regular community pharmacist) can ensure that supplies of medication are available when required, as the pharmacist is able to anticipate prescriptions and have all drugs to hand [50].

The problem of availability of medication becomes more acute outside normal working hours. This has been addressed in different ways across the country: by making palliative care drugs available at central "out-of-hours" medical locations, by using prefilled drug bags or boxes available either at the patients' home or at access points such as a deputising agency, hospice, or by using a network of dedicated on-call palliative care community pharmacists [51].

Prescribing and dispensing of controlled drugs

Controlled drugs (CDs) in the United Kingdom are subject to the requirements of the Misuse of Drugs Regula-

tions 2001 as amended [52] together with other local guidance. The legislation is split into five schedules. Schedule 1 lists drugs such as lysergic acid diethylamide, ecstasy-type substances, and cannabis, which have virtually no therapeutic use and have the strictest control imposed on them. Schedule 2 drugs include the principal opioids and major stimulants (e.g., amphetamine), while buprenorphine and most barbiturates fall into schedule 3. Schedule 4 drugs consist mainly of the benzodiazepines. Schedule 5 covers the low dose and dilute preparations of some of the schedule 2 drugs and has the lowest level of control. CDs are distinguished in the *British National Formulary* by the symbol CD. The status of compounds can be checked in the *Medicines, Ethics and Practice Guide* obtained online at the Royal Pharmaceutical Society Website www.rpharms.com [53].

The prescription

In the United Kingdom, regulations for prescribing CDs are under review. Medical and dental prescribers may prescribe all CDs in schedules 2–5 for the purpose of treating organic disease; nurse-independent prescribers may also prescribe CDs albeit from a limited list. At present, pharmacist-independent prescribers cannot prescribe CDs but may do so when acting as supplementary prescribers in partnership with an independent prescriber who is acting within a clinical management plan for a specific patient and with the patient's agreement. The Misuse of Drug Regulations are due to be amended to allow nurse- and pharmacist-independent prescribers extended permissions to prescribe CDs in schedules 2–5 for the purpose of treating organic disease or injury [54]. The regulations may be accessed at http://www.legislation.gov.uk/all?title=controlled%20drugs.

It is an offence for a prescriber to issue an incomplete prescription and it is illegal for a pharmacist to dispense a CD unless all the information required by law is given on the prescription. Failure to comply with the regulations (Box 22.3) will result in inconvenience to the patient and delay in supplying the necessary medicines.

The amended Misuse of Drugs Regulations 2001 may be accessed at http://www.legislation.gov.uk/uksi/2005/271/regulation/2/made.

Prescriptions for schedule 2 and 3 drugs (all strong opioids, barbiturates, and temazepam) must be completed as described in Box 22.3.

Alterations should be avoided but if an error is made, best practice is to cross out the error, initial and date this, and then write the correct information.

> ## Box 22.3 Details required for a CD prescription in schedule 2 or 3 (except temazepam)
>
> - The name and address of the patient (the age if under 12 years old).
> - Prescriptions ordering CDs must be signed by hand by the prescriber and specify the prescriber's registration number and address (which must be in the United Kingdom).
> - The date of prescribing should be included (but need not be in the prescriber's handwriting).
> - In the case of preparations, the form (i.e., tablets, capsules, and mixture) and the appropriate the strength (where there is more than one strength available) of the preparation.
> - The total quantity of the preparation, or the number of dosage units, in both words and figures (i.e., number of millilitres of liquid, number of tablets, patches, or ampoules rather than the total milligram of the drug).
> - The specified dose: for example, the instruction "one as directed" constitutes a dose but "as directed" does not indicate the specific dose.
> - The prescription may be computer generated but does not have to be computer generated. While the prescription may be "written in any form" if these other details on the prescription are handwritten, good practice would indicate that they are handwritten by the prescriber but if not, the prescription should only be written by a health-care professional.

It is good practice to supply only an appropriate amount for the needs of the patient and if more than 30 days' supply is given, then a note to justify the reason should be included in the patient records.

Prescriptions are valid for a period of 28 days (including those for temazepam, midazolam, and schedule 4 CDs). The prescriber may specify a second supply date in addition to the date of signing. The prescription is valid for 28 days from the latest of these two dates.

An example of a CD prescription is given in Figure 22.3.

Standardised private prescriptions for CDs

All private prescriptions for schedules 2 and 3 CDs including temazepam that are presented for dispensing in the community must be written on a standard prescription form which is either a personalised FP10(PCD) NC (which has the prescribers details already printed on) or a nonpersonalised FP10(PCD) SS (which is not preprinted). These prescription forms must include a unique six-digit identifier that is issued to the prescriber solely for the purpose of private prescribing.

Taking CDs abroad

If a patient travelling abroad from the United Kingdom needs to take more than three calendar months supply of CD, the licencing law required the patient to seek a licence from the Home Office. An application must be made in writing to the Home Office to include the following information:
- patient's full name and address and date of birth;
- country or countries of destination;
- departure date from and return date to the United Kingdom; and
- a letter from the prescribing doctor confirming details, including name, form (e.g., liquid or capsule), strength, and total quantity of each CD to be taken out of the United Kingdom.

Further information can be found at: http://www.homeoffice.gov.uk/drugs/licensing/personal/.

The application should be made at least 10 days before the intended day of departure from the United Kingdom.

If the amount of CDs to be taken out of the country is within the limits, or a licence has been obtained from the Home Office, then there is no need to declare the medicines to UK customs. The licence however has no legal status outside the United Kingdom and does not ensure safe passage through the customs of the country of destination. The patient must contact the Embassy or High Commission in the United Kingdom to clarify the requirements for taking CDs through the customs of the destination country or countries.

Unwanted medicines or disposal of CDs after a death at home

A patient or their representative may return unwanted medicines, including CDs, to any pharmacist for destruction. Since 2007 the UK Department of Health have issued new guidance on the destruction on CDs [54]. Destruction of stocks of CD held by an institution is regulated and may only be destroyed in the manner directed under the current Misuse of Drugs Regulations. Under the original regulations, the Secretary of State for Health authorised groups of people who could witness the destruction of stocks of CDs held by institutions. The Health Act

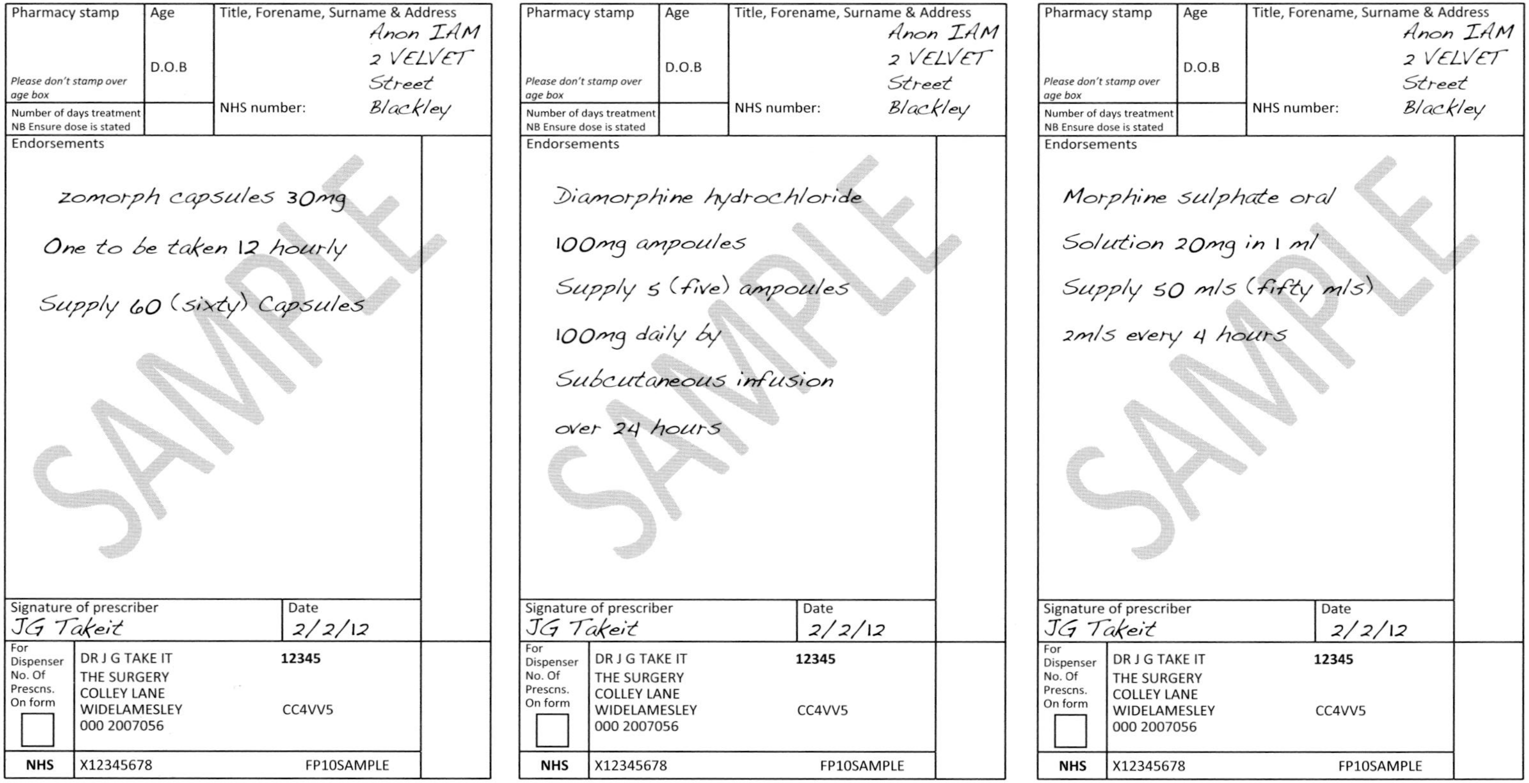

Prescription 1

Pharmacy stamp | Age | Title, Forename, Surname & Address
Anon IAM
2 VELVET
Street
Blackley

D.O.B

NHS number:

Please don't stamp over age box

Number of days treatment
NB Ensure dose is stated

Endorsements

zomorph capsules 30mg

One to be taken 12 hourly

Supply 60 (sixty) Capsules

Signature of prescriber
JG Takeit

Date 2/2/12

For Dispenser
No. Of Prescns.
On form

DR J G TAKE IT
THE SURGERY
COLLEY LANE
WIDELAMESLEY
000 2007056

12345

CC4VV5

NHS X12345678

FP10SAMPLE

Prescription 2

Pharmacy stamp | Age | Title, Forename, Surname & Address
Anon IAM
2 VELVET
Street
Blackley

D.O.B

NHS number:

Please don't stamp over age box

Number of days treatment
NB Ensure dose is stated

Endorsements

Diamorphine hydrochloride

100mg ampoules

Supply 5 (five) ampoules

100mg daily by

Subcutaneous infusion

over 24 hours

Signature of prescriber
JG Takeit

Date 2/2/12

For Dispenser
No. Of Prescns.
On form

DR J G TAKE IT
THE SURGERY
COLLEY LANE
WIDELAMESLEY
000 2007056

12345

CC4VV5

NHS X12345678

FP10SAMPLE

Prescription 3

Pharmacy stamp | Age | Title, Forename, Surname & Address
Anon IAM
2 VELVET
Street
Blackley

D.O.B

NHS number:

Please don't stamp over age box

Number of days treatment
NB Ensure dose is stated

Endorsements

Morphine sulphate oral

Solution 20mg in 1 ml

Supply 50 mls (fifty mls)

2mls every 4 hours

Signature of prescriber
JG Takeit

Date 2/2/12

For Dispenser
No. Of Prescns.
On form

DR J G TAKE IT
THE SURGERY
COLLEY LANE
WIDELAMESLEY
000 2007056

12345

CC4VV5

NHS X12345678

FP10SAMPLE

Figure 22.3 A specimen CD prescription as used in the United Kingdom.

2006 allowed strengthened governance and monitoring of CDs and required institutions and designated bodies to appoint "accountable officers" to oversee this task. Accountable officers may appoint authorised persons with appropriate training to witness destruction of stocks of CDs. Under UK law, however, CDs returned by a patient can be destroyed without the presence of an "authorised person." Good practice suggests that doctors and nurses should have a witness when destroying CDs that a patient has returned or no longer needs. It is also advised that a written record is made by those health professionals of the nature and quantity of the drugs that have been destroyed, how they were destroyed, and who was present. Preferably, because CDs are the property of the patient, they should, where possible, be returned for destruction by the patient or the patient's representative.

Pharmacy and palliative care: the future

Advances in oncological treatment mean patients encountered by palliative care have increasingly complex needs, with similarly complicated medication regimes. Furthermore, the proportion of patients seen by palliative care teams with a variety of nonmalignant conditions is increasing. This will only consolidate the valuable contribution of the pharmacist, within the palliative care team setting.

In the United Kingdom, there is impetus to maximise provision of patient care in the community setting, with initiatives to recognise patients who may be approaching the end of their life and projects to achieve preferred place of care in patients with a life-limiting illness. This is likely to lead to an increase in workload for community palliative care teams that will require the support of community pharmacists. Further training of interested community pharmacists in palliative care would be essential to ensuring effective patient care [55].

References

1. World Health Organization. *National Cancer Control Programmes. Policies and Managerial Guidelines*, 2nd edition. Geneva: WHO, 2002.
2. National Institute for Clinical Excellence. *Improving Supportive and Palliative Care for Adults with Cancer*. London: NICE, 2004.
3. McPherson ML. Preface. *Prog Palliat Care* 2010; 18(3): 130–131.
4. Walker K, Scarpaci L, and McPherson ML. Fifty reasons to love your palliative care pharmacist. *Am J Hosp Palliat Care* 2010; 27: 511–513.
5. McPherson ML and Holmes H. Precision pharmacopalliation: the Goldilocks' approach to medication management at end of life. *Prog Palliat Care* 2010; 18(3): 140–146.
6. Zeppetella G. How do terminally ill patients at home take their medication?. *Palliat Med* 1999; 13(6): 469–475.
7. Thompson CA. Palliative care pharmacists consider patients' psychosocial issues. *Am J Health Syst Pharm* 2008; 65(6): 500–501.
8. Snapp J, Kelley D, and Gutsgell TL. Creating a hospice pharmacy and therapeutics committee. *Am J Hosp Palliat Care* 2002; 19(2): 129–134.
9. Atkinson C and Kirkham S. Unlicensed uses for medication in a palliative care unit. *Palliat Med* 1999; 13: 145–152.
10. Todd J and Davies A. Use of unlicensed medication in palliative medicine. *Palliat Med* 1999; 13: 466.
11. Poole SG and Dooley MJ. Off-Label prescribing in oncology. *Support Care Cancer* 2004; 12: 302–330.
12. Joint Working Party of the Association for Palliative Medicine and the Pain Society. *The Use of Drugs Beyond Licence in Palliative Care and Pain Management*. London: Pain Society, 2002.
13. Williams NT. Medication administration through enteral feeding tubes. *Am J Health Syst Pharm* 2008; 65: 2347–2357.
14. White R and Bradnam V. *Handbook of Drug Administration via Enteral Feeding Tubes*. London: Pharmaceutical Press, 2007.
15. Aronson J. Compliance, concordance, adherence. *Br J Clin Pharmacol* 2007; 63(4): 383–384.
16. Bergman-Evans B. AIDES to improving medication adherence in older adults. *Geriatr Nurs* 2006; 27: 174–182.
17. Lecouturier J, Cunningham B, Campbell D, et al. Medication compliance aids: a qualitative study of users' views. *Br J Gen Pract* 2011; 61(583): 93–100.
18. Cramer J. Enhancing patient compliance in the elderly: role of packaging aids and monitoring. *Drugs Aging* 1998; 12(1): 7–15.
19. Russell PSB. Analgesia in terminal malignant disease. *BMJ* 1979; 1: 1561.
20. Dickinson RJ, Howard B, and Campbell J. The relief of pain by subcutaneous infusion of diamorphine. In: Wilkes E and Lenz J (eds), *Advances in Morphine Therapy*. The 1983 International Symposium on Pain Control. Royal Society of Medicine International Symposium series, no. 64. London: Royal Society of Medicine, 1984, pp. 105–110.
21. Oliver DJ. The use of the syringe driver in terminal care. *Br J Clin Pharmacol* 1985; 20: 515–516.
22. Coyle N, Mauskop A, Maggard J, et al. Continuous subcutaneous infusions of opiates in cancer patients with pain. *Oncol Nurs Forum* 1986; 13: 53–57.

23. Beswick DT. Use of syringe driver in terminal care. *Pharm J* 1987; 239: 656–658.

24. Burera E, Brenneis C, Michaud M, et al. Continuous subcutaneous infusion of narcotics using a portable disposable device in patients with advanced cancer. *Cancer Treat Rep* 1987; 71: 635–637.

25. Bottomley DM and Hanks GW. Subcutaneous midazolam infusion in palliative care. *J Pain Symptom Manage* 1990; 5(4): 259–261.

26. National Patients Safety Agency. December 2010. Available at: http://www.nrls.npsa.nhs.uk/alerts/?entryid45=92908 (accessed on June 14, 2011).

27. Twycross R and Wilcock A. *Palliative Care Formulary*, 3rd edition. Oxford: Radcliffe Medical Press, 2011. Available at: www.palliativedrugs.com (accessed on May 15, 2012).

28. Dickman A, Schneider J, and Varga J. *The Syringe Driver: Continuous Subcutaneous Infusions in Palliative Care.* Oxford: Oxford University Press, 2005.

29. SIGN Guideline 106. 2008. Control of pain in adults with cancer: Scottish Intercollegiate Guidelines Network, Scottish Cancer Therapy Network. Available at: www.sign.ac.uk (November 2008).

30. Back I. www.pallmed.net Drug compatibility database. 2011.

31. O'Doherty C, Hall E, Schofield L, et al. Drugs and syringe drivers: a survey of adult specialist palliative care practice in United Kingdom and Eire. *Palliat Med* 2001; 15: 149–154.

32. Johnson I and Patterson S. Drugs used in combination in the syringe driver—a survey of hospice practice. *Palliat Med* 1992; 6: 125–130.

33. Wilcock A, Jacob J, Charlesworth S, et al. Drugs given by a syringe driver: a prospective multicentre survey of palliative care services in the UK. *Palliat Med* 2006; 20: 661–664.

34. MHRA. Public consultation (MLX356); Proposal for amendments to medicines legislation to allow mixing of medicines in palliative care. 2009. Available at: http://www.mhra.gov.uk/Publications/Consultations/Medicines consultations/MLXs/CON033523 (accessed on May 15, 2012).

35. Allwood MC. Diamorphine mixed with antiemetic drugs in plastic syringes. *Br J Pharm Pract* 1984; 6: 88–90.

36. Collins AJ, Abethell JA, Holmes SG, et al. Stability of diamorphine hydrochloride with haloperidol in prefilled syringes for subcutaneous infusion. *J Pharm Pharmacol* 1986; 38(Suppl.): 51.

37. Regnard C, Pashley S, and Westrope E. Anti-emetic/diamorphine compatibility in infusion pumps. *Br J Pharm Pract* 1986; 8: 218–220.

38. Allwood MC. The compatibility of high dose diamorphine with cyclizine or haloperidol in plastic syringes. *Int J Pharm Pract* 1991; 5: 120.

39. Allwood MC. The stability of diamorphine alone and in combination with antiemetics in plastic syringes. *Palliat Med* 1991; 5: 330–333.

40. Allwood MC, Brown PC, and Lee M. Stability of injections containing diamorphine and midazolam in plastic syringes. *Int J Pharm Pract* 1994; 3: 57–59.

41. Fielding H, Kyaterekera N, Skellern G, et al. The compatibility and stability of octreotide acetate in the presence of diamorphine hydrochloride in polypropylene syringes. *Palliat Med* 2000; 14: 205–207.

42. Smith J, Hirsch C, Marriott J, et al. The stability of diamorphine and glycopyrrolate in PCA syringes. *Pharm J* 2000; 265: R69.

43. Negro S, Reyes R, Azuara M, et al. Morphine, haloperidol, hyoscine N-butylbromide combined in s.c. infusion solutions: compatibility and stability. *Int J Pharm* 2006; 307: 278–284.

44. Grassby PF and Hutchings L. Drug combinations in syringe drivers: the compatibility and stability of diamorphine with cyclizine and haloperidol. *Palliat Med* 1997; 11: 217–224.

45. Fawcett JP, Woods DJ, Munasiri B, et al. Compatibility of cyclizine lactate and haloperidol lactate. *Am J Hosp Pharm* 1994; 51: 2292.

46. Grassby PF. Personal communication, 1996.

47. Gardiner PR. Compatibility of an injectable oxycodone formulation with typical diluents, syringes, tubings, infusion bags and drugs for potential co-administration. *Hosp Pharm* 2003; 10: 354–361.

48. Mitten T. Subcutaneous infusions: a review of problems and solutions. *Int J Palliat Nurs* 2001; 7(2): 75–85.

49. Reymond L, Charles MA, Bowman J, et al. The effect of dexamethasone on the longevity of syringe driver subcutaneous sites in palliative care patients. *Med J Aust* 2003; 178: 486–489.

50. Thomas K. Out-of-hours palliative care in the community. Continuing care for the dying at home. London: Macmillan Cancer Relief, 2001. Available at: http://www.epolitix.com/Resources/epolitix/Forum%20Microsites/Macmillan%20Cancer%20Relief/ooh-report-1.pdf (accessed on May 16, 2012).

51. Hirsch C, Hayer B, Salih Z, et al. Access to palliative care drugs 'out of hours': a preliminary evaluation of two West Midlands models. *International Journal of Pharmacy Practice* 2009; 17: B80–B81.

52. Misuse of Drugs Regulations. 2001 (SI 3998). Available at: www.opsi.gov.uk/si/si2001/20013998.htm (accessed on May 15, 2012).

53. The Royal Pharmaceutical Society. www.rpharms.com/legal-classification-of-medicines/legal-classification-of-medicines.asp (Accessed on July 15, 2011).

54. National Prescribing Centre. *A guide to Good Practice in the Management of Controlled Drugs in Primary Care*, 3rd edition. England: National Prescribing Centre, 2009. www.npc.nhs.uk/controlled_drugs/resources/controlled_drugs_third_edition.pdf (accessed on May 15, 2012).

55. Needham DS, Wong IC, Campion PD, et al. Evaluation of the effectiveness of UK community pharmacists' interventions

in community palliative care. *Palliat Med* 2002; 16: 219–225.

56. Jones VA, Murphy A, and Hanks GW. Solubility of diamorphine. *Pharm J* 1985; 235: 426.

57. Walker SE and Lau DWC. Compatibility and stability of hyaluronidase and Hydromorphone. *Can J Hosp Pharm* 1992; 45: 187–192.

58. Bruera E, Fainsinger R, Moore M, et al. Clinical note: local toxicity with subcutaneous methadone. Experience of two centres. *Pain* 1991; 45: 141–143.

59. Fainsinger R, Schoeller T, and Bruera E. Methadone in the management of cancer pain: a review. *Pain* 1993; 52: 137–147.

60. Luczak J, Dickenson AH, and Kotlinska-Lemieszek A. The role of Ketamine, an NMDA receptor antagonist, in the management of pain. *Prog Palliat Care* 1995; 3: 127–134.

61. Mercadante S. Ketamine in cancer pain: an update. *Palliat Med* 1996; 10: 225–230.

62. Bell RF, Eccleston C and Kelso EA. Ketamine as an adjuvant to opioids for cancer pain. *Cochrane Database Syst Rev* 2003; (1): CD003351. doi:10.1002/14651858.CD003351.

63. Bleasel MD, Peterson GM and Dunne PF. Plasma concentrations of Midazolam during continuous subcutaneous administration in palliative care. *Palliat Med* 1994; 8: 231–236.

Further reading

Bernard SA and Bruera E. Drug interactions in palliative care. *J Clin Oncol* 2000; 18(8): 1780–1799.

British National Formulary. Guidance on prescribing in terminal care (in the first section of the book).

Centre for Palliative Care Research and Education. Queensland health. In: *Guidelines for Subcutaneous Device Management in Palliative Care*, 2nd edition. Australian Government Department of Health and Ageing, 2010. Available at: www.health.qld.gov.au/cpcre (accessed on May 15, 2012).

NHS Scotland. Palliative Care Guidelines – Subcutaneous infusion of medication via a McKinley Pump or syringe driver, 2010. Available at: http://www.palliative careguidelines.scot.nhs.uk/documents/Syringe%20driver .pdf (accessed on May 15, 2012).

Trissel LA. *Handbook on Injectable Drugs*, 16th edition. Houston, TX: American Society of Health System Pharmacists Inc., 2011.

Urie J, Feilding H, McArthur D, et al. Palliative care. *Pharm J* 2000; 256: 603–614.

Watson M, Lucas C, Hoy A, et al. Palliative Care Guidelines Plus, 2011. Available at: http://book.pallcare.info/index.php (accessed on May 15, 2012).

23 Complementary Approaches to Palliative Cancer Care

Elizabeth Thompson[1], Catherine Zollman[2]

[1] University Hospitals Bristol NHS Foundation Trust, Bristol Homoeopathic Hospital, Bristol, UK
[2] Penny Brohn Cancer Care, Bristol, UK

Introduction

The past 25 years have seen an increase in the use of complementary therapies (CTs) with palliative care settings appearing to be no exception to this observation. The only published survey of UK hospices in 1992 showed 70% of respondents offering massage and aromatherapy services [1]. Of 55 oncology departments surveyed in England and Wales in 1998, 38 were offering at least one CT [2]. In Washington State, 86% of hospices surveyed by phone interview offered CT to their patients and with such widespread use the authors suggested CT reimbursement schedules should be integrated into hospice care [3]. Of the total number of women with breast cancer in the United Kingdom in the year 2000, 31.5% had consulted a CT practitioner since diagnosis [4]. The vast majority of patients and service providers use a combination of complementary approaches and orthodox palliative care, and there are similarities between these two approaches that make the resulting package of care potentially attractive. This chapter will explore these similarities and show how CT and orthodox palliative medicine might truly "complement" each other.

There is sometimes confusion around the terminology and concepts of "CTs" with other terms being used interchangeably. Useful distinctions and other important points are summarised in Table 23.1. One suggested definition of Complementary Medicine is:

> Areas of medicine that are generally outside current accepted medical thought, scientific knowledge or university teaching [7].

For clarity, the term "CTs" will be used throughout this chapter. However defined, the term CT describes a very heterogeneous group of approaches, some of which have features in common, while others have conflicting theories and practice. A newer term "integrated" or "integrative medicine" describes a whole person approach, which emphasises the importance of physical, psychological, social, and spiritual aspects of care and combines conventional and complementary interventions in the most appropriate way for the individual patient. For the purpose of this chapter, we have not considered psychotherapy, cognitive/behavioural approaches, or counselling under our definition of CT.

Similarities between complementary therapies and holistic palliative care

Palliative care acknowledges that a patient's physical symptoms cannot be fully understood or helped without an appreciation of emotional, psychological, and social factors. Likewise, many CT practitioners claim to have a holistic perspective. The central tenets of anthroposophy, a philosophical and therapeutic system developed by Rudolf Steiner, are a good example of this approach (see Box 23.1).

Palliative care and CT disciplines are person-centred rather than disease-centred and both have strategies that ensure it is never the case that "there is nothing more to be done." Many CT treatments also focus on well-being and contribute to a pleasurable sense of being cared for, thereby improving quality of life. Patients' symptoms can

Handbook of Palliative Care, Third Edition. Edited by Christina Faull, Sharon de Caestecker, Alex Nicholson and Fraser Black.
© 2012 by John Wiley and Sons, Inc. Published 2012 by John Wiley & Sons, Inc.

Table 23.1 Assumptions about CTs.

Statement	Comments
Alternative	Implies used instead of orthodox treatment. In fact, the majority of CT users appear not to have abandoned orthodox medicine
Not provided by the NHS	CT is increasingly available on NHS. Of the total number of GP practices in the United Kingdom, 39% provide access to CT for NHS patients [5]
Unregulated	Osteopaths and chiropractors are now state registered and regulated. Other CT disciplines will probably soon follow
Natural	Many conventional pharmacological products are derived from natural products, for example, plants and minerals. Conversely CT can involve unnatural practices
Holistic	As in conventional medicine, there are practitioners who take a holistic approach to their patient and there are those who are more reductionist in outlook
Unproven	There is a growing body of evidence that supports the claim that certain types of CTs are effective in certain clinical conditions
Irrational—no scientific basis	Basic science research is beginning to give an understanding of the mechanisms of some types of CT (e.g., acupuncture, hypnosis [6,9])
Harmless	There are reports of rare but serious adverse effects associated with some CT use [51]

be improved, relationships healed, and preparations for death embraced. Realistic hope can sustain people. Existential questions and concerns form a regular feature of work with people with advanced disease. Some CT disciplines include a spiritual dimension and can recognise and address symptoms at this level. As with the best of palliative care nursing, many CT approaches involve practitioners and patients in a degree of physical contact that legitimises touch and human contact.

The benefit of any intervention, particularly in advanced illness, must clearly outweigh any harm. Except for some notable exceptions (see later sections), CT approaches have very few harmful effects if used appropriately.

Most palliative care units have a "low-tech" atmosphere where patients are helped to feel at home. Most CT approaches require a minimum of equipment and can be readily practiced by the bedside, at home, or in a day-care centre. Techniques can even be taught to relatives or patients themselves as well as volunteers and medical and nursing staff.

The above features, common to many CTs and to holistic palliative care, have led many patients with cancer to seek out complementary treatments. They have also led many existing palliative care services to incorporate a range of these approaches. The rest of this chapter will describe some of the treatments most commonly used and encountered in these settings, considering the background to each therapy as well as the research evidence, indications, and contraindications for its use. We will then consider some of the problems patients may experience related to their use of CT, and discuss ways in which these can be minimised by appropriate advice and involvement from the palliative care team.

Box 23.1 Central tenets of anthroposophy

- Each individual is unique.
- Scientific, artistic, and spiritual insights may need to be applied together to restore health.
- Life has meaning and purpose—the loss of this sense may lead to a deterioration in health.
- Illness may provide opportunities for positive change and a new balance in our lives.

The CTs discussed in this chapter are considered in alphabetical order.

Acupuncture

Acupuncture, the ancient Chinese art of healing using the insertion of fine needles, has origins dating back to at least 2500 BC. The *Yellow Emperor's Classic of Internal Medicine* [8] describes, among other concepts, an elaborate system of diagnosis based on vital energy, or "Qi," and meridians, which are a series of invisible lines joining acupuncture points together.

The patient is treated using thin needles inserted in a carefully chosen combination of specific acupuncture points. The needles are left *in situ* or stimulated by hand for up to 20 min. In addition, some needles are stimulated using electroacupuncture equipment, using "moxibustion" (a technique involving heat and herbs), or given painless stimulation using low-level laser therapy.

Over the past 30 years, evidence has accumulated on many of the basic mechanisms of action of acupuncture, for example, modulation of neural responses, stimulation of multiple endogenous opioids, release of serotonin (which can influence mood), autonomic effects, alteration in blood supply, and increased production of corticosteroids [9]. One study concluded that acupuncture is underutilised in hospice and palliative medicine with 23 out of 27 randomised controlled clinical trials investigating dyspnoea, nausea and vomiting, pain, and xerostomia reporting significant outcomes in favour of acupuncture [10].

Indications for acupuncture

Acupuncture is used for a wide variety of problems and symptoms, and the WHO has published a list of common conditions helped by acupuncture [11].

Painful conditions

Uncontrolled studies in patients with malignancy show that a reduction in consumption and side effects of conventional analgesics is sometimes possible using acupuncture to treat bone pain, nerve pain, and pain due to soft tissue disease [12]. However, pain relief for malignant conditions is generally of shorter duration than for nonmalignant conditions and tolerance to the effects of acupuncture may be more of a problem in the former. If disease progression occurs, duration of pain relief can decrease. Acupuncture can also be helpful for syndromes including postsurgical and postradiotherapy pain syndromes.

Breathlessness

In a series of 20 patients with disabling, advanced cancer-related breathlessness, use of acupuncture was associated with clinical improvements measured both subjectively and objectively [12]. However, a systematic review of interventions for alleviating cancer-related dyspnoea concluded that acupuncture was not beneficial [13] and a previous Cochrane review of five trials of acupuncture and acupressure had suggested evidence for a clinical effect was limited [14].

Nausea and vomiting

Nausea and vomiting (including chemotherapy-induced symptoms) have been reduced by acupuncture and TENS, and these effects appear to be reproducible. A systematic review of acupuncture antiemesis found that 11 out of 12 good-quality, randomised, placebo-controlled trials favoured acupuncture [15].

Hot flushes

Although observational data suggest a benefit using acupuncture for vasomotor symptoms both in prostate cancer and in breast cancer [16–18], randomised controlled trials have shown conflicting results with one trial suggesting a clear difference between sham and verum acupuncture for postmenopausal women and another no difference for women with breast cancer on tamoxifen [19,20].

Xerostomia

One study evaluating acupuncture-like transcutaneous nerve stimulation in the treatment of radiation-induced xerostomia in patients with head and neck cancer treated with radical radiotherapy showed improved whole saliva production and related symptoms that were sustained at 6 months [21]. Another investigated acupuncture for 117 hospice patients with xerostomia over 2 years and although symptoms were improved a 5-week acupuncture intervention study was not feasible as patients were too near death [22].

Safety, adverse effects, and recommended contraindications

Generally, acupuncture has a low side effect profile. Many patients feel very relaxed and some feel slightly drowsy after their first acupuncture treatment. Patients can be treated lying down or sitting up. They often feel a combination of sensations such as heaviness, numbness, tingling, and soreness around the needles, a phenomenon called "de Qi" (pronounced "ter chi"). Disposable needles should be used to prevent the risk of infection to patients. Acupuncture should not be used for patients with significantly impaired clotting. Needles should not be used in a lymphoedematous limb. Patients with an unstable spine should not have treatment over the spine. Patients fitted with pacemakers should not have electroacupuncture.

Dietary interventions

Although "healthy eating" advice is a mainstay of general health promotion and disease prevention strategies, the use of diet as a "treatment" for established disease (other than certain well-defined deficiency or intolerance syndromes) is rare in contemporary Western medicine. CT encompasses a wide spectrum of possible dietary interventions (Table 23.2). Patients with cancer may use these interventions with a variety of aims in mind (Table 23.3). The link between various dietary factors and development of certain cancers in humans seems well established [23,24]; however, the evidence for dietary approaches in the management of established cancer remains less clear. One pilot study investigated 3 months of a package of intensive lifestyle changes (involving dietary change to a mainly plant-based diet, regular exercise, stress management, and regular participation in a psychological and emotional cancer support group). Telomere shortness has been discovered as a marker for premature mortality from cancer, and in this study, telomerase activity and therefore maintenance of chromosomal health was demonstrated offering a potentially preventative impact [24]. The evidence for dietary approaches in the management of established cancer remains less clear. Interesting data have emerged using the same intensive lifestyle changes for a group of men who had already chosen not to undergo conventional treatment for their prostate cancer. Data showed a decrease in prostate-specific antigen (PSA) levels and LNCaP growth (a prostate tumour cell line), and these changes were proportional to the degree of changes individuals could make in diet and lifestyle [25]. Larger randomised controlled trials are needed to follow-up this preliminary data. The scope of this chapter precludes a detailed review [26] but the tables below give an idea of the types of intervention, their possible adverse effects, and some examples of relevant research findings.

With terminally ill patients, it is particularly important to balance realistic chances of benefit with the likely adverse effects. While most dietary interventions are safe and well tolerated, complete dietary regimes can be arduous, prolonged, nutritionally unbalanced, or inadequate, and involve an upheaval of daily life. However, playing an active part by choosing and maintaining a dietary intervention can be, for some, an important self-help coping strategy.

Healing

Spiritual healing is a process whereby a practitioner focuses intention to produce a change in another living system. Although viewed by many orthodox practitioners as one of the "fringe" CTs, patients find healing acceptable and helpful with few, if any, side effects. It is not necessary for patients or healers to hold any particular religious or spiritual belief.

Healing is practised under various names (therapeutic touch, nonmanual touch therapy, psychic healing, and so on) but can be broadly classified into two differing approaches:

1. *Laying on of hands*—where the healer's hands are placed gently on or near the body of the patient with a "healing intention." The process usually takes 15–20 min. Patients may experience warmth, tingling, or relaxation during or immediately after the procedure. Reiki is a distinct form of healing originating in Japan. It involves the laying on of hands in a particular routine, which is thought to channel energy into the patient and increase their own healing energy in a way that is both relaxing and health promoting. There are many accounts of Reiki being beneficial in a palliative care setting [37] but no systematic studies are available.

2. *Distance healing*—where the patient and healer(s) may be physically separated by large distances and where meditation, prayer, or other focused intent is used by the healer(s). The patient may not necessarily know that healing is taking place.

Both approaches may involve visualisation techniques such as seeing patients surrounded in light, picturing them fit and well, or clearing images of disease from their bodies.

Evidence for the effectiveness of healing

One study in the palliative care setting showed that for ten patients who had three noncontact therapeutic touch sessions, the sensation of well-being increased as measured by the Well-being Scale [38]. Despite the lack of a clear mechanism of action, there is a body of evidence that suggests that healing can have statistically significant effects. Two examples of distance healing are given here. In the first example, 393 patients admitted to a coronary care

Table 23.2 Types of dietary intervention relevant to palliative care.

Type of intervention	Principles on which intervention is based	Details of intervention	Potential adverse effects of intervention
Ingestion of nutritional supplements (vitamins, minerals, and so on normally found in the diet): different philosophies	1. Ingestion at recommended daily allowances (RDA) prevents deficiency due to inadequate dietary consumption, for example, treatment- or disease-related anorexia 2. Ingestion at doses higher than RDA used to compensate for increased nutritional need, for example, during cancer treatment, postoperative 3. Ingestion at megadoses uses supplements as pharmacological agents to treat disease	For example, vitamin C, β-carotene, vitamin B complex, CoQ10, selenium, zinc, evening primrose oil, and vitamin E Supplements often available in liquid or powder preparations Can involve taking more than 18 tablets a day at doses such as 8 mg vitamin C per day	None Evening primrose oil can exacerbate temporal lobe epilepsy Tablet fatigue:. Megadose vitamin C can cause diarrhoea. Hypervitaminosis A occasionally in prolonged use, especially if liver function deranged. Copper deficiency with prolonged zinc supplementation. High-dose folic acid may antagonise methotrexate; very high dose vitamin C may increase methotrexate toxicity
Ingestion of nutritional products or extracts	Taking supplements of food constituents at doses higher than normally ingested in the diet	For example, green tea extract, curcumin (from turmeric), indole-3-carbinol (found in cruciferous vegetables) For example, omega 3 fish oil	Usually well tolerated. Very high doses may cause adverse effects, such as GI upset, caffeine-related toxicity (with green tea extract) and reversible hepatotoxicity Supplements can reverse weight loss and increase survival in patient with advanced cancer [27]
Ingestion of other products or extracts for their purported anticancer activity	Eating substances that are not a normal dietary constituent. (NB much overlap with herbal medicine products.)	For example, melatonin, laetrile extract from apricot kernels, shark's cartilage	Melatonin at doses of 20 mg/day is being used in some US settings with apparent survival benefits and little toxicity in advanced solid cancers. Melatonin inhibits cancer cell growth *in vitro*. Formal human studies are lacking [28]. Laetrile has considerable toxicity Most products are expensive and unproven

(*continued*)

Table 23.2 (*Continued*)

Type of intervention	Principles on which intervention is based	Details of intervention	Potential adverse effects of intervention
Complete dietary regimes	Dietary regimes used as complete treatments for disease, for example, the metabolic therapy described by Dr Max Gerson in the 1950s; Livingstone-Wheeler regime; macrobiotic diet, and so on	*Gerson*—strict vegetarian diet; salt, alcohol and nicotine excluded; freshly pressed vegetable juices, coffee enemas, potassium supplements and enzymes *Livingstone-Wheeler*—diet as above plus vaccine prepared from patient's own blood	Lifestyle disruption: some regimes are time-consuming and arduous. Malnutrition has been described anecdotally in patients with advanced disease on strict anticancer dietary regimes

unit (CCU) were randomly allocated to receive intercessory prayer (IP) from a group of Christians based outside the hospital, or to receive no distant healing. Patients and assessors were unaware of the treatment allocation. Treatment group patients had significantly fewer complications (cardiac arrest, pneumonia, intubation, requirement for antibiotics, or diuretics) during their CCU stay [39].

The second example concerns studies in psychiatric and hospitalised patients. These have demonstrated significant anxiolytic effects of healing when compared to sham or placebo procedures [40]. However, a Cochrane review of trials of IP felt results from the 10 trials involving 7,646 patients were equivocal and research monies could be spent investigating other interventions [41].

Adverse effects and safety issues

There are no published reports of adverse reactions to the procedure of healing itself, although there are anecdotal reports of patients stopping necessary medication after seeing faith healers. The Confederation of Healing Organisations, which represents healers in the United Kingdom, has published a code of conduct for members, which advises them against making diagnoses and giving medical advice.

Provided that practitioners and patients are clear about the limitations of therapy, and there is regular reassessment by medically trained professionals, healing can be considered a very safe therapy. However, sensitivity concerning the religious beliefs and customs of the patient is necessary.

Herbalism

Herbalism, or phytotherapy, is the study and practice of using plant material for medicinal and health promotion purposes. Much of modern pharmacological prescribing has its roots in ancient herbal traditions. However, herbalists hold that isolation and extraction reduce efficacy and increase toxicity. They believe in a wider and more balanced pharmacology of plants, and therefore prefer to use organically grown, whole plant preparations.

For clarity, we can divide the topic into its main branches: Chinese herbalism, Western herbalism, and specific herbal "cures."

Chinese herbalism

Chinese herbalists use a traditional system of diagnosis, observing the pulse and the tongue, to decide on an individual prescription, often containing a number of herbs. They may combine this with acupuncture treatment.

Western herbalism

A Western herbalist takes a case history, exploring physical, psychological, and emotional dimensions, that centres on looking for a pattern of disturbance or disease. Individualised prescriptions are determined by key symptoms thought to correspond to dysfunction in certain organs. Herbs are usually administered as tinctures or alcohol–water extracts, but elixirs, pills, ointments, pessaries, and suppositories are also used. Experienced

Table 23.3 Range of reasons why patients may use dietary interventions and examples of related evidence.

Reasons why patients may try dietary intervention as part of cancer care	Examples of interventions used for this purpose	Examples of relevant research evidence
Improving immune function	IP6	Phytic acid active ingredient of high-fibre diet significantly inhibited DMBA, rat mammary cancer *in vivo* RCT ($n = 14$) showed reduction in side effects and preservation of quality of life [29]
	MGN-3	Early studies of MGN-3 (rice bran extract) supplementation show enhanced lymphocyte NK cell activity
Reducing risk of cancer (primary prevention)	Supplementation above RDA	Antioxidant vitamin supplementation shown to reverse precancerous changes, but possibly only in populations where vitamin deficiency is endemic
		RCT of supplementation with vitamin D + calcium showed reduced risk of breast cancer. RR of 0.23 compared to placebo [30]
		Studies showed unexpected increase of lung cancer among smokers and ex-smokers who received β-carotene (20 mg/day) compared with those who did not [31]
Reducing risk of cancer recurrence or spread (secondary prevention)	Change to more healthy eating pattern	Fat intake negatively correlated with disease-free survival in breast cancer. Diet high in fruit and vegetables coupled with physical exercise increases survival [32]
Improved survival	Megadose vitamin supplementation	High-dose vitamin C trials seem on balance to show no benefit although methodological disputes are ongoing
		Breast cancer-specific survival were not improved for a megadose vitamin and mineral supplemented group compared with matched controls [33]
	Nutritional products such as green tea or laetrile (apricot kernel extract)	Five cups green tea associated with reduced recurrence rates in Japanese women with Stage 1 & 2 breast cancer [34]
		Controlled trials of laetrile show no benefits
	Complete dietary regimes	Gerson [35]
	Dairy free	Relationship between IGF-1 present in high levels in dairy produce that is known to enhance tumour cell proliferation. Higher circulating levels of IGF-1 have been associated with increased risk of prostate cancer [36]

herbalists anecdotally report success in treating nausea in the terminally ill patient when other conventional methods have failed.

Specific herbal "cures"

Some individual herbal preparations are purported to have anticancer effects or to enhance conventional cancer treatments by reducing toxicity or increasing efficacy. They can be used singly or as part of regimes, such as the Gerson therapy. Some commonly encountered remedies are the following:

• Iscador, a preparation, of the mistletoe plant, is part of a wider medical approach known as anthroposophy, founded by Rudolf Steiner in 1920.

• "Essiac" (burdock, sheep sorrel, turkey rhubarb, and slippery elm bark).
• *Astragalus membranaceus* or "huang qi," from the root of the milk vetch plant—claimed to have tonic and immunostimulant properties.
• "Kombucha"—a mixture of bacteria and yeast grown in birch leaf tea.

Evidence for effectiveness of herbal medicine

Iscador has been shown to have immunostimulatory properties and to increase natural killer cell activity [42]. Reduction of radiotherapy-induced T-cell suppression has been seen in mice. A retrospective cohort study of women with breast cancer treated postoperatively with mistletoe extract showed that adverse effects of orthodox treatment, quality of life, and relapse-free intervals were all improved compared to standard treatment-matched controls [43]. Systematic reviews of trials of mistletoe overall suggest quality of trial design is variable and therefore evidence for mistletoe therapy is inconclusive [44]. However, data are suggestive of an impact on quality of life and possibly survival for patients with cancer using mistletoe and more high quality trials are needed to explore these findings further [45].

A meta-analysis of 34 trials of *Astragalus* with chemotherapy for non-small cell lung cancer suggests improved tumour response and less toxicity with the combination [46]. Other studies show that adjuvant *Astragalus* improves efficacy and reduces toxicity when given with platinum-based chemotherapy or with radiotherapy [47].

A meta-analysis of randomised clinical trials comparing *Hypericum* (St. John's wort) with conventional antidepressants in mild depression showed similar efficacy with considerably lower toxicity for the herbal product [48].

There is increasing interest in the potential role of certain medicinal mushrooms, already widely used in Asia in cancer treatment, and *in vitro* work shows antitumour and apoptotic induction activity [49].

Adverse effects

Although an extensive review of herbal safety published in the *Food and Drug Law Journal* in 1992 states that "there is no substantial evidence that specific toxic reactions to herbal products are a major source of concern" [50], an important issue is the potential for drug–herb interactions, for example, the cytochrome P450 enzyme inducing effects of St. John's wort. Care needs to be exercised especially in the palliative care setting where patients are often on multiple drug treatments and where they may have diminished renal and/or hepatic function. There have since been a few reports of severe idiosyncratic reactions such as acute hepatitis and irreversible rapidly progressive interstitial renal fibrosis following the ingestion of traditional Chinese herbs [51]. Side effects of Iscador are similar to those of Interferon, with high fever, headaches, and muscle pains; liver pain has been observed in patients with liver metastases.

Given the large number of people using herbal remedies, there are very few reports of serious adverse effects. A recent cross-sectional survey of patients attending the outpatient department at a specialist cancer centre identified potential risks of herbal products and supplements and issued a health warning in 20 cases (12.2%) [52]. The National Poisons Unit and other databases are establishing a list of known herb–drug interactions and validated reports of adverse events attributed to herbal products.

Homoeopathy

Homoeopathy from the Greek "homeo" similar, plus "pathos" illness, is based on the "law of similars." This is the principle of treating like with like where symptoms of disease are treated with medicines capable of producing similar symptoms when given to healthy individuals. Information about each remedy is built up from toxicology, proven evidence of the remedy on healthy volunteers, or through clinical cases where outcome has been good.

The homoeopathic method was described in 1790 by the German physician Samuel Hahnemann who conducted the first proving or trial of a medicine from cinchona, the Peruvian bark. During experiments to reduce adverse effects, he discovered that serial dilution made medicines less toxic but paradoxically more active, particularly when dilution was combined with vigorous shaking known as succussion. This process to create a highly succussed solution is called "potentisation" and is considered to increase the therapeutic action of the remedy by a mechanism not presently understood. The remedies are thought to stimulate a self-repair, self-regulating response within the body.

The homoeopath identifies patterns emerging from a holistic clinical history and matches these with features of known homoeopathic remedies to make an individual prescription. Case studies suggest that one remedy may not produce any response whereas another, which fits the symptom pattern more closely, may be followed by dramatic improvement in key symptoms as well as nonspecific improvements in anxiety and psychological adjustment. Remedies can be prescribed in tablet or liquid form and are easily administered in the terminal phase without interfering with other medications.

Evidence and indications for homoeopathy

Controversy exists over whether the clinical effects seen with homoeopathic care are due to placebo responses alone [53]. Basic science is investigating highly succussed dilutions. For example, one study showed that low-dose cytokines, which have undergone "sequential kinetic activation," were active in a mouse asthma model and the antiasthma activity was confirmed on histology [54]. Many clinical trials of homoeopathy have been carried out and when systematically reviewed clinical effects appear to be due to more than a placebo response [55,56]. Published work has shown homoeopathy to be useful for a range of symptoms in the diagnosis of cancer in particular fatigue, hot flushes, mood disturbance, and chemotherapy-induced stomatitis [57–59]. A Cochrane review suggested trial results were encouraging and more research was needed in this important clinical area [60]. When investigating hot flushes although observational data showed promising results, randomised controlled trials have failed to prove these changes were due to more than a placebo response [61,62]. Some authors have described the placebo response as being made up of many nonspecific effects [63]. As with some of the acupuncture research, there is evidence for real improvements with these interventions but as yet it is not understood whether effects are all nonspecific or whether in a trial design a constructive therapeutic encounter may be masking some of the specific effects of needling or the homoeopathic medicine.

Adverse effects

There are no known toxic effects of homoeopathy. However, patients and homoeopaths describe a number of remedy reactions suggestive of a shift within the self-regulating mechanism thought to orchestrate the body. These include the transient development of new symptoms or a worsening of existing symptoms called a homoeopathic aggravation. In one audit of 116 patients in routine outpatient practice [64], a third of the patients described aggravations and new symptoms and 5 patients regarded the aggravation as adverse. These reactions are transient and respond quickly to decreasing the frequency or stopping the remedy.

Betty's story

Betty is 78 and was referred by her general practitioner in October 2008 with metastatic gastric carcinoma and difficult symptoms of abdominal pain and anxiety. Having been independent, she had lost much of her confidence. We took time to build a detailed profile of her as an individual and prescribed a number of homoeopathic and herbal medicines: *Natrum phosphoricum*, an individualised homoeopathic medicine as a liquid daily; *Cuprum metallicum*, a local homoeopathic medicine as a tablet for night-time cramping; and Iscador, a herbal preparation of mistletoe in low dose by mouth for immune support. This is how Betty summarised things. "*In January 2008 I was diagnosed with stomach cancer. After receiving chemotherapy, a gastrectomy and chemotherapy and radiotherapy, in March 2009 I was told nothing more could be done as my cancer had returned. Giving me a life expectancy of 2 months I was discharged from oncology back to my GP and the Palliative Care Team. Grasping at straws I asked my GP if he could refer me to the BHH and here I am 2 years later to say how life and faith has been restored to me. Even after contracting shingles Christmas 2009, homoeopathy came to my rescue to rid me of the terrible discomfort of the aftermath. Homoeopathy has not only helped my body cope with cancer and its initial invasive treatment but has given me a new lease of life and boosted my confidence.*"

Massage, aromatherapy, and reflexology

The use of touch to relieve discomfort is probably one of the most instinctive and oldest therapies in existence.

Massage, which can be defined as therapeutic soft tissue manipulation, is a component of many traditional systems of medicine. Swedish massage is the form on which most current European techniques are based. Indian head massage is a type of head and shoulders massage often given without undressing the client. It is adapted from traditional Indian Ayurvedic practice and may be particularly suited to situations where a full body massage is impractical.

Aromatherapy is massage using essential oils— aromatic plant extracts prepared by distillation— which are said to have different properties (relaxing, invigorating, antiseptic, purifying, and so on). A combination of diluted essential oils will be selected to suit the preference and nature of the patient.

Reflexology is a technique whereby the feet are massaged in a way that is claimed to affect the functioning of the organs of the body. Specific areas of the feet (reflex zones) are said to correspond to individual organs, and massaging these areas can either give the therapist diagnostic information or lead to therapeutic change in the corresponding organ.

Massage techniques have been extensively employed in palliative care settings [1] and have been adapted for these circumstances; for example, using gentle massage strokes to avoid overtreating frail patients. Treatments can be given by independent massage therapists but increasingly trained nurses, physiotherapists, and occupational therapists are providing massage and aromatherapy. If essential oils are used, they must be diluted with a carrier oil (e.g., sweet almond oil) and can be used singly or in established combinations of four to five low-toxicity oils.

Indications and effects of massage therapies

Practitioners using massage in palliative care settings have reported psychological, emotional, and physical benefits for patients and staff. The research base is rigorously and extensively reviewed elsewhere [65]. Key points emerging are summarised as follows.

Psychological effects: A small number of well-conducted randomised controlled trials support the claim that massage is effective in relieving anxiety in institutional settings. Effects on depression are less clear.

Emotional effects: The pampering and pleasure received during a massage can be one of the few positive physical experiences for a patient with advanced disease. In the words of one patient: "it was done so lovingly and gently. The whole experience has made me feel I was worth caring about" [66]. Practitioners also report an effect of massage in improving the body image of patients who have undergone mutilating surgery. Massage may lead to emotional release although patients can be nurtured and supported without feeling they have to "open up" and talk.

Physical effects: Massage is frequently used for pain relief, perhaps alleviating pain through reduction in anxiety and muscle tension, although there are almost no reliable research data on the subject. Lymphoedema is now widely treated by using specialist massage and bandaging techniques.

There are also anecdotal reports describing improvements in sleep patterns, lethargy, fatigue, terminal agitation, and restlessness after massage.

Interpersonal significance: Massage gives staff and relatives a way of spending time and being with the dying patient.

Use among staff: Staff support systems sometimes include massage, and practitioners report that these sessions are used to "unload" problems. As one member of staff puts it: "Massage allows me to 'take in' so that I can 'give out.'" [65].

Evidence comparing the different massage therapies

Randomised trials comparing aromatherapy massage with massage using carrier oil alone [66,67] have provided results that are difficult to interpret owing to a number of methodological flaws. There seems at least to be a suggestion that essential oils may augment the effects of massage in reducing anxiety and some physical symptoms. One study compared aromatherapy massage with cognitive behavioural therapy for emotional distress in patients recruited from oncology outpatient clinics [68]. Significant improvement in anxiety and depression was seen for both groups with greater preference for aromatherapy massage.

Reflexology has been researched across a range of clinical conditions and there is some evidence from high-quality trials that reflexology can improve quality of life [69].

Adverse effects and recommended contraindications

Providing massage is gentle and care is taken in moving and lifting patients, adverse effects are rare. As with other complementary disciplines, contraindications reflect established practise rather than documented side effects. No serious adverse events with aromatherapy have been documented.

Limbs affected by deep vein thrombosis should not be massaged, and extreme caution should be exercised when massaging close to bone metastases. Skin recovering from radiotherapy should generally be avoided. Patients with abnormal clotting or platelets should be massaged with great care.

The variety and concentration of aromatherapy oils is limited to avoid theoretical risks of overexposure or interaction with concurrent medication. Although vigorous massage close to active tumour sites is generally avoided, there are no known reports of metastatic spread being promoted by massage.

Mind–body techniques: hypnosis, meditation, relaxation, and visualisation

Mind–body medicine encompasses a wide range of therapeutic interventions that address psychological and emotional issues with the aim of altering physical symptoms and possibly disease processes.

Techniques encompassed by the term "mind–body approaches" include counselling, psychotherapy, therapy involving hypnosis, cognitive-behavioural techniques, NLP, relaxation, yoga, visualisation, and meditation. We will not consider psychotherapy, cognitive-behavioural approaches, or counselling within the scope of this chapter.

Hypnosis

Hypnotic techniques increase a patient's suggestibility and responsiveness to psychological approaches by using an altered state of consciousness, or "trance." Hypnotic techniques can be used to augment any number of psychotherapeutic or psychological techniques, from hypnoanalysis to cognitive behavioural techniques. A recent meta-analysis of trials comparing identical cognitive-behavioural interventions delivered alone or with hypnosis showed a substantial enhancement in treatment outcome with adjunctive hypnosis [70]. One hospice reports the use of a retrospective questionnaire to evaluate hypnotherapy in a day care setting. Out of 256 patients who had hypnotherapy, 52 surviving patients were sent the questionnaire. Forty-one patients responded and 61% of these patients reported improved coping.

Meditation

Meditation is a process by which the mind is stilled to facilitate a calm and pleasant experience of the present moment. It may also, but does not necessarily, have a spiritual dimension (Table 23.4).

Visualisation and imagery

Imagined scenes, objects, places, or people are used in many mind–body techniques to enable a change in subjective experience. A favourite beach or beautiful gardens are popular images. Most of these techniques can be taught

---

Table 23.4 Categories of meditation techniques.

Concentrative meditation
Involves focusing the mind on the breath, an image (real or imagined), or a sound (often repeated). Through this concentration, the mind becomes more tranquil and aware

Mindfulness meditation
Attention is opened to whatever enters the mind without judgement or worries, so that eventually the mind becomes more calm and clear

---

and applied in one-to-one sessions or facilitated groups by therapists or doctors and nurses with appropriate training. Using audiotapes and headphones, patients can practice the technique anywhere, at home or in hospital, and many learn to "customise" the methods to suit themselves.

Indications and effects of mind–body techniques

Mindfulness-Based Stress Reduction (MBSR) has been reported to improve anxiety and changes within the brain responsible for emotional regulation have now been identified after just 16 weeks of MBSR [71]. Studies have indicated efficacy of mind–body techniques in certain situations. For example, the pain of oral mucositis was much reduced in patients undergoing bone marrow transplantation who had relaxation and imagery training [72] and pain in patients with advanced cancer was reduced by deep-breathing, progressive muscle relaxation, and imagery training [73]. Several studies have demonstrated that anxiety and nausea related to chemotherapy respond well to mind–body approaches, especially in children and adolescents. Anticipatory nausea and vomiting have been helped by hypnosis [74].

Altering the course of the disease

A few studies have examined the effects of mind–body interventions on the progression of cancer. Results are contradictory and it is still difficult to draw definite conclusions in this controversial area [75].

Carl Simonton encouraged patients with cancer to use images such as sharks eating cancer cells or armies of soldiers in battle, to enhance immune function, and augment the effect of conventional treatment. An uncontrolled study in 225 selected patients with cancer reported survival figures "as much as twice as long" as national averages [76]. However, the study had profound methodological flaws, such as a nonrepresentative sample and lack of any staging or prognostic data.

Spiegel and co-workers, while conducting a randomised study of a 12-month psychosocial group intervention to improve quality of life in patients with metastatic breast cancer, found a clinically and statistically significant survival advantage in intervention patients compared with controls [77]. A study using a structured psychological intervention in melanoma patients showed reduced recurrence and improved survival at 6 and 10 years [78]. The multiapproach lifestyle package that Ornish has used has shown changes in gene expression suggestive that changes in survival could be possible [79]. Further work has suggested that it is the application of such psychological interventions that may be the key to improving survival [80].

Adverse effects and contraindications

Providing that any therapist who employs hypnotic techniques has the appropriate training and background experience, mind–body therapies are generally very safe. Therapists need to be aware of the psychological vulnerability of patients with cancer and the limited time available for patients with terminal illness to deal with deep trauma or ingrained patterns of behaviour. Realistic goals of therapy need to be agreed and often techniques used symptomatically are more appropriate than an analytic approach.

The WHO cautions that hypnosis should not be used in patients with psychosis, organic psychiatric conditions, or antisocial personality disorders.

Documented adverse effects of sustained meditation include grand mal seizures in established epileptics and acute psychosis in individuals with a history of schizophrenia.

Robert was initially diagnosed in March 1996 with adenoid cystic cancer (of the tongue), and in January 1997 scans revealed secondaries on his liver and both lungs. He attended the Bristol Cancer Help Centre (now the Penny Brohn Cancer Care Centre) and describes "*a typical day's holistic treatment (mind, body and spirit) included individual sessions with the doctor, counsellor, nutritionist, art therapist and healer and group sessions on guided meditation and relaxation. There was also empowering, informal interaction with other patients. I remember saying to my wife that I would always appreciate their CT for helping me to live with cancer, even if I lived no longer than forecast.*" With visualisation "*my imagination runs riot with a rich mixture of themes including peace, war and humour. The regular hero is my immune system known affectionately as 'Baldrick' because of his indefatigable optimism and cunning plans. I discovered how to graft my wicked sense of humour onto their creative therapies in order to ensure that my cancer cells die laughing. At first the techniques such as meditation and visualisation seemed to be separate, until I quickly discovered how they inter-relate: for example I have powerful visualisations during healing sessions.*"

Potential problems with CT approaches in palliative care settings

Guilt and responsibility

One of the most important potential adverse effects of CT that has been observed is the generation of guilt. Many CT disciplines support the belief that the way people behave

and look after their bodies influence their state of health. They also place great emphasis on the role of self-healing. These two axioms can develop into a two-edged sword. On the one hand, they can promote greater independence and self-esteem by reversing the patient's traditional role of sitting back and letting the doctors do the work. On the other hand, they can create a burden of responsibility and guilt in patients who come to believe that they are the cause of their own illness and that the reason they are not getting better is because they are not trying hard enough, eating well enough, or being good enough to people. CT practitioners, particularly those who are unused to working with patients with a terminal disease, must be very aware of these risks.

Increasing denial

CT can be used as a psychological or emotional support in the face of progressing disease or impending death. However, there is a fine line between this and a potential for increasing an unhelpful pattern of denial, which can risk delaying or even preventing appropriate adjustment and acceptance. This is not unique to CT. Inappropriate use of conventional oncological treatments may have similar effects.

Masking important symptoms

Use of CT can mask or disguise the development of complications that require urgent conventional medical treatment (e.g., incipient cord compression). It may also mask disease progression for which further conventional symptomatic treatment is superior (e.g., radiotherapy to bony metastases). Regular medical reassessment of all patients with new or persistent symptoms is mandatory.

Antagonism and communication difficulties

There is often an element of faith in some of the principles of CT, and disagreement about the effectiveness of various techniques. It is possible that those who do not share these beliefs (either family members or conventional medical carers) will feel antagonised by a patient's decision to seek CT treatments. This can lead to isolation and fragmentation of care, placing patients in the difficult position of having to choose between conflicting advice.

Financial

The financial implications of CT for both patient and health service purchasers need to be carefully considered. Complementary treatments are labour intensive but generally cost little in terms of medication or equipment. Cost effectiveness is not established.

Supervision and responsibility

CT practitioners will often be working outside the conventional management structures of the NHS. Some may be working as volunteers. Job descriptions, limits to practice, review procedures, lines of clinical and management responsibility, and codes of conduct all need to be clearly and carefully defined. In the United Kingdom, standards for certain aspects of CT provision have recently been published within the *Manual of Cancer Services* [81], which is linked to the National Cancer Peer Review process. This first set of standards includes measures related to the following areas:

- Practitioners' employment within the NHS.
- A requirement for evidence of appropriate and recognised qualifications.
- The provision of written information to patients about the therapies being offered.
- The need for seeking and recording that informed consent has been sought from patient for treatment being offered.
- Standards related to the sterility and safety of equipment and substances used in CT practice.

Interprofessional issues

Many conventional health-care professionals have undergone CT training but other CT practitioners will have trained outside the multiprofessional environment of an NHS hospital. The language they use and the way in which they conduct their practice may therefore be unfamiliar to medical, nursing, and other health-care professionals. This can lead to misunderstandings and frustration. The presence of CT practitioners at multidisciplinary team (MDT) meetings can be problematic initially, but with time, familiarity and mutual respect can develop.

Conclusions

This chapter has begun to explore the similarities between palliative care and complementary approaches, and to examine the relevance of individual CTs to the palliative care setting. As practitioners individualise their patients' care, they may be asked about therapies with which they are unfamiliar and inexperienced. Although there is no evidence that any of the complementary approaches can cure cancer, there is much that demonstrates their ability to improve symptoms and quality of life, and patient satisfaction with these approaches is high. Discussing the relevance of CTs in individual cases openly, and with an awareness of this evidence, may facilitate a profound and therapeutic patient/carer relationship.

By integrating the best of orthodox and complementary care, it may be possible to meet more of the needs of palliative care patients. However, well-designed research is necessary to establish the most appropriate strategy for future developments [82].

References

1. Wilkes E. *Complementary Therapy in Hospice and Palliative Care.* Sheffield: Trent Palliative Care Centre, 1992.
2. White P. Complementary medicine treatment of cancer a survey of provision. *Compl Ther Med* 1998; 6: 10–13.
3. Kozak LE, Kayes L, McCarty R, et al. Use of complementary and alternative medicine (CAM) by Washington State hospices. *Am J Hosp Palliat Care* 2008; 25(6): 463–468.
4. Rees R, Feigel I, Vickers A, et al. Prevalence of complementary therapy use by women with breast cancer: a population-based survey. *Eur J Cancer* 2000; 36: 1359–1364.
5. Thomas K, Fall M, Parry G, et al. *National Survey of Access to Complementary Health Care via General Practice.* Sheffield: Medical Care Research Unit, 1995.
6. Crawford HJ and Gruzelier JH. A midstream view of the neuropsychophysiology of hypnosis: recent research and future directions. In: Fromm E and Nash MR (eds), *Contemporary Hypnosis Research.* New York: Guilford Press, 1992, pp. 227–266.
7. Ernst E and Henstschel C. Diagnostic method in complementary medicine. Which craft is witchcraft? *Int J Risk Safety Med* 1995; 7: 55–63.
8. Veith I. *The Yellow Emperor's Classic of Internal Medicine.* Berkeley: University of California Press, 1972.
9. Bai L, Tian J, Zhong C, et al. Acupuncture modulates temporal neural responses in wide brain networks: evidence from fMRI study. *Mol Pain* 2010; 6: 73. doi: 10.1186/1744-8069-6-73.
10. Standish LJ, Kozak L, and Congdon S. Acupuncture is under-utilized in hospice and palliative medicine. *Am J Hosp Palliat Care* 2008; 25(4): 298–308.
11. Bannerman R. Acupuncture: the World Health Organisation view. *World Health* 27/28 December 1979: 24–29.
12. Thompson JW and Filshie J. Transcutaneous electrical nerve stimulation (TENS) and acupuncture. In: Doyle D, Hanks G, McDonald N (eds), *The Oxford Textbook of Palliative*

Medicine, 2nd edition. Oxford: Oxford University Press, 1997, pp. 421–437.

13. Ben-Aharon I, Gafter-Gvili A, Paul M, et al. Interventions for alleviating cancer-related dyspnea: a systematic review. *J Clin Oncol* 2008; 26(14): 2396–2404.

14. Bausewein C, Booth S, Gysels M, et al. Non-pharmacological interventions for breathlessness in advanced stages of malignant and non-malignant diseases. *Cochrane Database Syst Rev* 2008; (2): CD005623.

15. Vickers AJ. Can acupuncture have specific effects on health? A systematic literature review of acupuncture anti-emesis trials. *J R Soc Med* 1996; 89(6): 303–311.

16. Porzio G, Trapasso T, Martelli S, et al. Acupuncture in the treatment of menopause-related symptoms in women taking tamoxifen. *Tumori* 2002; 88(2): 128–130.

17. Hammar M, Frisk J, Grimas O, et al. Acupuncture treatment of vasomotor symptoms in men with prostatic carcinoma: a pilot study. *J Urol* 1999; 161(3): 853–856.

18. de Valois BA, Young TE, Robinson N, et al. Using traditional acupuncture for breast cancer-related hot flashes and night sweats. *J Altern Complement Med* 2010; 16(10): 1047–1057.

19. Sunay D, Ozdiken M, Arslan H, et al. The effect of acupuncture on postmenopausal symptoms and reproductive hormones: a sham controlled clinical trial. *Acupunct Med* 2011; 29(1): 27–31.

20. Liljegren A, Gunnarsson P, Landgren BM, et al. Reducing vasomotor symptoms with acupuncture in breast cancer patients treated with adjuvant tamoxifen: a randomized controlled trial. *Breast Cancer Res Treat* 2010. doi: 10.1007/s10549-010-1283-3.

21. Blom M, Dawidson I, Fernberg JO, et al. Acupuncture treatment of patients with radiation induced xerostomia. *Eur J Cancer B Oral Oncol* 1996; 32B(3): 182–190.

22. Meidell L and Holritz RB. Acupuncture as an optional treatment for hospice patients with xerostomia: an intervention study. *Int J Palliat Nurs* 2009; 15(1): 12–20.

23. Doll R. *Causes of Cancer*. Oxford: Oxford University Press, 1981.

24. Ornish D, Lin J, Daubenmier J, et al. Increased telomerase activity and comprehensive lifestyle changes: a pilot study. *Lancet Oncol* 2008; 9(11): 1048–1057.

25. Ornish D, Weidner G, Fair WR, et al. Intensive lifestyle changes may affect the progression of prostate cancer. *J Urol* 2005; 174(3): 1065–1069.

26. Butler E. Nutrition. In: Barraclough J (ed.), *Enhancing Cancer Care: Complementary Therapy and Support*. Oxford: OUP, 2007, Chap 20.

27. Barber MD. Cancer cachexia and its treatment with fish-oil-enriched nutritional supplementation. *Nutrition* 2001; 17(9): 751–755.

28. Cutando A. Melatonin and cancer: current knowledge and its application to oral cavity tumours. *J Oral Pathol Med* 2011; 40(8): 593–597. doi: 10.1111/j.1600-0714.2010.01002.x.

29. Bacic I, Druzijanic N, Karlo R, et al. Efficacy of IP6 +inositol in the treatment of breast cancer patients receiving chemotherapy: prospective, randomized, pilot clinical study. *J Exp Clin Cancer Res* 2010; 29(12):0392–9078, 1756–9966.

30. Lappe JM, Travers-Gustafson D, Davies KM, et al. Vitamin D and calcium supplementation reduces cancer risk. *Am J Clin Nutr* 2007; 85(6): 1586–1591.

31. Albaneset AL. The effect of Vitamin E and beta-carotene on the incidence of lung cancer and other cancers in male smokers. *New Eng J Med* 1994; 330(15): 1029–1035.

32. Pierce JP, Stefanick ML, Flatt SW, et al. Greater survival after breast cancer in physically active women with high vegetable-fruit intake regardless of obesity. *J Clin Oncol* 2007; 25(17): 2345–2351.

33. Lesperance ML, Olivotto I A, Forde N, et al. Mega-dose vitamins and minerals in the treatment of non-metastatic breast cancer: an historical cohort study. *Breast Cancer Res Treat* 2002; 76(2): 137–143.

34. Seely D, Mills EJ, Wu P, et al. The effects of green tea consumption on incidence of breast cancer and recurrence of breast cancer: a systematic review and meta-analysis. *Integr Cancer Ther* 2005; 4(2): 144–155.

35. Hildenbrand GL, Hildenbrand LC, Bradford K, et al. Five-year survival rates of melanoma patients treated by diet therapy after the manner of Gerson: a retrospective review. *Altern Ther Health Med* 1995; 1(4): 29–37.

36. Oliver SE, Gunnell D, Donovan J, et al. Screen-detected prostate cancer and the insulin-like growth factor axis: results of a population-based case-control study. *Int J Cancer* 2004; 108(6): 887–892.

37. Demmer C and Sauer J. Assessing complementary therapy services in a hospice program. *Am J Hosp Palliat Care* 2002; 19(5): 306–314.

38. Giasson M and Bouchard L. Effect of therapeutic touch on the well-being of persons with terminal cancer. *J Holist Nurs* 1998; 16(3): 383–398.

39. Byrd RC. Positive therapeutic effects of intercessory prayer in a coronary care unit population. *South Med J* 1988; 81(7): 826–829.

40. Simington JA and Laing GP. Effects of therapeutic touch on anxiety in the institutionalised elderly. *Clin Nurs Res* 1993; 2(4): 438–450.

41. Roberts L, Ahmed I, Hall S, et al. Intercessory prayer for the alleviation of ill health. *Cochrane Database Syst Rev* 2009; (2): CD000368.

42. Hajto T. Immunomodulatory effects of Iscador: a viscum album preparation. *Oncology* 1986; 43(Suppl. 11): 51–65.

43. Schumacher K, Schneider B, Reich G, et al. Influence of postoperative complementary treatment with lectin-standardized mistletoe extract on breast cancer patients. A controlled epidemiological multicentric retrolective cohort study. *Anticancer Res* 2003; 23(6): 5081–5088.

44. Horneber MA, Bueschel G, Huber R, et al. Mistletoe therapy in oncology. *Cochrane Database Syst Rev* 2008; (2): CD003297.

45. Ostermann T, Raak C, and Bussing A. Survival of cancer patients treated with mistletoe extract (Iscador): a systematic literature review. *BMC Cancer* 2009; 9: 451. doi: 10.1186/1471-2407-9-451.

46. McCulloch M, See C, Shu XJ, et al. Astragalus-based Chinese herbs and platinum-based chemotherapy for advanced non-small-cell lung cancer: meta-analysis of randomized trials. *J Clin Oncol* 2006; 24(3): 419–430.

47. Qi F, Li A, Inagaki Y, et al. Chinese herbal medicines as adjuvant treatment during chemo- or radiotherapy for cancer. *Biosci Trends* 2010; 4(6): 297–307.

48. Linde K, Ramirez G, Mulrow CD, et al. St John's wort for depression: an overview and meta-analysis of randomised clinical trials. *BMJ* 1996; 313(7052): 253–258.

49. Jiang J and Sliva D. Novel medicinal mushroom blend suppresses growth and invasiveness of human breast cancer cells. *Int J Oncol* 2010; 37(6): 1529–1536.

50. McCaleb RS. Food ingredient safety evaluation. *Food Drug Law J* 1992; 47: 657–665.

51. Vanherweghem JL, Depierreux M, Tielemans C, et al. Rapidly progressive interstitial renal fibrosis in young women: association with slimming regimen including Chinese herbs. *Lancet* 1993; 341(8842): 387–391.

52. Werneke U, Earl J, Seydel C, *et al* Potential health risks of complementary alternative medicines in cancer patients. *Br J Cancer* 2004; 90(2): 408–413.

53. Shang A, Huwiler-Muntener K, Nartey L, et al. Are the clinical effects of homoeopathy placebo effects? Comparative study of placebo-controlled trials of homoeopathy and allopathy. *Lancet* 2005; 366(9487): 726–732.

54. Gariboldi S, Palazzo M, Zanobbio L, et al. Low dose oral administration of cytokines for treatment of allergic asthma. *Pulm Pharmacol Ther* 2009; 22(6): 497–510.

55. Kleijnen J, Knipschild P, and ter Riet G. Trials of homeopathy. *BMJ* 1991; 302(6782): 316–323.

56. Linde K, Clausius N, Ramirez G, et al. Are the clinical effects of homeopathy placebo effects? A meta-analysis of placebo-controlled trials. *Lancet* 1997; 350(9051): 834–843.

57. Thompson E and Reilly D. The homeopathic approach to symptom control in the cancer patient: a prospective observational study. *Palliat Med* 2002; 16(3): 227–233.

58. Thompson E and Reilly D. The homeopathic approach to the treatment of symptoms of oestrogen withdrawal in breast cancer patients. A prospective observational study. *Homeopathy* 2003; 92(3): 131–134.

59. Oberbaum M, Yaniv I, Ben-Gal Y, et al. A randomized, controlled clinical trial of the homeopathic medication TRAUMEEL S in the treatment of chemotherapy-induced stomatitis in children undergoing stem cell transplantation. *Cancer* 2001; 92(3): 684–690.

60. Kassab S, Cummings M, Berkovitz S, et al. Homeopathic medicines for adverse effects of cancer treatments. *Cochrane Database Syst Rev* 2009; (2): CD004845.

61. Jacobs J, Herman P, Heron K, et al. Homeopathy for menopausal symptoms in breast cancer survivors: a preliminary randomized controlled trial. *J Altern Complement Med* 2005; 11(1): 21–27.

62. Thompson EA, Montgomery A, Douglas D, et al. A pilot, randomized, double-blinded, placebo-controlled trial of individualized homeopathy for symptoms of estrogen withdrawal in breast-cancer survivors. *J Altern Complement Med* 2005; 11(1): 13–20.

63. Di Blasi Z, Harkness E, Ernst E, et al. Influence of context effects on health outcomes: a systematic review. *Lancet* 2001; 357(9258): 757–762.

64. Thompson E, Barron S, and Spence D. A preliminary audit investigating remedy reactions including adverse events in routine homeopathic practice. *Homeopathy* 2004; 93(4): 203–209.

65. Vickers A. *Massage and Aromatherapy: A Guide for Health Professionals*. London: Chapman & Hall, 1996.

66. Corner J, Cawley N, and Hildebrand S. An evaluation of the use of massage and essential oils on the wellbeing of cancer patients. *Int J Palliat Nurs* 1995; 1(2): 67–73.

67. Wilkinson S. Aromatherapy and massage in palliative care. *Int J Palliat Nurs* 1995; 1(1): 21–30.

68. Serfaty M, Wilkinson S, Freeman C, et al. The ToT Study: Helping with Touch or Talk (ToT): a pilot randomised controlled trial to examine the clinical effectiveness of aromatherapy massage versus cognitive behaviour therapy for emotional distress in patients in cancer/palliative care. *Psychooncology* 2011; 21(5): 563–569. doi:10.1002/pon.1921.

69. Ernst E, Posadzki P, and Lee MS. Reflexology: an update of a systematic review of randomised clinical trials. *Maturitas* 2011; 68(2): 116–120.

70. Kirsch I, Montgomery G, and Sapirstein G. Hypnosis as an adjunct to cognitive behavioural psychotherapy: a meta-analysis. *J Consult Clin Psychol* 1995; 63(2): 214–220.

71. Holzel BK, Carmody J, Vangel M, et al. Mindfulness practice leads to increases in regional brain gray matter density. *Psychiatry Res* 2011; 191(1): 36–43.

72. Syrjala KL, Donaldson GW, Davis MW, et al. Relaxation and imagery and cognitive-behavioural training reduce pain during cancer treatment: a controlled clinical trial. *Pain* 1995; 63(2): 189–198.

73. Sloman R, Brown P, Aldana E, et al. The use of relaxation for the promotion of comfort and pain relief in persons with advanced cancer. *Contemp Nurse* 1994; 3(1): 6–12.

74. Redd WH, Andresen GV, and Minagawa RY. Hypnotic control of anticipatory emesis in patients receiving cancer chemotherapy. *J Consult Clin Psychol* 1982; 50(1): 14–19.

75. Astin JA, Shapiro SL, Eisenberg DM, et al. Mind-body medicine: state of the science, implications for practice. *J Am Board Fam Prac* 2003; 16(2): 131–147.

76. Simonton OC, Matthews-Simonton S, and Sparks TE. Psychological intervention in the treatment of cancer. *Psychosomatics* 1980; 21(3): 226–233.

77. Spiegel D, Bloom JR, Kraemer HC, et al. Effects of psychosocial treatment on survival in patients with metastatic breast cancer. *Lancet* 1989; 2(8668): 888–891.

78. Fawzy FI, Fawzy N, Hyun CS, et al. Malignant melanoma: effects of an early structured psychiatric intervention, coping and affective state on recurrence and survival 6 years later. *Arch Gen Psychiatry* 1993; 50(9): 681–689.

79. Ornish D, Magbanua MJ, Weidner G, et al. Changes in prostate gene expression in men undergoing an intensive nutrition and lifestyle intervention. *Proc Natl Acad Sci USA* 2008; 105(24): 8369–8374.

80. Cunningham AJ, Edmonds CV, Phillips C, et al. A prospective, longitudinal study of the relationship of psychological work to duration of survival in patients with metastatic cancer. *Psychooncology* 2000; 9(4): 323–339.

81. Department of Health. *Manual for Cancer Services 2008: Complementary Therapy (Safeguarding Practice) Measures.* London: Department of Health, 2009.

82. Ernst E, Filshie J, and Hardy J. Evidence-based complementary medicine for palliative cancer care: does it make sense? *Palliat Med* 2003; 17(8): 704–707.

Further reading

Barraclough J (ed). *Enhancing Cancer Care: Complementary Therapy and Support.* Oxford: OUP, 2007.

Research Council for Complementary Medicine. *Defining the Question: Research Issues in Complementary Medicine, Parts I & II.* London: Research Council for Complementary Medicine, 1997.

Macmillan Cancer Relief. *Directory of Complementary Therapy Services in UK Cancer Care.* London: Macmillan Cancer Relief.

Lerner M. *Choices in Healing.* Cambridge, MA: MIT Press, 1996.

Tavares M. *National Guidelines for the Use of Complementary Therapies in Supportive and Palliative Care.* London: Foundation of Integrated Health and National Council for Hospice and Specialist Palliative Care.

Acknowledgements. We would like to thank Dr Jacqueline Filshie of the Royal Marsden Hospital, Sutton for her contributions to the section on acupuncture and Keith Robertson, Director of Education, Scottish School of Herbal Medicine. We also thank "Betty" and "Robert" for consenting to the use of their case histories.

24 Spirituality in Palliative Care

Megory Anderson[1], Christina Faull[2]

[1] Sacred Dying Foundation, San Francisco, USA
[2] University Hospitals of Leicester and LOROS, The Leicestershire and Rutland Hospice, Leicester, UK

Introduction

Two things are certain about spirituality at the end of life: it is not easy to define but it is interwoven into every experience of the dying person, from pain management to family dynamics to questioning the ultimate meaning of life and the impending death.

A framework for the spiritual care of those that are dying is as important as the medical aspects of their care. What is somewhat different about spiritual care is that our task as care professionals (CPs) is not the one based on a body of expert knowledge but more that of facilitator. The framework for spiritual care starts with assessment and proceeds to respond to the individual's experience of dying. The dying person ultimately determines his or her own spiritual course of action but may need help in finding that course through provision of support, information, exploration with others, and signposting to key advisors:

> Death is not primarily a medical event. Death is a personal, relational and spiritual event yet the majority of professional effort is concerned with the medical aspects of the end of life, often to the neglect of more pertinent issues facing the dying patient and their family. [1]

Most care practitioners assume that spiritual needs fall *solely* under the jurisdiction of the religious or pastoral care leaders. However, the interconnectedness of spiritual meaning and physical, psychological, and social expression makes this an ineffective strategy. In the case narrative (Box 24.1), the patient was distressed and was not responding to initial interventions. Eventually the team gained some understanding of her fears; of what may be to come after she had died. The care she received from her professional team needed to integrate a response to this in order to be most effective. It was indeed the care team's

Box 24.1 Case narrative

Eighty-two-year-old Mrs. Browning, in the advanced stages of illness and, although alert, was becoming more agitated and rambling in her speech. Her physician prescribed medication and recommended the social worker speak to her. The social worker gleaned little information, but noted several references to God. She immediately called in the chaplain, who, also somewhat at a loss as to what best to help, laid hands on Mrs. Browning and said some prayers.

A long-time friend and lay person from the church came by for a visit and noticed the change in her friend. She sat and listened to the ramblings. As the nurse began her care, she commented to the friend that Mrs. Browning was "in her own world now." To which the friend responded, "She's actually talking to her father. He was very strict, you know, especially about religion. I can see she's upset, and I can guess why. She must be afraid of what he'll do to her."

The nurse listened for a moment, and suggested to the friend, "Then why don't we give something to comfort her?" She fetched a small pillow, wrapped a cloth around it, and put it into Mrs. Browning's arms.

"There you go, darling. Mummy's right here. Hold tight and you'll be just fine." Her hand started stroking the pillow, and within minutes, she was calm. The friend smiled, thanking the nurse. "I knew the idea of her father would upset her. I'm glad you sorted out how to give her back her mother."

job not only to assess the symptom and its causes but also to make and enact an appropriate care plan. The whole person and his or her dying experience is a spiritual integration. In many traditions, it is just as the body begins to shut down that the spiritual self emerges in response. At this point in a person's life however, a shift in care is

---

Handbook of Palliative Care, Third Edition. Edited by Christina Faull, Sharon de Caestecker, Alex Nicholson and Fraser Black.
© 2012 by John Wiley and Sons, Inc. Published 2012 by John Wiley & Sons, Inc.

required which explicitly recognises this interconnectedness, and integrates it as a key part of everyone's role.

Spirituality and the need for spiritual care

The European Association for Palliative Care (EAPC) has an active task force looking at spiritual care in palliative care. The agreed working definition of spirituality is given here.

> Spirituality is the dynamic dimension of human life that relates to the way persons (individual and community) experience, express and/or seek meaning, purpose and transcendence, and the way they connect to the moment, to self, to others, to nature, to the significant and/or sacred [2].

These aspects of spirituality include (but are not limited to):

- religious practices and beliefs in God or a transcendent power;
- ultimate meaning of life and death;
- understanding of self and values;
- relationships with family and loved ones;
- quality of life in the midst of illness, including suffering, pain, loss, and distress; and
- hope in the midst of illness, including afterlife, peaceful resolution, legacy.

> The terms "spirituality" and "religion" are sometimes used interchangeably in the literature and older studies tend to use "religious" as the preferred term. While the two terms are clearly interconnected, "religion" refers to the practices associated with organised religion and their beliefs and "spirituality" is the wider umbrella term that includes individual concerns, general beliefs about the meaning of life and death, and the transcendent (beyond earthly/embodied life).

In the UK 2011 census, 29% of people declared themselves as "agnostic" or "unsure." A lack of or being without overt or articulated religious or spiritual beliefs does not negate the fact that being human has a spiritual dimension. The search for meaning is an almost intrinsic part of being human [3] and, at the end of life, sometimes a void in this can be more distressing than those who have well rehearsed and articulated answers to the issues raised by mortality.

Issues related to spirituality and the potential need for support emerge from the first diagnosis of a terminal illness to imminent dying and death, and beyond (see Figure 24.1). An early assessment of personal religious and spiritual "history" should determine in what ways the person finds hope, is challenged by questioning or despair, and will find meaning in the midst of this experience. Spiritual care must be integrated with each step along the way. It does not end even when death occurs as for most people, religious and cultural traditions honour postdeath rituals around the body and in a period of grieving and celebration.

Who provides the spiritual care?

In traditional societies throughout the world, spiritual customs, practices, and beliefs were intimately tied to the care of all the sick, most especially those suffering pain-filled illnesses, and those preparing for death. It would have been unusual to consider the role of religion and/or spirituality as a separate charge in caring for the sick and dying. The social dimension of spiritual practices is pervasive in most if not all traditional cultures. Religious representatives from the community would naturally be at the bedside of the sick and dying. Rituals were performed by both clergy and family members; it was understood that "doctor" and "priest" stood side by side at the deathbed.

Beginning a few centuries ago in the Western world, religion became much less a part of everyday social living and religious rites much less observed. However, as Grant et al. discuss: "Despite the decline of formal religion, many people still regard the idea of spirituality as essential to their sense of self, especially at times of inner turbulence" [5]. A reliance, however, on simply calling in the local clergy to "handle" this aspect of patients and families experiences is not an appropriate approach. Many patients will decline to see the local 'vicar' or hospital 'chaplain' as they have seldom set foot in a church and do not recognise the religious structure as a valid response to their spiritual anxiety. Thus, the care team must realise that any type of spiritual questions, concerns, and conversation may come their way. They should also consider that if they do not assess the patient's spiritual concerns then they may not be considered by anyone, leaving huge potential for ongoing distress.

The reality is that the people who care for the patient are the vital life connections he or she experiences most closely and most often. Doctors, nurses, care assistants, and social workers provide information, comfort, and physical care. They are among the most frequent faces the patient sees, and this social dynamic also makes them spiritual caregivers by default.

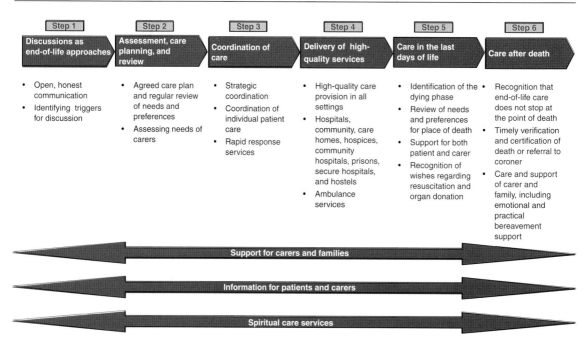

Figure 24.1 Spiritual care must be integrated throughout the "steps" of end-of-life care. (Reproduced from Reference 4.)

While all professional carers need to be open to considering and discussing a patient's spiritual needs, Walter questions the assumption that all care team members should be responsible for spiritual care of the patient and asks the question, "Can all staff provide spiritual care to all patients who are searching for meaning?" [6]. While professionals offer medical, psychosocial, and spiritual support and presence as the patient makes the "journey" through illness and the dying experience, the lenses and experiences they bring to the patient often conflict with the belief system the patient holds. The patient may well need access to specific support to address their spiritual needs more effectively.

Impact of providing spiritual care on members of the professional care team

Addressing individual spiritual experiences can be a particularly challenging role for the team members to embrace. After all, we are all human beings with our own thoughts, opinions, doubts, hopes, and feelings that shape spiritual issues. All these aspects come into play when we try to support patients and families in their spiritual searching or distress. When a patient asks during a bedside visit, "Has my life been a waste? What will happen to me after death?" there is no way to avoid or disregard our own mortality in dealing with someone else's—this is a fact to be accepted up front. Depending on our own relationship to religion and spirituality, these questions may trigger our own:

- Doctrinal beliefs (or lack thereof)
- Hopes
- Fears
- Doubts
- Family "baggage"
- Many related intellectual, emotional, and visceral responses.

Extending widely, far beyond theology and religious ritual, these issues are the stuff of contemplation for everyone in the dying process. Attention must be paid to the gravity of these issues in our own lives to be conscious of how they will impact the patient under our care. Encounter with them is inevitable and often.

What is central here is our common humanity, and an embracing of the concept that out of empathy as fellow humans, we can and should assist in the spiritual aspect of palliative care, taking into account but keeping discrete our own relationship to religion or spirituality. In a changing world we can help to achieve the goal set forth by the *Dying Matters* coalition in the United Kingdom "...so that dying, death, and bereavement will be accepted as a natural part of everybody's life cycle" [7]. A major figure in the history of palliative care is Dame Cicely Saunders, founder of the modern-day hospice movement. She is best known for her concept of total pain—often known as Total Suffering—that encompasses the full range of pain a person can endure: physical, emotional, psychological, spiritual, and so on. Thus, palliative care must address all of these levels, not just the physical, to be effective. In particular, Dame Cicely was aware of spiritual pain, and the current addressing of the spiritual aspect of palliative care is due in large part to her pioneering efforts [8].

Strategies for addressing the spiritual aspect of palliative care

The essential skill sets in addressing the spiritual aspects of palliative care for patients and families are as follows:
- Assessment
- Listening
- Responding
- Teamwork.

Assessment
It is often hard to begin a discussion of meaning and beliefs with patients. It can feel strangely more personal than other aspects of an assessment and may seem to appear nosey or intrusive. It can also be somewhat difficult to know the language of formal religions, and how to ask about specifics without appearing rude or ignorant. Many aspects of the communication skills described in Chapter 6, *Communication Skills in Palliative Care*, will help develop a degree of comfort in this. Box 24.2 lists some questions to support a spiritual care assessment.

The spiritual needs of the patient are diverse. Questions that may arise for any of the team members from patients include the following:
- Is dying going to hurt?
- Why did I get this disease?
- Did I do something wrong? Am I being punished?
- I'm afraid of being alone.
- I feel bad about some of the things I have done.
- What will happen when I'm gone?

Puchalski and Romer provide examples of patient statements that reflect spiritual concerns [10] (Box 24.3). As death approaches, and as the patient focus moves inward, the questions grow more personal and reflective, many are fear based. Many are directed toward "God." The patient will turn to the nurse, the care assistant,

---

Box 24.2 Example questions for a spiritual assessment

- What things do you enjoy doing? Are you doing them now?
- Where does your sense of what to do come from?
- Do you have someone you talk to for [spiritual/religious] guidance [matters]?
- What gives your life meaning?
- What sustains you during difficult times?
- What do you hope for?
- Are you part of a religious or spiritual community? Is it a source of support? In what ways?
- What aspects of your religion/spirituality would you like me to keep in mind as I care for you?
- Do your religious or spiritual beliefs influence the way you look at your disease and the way you think about your health?
- As we plan for your care, how does your faith impact on your decisions?

Source: Reproduced from Reference 9.

---

the specialist—whomever the patient feels a connection to—for responses to those spiritual concerns.

Sometimes spiritual distress can be recognised more from behaviour than from the words patients use, such as in the case narrative in Box 24.4.

Assessment tools have emerged as a feature of each cultural and national group:
- *The United Kingdom*: The Liverpool Care Pathway (LCP) for the Dying Patient is now used extensively [11].
- *North America*: Puchalski and Ferrell give examples of several instruments from the North American context, including the widely used Faith and Belief/Importance/Community/Address, Action in Care [12].
- *Europe*: The EAPC is currently developing resources for definitions and assessments [1].
- *Australia*: Deborah O'Connor and Bruce Rumbold report on Australian efforts to more firmly establish the spiritual aspects of palliative care [13].
- *Cross-cultural*: Lucy Selman et al. have developed a cross-cultural review of tools for the measurement of spirituality [14].

Listening
Perhaps the most human part of the entire process is listening. People like to be heard, to be paid attention to and valued, all their lives. This principle is all the more important during times of pain and dying. Caregivers

Box 24.3 Patient statements that reflect spiritual concerns

Lack of meaning/existential concerns	My life is meaningless. I feel useless.
Abandonment by God and others/loneliness	God has abandoned me. No one comes to see me. I am so alone.
Anger/inability to forgive	Why would God take my child?. . . It is not fair.
Relationship with deity	I want to have a deeper relationship with God. I want to understand my spirituality more.
Conflicts about belief system	I am not sure whether God is with me anymore. I question all I used to hold as meaningful.
Despair	Life is being cut short. There is nothing left for me to live for.
Grief/Loss	I miss my loved one so much. I wish I could run again.
Guilt/shame	I do not deserve to die pain-free.
Reconciliation	I need to be forgiven for what I did. I would like my wife to forgive me.
Isolation	Since moving to assisted living, I am not able to go to my church anymore. I have moved and can no longer attend my support group meeting.
Religious rituals needs	I just cannot pray anymore.
Loss of faith or meaning	What if all that I believe is not true?

Source: Reproduced from Reference 10.

Box 24.4 Case narrative

Mr. Blair was not yet 60, the father of two sons at university, and divorced from his wife of 23 years. He had fought hard against pancreatic cancer but was now in the advanced stages of disease, barely resigned to the fact that he was not going to live much longer. He was angry and discouraged. The chaplain was a young interfaith chaplain who tried to speak with him on several occasions. Her quiet demeanour was not a match for his anger, and on one visit, he became visibly hostile. "I don't want any talk of dying," he shouted, "It's bad enough they put me in this place."

Increasingly, Mr. Blair expressed his anger to the staff, sometimes refusing medication. His nurse, an experienced man in his 50s, decided to spend a few moments talking to him. He closed the curtain around him and just sat, looking at him straight in the eye.

"You have been behaving very badly," he told his patient. There was silence.

"Tell me why you want to bully us all," said the nurse.

Mr. Blair kept silent for another few moments, and then turned his head into the pillow. "It's no good now. I've mucked everything up." More silence, and then he quietly said, "The divorce, you see, and then the kids are angry with me. And now this. I did everything wrong, and now I get this. I must be a pretty horrible person for it all to end up this way."

The nurse kept quiet for a moment and then said, "I can see how that looks. Perhaps we can find a way for you to put some of those things right. It won't cure the cancer, mind you, but you might have peace of mind if you say you're sorry."

Mr. Blair nodded his head, almost imperceptibly, and the two men made plans for the next day.

must become comfortable listening as attentively to spiritual issues as they would to medical issues. Listening (and true hearing with intentionality) is nonjudgemental, open, loving and, many times, intuitive.

If the caregiver wishes to, and the patient and/or family are amenable, one could even establish a "Sacred Space," for listening by means of introductory silence, playing music that calms the patient, and so on. The Chaplain or religious advisor may be able to offer suggestions. Not that this is intended as a substitute to sacred spaces of organised religions, but simply as a method for helping the patient and carer enter into something deeper and more significant than ordinary conversation.

Responding

This may, for some CPs, be the most challenging aspect of the process. Here are some thoughts:

Clergy request: If the patient or family have requested a clergy person be called, whether a specific member of religious clergy (such as their rabbi, pastor, and imam), or simply a representative of a particular faith tradition, every effort should be made to make this contact as quickly as possible, and to facilitate these visits.

Nonreligious: CPs are not being asked to become instant theologians or pastoral counsellors. Responses can be personal, but not dogmatic. For example, if a patient asks "What do you think will happen to me after death?" A perfectly good response could be, "Tell me what you think will happen" or "Were you brought up to believe a certain way?" This could begin a process of self-examination for the patient and subsequent sharing.

Coreligionists: If, by chance, the CP and patient share a common faith tradition, then there is no problem in sharing and participating in shared spiritual traditions, such as the Rosary for Roman Catholics or the Twenty-Third Psalm for Christians or Jews; however, these should never be imposed on the patient or family. When the CP is invited to participate in a shared spiritual tradition, that is, with suitable caution, fine.

No shared traditions: If, as may well be the case today, the patient and CP have no shared spiritual or religious traditions, remember that you share a common humanity, and your presence, loving attentiveness, and nondogmatic responses will be effective in the process. Spirituality transcends denominational differences.

Respond to what is asked: On the basis of effective listening, we help and support the patient in expressing their thoughts, fears, and concerns (they may not always be clear themselves of what these are and will need to be allowed time and space to consider). We then make sure we respond to what the patient is asking for, fulfilling the requested need as well as possible. An example for thought is in Box 24.5.

There is increasing availability of quality materials to support individual and team development in managing spiritual care. The Additional Resources section lists articles from several English-language cultural situations that could form the basis of ongoing group discussions. Puchalski and Ferrell's *Making Heath Care Whole: Integrating Spirituality into Patient Care* is an excellent exam-

ple of the evolving North American approach to this area [12].

Box 24.5 Case narrative

Mrs. Cooper was an 88-year-old woman with advanced illness. A scientist by training, she had little time or regard for religion in general. She politely declined a visit from the staff chaplain. In the night, when she was in pain, her nurse would often sit with her until the medications took effect. They would talk.

"I know there is nothing after I die; I reconciled myself to that a long time ago."

The nurse paused for a moment and then asked, "But your family and friends will keep part of you alive, don't you think?"

Mrs. Cooper half laughed, "I expect they will tell some tales after I'm gone."

"How do you want them to carry your legacy forward?"

"It's not up to me," Mrs. Cooper replied.

The nurse spoke to the social worker the next day, who spoke to Mrs. Cooper's family. They gathered together the following Sunday, three generations of children, grandchildren, and great-grandchildren. Each had brought in a picture of their mother, grandmother. Each had a story to tell. It was not a story of "remember when we had Christmas dinner and you forgot the roast beef." This was a storytelling of what they had learned from their grandmother. "You taught me to not hold back in school," one granddaughter said, "I was best in my class because of you, Granny. I knew I was smarter than the boys, and I worked hard to stay in front. Thank you for telling me I could do it."

Her son told her that they were going to give some money to the local research clinic. "We are naming a project after you, Mum. They'll do good science in your name. Other people will want to give, too. You'll be proud."

One by one, the family let their mother know how much she meant to all of them and how much her life had counted for something good.

Spirituality and liminal time

Liminality is a term from anthropology used to describe the transition from one stage of life, or state of being, to another, and for the actively dying person, it is that in-between state, with one foot in this life and one in the next [15]. Many physical and spiritual things occur within this liminal time, an experience that is quite commonplace for hospice nurses. There are conversations with deceased family members, visions (usually in the upper corners of the room) of saints, angels, and holy figures. There is a change of light or sound in the room, along with perhaps a perfectly lucid moment immediately before the moment of death.

This liminal state may be the time when the actively dying person is offered the Last Rites, anointing, or is encouraged to recite the Hebrew prayer the *Vidui*, or the *Shahadah* in Arabic. Religious traditions honour this time just preceding death (and just following) as extremely holy.

This may be a time when CPs feel helpless and unsure of how to support the dying patient and, in particular, a mourning family member. So, how can care teams, family physicians, and care institutions participate in honouring the spiritual process of dying in liminal time?

- Create sacred space
  - Allow the dying person as much privacy as possible. Place a sign on the door or curtain that says "This person is dying. Please respect this space and what is happening here."
  - Use soft music, flowers, items from home to create a sense of peace and the comfort of the familiar.
- Allow for religious traditions to take precedence
  - The physical shutting-down process is naturally unfolding. Recognise that the spiritual dynamics may be more important to the dying person and the family. Step back and allow room for ritual and prayer to happen.
- Set up vigiling teams
  - To vigil means to sit and keep watch with a dying person until death. Many people die alone. Assemble teams of volunteers to sit quietly with the dying person to provide comfort and a calming presence. Their presence also holds that space sacred for the dying person and loved ones.
- Honour the liminal experiences
  - If the dying person is having a conversation with her mother, who has come to take her "home," acknowledge this moment as a window into mystery rather than dismissing it as cognitive error.
- Recognise that aftercare is equally as important to family as care before the death.
  - Many religious traditions include washing and caring for the body immediately after death occurs, sometimes placing the body on the floor or facing East. There are also rituals that can be performed lovingly in a more general spiritual framework. Respect for the body and how it has served the person is a powerful spiritual insight in physical form. If unsure of rituals and practices of significance to the patient, do not be afraid to ask the family. There is some reference to such practices included in Chapter 21, *Terminal Care and Dying*.

Teamwork

In the process of addressing the spiritual aspects of palliative care, just as in all of the other aspects, a team approach is very helpful. Self-awareness, however, is a useful starting point. To have some insight into our own spirituality, the way we make sense of meaningful events for ourselves and the significance we place on them can be a powerful "gift" we give to ourselves and ultimately to the teams we work in as a means of fostering a holistic approach to care and promoting a recognition of the importance of the spiritual domain of care across the team. While respecting patient privacy, share experiences with your team members, and propose possible responses and best practices. This aspect of care can make us feel especially humble, helpless and inspired, and it is very important to share and support experiences so that the team develops and remains strong. See the work of Gillian White for a useful guide as to how such an approach could be implemented within your team [16].

Conclusion

Death is not primarily a medical event. Spirituality at the end of life has a great importance for patients, including those who have no religious or faith-based belief. Many of these patients will have an element of spiritual distress as they face the ending of a life that may or may not have been well spent, reflection on things finished and unfinished, and the prospect of something or nothing after the death of the body.

Spiritual care needs to become a far more conscious and purposeful part of the role of the broad care team. Using the tools and skills presented in this chapter, together with the reflections and studies presented, caregiver teams should feel more confident that they can assess and respond to the spiritual aspects of patients' needs with the same professionalism and excellence as for all other aspects of care.

References

1. Watson M. Spiritual aspects of advance care planning. In: Thomas K and Lobo B (eds), *Advance Care Planning in End of Life Care*. Oxford: Oxford University Press, 2010.
2. Nolan S, Saltmarsh P, and Leget C. Spiritual care in palliative care: working towards an EAPC task force. *Eur J Palliat Care* 2011; 18: 86–89.
3. Frankl V. *Man's Search for Meaning*. Boston, MA: Beacon Press, 2006.
4. Department of Health. *End of Life Care Strategy*. London: DH, 2008.
5. Grant L, Murray SA, and Sheikh A. Spiritual dimensions of dying in pluralist societies. *BMJ* 2010; 341: 659–662.
6. Walter T. Spirituality in palliative care: opportunity or burden? *Palliat Med* 2002; 16: 133–139.
7. Seymour JE, French J, and Richardson E. Dying matters: let's talk about it. *BMJ* 2010; 341: 646–648.
8. Du Boulay S. *Cicely Saunders: The Founder of the Modern Hospice Movement*. London: Hodder and Stoughton, 1984.
9. Skalla K. Spiritual assessment. In: *Spiritual Care SIG Toolkit*. Oncology Nursing Society, 2005. Available at: http://wwwnew.towson.edu/sct/assessment.htm (accessed on October 17, 2011).
10. Puchalski C and Romer AL. Taking a spiritual history allows clinicians to understand patients more fully. *J Palliat Med* 2000; 3: 129–137.
11. The Liverpool Care Pathway for the Dying Patient. Available at: http://www.liv.ac.uk/mcpcil/liverpool-care-pathway (accessed on October 27, 2011).
12. Puchalski CM and Ferrell B. *Making Health Care Whole: Integrating Spirituality into Patient Care*. West Conshohocken, PA: Templeton Press, 2010.
13. O'Connor D and Rumbold B. A spiritual core for palliative care. *Aus J Pastoral Care and Health* 2011; 5. Available at: http://sca.mintleaf.net/2011/03/a-spiritual-core-for-palliative- care/ (accessed on October 27, 2011).
14. Selman L, Harding R, Gysels M, et al. The measurement of spirituality in palliative care and the content of tools validated cross-culturally: a systematic review. *J Pain Symptom Manage* 2011; 41: 728–753.
15. Anderson M. Spiritual journey with the dying, liminality, and the nature of hope. *Liturgy* 2007; 22: 41–47.
16. White G. *Talking About Spirituality in Health Care Practice: A Resource for Health Professionals Working in Multidisciplinary Teams*. London: Jessica Kingsley, 2006.

Further reading

Ariès P. *The Hour of Our Death*. New York: Oxford University Press, 1991.

Barclay S and Maher J. Having the difficult conversations about the end of life. *BMJ* 2010; 341: 653–655.

Boyd K and Murray SA. Recognising and managing key transitions in end of life care. *BMJ* 2010; 341: 649–652.

Ong CK and Forbes D. Embracing Cicely Saunders's concept of total pain. *BMJ* 2005; 331: 576.

Chochinov HM and Cann BJ. Interventions to enhance the spiritual aspects of dying. *J Palliat Med* 2005; 8(Suppl 1): S103–S116.

Cohen AB and Koenig HG. Spirituality in palliative care. *Geriatric Times* 2002; 3(6). Available at: http://palliativecare.medicine.duke.edu/modules/news/article.php?storyid=1 (accessed on October 27, 2011).

Edwards A, Pang N, Shiu V, et al. The understanding of spirituality and the potential role of spiritual care in end-of-life and palliative care: a meta-study of qualitative research. *Palliat Med* 2010; 24: 753–770.

Ellershaw J, Dewar S and Murphy D. Achieving a good death for all. *BMJ* 2010; 341: 656–658.

Mitchell D and Gordon T. *Spiritual & Religious Care Competencies for Specialist Palliative Care*. London: Marie Curie Cancer Care, 2003.

Speck P, Higginson I, and Addington-Hall J. Spiritual needs in health care. *BMJ* 2004; 329: 123–124.

Stanworth R. *Recognizing Spiritual Needs in Patients who are Dying*. Oxford: Oxford University Press, 2004.

Tan H, Wilson A, Olver I, et al. The experience of palliative patients and their families of a family meeting utilised as an instrument for spiritual and psychosocial care: a qualitative study. *BMC Palliat Care* 2011; 10(7).

Index

Note: Page number followed by b, f, and t indicates box material, figure and table respectively.

Handbook of Palliative Care, Third Edition. Edited by Christina Faull, Sharon de Caestecker, Alex Nicholson and Fraser Black.
© 2012 by John Wiley and Sons, Inc. Published 2012 by John Wiley & Sons, Inc.

13-72